Modern Pharmaceutics

DRUGS AND THE PHARMACEUTICAL SCIENCES
A Series of Textbooks and Monographs

Executive Editor

James Swarbrick
PharmaceuTech, Inc.
Pinehurst, North Carolina

Advisory Board

FIFTH EDITION

Modern Pharmaceutics

Volume 1
Basic Principles and Systems

edited by

Alexander T. Florence
The School of Pharmacy
University of London
London, UK

Juergen Siepmann
College of Pharmacy
Université Lille Nord de France
Lille, France

informa
healthcare

New York London

Informa Healthcare USA, Inc.
52 Vanderbilt Avenue
New York, NY 10017

© 2009 by Informa Healthcare USA, Inc.
Informa Healthcare is an Informa business

International Standard Book Number-10: 1-4200-6564-5 (Hardcover)
International Standard Book Number-13: 978-1-4200-6564-0 (Hardcover)

Library of Congress Cataloging-in-Publication Data

Modern pharmaceutics / edited by Alexander T. Florence, Juergen
Siepmann.—5th ed.
        p. ; cm.—(Drugs and the pharmaceutical sciences ; v. 188-)
    Includes bibliographical references and index.
    ISBN-13: 978-1-4200-6564-0 (hb : alk. paper)
    ISBN-10: 1-4200-6564-5 (hb : alk. paper) 1. Drugs—Dosage forms. 2.
Pharmacy. 3. Biopharmaceutics. 4. Drugs—Administration. I.
Florence, A. T. (Alexander Taylor) II. Siepmann, Juergen. III. Series:
Drugs and the pharmaceutical sciences ; v. 188.
    [DNLM: 1. Dosage Forms. 2. Biopharmaceutics. 3. Drug Delivery
Systems. 4. Pharmaceutical Preparations—administration & dosage. 5.
Pharmacokinetics. W1 DR893B v.188 2009 / QV 785 M6895 2009]
    RS200.M63 2009
    615′.1—dc22

                                                                    2009002881

For Corporate Sales and Reprint Permissions call 212-520-2700 or write to: Sales Department, 52 Vanderbilt Avenue, 16th floor, New York, NY 10017.

**Visit the Informa Web site at
www.informa.com**

**and the Informa Healthcare Web site at
www.informahealthcare.com**

Preface

Modern Pharmaceutics edited by Gilbert Banker and Christopher Rhodes has become a classic in the field. It is well known and has been well received on an international basis, necessitating the publication of this fifth edition. The present editors took on the difficult task of following in the footsteps of the founding editors and their associates with some trepidation. It has been several years since the last edition, and on realizing that Dr. Banker and Dr. Rhodes wanted to pass on the editorship, we accepted the mantle.

Given the passage of time and the growth and change in the field, the book has been divided into two volumes: *Basic Principles and Systems* and *Applications and Advances*. There have been so many exciting developments which impinge on pharmaceutics that it was time to reconsider the content of the book.

Basic Principles and Systems is principally a textbook and advanced reference source of pharmaceutics, which focus on the core of the subject that is key to pharmacy. We define pharmaceutics as encompassing the design, formulation, manufacture, assessment and determination of the quality of pharmaceutical products, and also the quality of effect in patients as the guiding principles. We have therefore continued only with chapters that fall within these criteria.

We have added chapters on in vivo imaging of dosage forms, surfactant systems, and the solid state. In each of these fields there have been significant advances. In vivo imaging is a powerful adjunct to biopharmaceutical studies, providing evidence of the spatial distribution of dose forms, which is vital in site-specific therapies. Surfactant systems, aspects of nanotechnology before this became a vogue, are now used with more sophistication than in the past and provide a wide variety of means of administration of drugs. Techniques for investigating the solid state have become more abundant and shed more light on crystal forms, key to the optimal design of delivery systems and choice of drug salt or form.

This volume opens with an essay on new challenges and paradigms in pharmaceutics and follows with updated chapters on drug absorption, pharmacokinetics, bioavailability, and route of administration, the starting points for the design of systems. Chemical kinetics and drug stability, excipient design and characterization as well as preformulation along with a chapter on optimization techniques further treat these fundamentals of pharmaceutics. Chapters on disperse systems, tablets, hard and soft capsules, and parenteral products complete *Basic Principles and Systems*.

Many of these chapters are written by their original authors. We are grateful for their enterprise, enthusiasm, and time and also thank those authors who wished to stand down. They have allowed the new authors to draw heavily on their original material, which has eased the process and has allowed us to retain the essence of the earlier volumes.

We thank Sandra Beberman of Informa Healthcare USA for her patience with new editors and her encouragement, and all the staff at Informa Healthcare USA who have nursed these two volumes through to press. We also thank of course all who have devoted time in preparing material for this new edition of *Modern Pharmaceutics*.

We trust that *Basic Principles and Systems* and its companion *Applications and Advances* will satisfy the needs of a wide range of colleagues who have an interest or indeed passion for pharmaceutics. If there are lacunae, perhaps this will lead readers to research these areas.

Alexander T. Florence
Juergen Siepmann

Contents

Contributors

David Attwood   School of Pharmacy and Pharmaceutical Sciences, University of Manchester, Manchester, U.K.

Larry L. Augsburger   University of Maryland, School of Pharmacy, Department of Pharmaceutical Sciences, Baltimore, Maryland, U.S.A.

David W. A. Bourne   College of Pharmacy, University of Oklahoma, Oklahoma City, Oklahoma, U.S.A.

James C. Boylan   Pharmaceutical Consultant, Gurnee, Illinois, U.S.A.

Graham Buckton   School of Pharmacy, University of London, London, and Pharmaterials Ltd., Reading, U.K.

Maureen D. Donovan   Division of Pharmaceutics, University of Iowa, Iowa City, Iowa, U.S.A.

Alastair J. Florence   Strathclyde Institute of Pharmacy and Biomedical Sciences, University of Strathclyde, Glasgow, U.K.

Alexander T. Florence   Centre for Drug Delivery Research, The School of Pharmacy, University of London, London, U.K.

Gavin W. Halbert   Cancer Research UK Formulation Unit, Strathclyde Institute of Pharmacy and Biomedical Sciences, University of Strathclyde, Glasgow, U.K.

Zheng-Rong Lu   Department of Pharmaceutics and Pharmaceutical Chemistry, College of Pharmacy, University of Utah, Salt Lake City, Utah, U.S.A.

Michael Mayersohn   College of Pharmacy, Department of Pharmacy Practice and Science, University of Arizona, Tucson, Arizona, U.S.A.

Steven L. Nail   School of Pharmacy, Purdue University, West Lafayette, Indiana, U.S.A.

Ornlaksana Paeratakul   Faculty of Pharmacy, Srinakharinwirot University, Nakhon Nayok, Thailand

Rolland I. Poust   College of Pharmacy, University of Iowa, Iowa City, Iowa, U.S.A.

Wandee Rungseevijitprapa   Faculty of Pharmaceutical Sciences, Ubon Ratchathani University, Ubon Ratchathani, Thailand

Adel Sakr   College of Pharmacy, University of Cincinnati, Cincinnati, Ohio, U.S.A.

Juergen Siepmann   Department of Pharmaceutical Technology, College of Pharmacy, Université Lille Nord de France, Lille, France

Florence Siepmann   Department of Pharmaceutical Technology, College of Pharmacy, Université Lille Nord de France, Lille, France

Murat Turkoglu   Department of Pharmaceutical Technology, Marmara University, Istanbul, Turkey

1

Pharmaceutics: New Challenges, New Paradigms

Alexander T. Florence
*Centre for Drug Delivery Research, The School of Pharmacy,
University of London, London, U.K.*

Juergen Siepmann
*Department of Pharmaceutical Technology, College of Pharmacy,
Université Lille Nord de France, Lille, France*

INTRODUCTION

Background

The essence of pharmaceutics, as many of the chapters in the two volumes of this book illustrate, is the amalgamation of physical science (physical pharmacy) with aspects of biological science. It is a distinct discipline quite different from biophysics or chemical biology because at its center is not only the dosage form with its active and inactive ingredients but also the behavior of the ensemble in the environment in which these medicines are used, generally in human subjects. Pharmaceutics has existed as a discipline within pharmacy and the pharmaceutical sciences for a long time. It is difficult to discern the origins of the term, although one can deduce from the evolution of textbooks of pharmaceutics something about its development. From the early days of the 20th century to the mid-1950s, it was concerned primarily with the science and practice of the manufacture of medicines (dosage forms) on small and large scales and the preparation of galenicals. It was viewed sometimes as a discipline without much regard to the fate of the dosage form in vivo. However, this is not really the case. For example, the 1924 edition of Martindale and Wescott's *The Extra Pharmacopeia* (1) discusses enteric coating of tablets to minimize the effects of drugs on the intestinal mucosa in the following words:

> Various substances have been proposed for the coating of pills, tablets and capsules to render them insoluble in the stomach but soluble in the intestines, i.e. on reaching the duodenum. Drugs, for example, which irritate the mucous membrane and the administration of which is liable to induce vomiting, and substances intended to act solely on the intestines and the anthelmintic drugs, have been so given. Keratin, as usually employed, seldom brings about the desired effect.

1

Here there is clear concern for the usefulness of formulations and the therapeutic consequences of their composition. The use of keratin-coated pills is reported in a Lancet paper in 1893 (2), but the process is accredited to a German, Dr Unna, who first marketed such products (3). There were concerns about the quality of such systems, particularly product ageing, and it is interesting that as early as 1938, an X-ray study was carried out on the disintegration in vivo of keratin-coated systems (4). The first commercial sustained-release preparations emerged in the late 1940s with the Spansule™, which contained wax-coated beads with different release properties in a soluble capsule, thus controlling release of the drug in the GI tract.

The term *biopharmaceutics* was an invention of the 1960s. The nature of the dosage form was from then on inextricably linked with its performance in patients. Micro-encapsulation of drugs, encouraged by the National Cash Register Company (NCR) patents on carbonless copy paper at the time (5), was adapted to the development of controlled- or sustained-release products, and this has more recently evolved into nanotechnological approaches. Nanotechnology began in the pharmaceutical domain, much before the current vogue for all things "nano," with Peter Speiser and his coworkers in the 1970s in Zurich developing "nanoparts" and nanocapsules (6). Pharmaceutical nanotechnology, therefore, is not as new as some of its proponents would have us to believe. Table 1 is a brief summary of just some of the key events in pharmaceutical technology.

Table 1   Key Development of Controlled-Release Systems[a]

Date	System	Remark
1867	Collodion coating	Delayed-release coating for pills
1884	Keratin coating	Enteric-coated pills prepared with keratin (Unna)
1887	Salol coating	As an enteric coating material (Ceppi)
1929	Coacervation	Bungenberg de Jong and Kruyt
1936	Stearic acid coating	Stearic acid and waxes and mixtures for release control
1945	CAP	Cellulose acetate phthalate as enteric coating material
1945	Spansule™	Wax-coated and uncoated drug beads in a capsule (SKF)
1950	Lontab™	Lontab tablets (Ciba)
1953	Microencapsulation	NCR patent for carbonless copy paper
1959	Duplex™	Film-coated tablet between the core and external layer
1959	Duretter™	Plastic matrix dosage forms (Durules)
1962	Liposomes	Bangham's discovery
1973	Nanoparticles	Nanoencapsulation (Speiser et al., ETH Zurich)
1974	Ocusert™	Delivery to conjunctival sac (Alza)
1975	Silicone implants	Silicone implants for slow release (Folkman)
1975	Oros™	Oral osmotic pump (Alza)
1979	Transdermal patch	Scopolamine patch approved by the FDA
1981	Zoladex™	Poly(lactide) implants for polypeptide delivery (ICI)
1982	Dendrimers	Synthesized by Tomalia
1988	Stealth liposomes	Gabizon and Papahadjopolous; Allen et al., 1989
1989	Lupron Depot™	TAP launches leuprorelin PLGA microsphere SR product
1990	Liposome	First liposome product to gain approval (Ireland)
1994	Stealth liposome	LTI seeks approval of doxorubicin stealth liposome (Caelyx)
2003	Drug-eluting stents	First FDA approval (Cypher™ sirolimus)
2006	Dendrimer product	First dendrimer pharmaceutical (VivaGel™ Star Pharma)

[a]Dates are approximate.
Abbreviations: CAP, Cellulose acetate phthalate; SKF, SmithKline French; NCR, National Cash register Company; ICI, Imperial Chemical Industries; TAP, Takeda Abbot Pharmaceutical Company; SR, Sustained release; LTI, Liposome Technology Incorporated.

Means for the production and the design of refined controlled-release systems was advanced by the development of biodegradable polymers, the three archetypal polymers being poly(lactic acid–glycolic acid) (PLGA), poly(lactic acid) (PLA), and poly (glycolic acid) (PGA). Now there are many other polymers and copolymers that act as carriers for drugs. Lipid-based delivery systems, most notably liposomes, discovered by Bangham in the 1960s, led to the marketing, some 20 to 25 years later, of liposome-based doxorubicin and amphotericin products. The list of liposomal products is now impressive, but the gestation time was long as more was learned about the behavior of dosage forms in the body and about their stability, their interaction with proteins, uptake by the reticuloendothelial system, and extravasation, not to mention diffusion and uptake into diseased sites. Dendrimers, spherical or starburst polymers first synthesized by Tomalia and coworkers (7) in the early 1980s, are also now finding their niche along with a variety of other nanoconstructs, but the period from the first concept to the clinic is still proving tortuous. Many polymer micro- and nanoparticles have random polymeric internal and surface structures. So, in theory, the ability to synthesize dendrimers with their precise architectures and controlled arrangement of surface groups allows the practice of true molecular pharmaceutics, with precisely positioned ligands and other agents.

In a relatively short period of time, pharmaceutics has moved from the macroscopic through the microscopic to the nanoscopic domain and from the more empiric to the more quantitative. It has long been intertwined with colloid science typically in relation to the formulation of micellar-solubilized products and the stabilization of suspensions and emulsions; the application of colloid science to nanosystems is more vital than ever, as discussed in chapter 12, volume 2.

In many experimental systems, for example, with dendrimers (2.5 to 10 nm in diameter) and carbon nanotubes as vehicles for delivery, the drug has dimensions in the same range as these putative carriers. This is an inevitable consequence of the fact that not only have such dosage forms become smaller but also the average size of therapeutic molecules has grown with the use of more biologicals. New or reinvented approaches to the interactions between a carrier and a drug need to be applied. A deal of effort has been addressed to the topic of carrier-mediated drug targeting, perhaps at the expense of the physical, pharmaceutical, and technological aspects of the task, but there is a growing realization that the neglect of the fundamental physical aspects of pharmaceutics is a mistake. Particulate delivery systems once administered are placed in new thermodynamic situations, which we must model and predict and thus design products that are colloidally stable yet labile enough to deliver their loads and be excreted.

NEW PARADIGMS

According to one dictionary, a paradigm is "a philosophical and theoretical framework of a scientific school of discipline within which theories, laws and generalizations and the experiments performed in support of them are formulated," but a simpler definition of "a generally accepted perspective of a particular discipline at a given time" is apposite too. Pharmaceutics is espousing new paradigms. The concept of the carrier system, traditionally tablets, capsules, suppositories, or the like with the drug internalized, has changed as the actives such as DNA and other macromolecules may not be internalized but may be intertwined with the complexing molecules, as hinted above, to form the delivery vector, usually leading to condensation. Active molecules may be adsorbed to the surface of nanoparticles. Products such as drug-releasing coated stents present new challenges, not least in quality control.

A More Predictive Science?

Reflecting on past decades of research in pharmaceutics, drug delivery, and drug targeting, one can detect a certain lack of an overall ability to predict the ultimate behavior of systems, not only but especially at the early formulation stage, and with behavior in vivo. Is pharmaceutics still too empirical, a shadow that has held the subject back for many years? There has been success in drug solubility prediction, as the work of Peterson (8) and others (9) has demonstrated, but in a related field, that of the micellar solubilization of drugs by surfactants, in spite of decades of research, it is not an easy task to predict the solubilization potential of a given surfactant system for a given drug molecule. In the same way, more recent research in gene delivery employing cationic complexing polymers, lipids or dendrimers to condense the DNA, has led to transfection of cells in culture with varying degrees of success, but there is no consensus yet as to the optimum size, shape, charge, or other characteristics of the gene construct to achieve maximal cell penetration, nor has it been possible to predict a priori the effectiveness of a given construct on a particular cell line.

Pharmaceutics has come a long way since its focus mainly on physical systems, but there must be a fresh look at the type of research problems that are tackled if we are to achieve a more predictive science. Not only this, but it seems a long time since new equations entered pharmaceutics' basic pantheon. It is several decades since Takeru Higuchi developed the equations for the diffusion of drugs in, and release from, complex systems (10). There is a need to explore new areas of pharmaceutics, to explain phenomena that otherwise will not be treated theoretically. Issues of adhesion, including mucoadhesion, film coating, tack, and cracking in films, are but some of the areas that require a greater theoretical approach after considerable amounts of phenomenological research has been published.

The study of the behavior of dosage forms in vivo, not least of nanosystems, is desperately short of a comprehensive theoretical base, which will relate properties, both physical and biological, not only to the size of particulate systems but also to their surface characteristics. On the other hand, while pharmaceutics must continue to reinvent itself, all those involved in medicines development and drug delivery and targeting must be acquainted and absorb the canon of pharmaceutics that already exists. This centers around the quality, pharmacy, and standards of products, modes of production and sterilization and characterization, their reproducibility, their quality (both intrinsic and quality related to activity), as well as studies of the potential of products themselves to cause harm. All this is a unified holistic approach. It is little use concentrating on the fabrication of physical devices if these are not able to be manufactured, or are not stable and not safe. This must be balanced by the imperative to carry out research that explores new materials and ideas whether or not we have all the requisite information that might be required ultimately for their conversion to dosage forms.

In drug targeting, much effort goes into the design of nanoparticles (although here again the approach is often necessarily empirical when there should be a more comprehensive understanding of, say, drug- or protein-polymer interactions), but little attention is paid, other than in a descriptive sense, to the issues surrounding the flow and movement of nanoparticles toward their distant targets and destinations. The nature of the flow of nanoparticles in vivo has been largely neglected, yet it is a branch of pharmaceutical engineering science. Flow, interactions between particles, and interactions of particles with blood components, erythrocytes, and proteins must be addressed in a unified manner before there can be any major advance in the predictability or, indeed, the reality of targeting, especially with nanoparticles decorated with ligands intended to interact with epithelial receptors. The flow of asymmetric carbon nanotubes in blood can be predicted to an extent by extant equations linking viscosity to axial ratio, but experimental proof is required.

This introductory chapter explores some areas of pharmaceutics and also the academic and educational aspects of the discipline. If we are to attract the best scientists into the field, the subject must be presented at undergraduate levels in an exciting and relevant manner. It must show the promise of controlling drug and therapeutic agents and the fact that that there is still much to do. Above all, it must demonstrate connections to avoid insularity and isolation as a discipline while remembering its heartland.

Connections

Connections between research in pharmaceutics and education in pharmacy are vital, but so too are the connections not only between the different types of research but also between different disciplines that can underpin pharmaceutics. Perhaps pharmaceutics could benefit from more research for its own sake, with less directed research aimed at the production of marketable dosage forms. Research on phenomena that are interesting in themselves, research into potential situations (what if?), and research into real systems and situations to answer the question "How does this work?" or "What causes this system to behave as it does?" are all legitimate. Some of these connections are illustrated in Figure 1, some being vital in the educational process.

Pharmaceutics as such is a distinct subject professed within schools of pharmacy worldwide. With the increasing trend toward a more clinical orientation of pharmacy graduates, as already has been achieved in the United States, there may be diminished attention paid to the teaching of pharmaceutics. As in research, there must be a greater effort to present the subject not only in its physicochemical envelope but to demonstrate the importance of the subject matter ultimately in the clinic. As examples, consider the

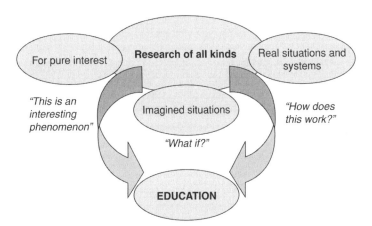

Figure 1   The connections between research of all types in pharmaceutics from the real to the imagined and the link to education. Education must inspire a questioning attitude in students and stimulate them about a subject, pharmaceutics, that continues to adapt and to evolve.

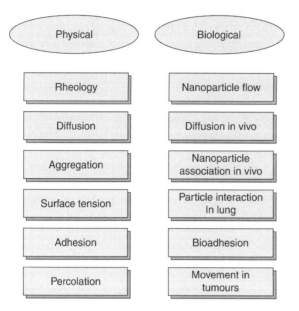

Figure 2 Examples of the connections between phenomena known in physical pharmacy and biological events using the examples of rheology, diffusion, aggregation, surface tension, adhesion, and percolation, and their biological importance in particulate systems as an example.

connections in Figure 2 between the physical phenomena of rheology, diffusion, aggregation, surface tension, adhesion, and percolation, some of the staples of physical pharmacy, to the behavior of systems in vivo.

These topics might be thought of as biopharmaceutics, but they are more than this. They are about the relevance of physicochemical phenomena in all aspects of therapy: rheology relating to blood flow and joint lubrication, crystallization as relevant to crystalluria and drug precipitation from formulations, surface tension and lung surfactant expansion and solubilization of drugs, colloidal interactions and interactions between nanoparticles and surfaces in vivo, and so on. This is what we might call *clinical pharmaceutics*. Clinical pharmaceutics also deals with the adverse effects of dose forms, induced by their excipients and by colors, flavors, tonicifiers, or impurities (11). It also concerns the beneficial influence of dose forms and modes of delivery on clinical outcomes.

Pharmaceutics faces two challenges in schools of pharmacy, one from the clinical impetus that exists and one from the need to maintain the basic and fundamental science in the subject, one which is distinctively pharmaceutics. The latter is not for its own sake, but because the combination of physical, chemical, and biological knowledge that the subject encompasses is vital for improved therapy and the development of safe and novel systems. It could be argued that while there has been progress in the subject in controlled-release technologies with direct patient benefit, pharmaceutical nanotechnology, and aspects of drug targeting, the study of basic phenomena perhaps deserves reinforcement. In particular, we require the application of physical pharmacy concepts to delivery and targeting issues. One example would be the interaction between a nanoparticle and a cell surface as characterized by Sun and Wirtz (12) in Figure 3A. This has clear analogies to, say, indentation testing of pharmaceutical materials shown in Figure 3B, two widely separated topics. Such connections or analogies are intriguing as well as useful.

(A)

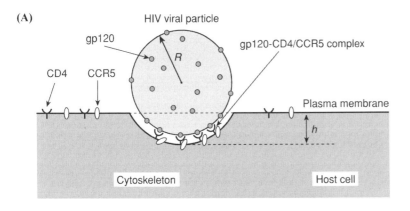

(B)

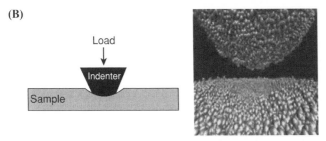

Figure 3 Analogies I. (**A**) Comparison between a diagram from Sun and Wirtz (12) on the interaction of a viral particle with a plasma membrane and (**B**) an illustration demonstrating an indentation measurement on a solid. (**A**) R = radius of the particle and h = the depth of "indentation" of the viral particle. Various receptor and ligand molecules are denoted in addition to ligand-receptor complexes. Sun and Wirtz invoke Young's modulus and other physical terms to describe the interaction. Hiestand and Smith (13) cite Tabor's (14, 15) equation for indentation hardness P, obtained using a pendulum indenter (which actually might be a relevant model for particle-receptor interactions during flow):

$$P = \left[\frac{4mgrh_r}{\pi a^4}\right]\left[\frac{h_i}{h_r} - \frac{3}{8}\right]$$

where m is the mass of the indenter, g is the gravitational constant, r is the radius of the spherical indenter, a is the chordal radius of the dent produced on impact, and h_i is the initial height of the indenter, whereas h_r is the rebound height of the indenter.

NEEDS

There are still urgent needs in the field of pharmaceutical nanotechnology, which are posited below (16), but these might also be suitably modified for many delivery systems.

1. The relevance to the whole animal of in vitro tests of activity, selectivity, uptake, and toxicity of nanoparticulate carrier systems.

    In vitro systems are generally static, whereas most interactions between particles and ligands on cell surfaces occur under dynamic conditions. Flow of blood in which nanosystems move generally decreases the interaction between carrier and target, through shear forces at surfaces. Laminar and nonlaminar flow in vessels and other tubules is determined by the variable velocity and velocity gradients in blood vessels (17). Dilution effects and the propensity of nanoparticles to interact with proteins in the blood affect the translation from cell culture to living animal.

2. Scaling factors in animal models and the extrapolation of results to human subjects.

    The relevance to the human subject of animal studies, which form the greatest number of sources of data to date, is obscure. Does a 100-nm particle behave in the same way in a mouse and in a human? What is the importance of the distance traveled between the point of entry and the point of interaction with target? How does the physiology of various species influence interpretation of data? Kararli (18) reviewed aspects of the physiological differences between a variety of experimental animals and human subjects in relation to drug absorption. A similar exercise is necessary to determine the influence of species differences on nanocarrier behavior and fate.

3. The causes of the differential uptake and transport of particles in different cell lines in vitro and tissues in vivo.

    Studies of transfection of a variety of cell lines with a particular DNA-complexing agent have frequently shown very marked differences in effectiveness. For example, in the case of dendriplexes (dendrimer-DNA complexes), Bayele et al. (19) have shown 1000-fold differences in transfection. These variations have been confirmed by many researchers. Is this due to cell size (i.e., the distance to be traveled), membrane differences, cell culture media, differences in cell division rate, or the nature of the nucleus and cytoplasm of each cell type? Is there a physical cause, rather than a fundamental biological problem? Diffusion in the cytoplasm is, in part, a purely physical phenomenon; the process is akin to diffusion in a complex gel, strongly dependent on the radius of the particle and the "pore size" of the gel as well as the volume fraction of the gelator. Both obstruction effects and adsorption can occur, so that diffusion is slow, and above critical particle radius ceases altogether. With biological therapeutics, their size often controls their release from delivery systems and certainly their escape into and diffusion in tissue.

4. The influence of the nature of the polymer or other construction material in the manufacture of nanosystems on their biological and colloidal behavior.

    It is one thing to formulate a protein in a polymeric carrier and another to be able to *predict* the miscibility of that protein with the polymer and its potential distribution within the matrix of the polymer. Does phase separation occur as the mixing of two macromolecules is not a simple process thermodynamically? Phase separation can lead to rapid release of active. There has been significant concentration on the effect of the size of nanoparticles on physical and biological behavior but perhaps less on the nature of the polymer in as far as this affects the capacity of the system to encapsulate therapeutic agents or the potential to influence particle flocculation and the vital interactions at close approach of the nanoparticles and cell surface receptors. The Hamaker constants (see chap. 11) are fundamental for assessing the attractive forces between surfaces, and for different polymeric materials can be quite different (20,21), as shown in Table 2.

Table 2 Hamaker Constants (in vacuo) for Some Polymers

Polymer	A ($\times 10^{20}$ J)
Polyvinyl chloride	10.8, 7.5
Polyethylene	10.0
Polystyrene	9.8, 6.6, 6.4, 7.8
PVAc	8.9
PVA	8.8
Polyethylene oxide	7.5
PMMA	6.3
PDMS	6.3
PTFE	3.8

van der Waals attraction between two particles at a distance S
(i) for two spheres of equal radius r is $-Ar/12S$, and
(ii) for two spheres of unequal radii r_1 and r_2 is $-Ar_1r_2/6S(r_1+r_2)$.
Source: Adapted from Refs. 20 and 21.

5. Analysis of the colloidal behavior of nanoparticles and especially the influence of surface ligands on this behavior.

   As suggested above, the addition of specific ligands to the surface of nanoparticles, whether by covalent attachment or by adsorption, does not always lead to improved targeting in animals. Thus, the manner in which the ligands affect the physical stability and interactions of nanosystems is a worthy goal to elucidate the optimal conformation and configuration of adsorbed ligands.

6. Nanoparticle navigation in complex biological networks.

   A better understanding of the movement of nanoparticles in the complex environment in which they are deposited in tissues, in tumors, and in blood, lymph, and the extracellular matrix is essential for prediction of behavior. The influence of particle size, shape, and flexibility on such movement is key (22). Does shape matter? If flow matters, then asymmetric particle flow is clearly different from the flow of spherical particles. Hence, there is a need for better comprehension of such behavior, particularly with the advent of carbon nanotubes whose rheological and diffusional properties will differ from those of spherical systems.

7. Analysis of published data to move pharmaceutical nanotechnology toward greater predictability of nanoparticle behavior.

   Targeting activity is essential in the design of many delivery systems, vaccines, and gene delivery vectors, hence collating the already voluminous material that has been published and finding common threads to improve predictive powers are important. One of the difficulties here is the variation in size measurement techniques and their interpretation, as has been emphasized in two recent publications (23,24), one going so far as to suggest that 90% of published measurements are faulty. Accurate size measurements are essential. If size is key to access to targets or interactions with receptors, then the width of the particle size distribution must be known. Figure 4 illustrates this in a general way. If the optimal size range is as shown, then particles in region A will no doubt have access but will have different flow characteristics, particles in B will be in the desired range, while those in C will not access the target. It may be that particles in category D will, in fact, exhibit toxicity. It is perhaps

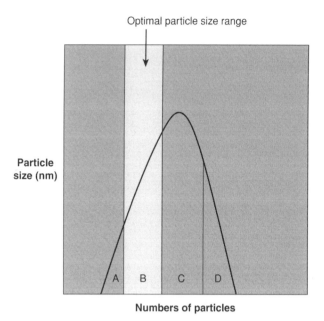

Optimal particle size range

Particle
size (nm)

Numbers of particles

Figure 4 A diagrammatic particle size distribution with a hypothetical optimum-size band for biological activity, extravasation, transport, and receptor interactions. Zones A to D are discussed in the text.

timely to explore a "gold standard" for particle sizing so that all laboratories routinely use and cite the values they obtain with their equipment using a standard material, for example, a gold sol. After all, this is a common practice in surface science, where the surface tension of water is routinely cited as a marker of accuracy and precision.

8. Pharmaceutical aspects of nanotoxicology or nanosafety.

The study of nanotoxicology has been referred to by the Oberdösters in a review (25), which will repay reading as a discipline emerging from studies of ultrafine particles. Nanoparticles, unlike the majority of microparticles, can penetrate the body in a variety of ways and can be absorbed and translocated to organs such as the liver and spleen. It is clear that we must have more specific information on the safety of nanosystems, the influence of the nature of their surfaces and the material of which they are composed, and the influence of porosity, size, and shape.

9. Pharmacokinetics of drugs and other agents encapsulated in nanosystems and more studies on the kinetics of distribution of carriers in vivo.

This is a fairly self-evident need. It is important that we distinguish between the pharmacokinetics of drug that is released from the carrier and the biokinetics of the carriers themselves (i.e., carrier kinetics). It is wrong etymologically to discuss the pharmacokinetics of vectors.

10. The physical chemistry of peptide, protein, or macromolecule—polymer miscibility in relation to the incorporation of these molecules in polymer nanoparticles, microparticles, and implants, their stability, and release.

Given sometimes overwhelming biological interests, the pharmaceutical and physicochemical issues in formulation must not be underestimated. One lack seems to be a systematic study of the interactions between peptides, proteins, and DNA and the variety of polymers used in the construction of nanosystems. The basic thermodynamics of mixing under the conditions of preparation will yield valuable data. Gander et al. (26) have approached this subject in relation to the microencapsulation of proteins by PLGA spheres by spray drying and sought correlations between Hildebrand constants, partial Hansen solubility parameters, and other thermodynamic measures. They were able to conclude that encapsulation efficiency is increased and burst release reduced if polymer-drug interactions are dominant and polymer-solvent and drug-solvent interactions are reduced. The same authors also studied the thermodynamics of interactions in the preparation of microcapsules (27). More studies of this kind are important especially when polymer mixtures are used and polymer-polymer interactions turn out to be complex. Figure 5 illustrates a study of protein-polysaccharide interactions (28), which points out regions of compatibility and incompatibility in the phase diagram.

The above subject areas are possibly an idiosyncratic and certainly an incomplete list of topics in nanotechnology. They arise from the need to counteract the exaggerated claims for nanosystems in drug delivery and targeting by addressing the core factors which prevent quantitative delivery of therapeutic agents to complex targets such as tumors and sites of inflammation.

Some phenomena are extremely difficult, if not impossible, at present to investigate in vivo; hence, there needs to be a theoretical approach to many of the phenomena we invoke to explain delivery and targeting with nanoparticles. The stochastic nature of many interactions must be incorporated into predictions. While we are studying the biological barriers to delivery and targeting, we should devise new systems, which are better able to

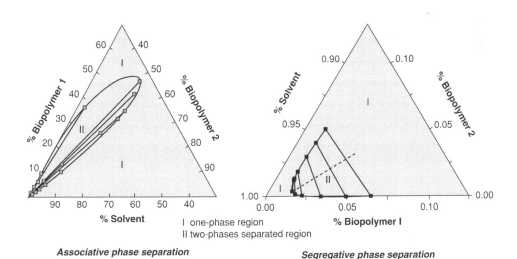

Figure 5 Phase diagrams for biopolymer 1–biopolymer 2 solvent systems from Doublier et al. (28). Not shown is the Flory-Huggins lattice model for predicting experimental tie lines, whose equations exhibit enthalpic and entropic terms. The diagram on the right illustrates the most common form of thermodynamic incompatibility or "segregative phase separation" where solvent–biopolymer 1 interactions are favored over biopolymer 1–biopolymer 2 interactions and solvent-solvent interactions, hence demixing. In the associative phases separation, interactions between the two biopolymers are favored (e.g., because of interactions between a positively and a negatively charged molecule).

take their load quantitatively to their targets yet release them in a predictable manner when and only when they reach their site of action. A tall order.

Nanotechnology offers the opportunity not only to enhance delivery and targeting but also to produce new material and devices: in the formation of fine membranes, meshes, lubricant material for fine valves, and so on. There is also the recognition of the potential of the toxicity of materials such as titanium dioxide, used not as a carrier but as an excipient in tablets. Titanium dioxide is absorbed from the GI tract in the form of rutile, some 50 nm in diameter (29), and particles of 2 to 5 nm after inhalation (30). The ever present possibility of aggregation and its influence on interpretation of nanoparticle toxicity has been discussed (31).

Fundamental Topics

The late Nobel laureate in physics Pierre-Gilles de Gennes, for much of his research career, worked in the field of soft matter, which has so much significance in pharmaceutical systems. In his 1994 Dirac Memorial Lecture (32) given in Cambridge, he ranged widely over topics such as the dynamics of partial and complete wetting, principles of adhesion and tack, and polymer/polymer welding. "Compared to the giants of quantum physics," de Gennes wrote modestly, "we soft-matter theorists look like the dwarfs of German folk tales. These dwarfs were often miners or craft-workers: we, also, are strongly motivated by industrial purposes. *We see fundamental problems emerging from practical questions.*" It is this last sentence that is especially relevant to pharmaceutics, where the issues of compaction, flow, film formation, wetting, and adhesion and tack can be of industrial relevance but are incompletely understood. Yet there are pressing issues raised by the necessity to formulate and deliver drugs that are macromolecules or labile and which possess the "wrong" physical and chemical characteristics as drug molecules. The objective de Gennes proposes is that we need to obtain "simple impressionistic visions of complex phenomena, ignoring many details, actually in many cases operating only at the level of scaling laws."

Pharmaceutical formulations and systems are frequently, and possibly usually, extremely complex. We use multicomponent systems, polymers of varied molecular weight, surfactants, products of polymerization processes, which are impure, particles of a wide distribution of sizes and shapes, and processes that are themselves often complex and ill defined at a molecular level. Then we administer these systems to a complex biological environment. We are a long way from a pharmaceutical theory of everything. To return to an earlier theme, we need the theoretical bases on which to become less empirical. This present book contains a chapter by Frenning and Alderborn (chap. 11, vol. 2) on aspects of pharmaceutical physics, written to illustrate the approaches that can be made to complex fields in pharmacy. Some of the topics once of great interest in pharmaceutics laboratories, say in the domain of powder technology, are still pursued elsewhere, for example, in physics. As an example, a paper on the wet granular pile stability recently tackled problems of spherical and nonspherical particle mixing and agglomeration (33).

Other Topics

Aqueous Interaction with Solids: Wetting and Dewetting

Water repellency (34) is relevant to pharmaceutical systems. With porous dosage forms, there is generally a desire to *avoid* water repellency to allow ingress of water. A

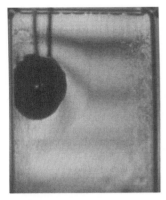
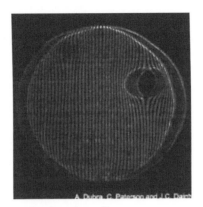

A soap film bursting   ▲ Breakup of tear film

Figure 6 Analogies II. (*Left*) A film of sodium dodecyl sulfate in air a few microseconds after a spark bursts the film and causes rapid contraction of the surfactant layers with thickening in the so-called aureole region around the hole. (*Right*) An image of tear film rupture on a solid surface. *Source*: Left figure from A. T. Florence and K. J. Mysels, 1967 (unpublished photograph); right figure from the laboratory of A. Dubra (38), Imperial College London.

possibility of reversible repellency might be of advantage in controlling release of drugs by first inhibiting uptake of water and then allowing it. Indeed, the wettability of textured materials can be tuned rapidly with an electric field, for example (35), leading to the possibility of pulsed release from dose forms as the systems are tuned and detuned. Dewetting is also related to issues of water repellency and is important in some biological situations. In xerophthalmia (dry eye), the dewetting of the cornea through the breakup of the tear film leads to dry spots. Studies on dewetting of polymer films on mica or viscous fluids or surfactant films or solutions can lead to understanding of many physical and biological processes. Photographs of thin surfactant film breakup obtained many years ago (36,37) in the late Karol Mysels' laboratory (Fig. 6) bear a remarkable similarity to recent work by Dubra et al. (38) on tear film breakup.

Flow of Complex Liquids

In Balaz's paper on the flow of complex liquids (such as binary fluids) through heterogeneous channels (39), it is argued that the dynamic behavior of complex fluids in confined geometries is vital if we are to understand a range of topics from the processing of polymeric materials to the flow of blood in confined spaces. Not least, the work has provided basic information and the optimal configurations for the production of emulsions having well-controlled structures. The molecular dynamics of sorbed fluids in mesoporous materials (40) are relevant to the understanding of hysteresis in porous systems, important in some pulsatile hydrogel delivery systems, which display considerable hysteresis, which may only be in part due to the mechanics of the polymer chains.

The chapter by Anthony Hickey (chap. 5, vol. 2) on inhalational delivery of drugs exemplifies the theory that has been derived to understand the processes of lung deposition so far. Nanoparticulate interaction with the lung surfactant layer has been discussed and a three-dimensional cellular model devised to study these processes (41).

Boundary Lubrication, Splashes, and Turbulence

Boundary lubrication under water discussed by Briscoe et al. (42) is relevant to particles with surfactant layers. They state,

> Boundary lubrication, in which the rubbing surfaces are coated with molecular monolayers, has been studied extensively for over half a century. Such monolayers generally consist of amphiphilic surfactants anchored by their polar headgroups; sliding occurs at the interface between the layers, greatly reducing friction and especially wear of the underlying substrates. This process, widespread in engineering applications, is also predicted to occur in biological lubrication via phospholipid films, though few systematic studies on friction between surfactant layers in aqueous environments have been carried out. Here we show that the frictional stress between two sliding surfaces bearing surfactant monolayers may decrease, when immersed in water, to as little as one per cent or less of its value in air (or oil). We attribute this to the shift of the slip plane from between the surfactant layers, to the surfactant/substrate interface. The low friction would then be due to the fluid hydration layers surrounding the polar head groups attached to the substrate. These results may have implications for future technological and biomedical applications.

Investigation of splashes (43,44) might seem abstruse pharmaceutically, but such work would be of relevance to the nature of micro- and nanoparticle interaction with alveolar fluids from the airways: hydrophilic spheres have been shown to enter liquid surfaces without commotion, while hydrophobic particles cause a splash. Problems of turbulence (45), aspects of mixing (46), and the nature of complex liquids, inter alia, are studies on apparently nonpharmaceutical systems which nevertheless have or may have relevance to a theoretically based approach to pharmaceutical design and manufacture and thus a deeper understanding of product performance.

The Pharmaceutics of Cell Therapy

Pharmaceutics has progressed as drugs have developed first from natural product extracts, through synthetic and generally small molecules to peptides, proteins, and oligonucleotides and DNA itself, into the beginning era of cell-based therapies. Cell therapy, whether with stem cells, dendritic cells, or pancreatic cells, involves a host of pharmaceutical issues: of dose, of quality, of consistency, and of accurate delivery to specific sites. Several means of delivery cells have been explored, including direct intramuscular injection (e.g., into cardiac muscle) (47) and intravenous administration. It has been reported that stem cells when injected directly into the blood are able to locate myocardial infarctions by the process of cell homing (48). Cell-collagen composites have been employed (by implantation) for the repair of tendon injuries (49), biodegradable alginate beads for delivery of bone cells and antibiotics (50), and PEGylated fibrin patches for mesenchymal stem cell delivery (51). Clearly, the route of administration is key to determining the distribution of injected dendritic cells (52): intravenously administered cells accumulate in the spleen, whereas intramuscularly injected cells accumulate in the T-cell regions of lymph nodes, results confirmed by Morse et al. (53), who found intravenously administered dendritic cells localized first in the lungs and then distributed to liver, spleen, and bone marrow. Data on the biodistribution of nanoparticles are relevant to an understanding of some of the issues in cell-based therapeutics, while efficient delivery matrices are also key.

Guidelines of human somatic cell therapy developed by the FDA in the United States and by the EU's Committee for Medicinal Products for Human Use (CHMP) both address the triad of safety, quality, and efficacy that have been applied routinely to conventional therapeutic agents (54).

MATHEMATICAL MODELING

To be a more predictive science, pharmaceutics needs to embrace mathematical modeling of systems, however complex they may be. Mathematical modeling is one area that holds much promise for estimating the behavior of dose forms, such as in the release and diffusion of drugs in brain tissue (55). A thorough theoretical analysis can provide major benefits, including the following:

1. It can help to *understand how the dose forms work*, for example, why the drug is released at a particular rate from a controlled delivery system (56–58). The underlying mass transport mechanisms can be elucidated, and most importantly, the dominant physicochemical processes can be identified (59). Often a significant number of phenomena are involved, such as the wetting of a device's surface, water penetration into the dose form, drug dissolution, swelling of polymeric excipients, glassy to rubbery phase transitions, drug and excipient diffusion out of the dose form, polymer dissolution and/or degradation, and drug-polymer interactions, to mention just a few. Chapter 11 in volume 2 gives a detailed description of a number of these phenomena. If several of these processes occur in sequence and significantly differ in velocity, the much faster ones can be neglected. In the case where certain processes in the sequence are much slower than all the others, then these are release rate limiting.

   It is valuable to know which phenomena are dominant in a particular system, because this knowledge simplifies device optimization and trouble-shooting during product development, scale-up, and production. It has to be pointed out that the type of dose form, type and amount of drug and excipients, and even the type of preparation technique can significantly alter the relative importance of the involved physicochemical phenomena. Chapter 1 in volume 2 on sustained- and controlled-release drug delivery systems provides an overview on the most frequently used control mechanisms in advanced drug delivery systems, including matrix tablets for oral administration and biodegradable microparticles for parenteral use. Furthermore, a theoretical analysis based on comprehensive experimental in vivo results can give valuable insight into the phenomena that are governing the fate of the drug once it released into the human body. Obviously, this knowledge—the thorough understanding of the processes occurring within the dose form as well as within the living organism—provides the basis for an efficient improvement of the safety of the respective drug treatment, especially in the case of highly potent drugs with narrow therapeutic windows.

2. Mathematical modeling can significantly *facilitate the development of new products* and the optimization of existing ones. An appropriate mathematical theory allows for a quantitative prediction of the effects of different formulation and processing parameters on the resulting properties of the dose form, for example, the release rate of an incorporated drug. Figure 7 shows an example for such a simulation: the effects of the initial radius of propranolol HCl–loaded, hydroxypropyl methylcellulose (HPMC)-based

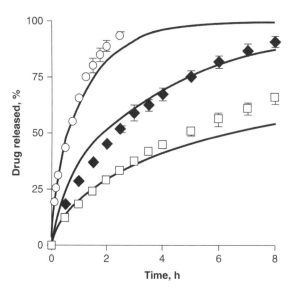

Figure 7 Theoretical prediction (*curves*) of the effects of the initial radius of hydroxypropyl methylcellulose–based matrix tablets containing 5% propranolol HCl on the resulting drug release kinetics in phosphate buffer pH 7.4. The symbols represent independent experimental results, confirming the theoretical calculations. The initial tablet height is 2.6 mm, the initial tablet radius is varied from 1.0 to 2.5 to 6.5 mm (corresponding to the *upper curve—open circles*; *middle curve—filled diamonds*; and *lower curve—open squares*). *Source*: From Ref. 60.

matrix tablets on the resulting drug release kinetics in phosphate buffer pH 7.4 are shown (curves) (60). The initial tablet height was constant (2.6 mm), whereas the initial tablet radius was varied from 1.0 to 6.5 mm (corresponding to the curves at the top to the bottom). Clearly, the resulting relative release rate significantly decreases when increasing the initial tablet radius, which can at least partially be attributed to the decreasing "surface area:volume ratio" of the system (and thus decreased relative surface area available for diffusion). The symbols in Figure 7 represent the independently determined experimental drug release kinetics from these matrix tablets. The good agreement between theory and experiment serves as an indication for the validity of this model for this type of drug delivery system. But also, the effects of other formulation and processing parameters on the resulting system properties can be theoretically predicted, including the initial drug and polymer content, type and amount of plasticizer, as well as size and shape of the dose form (61,62).

In silico simulations can, thus, be used to effectively replace or minimize the series of cost- and time-intensive "trial-and-error" experiments during product development. This is particularly useful in the case of controlled drug delivery systems with long-term release kinetics, for example, implants that are intended to provide appropriate drug levels during several months or years.

Two types of mathematical theories can be distinguished: *empirical models* and *mechanistic realistic models*. Empirical models are purely descriptive and do not allow for a better understanding of the underlying physical, chemical, and/or biological phenomena. Furthermore, they cannot be used to quantitatively predict the effects of formulation and processing parameters on the resulting system properties. In contrast, mechanistic theories are based on real phenomena, such as diffusion, dissolution, swelling, and/or dissolution/erosion. They allow for the determination of realistic parameters characterizing the respective dose form, for example, the diffusion coefficient of the drug within a matrix former or the degradation rate constant of a polymeric excipient. On the basis of these parameters, further insight into the underlying mass transport phenomena can be gained. For instance, the relative importance of the involved processes can be determined.

Because of the large variety of drugs, excipients, and dose forms that are used, there is no universal mathematical theory valid for all types of systems. In each particular case, it must be determined which processes are involved and—if possible—which of them are dominant. This type of analysis must be based on comprehensive experimental results, otherwise, no reliable conclusions can be drawn. It has to be pointed out that obtaining good agreement between a *fitted* theory and a set of experimental results is not a proof for the validity of a mathematical theory. Fitting a model to experimental results implies that one or more model parameters are adjusted to obtain the least-deviations "theory-experiment." Especially if a significant number of parameters are simultaneously fitted to the same set of experimental data, caution has to be paid when drawing conclusions. To evaluate the validity of a mathematical model for a particular type of drug-loaded dose form, the theory should be used to predict the effects of different formulation and/or processing parameters on the resulting system properties and these theoretical predictions should be compared with independent experimental results. Also, care should be taken when applying a mathematical theory to a specific dose form so that no major assumptions on which the model is based are violated. As an example, the famous Higuchi equation (10) is unfortunately often misused and applied to drug delivery systems for which it is not valid.

Yet, there is a significant lack of mechanistic realistic mathematical theories, which appropriately describe both the physicochemical phenomena occurring within the dose form and the subsequent fate of the drug within the human body (55). This can at least partially be explained by the complexity of the resulting set of mathematical equations considering all the involved physical, chemical, and biological processes (63). Also, a large variety of phenomena can be of importance in vivo for the fate of the drug, including diffusion and convection within the extra- and intracellular space, reversible and irreversible binding to extracellular matrix, drug metabolism, passive and active uptake into living cells (e.g., by "simple" diffusion and/or by receptor-mediated internalization), release from endolysosomes into the cytosol of the cells, uptake into the cell nuclei, and uptake/elimination/distribution from/into the blood stream and/or lymphatic system. Figure 8 shows as an example some of the processes that can be decisive for the drug upon direct administration into brain tissue. Importantly, drug transport in vivo can be highly anisotropic (direction dependent), because the human organism is not one homogeneous mass. Major advances in this research area allowing for a better understanding of the underlying drug transport mechanisms have been achieved by the working groups of Nicholson (64) and of Haller and Saltzman (65,66). However, there is a significant need for comprehensive and mechanistic mathematical theories relating formulation and processing parameters of dose forms to the resulting drug concentrations at the site of action and the pharmacodynamic effects of the treatment.

An often underestimated aspect when characterizing dose forms in vitro is the importance of the type of environment the systems are exposed to. This includes, for instance, the physical state of the medium (liquid or gel), degree of agitation, pH and ionic strength of the medium, the maintenance or absence of sink conditions, the presence/absence of enzymes and/or macrophages, etc. For example, the drug release patterns from PLGA parenteral controlled drug delivery systems can strongly depend on the pH of the surrounding environment, because ester hydrolysis is catalyzed by

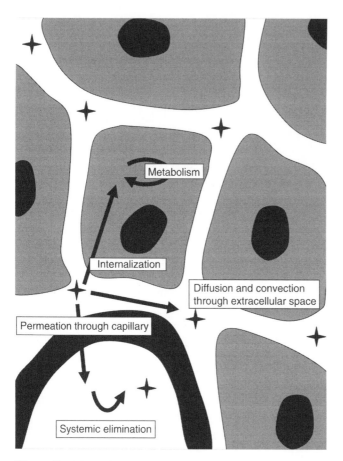

Figure 8 Schematic presentation of some of the processes that can be involved in drug transport within human brain tissue, including diffusion and convection through the extracellular spaces, permeation through capillaries, systemic elimination, internalization, and metabolism. The black circles represent drug molecules in the interstitial space. *Source*: From Ref. 63.

protons (67). Also, the osmotic pressure of the release medium can be of crucial importance for the drug release patterns from oral coated dose forms, in which crack formation is mandatory to allow for drug release. Appropriate mathematical modeling can be of great help in this perspective if the theory adequately takes into account the effects of the environmental conditions on the systems' properties. This allows for an appropriate correlation of the in vitro and in vivo results and thus for a significantly facilitated product development and improved safety of the drug treatment.

CONCLUSIONS

There can be no conclusions, only new challenges. This chapter, while it has not covered the whole gamut of possible topics or even all those described in this book, has attempted to show the connections between topics in a range of disciplines. It has always been the strength of pharmaceutics that perhaps it could not be defined, but we believe in its integrity and its ability to evolve and to have an important holistic view of medicines. This edition of *Modern Pharmaceutics*, following on from four editions edited by Gilbert

Banker and Christopher Rhodes, reflects the continual change and refinement in the subject and points the way to, and we hope encourages, further research, both applied and basic for the ultimate benefit of the patient.

REFERENCES

1. Martindale WH, Wescott WW. The Extra Pharmacopoeia. Vol 1, 18th ed. London: H. K. Lewis & Company, 1924:682–683.
2. Ritchie J. Brief notes of several cases of acute diarrhoea treated with keratin-coated carbolic acid pills. Lancet 1893; 142:1305–1306.
3. Dumez AG. A contribution to the history of the development of enteric capsules. J Am Pharm Assoc 1921; 10:372–376. Cited by: Jones BE. The history of the medicinal capsule. In: Podczeck F, Jones BE, eds. Pharmaceutical Capsules. 2nd ed. London: Pharmaceutical Press, 2004.
4. Gorley JT, Lee CO. A study of enteric coatings. J Am Pharm Assoc 1938; 27:379–384.
5. National Cash Register Company Patent 1953.
6. Kreuter J. Nanoparticles—a historical perspective. Int J Pharm 2007; 331:1–10.
7. Svenson S, Tomalia DA. Dendrimers in biomedical applications: reflections on the field. Adv Drug Deliv Rev 2005; 57:2106–2129.
8. Peterson DL, Yalkowsky SH. Comparison of two methods for predicting aqueous solubility. J Chem Inf Comput Sci 2002; 41:1531–1534.
9. Wassvik CM, Holmen AG, Bergstrom CA, et al. Contribution of solid-state properties to the aqueous solubility of drugs. Eur J Pharm Sci 2006; 29:294–305.
10. Higuchi T. Rate of release of medicaments from ointment bases containing drugs in suspensions. J Pharm Sci 1961; 50:874–875.
11. Florence AT, Salole EG, eds. Formulation Factors in Adverse Reactions. London: Wright, 1990.
12. Sun SX, Wirtz D. Mechanics of enveloped virus entry into host cells. Biophys J 2006; 90: L10–L12.
13. Hiestand HEN, Smith DP. Indices of tabletting performance. Powder Technol 1984; 38:145–159.
14. Tabor D. A simple theory of static and dynamic hardness. Proc R Soc Lond 1948; A192:247–274.
15. Tabor D. The Hardness of Metals. London: Oxford University Press, 1951.
16. Florence AT. Pharmaceutical Nanotechnology: more than size. Ten topics for research. Int J Pharm 2007; 339:1–2.
17. Florence AT. Nanoparticle flow: implications for drug delivery. In: Torchilin VP, ed. Nanoparticles as Drug Carriers. London: Imperial College Press, 2006:9–27.
18. Kararli TT. Comparison of the gastro-intestinal anatomy, physiology and biochemistry of humans and commonly used laboratory animals. Biopharm Drug Dispos 1995; 16:351–380.
19. Bayele H, Sakthivel T, O'Donell T, et al. Versatile peptide dendrimers for nucleic acid delivery. J Pharm Sci 2005; 94:446–457.
20. Parsegian VA. Van der Waals Forces. Cambridge: Cambridge University Press, 2006.
21. Morrison ID, Ross S. Colloidal Disperse Systems. New York: Wiley-Interscience, 2002: 358–359.
22. Geng Y, Dalheimer P, Cai S, et al. Shape effects of filaments versus spherical particles in flow and drug delivery. Nat Nanotechnol 2007; 2:249–255.
23. Gaumet M, Vargas A, Gurny R, et al. Nanoparticles for drug delivery@ the need for precision in reporting particle size parameters. Eur J Pharm Biopharm 2008; 69:1–9.
24. Keck CM, Muller RH. Size analysis of submicron particles by laser diffractometry—90% of the published measurements are false. Int J Pharm 2008; 355:150–163.
25. Oberdöster G, Oberdöster E, Oberdöster J. Nanotoxicology: an emerging discipline evolving from studies of ultrafine particles. Environ Health Perspect 2005; 113:823–839.

26. Gander B, Johansen P, Ho N-T, et al. Thermodynamic approach to protein microencapsulation into poly(D,L-lactide) by spray drying. Int J Pharm 1996; 129:51–61.

27. Gander B, Merkle HP, Nguyen VP, et al. A new thermodynamic model to predict protein encapsulation efficiency in poly(lactide) microspheres. J Phys Chem 1995; 99:16144–16148.

28. Doublier J-L, Garnier C, Renard D, et al. Protein-polysaccharide intercations. Curr Opin Colloid Interface Sci 2000; 5:202–214.

29. Florence AT, Jani PU, McCarthy D. Toothpaste and Crohn's disease. Lancet 1990; 336:1580–1581.

30. Grassian VH, O'Shaughnessy PT, Adamcakova-Dodd A, et al. Inhalation exposure study of titanium dioxide nanoparticles with a primary particle size of 2–5 nm. Environ Health Perspect 2007; 115:397–402.

31. Baveye P, Laba M. Aggregation and toxicology of titanium dioxide nanoparticles. Environ Health Perspect 2008; 116:A152.

32. de Gennes PG. Soft Interfaces: The 1994 Dirac Memorial Lecture. Cambridge: Cambridge University Press, 1997.

33. Scheel M, Seemann R, Brinkmann M, et al. Morphological clues to wet granular pile stability. Nat Mater 2008; 7:189–193.

34. Callies M, Quéré D. On water repellency. Soft Matter 2005; 1:55–61.

35. Krupenkin TN, Taylor JA, Schneider TM, et al. From rolling ball to complete wetting: the dynamic tuning of liquids on nanostructured surfaces. Langmuir 2004; 20:3824–3827.

36. Florence AT, Mysels KJ. Bursting of soap films VI. The effect of surfactant purity. J Phys Chem 1974; 78:234–235.

37. Florence AT, Frens G. Aureole profile in bursting soap films. Surface tension and surface relaxation in rapidly compressed monolayers. J Phys Chem 1972; 76:3024–3029.

38. Dubra A, Paterson C, Dainty C. Double lateral shearing interferometer for the quantitative measurement of tear film topography. Appl Opt 2005; 44:1101–1119.

39. Balazs AC, Verberg R, Pooley CM, et al. Modelling the flow of complex liquids through heterogeneous channels. Soft Matter 2005; 1:44–54.

40. Valiullin R, Naumov S, Galvosas P, et al. Exploration of molecular dynamics during transient sorption of fluids in mesoporous materials. Nature 2006; 443:965–968.

41. Rothen-Rutishauser BM, Kiama SG, Gehr P. A three dimensional cellular model of the human respiratory tract to study the interaction with particles. Am J Respir Cell Mol Biol 2005; 32:281–289.

42. Briscoe WH, Titmuss S, Tiberg F, et al. Boundary lubrication under water. Nature 2006; 444:191–194.

43. Eggers J. Coupling the large and the small. Nat Phys 2007; 3:145–146.

44. Duez C, Ybert C, Clanet C, et al. Making a splash with water repellancy. Nat Phys 2007; 3:180–183.

45. Grosiman A, Steinberg V. Elastic turbulence in a polymer solution flow. Nature 2000; 405:53–55.

46. Shinbrot T. Drat such custard. Nature 2005; 438:922–923.

47. Wold LE, Dai W, Sesti C, et al. Stem cell therapy for the heart. Congest Heart Fail 2004; 10:293–301.

48. Askari AT, Unzek S, Popovic ZB, et al. Effect of stromal-cell-derived factor 1 on stem cell homing and tissue regeneration in ischaemic cardiomyopathy. Lancet 2003; 362:697–703.

49. Awad HA, Boivin GP, Dressler MR, et al. Repair of patellar tendon injuries using a cell-collagen composite. J Orthop Res 2003; 21:420–431.

50. Ueng SW, Lee MS, Lin SS, et al. Development of a biodegradable alginate carrier system for antibiotics and bone cells. J Orthop Res 2007; 25:62–72.

51. Zhang G, Wang X, Wang Z, et al. A PEGylated fibrin patch for mesenchymal stem cell delivery. Tissue Eng 2006; 12:9–19.

52. Eggert AAO, Schreurs MW, Boerman OC, et al. Biodistribution and vaccine efficiency of murine dendritic cells are dependent on the route of administration. Cancer Res 1999; 59:3340–3345.

53. Morse MA, Coleman RE, Akabani G, et al. Migration of human dendritic cells after injection in patients with metastatic malignancies. Cancer Res 1999; 59:56–58.

54. Tsang L. Legal and ethical status of stem cells as medicinal products. Adv Drug Deliv Rev 2005; 57:1970–1980.

55. Siepmann J, Siepmann F, Florence AT. Local controlled delivery to the brain: mathematical modelling of the underlying mass transport mechanisms. Int J Pharm 2006; 314:101–119.

56. Siepmann J, Peppas NA. Modeling of drug release from delivery systems based on hydroxypropyl methylcellulose (HPMC). Adv Drug Deliv Rev 2001; 48:139–157.

57. Narasimhan B. Mathematical models describing polymer dissolution: consequences for drug delivery. Adv Drug Deliv Rev 2001; 48:195–210.

58. Raman C, Berkland C, Kim K, et al. Modeling small-molecule release from PLG microspheres: effects of polymer degradation and nonuniform drug distribution. J Control Release 2005; 103:149–158.

59. Siepmann J, Goepferich A. Mathematical modeling of bioerodible, polymeric drug delivery systems. Adv Drug Deliv Rev 2001; 48:229–247.

60. Siepmann J, Kranz H, Peppas NA, et al. Calculation of the required size and shape of hydroxypropyl methylcellulose matrices to achieve desired drug release profiles. Int J Pharm 2000; 201:151–164.

61. Siepmann F, Le Brun V, Siepmann J. Drugs acting as plasticizers in polymeric systems: a quantitative treatment. J Control Release 2006; 115:298–306.

62. Fan LT, Singh SK, eds. Controlled Release. A Quantitative Treatment. Berlin: Springer-Verlag, 1989.

63. Fung LK, Shin M, Tyler B, et al. Chemotherapeutic drugs released from polymers: distribution of 1,3-bis(2-chloroethyl)-1-nitrosourea in the rat brain. Pharm Res 1996; 13:671–682.

64. Nicholson C. Diffusion and related transport mechanisms in brain tissue. Rep Prog Phys 2001; 64:815–884.

65. Haller MF, Saltzman WM. Localized delivery of proteins in the brain: can transport be customized? Pharm Res 1998; 15:377–385.

66. Haller MF, Saltzman WM. Nerve growth factor delivery systems. J Control Release 1998; 53:1–6.

67. Lu L, Garcia CA, Mikos AG. In vitro degradation of thin poly(DL-lactic-co-glycolic acid) films. J Biomed Mater Res 1999; 46:236–244.

2

Principles of Drug Absorption

Michael Mayersohn
College of Pharmacy, Department of Pharmacy Practice and Science,
University of Arizona, Tucson, Arizona, U.S.A.

INTRODUCTION

Drug dosing most often involves the oral route of administration. The vast majority of drug dosage forms are designed for oral ingestion, primarily for ease of administration. It should be recognized, however, that this route may result in inefficient and erratic drug therapy. Whenever a drug is ingested orally (or by any nonvascular route), one would like it to have rapid and complete absorption into the bloodstream for the following reasons:

1. Assuming that there is some relationship between drug concentration in the body and the magnitude of the therapeutic response (which is often the case), the greater the concentration achieved, the larger the magnitude of response.
2. In addition to desiring therapeutic concentrations, one would like to obtain these concentrations rapidly. The more rapidly the drug is absorbed, in general, the sooner the pharmacological response is achieved.
3. In general, one finds that the more rapid and complete the absorption, the more uniform and reproducible the pharmacological response becomes.
4. The more rapidly the drug is absorbed, the less chance there is of drug degradation or interactions with other materials present in the gastrointestinal tract (GIT).

In a broad sense, one can divide the primary factors that influence oral drug absorption and thus govern the efficacy of drug therapy into the following variables: physicochemical, physiological, and dosage form. For the most part, these variables will determine the clinical response to any drug administered by an extravascular route. Although often the total response to a drug given orally is a complex function of the aforementioned variables interacting together, the present discussion is limited primarily to the first two categories involving physicochemical and physiological factors. Dosage form variables influencing the response to a drug and the effect of route of administration are discussed in chapters 4, 5 and 6.

The vast majority of drugs in current use and those under development are relatively simple organic molecules obtained from either natural sources or by synthetic methods. It is important to note, however, the virtual revolution in development of new therapeutic entities; those based upon the incredible advances being made in the application of molecular biology and biotechnology. These new drugs, especially peptides, proteins, and monoclonal antibodies are not the traditional small organic molecules stressed in this chapter. Indeed, those compounds have unique physicochemical properties, which are quite different from those of small organic molecules, and they offer remarkable challenges for drug delivery. As a result, new and more complex physical delivery systems are being designed in conjunction with an examination of other, less traditional routes of administration (e.g., nasal, pulmonary, transdermal). Because of issues of instability in the GIT and poor intrinsic membrane permeability, it appears unlikely that these new biologically-based drugs will employ the oral route for administration. Numerous strategies are being explored, but to date relatively little success has been achieved (1). One approach that shows promise involves conjugating a poorly absorbed compound to a so-called molecular transporter. The latter are oligomers of arginine that undergo active cellular uptake (2,3).

ANATOMICAL AND PHYSIOLOGICAL CONSIDERATIONS OF THE GASTROINTESTINAL TRACT

The GIT is a highly specialized region of the body whose primary functions involve the processes of secretion, digestion, and absorption. Since all nutrients needed by the body, with the exception of oxygen, must first be ingested orally, then processed by the GIT, and then made available for absorption into the bloodstream, the GIT represents a significant barrier and interface with the environment. The primary defense mechanisms employed by the gut to rid it of noxious or irritating materials are vomiting and diarrhea. In fact, emesis is often a first approach to the treatment of oral poisoning. Diarrhea conditions, initiated by either a pathological state or a physiological mechanism, will result in the flushing away of toxins or bacteria or will represent the response to a stressful condition. Indeed, the GIT is often the first site of the body's response to stress, a fact readily appreciated by students taking a final exam! The nearly instinctive gut response to stress may be particularly pertinent to patients needing oral drug therapy. Since stress is a fact of our daily lives, and since any illness requiring drug therapy may to some degree be considered stressful, the implications of the body's response to stress and the resulting influence on drug absorption from the gut may be particularly pertinent.

Figure 1 illustrates the gross functional regions of the GIT (4). The liver, gallbladder, and pancreas secrete materials vital to the digestive and certain absorptive functions of the gut. The lengths of various regions of the GIT are presented in Table 1. The small intestine, comprising the duodenum, jejunum, and ileum, represents greater than 60% of the length of the GIT, which is consistent with its primary digestive and absorptive functions. In addition to daily food and fluid intake (~ 1–2 L), the GIT and associated organs secrete about 8 L of fluid per day. Of this, only 100 to 200 mL of stool water is lost per day, indicating efficient absorption of water throughout the tract.

Stomach

After oral ingestion, materials are presented to the stomach, whose primary functions are storage, mixing, and reducing all components to a slurry with the aid of gastric secretions and then emptying these contents in a controlled manner into the upper small intestine (duodenum). All these functions are accomplished by complex neural, muscular, and hormonal processes. Anatomically, the stomach has classically been divided into three

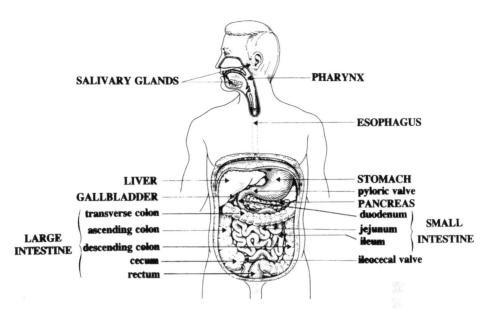

SALIVARY GLANDS — PHARYNX

ESOPHAGUS

LIVER — STOMACH
GALLBLADDER — pyloric valve
— PANCREAS
transverse colon — duodenum
ascending colon — jejunum — SMALL
LARGE — ileum — INTESTINE
INTESTINE — descending colon
cecum — ileocecal valve
rectum

Figure 1 Diagrammatic sketch of the gastrointestinal tract (and subdivisions of the small and large intestines) along with associated organs. *Source*: Modified from Ref. 4.

Table 1 Approximate Lengths of Various Regions of the Human Gastrointestinal Tract

Region	Length (m)
Duodenum	0.3
Jejunum	2.4
Ileum	3.6
Large intestine	0.9–1.5

parts: fundus, body, and antrum (or pyloric part), as illustrated in Figure 2 (5). Although there are no sharp distinctions among these regions, the proximal stomach, made up of the fundus and body, serves as a reservoir for ingested material and secretes acid, while the distal region (antrum), which secretes gastrin, is the major site of mixing motions and acts as a pump to accomplish gastric emptying. The fundus and body regions of the stomach have relatively little tone in their muscular wall and, as a result, can distend outward to accommodate a meal of up to 1 L.

A common anatomical feature of the entire GIT is its four concentric layers. Beginning with the luminal (i.e., inner or absorbing) surface these are the mucosa, submucosa, muscularis mucosa, and serosa. The three outer layers are similar throughout most of the tract; however, the mucosa has distinctive structural and functional characteristics. The mucosal surface of the stomach is lined by an epithelial layer of columnar cells, the surface mucous cells, which secrete mucous (mucopolysaccharides) that protects the epithelial surface from acid, enzymes, and pathogens. Covering the epithelial cell surface is a layer of mucous 1.0 to 1.5 mm thick. Along this surface are many tubular invaginations, referred to as gastric pits, at the bottom of which are found specialized gastric secretory cells. These secretory (parietal) cells form part of an

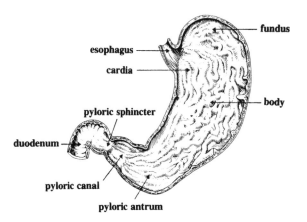

Figure 2 Diagrammatic sketch of the stomach and anatomical regions. *Source*: Modified from Ref. 5.

extensive network of gastric glands, which produce and secrete about 2 L of gastric fluid daily. The epithelial cells of the gastric mucosa represent one of the most rapidly proliferating epithelial tissues, being shed by the normal stomach at the rate of about a half-million cells per minute. As a result, the surface epithelial layer is renewed every one to three days.

The next region, the muscularis mucosa, consists of an inner circular and an outer longitudinal layer of smooth muscle. This area is responsible for the muscular contractions of the stomach wall needed to accommodate a meal by stretching and for the mixing and propulsive movements of gastric contents. An area known as the lamina propria lies below the muscularis mucosa and contains a variety of tissue types, including connective and smooth muscles, nerve fibers, and the blood and lymph vessels. It is the blood flow to this region and to the muscularis mucosa that delivers nutrients to the gastric mucosa. The major vessels providing a vascular supply to the GIT are the celiac and the inferior and superior mesenteric arteries. Venous return from the GIT is through the splenic and the inferior and superior mesenteric veins. The outermost region of the stomach wall provides structural support for the organ.

Small Intestine

The small intestine has the shape of a convoluted tube and represents the major length of the GIT. The small intestine, comprising the duodenum, jejunum, and ileum, has a unique surface structure, making it ideally suited for its primary role of digestion and absorption. The most important structural aspect of the small intestine is the means by which it greatly increases its effective luminal surface area. The initial increase in surface area, compared with the area of a smooth cylinder, is due to the projection within the lumen of folds of mucosa, referred to as the folds of Kerckring. Lining the entire epithelial surface are fingerlike projections, the villi, extending into the lumen. These villi range in length from 0.5 to 1.5 mm, and it has been estimated that there are about 10 to 40 villi/mm^2 of mucosal surface. Projecting from the villi surface are fine structures, the microvilli (average length 1 mm), which represent the final large increase in the surface area of the small intestine. There are approximately 600 microvilli protruding from each absorptive cell lining the villi. Relative to the surface of a smooth cylinder, the folds, villi, and microvilli increase the effective surface area by factors of 3, 30, and 600, respectively.

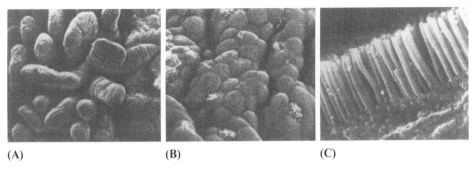

(A)   (B)   (C)

Figure 3 (**A**) Photomicrograph of the human duodenal surface illustrating the projection of villi into the lumen (magnification 75×). The goblet cells appear as white dots on the villus surface. (**B**) Photomicrograph of a single human duodenal villus illustrating surface coverage by microvilli and the presence of goblet cells (*white areas*) (magnification 2400×). (**C**) Photomicrograph illustrating the microvilli of the small intestine of the dog (magnification 33,000×). *Source*: From Ref. 6.

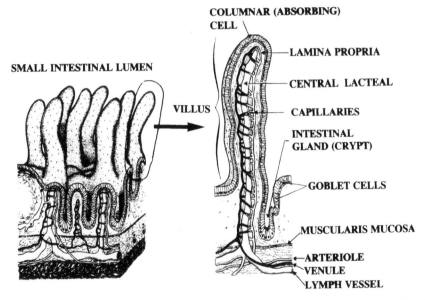

Figure 4 Diagrammatic sketch of the small intestine illustrating the projection of the villi into the lumen (*left*) and the anatomic features of a single villus (*right*). *Source*: Modified from Ref. 4 (see p. 439).

The resulting area represents a surface equal to about two-thirds of a regulation tennis court! These structural features are clearly indicated in the photomicrographs shown in Figure 3. A diagrammatic sketch of the villus is shown in Figure 4.

The mucosa of the small intestine can be divided into three distinct layers. The muscularis mucosa, the deepest layer, consists of a thin sheet of smooth muscle 3 to 10 cells thick and separates the mucosa from the submucosa. The lamina propria, the section between the muscularis mucosa and the intestinal epithelia, represents the subepithelial connective tissue space and together with the surface epithelium forms the villi structure. The lamina propria contains a variety of cell types, including blood and lymph vessels and nerve fibers. Molecules to be absorbed must penetrate into this region to gain access to the bloodstream.

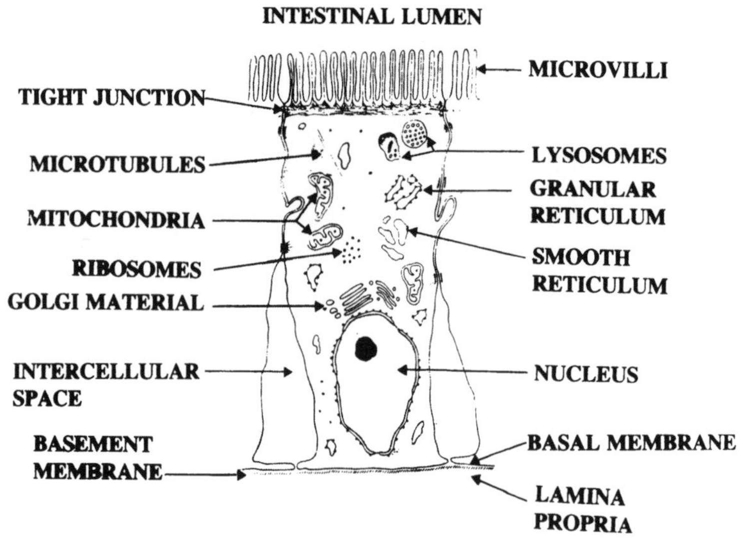

INTESTINAL LUMEN

Figure 5 Diagrammatic sketch of the intestinal absorptive cell. *Source*: Modified from Ref. 7.

The third mucosal layer is that lining the entire length of the small intestine and which represents a continuous sheet of epithelial cells. These epithelial cells (or enterocytes) are columnar in shape, and the luminal cell membrane, upon which the microvilli reside, is called the apical cell membrane. Opposite this membrane is the basal (or basolateral) plasma membrane, which is separated from the lamina propria by a basement membrane. A sketch of this cell is shown in Figure 5. The primary function of the villi is absorption.

The microvilli region has also been referred to as the striated or "brush" border. It is in this region where the process of absorption is initiated. In close contact with the microvilli is a coating of fine filaments composed of weakly acidic sulfated mucopolysaccharides. It has been suggested that this region may serve as a relatively impermeable barrier to substances within the gut such as bacteria and other foreign materials. In addition to increasing the effective luminal surface area, the microvilli region appears to be an area of important biochemical activity.

Consistent with the absorptive function of the GIT and, in addition to its large surface area, the enterocyte membrane contains proteins that are responsible for specialized (i.e., nonpassive) transport (influx) of certain molecules. In direct contrast with such processes but consistent with the GIT function as a barrier to the environment, there are also efflux transporters that move absorbed molecules back into the gut lumen. Complementing the efflux transporters is the metabolic activity of the enterocytes reflecting the high concentrations of cytochrome (phase I) and conjugating (phase II) enzymes. These enzymes are known to metabolize many drugs and form the basis for numerous drug-drug and drug-nutrient interactions. These factors are discussed in a later section.

The surface epithelial cells of the small intestine are renewed rapidly and regularly. It takes about two days for the cells of the duodenum to be renewed completely. As a result of its rapid renewal rate, the intestinal epithelium is susceptible to various factors that may influence proliferation. Exposure of the intestine to ionizing radiation and cytotoxic drugs (such as folic acid antagonists and colchicine) reduce the cell renewal rate.

Large Intestine

The large intestine, often referred to as the colon, has two primary functions: the absorption of water and electrolytes and the storage and elimination of fecal material. The large intestine, which has a greater diameter than the small intestine (~ 6 cm), is connected to the latter at the ileocecal junction. The wall of the ileum at this point has a thickened muscular coat called the ileocecal sphincter, which forms the ileocecal valve, whose principal function is to prevent backflow of fecal material from the colon into the small intestine. From a functional point of view the large intestine may be divided into two parts. The proximal half, concerned primarily with absorption, includes the cecum, ascending colon, and portions of the transverse colon. The distal half, concerned with storage and mass movement of fecal matter, includes part of the transverse and descending colon, the rectum, and anal regions, terminating at the internal anal sphincter (Fig. 1).

In humans, the large intestine usually receives about 500 mL of fluid-like food material (chyme) per day. As this material moves distally through the large intestine, water is absorbed, producing a viscous and finally a solid mass of matter. Because of efficient water absorption, of the 500 mL normally reaching the large intestine, approximately 80 mL are eliminated from the gut as fecal material.

Structurally, the large intestine is similar to the small intestine, although the luminal surface epithelium of the former lacks villi. The muscularis mucosa, as in the small intestine, consists of inner circular and outer longitudinal layers. Figure 6 (8) illustrates a photomicrograph and diagrammatic sketches of this region.

Pathways of Drug Absorption

Once a drug molecule is in solution, it has the potential to be absorbed. Whether or not it is in a form available for absorption depends on the physicochemical characteristics of the drug (i.e., its inherent absorbability) and the characteristics of its immediate environment (e.g., pH, the presence of interacting materials, and the local properties of the absorbing membrane). Assuming that there are no interfering substances present to impede absorption, the drug molecule must come in contact with the absorbing membrane. To accomplish this, the drug molecule must diffuse from the gastrointestinal (GI) fluids to the membrane surface. The most appropriate definition of drug absorption is the penetration of the drug across the intestinal "membrane" and the appearance of the unchanged form in the blood draining the GIT. The latter blood flow will drain into the portal circulation on the way to the liver. A clear distinction must be made between *absorbed* drug and *bioavailable* drug. The former was defined above; the latter refers to the appearance of unaltered drug in the systemic circulation (i.e., beyond the liver). There are two important points to this definition. First, it is often assumed that drug disappearance from the GI fluids represents absorption. This is true only if disappearance from the gut represents appearance in the blood stream. This may not be the case, for example, if the drug degrades in GI fluids or if it is metabolized within the intestinal cells. Second, the term intestinal membrane is rather misleading, since this membrane is not a unicellular structure but a number of unicellular membranes parallel to one another. In fact, relative to the molecular size of most drug molecules, the compound must diffuse a considerable distance. Thus, for a drug molecule to reach the blood, it must penetrate the mucous layer and brush border covering the GI lumen, the apical cell surface, the fluids within this cell, the basal membrane, the basement membrane, the tissue region of the lamina propria, the external capillary membrane, the cytoplasm of the capillary cell, and finally, the inner

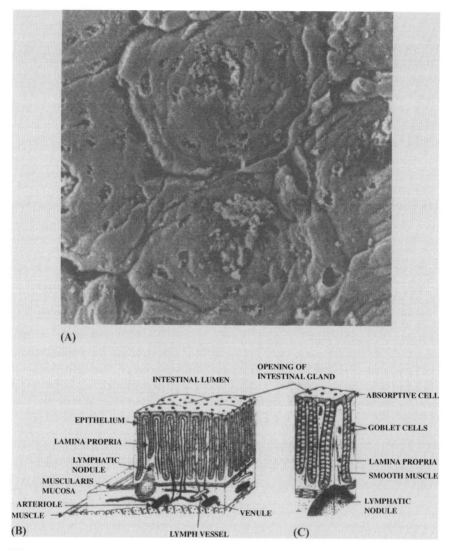

Figure 6 (**A**) Scanning electron micrograph of the luminal surface of the large intestine (transverse colon; magnification 60×). (**B**) Schematic diagram showing a longitudinal cross-section of the large intestine. (**C**) Enlargement of cross-section shown in (**B**). *Source*: Part A from Ref. 6 (see p. 135) and parts B and C modified from Ref. 8.

capillary membrane. Therefore, when the expression "intestinal membrane" is used, we are discussing a barrier to absorption consisting of several distinct unicellular membranes and fluid regions bounded by these membranes. Throughout this chapter the term intestinal membrane will be used in that sense.

For a drug molecule to be absorbed from the GIT and gain access to the portal circulation (on its way to the liver), it must effectively penetrate all the regions of the intestine just cited. There are primarily three factors governing this absorption process once a drug is in solution: the physicochemical characteristics of the molecule, the properties and components of the GI fluids, and the nature of the absorbing membrane. Although penetration of the intestinal membrane is obviously the first part of absorption, the factors controlling penetration are discussed in the following section. At this point, assume that the drug molecule has penetrated most of the barriers in the intestine and has reached the lamina propria region. Once in this region the drug may either diffuse through the blood capillary membrane and be carried away in the bloodstream or penetrate the central lacteal and reach the lymph. These functional units of the villi are illustrated in Figure 4. Most drugs reach the systemic circulation via the bloodstream of the capillary network in the villi. The primary reason for this route being dominant over lymphatic penetration is the fact that the villi are highly and rapidly perfused by the bloodstream. Blood flow to the GIT in humans is approximately 500 to 1000 times greater than lymph flow. Thus, although the lymphatic system is a potential route for drug absorption from the intestine, under normal circumstances it will account for only a small fraction of the total amount absorbed. The major exception to this rule will be drugs (and environmental toxicants, such as insecticides) that have extremely large oil/water partition coefficients ($K_{o/w}$ greater than about 10^5 or log partition of 5). By increasing lymph flow or, alternatively, reducing blood flow, drug absorption via the lymphatic system may become more important. The capillary and lymphatic vessels are rather permeable to most low-molecular-weight and lipid-soluble compounds. The capillary membrane, however, represents a more substantial barrier than the central lacteal to the penetration of very large molecules or combinations of molecules as a result of frequent separations of cells along the lacteal surface. The lymphatic route of movement is important, for example, for the absorption of triglycerides or emulsified fats in the form of chylomicrons, which are rather large (~ 0.5 µm in diameter). A recent study has concluded that effective lymphatic absorption of a drug depends not only on $K_{o/w}$ but also on the ability to partition into chylomicrons and long-chain triglycerides (9).

PHYSICOCHEMICAL FACTORS GOVERNING DRUG ABSORPTION

Oil/Water Partition Coefficient and Chemical Structure

As a result of extensive experimentation done in the early 1900s, it has been found that the primary physicochemical properties of a drug influencing its passive absorption into and across biological membranes are its $K_{o/w}$, extent of ionization in biological fluids determined by its pK_a value and pH of the fluid in which it is dissolved, and its molecular weight or volume. Passive absorption refers to a first-order kinetic process not having any membrane involvement (i.e., no energy is required or expended for transport to occur). The fact that these variables govern drug absorption is a direct reflection of the nature of biological membranes. The cell surface of biological membranes (including those lining the entire GIT) is lipid in nature; as a result, one may view penetration into the intestinal cells as a competition for drug molecules between the aqueous environment on one hand and the lipid-like materials of the membrane on the other. To a large extent, then, the principles of solution chemistry and the molecular attractive forces to which the drug molecules are exposed will govern movement from an aqueous phase to the lipid-like phase of the membrane.

At the turn of the last century, Overton examined the osmotic behavior of the frog sartorius muscle soaked in a buffer solution containing various dissolved organic compounds. He reasoned that, if the solute entered the tissue, the weight of the muscle would remain essentially unchanged, whereas, loss of weight would indicate an osmotic withdrawal of fluid and hence impermeability to the solute in solution. He noted that, in general, the tissue was most readily penetrated by lipid-soluble compounds and poorly penetrated by lipid-insoluble substances. Overton was one of the first investigators to illustrate that compounds penetrate cells in the same relative order as their $K_{o/w}$, suggesting the lipid-like nature of cell membranes. Using animal or plant cells, other workers provided data in support of Overton's observations. The only exception to this general rule was the observation that very small molecules penetrate cell membranes faster than would be expected based on their $K_{o/w}$ values. To explain the rapid penetration of these small molecules (e.g., urea, methanol, formamide), it was suggested that cell membranes, although lipid in nature, were not continuous but interrupted by small water-filled channels or "pores"; such membranes are best described as being lipid-sieve membranes. As a result, one could imagine lipid-soluble molecules readily penetrating the lipid regions of the membrane while small water-soluble molecules pass through the aqueous pores. Fordtran et al. (10) estimated the effective pore radius to be 7 to 8.5 and 3 to 3.8 Å in human jejunum and ileum, respectively. There may be a continuous distribution of pore sizes, a smaller fraction of larger ones and a greater fraction of smaller pores.

Our knowledge of biological membrane ultrastructure is the result of rapid advances in instrumentation. Although some controversy remains over the most correct biological membrane model, the concept of membrane structure presented by Davson and Danielli of a lipid bilayer is perhaps the one best accepted (11,12). The most current version of that basic model is illustrated in Figure 7 and is referred to as the "fluid mosaic" model of membrane structure (13). That model is consistent with what we have learned about the existence of specific ion channels and receptors within and along surface membranes.

Table 2 summarizes some literature data supporting the general dependence of the rate of absorption on $K_{o/w}$, as measured in the rat intestine (14,15). As with numerous other examples, as $K_{o/w}$ increases, the rate of absorption increases. However, note that this is seldom a simple linear relationship. For example, secobarbital has a value for absorption that is about three-times that of barbital; however, $K_{o/w}$ differs by 70-fold. One very extensive study (16–18) has examined in depth the physicochemical factors governing nonelectrolyte permeability for several hundred compounds. This study employed an in vitro rabbit gallbladder preparation, an organ whose mucosal surface is lined by epithelial cells. The method used to assess solute permeability is based upon

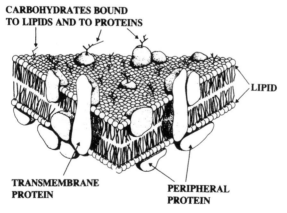

CARBOHYDRATES BOUND TO LIPIDS AND TO PROTEINS

LIPID

TRANSMEMBRANE PROTEIN

PERIPHERAL PROTEIN

Figure 7 Diagrammatic representation of the fluid mosaic model of the cell membrane. The basic structure of the membrane is that of a lipid bilayer in which the lipid portion (*long tails*) points inward and the polar portion (*round "head"*) points outward. The membrane is penetrated by transmembrane (or integral) proteins. Attached to the surface of the membrane are peripheral proteins (*inner surface*) and carbohydrates that bind to lipid and protein molecules (*outer surface*). *Source*: Modified from Ref. 13.

Table 2 Influence of $K_{o/w}$ on Absorption from Rat Intestine

Compound	$K_{o/w}$	Percentage absorbed
Olive oil/water		
Valeramide	0.023	85
Lactamide	0.00058	67
Malonamide	0.00008	27
Chloroform/water		
Hexethal	>100	44
Secobarbital	50.7	40
Pentobarbital	28.0	30
Cyclobarbital	13.9	24
Butethal	11.7	24
Allybarbituric acid	10.5	23
Phenobarbital	4.8	20
Aprobarbital	4.9	17
Barbital	0.7	12

Abbreviation: $K_{o/w}$, oil/water partition coefficient.

measurement of differences in electrical potential (streaming potentials) across the membrane. The more permeable the compound, the smaller the osmotic pressure it exerts and the smaller the osmotic fluid flow it produces in the opposite direction; this results in a small potential difference. If the compound is impermeable, it produces a large osmotic pressure and osmotic fluid flow, resulting in a large potential difference. Experimentally, one exposes the mucosal membrane surface to a buffer solution containing a reference compound to which the membrane is completely impermeable (e.g., mannitol) and measures the resulting potential difference. This is followed by exposing the same membrane to a solution of a test compound and again measuring the resulting potential difference. The ratio of the potential difference of the test compound to that of the reference compound is referred to as the reflection coefficient (σ). The σ is a measure of the permeability of the test compound relative to a reference solute with the particular membrane being used. The less permeable the test compound, the closer the σ approaches 1 ($\sigma = 1$); the more permeable the test compound, the closer the σ approaches 0 ($\sigma = 0$).

By using this method, Wright and Diamond were able to reach a number of important conclusions concerning patterns of nonelectrolyte permeability. In general, membrane permeability of a solute increases with $K_{o/w}$, supporting previous findings mentioned earlier. The two classes of exceptions to this pattern are highly branched compounds, which penetrate the membrane more slowly than would be expected on the basis of their $K_{o/w}$, and smaller polar molecules, which penetrate the membrane more readily than would be expected on the basis of their $K_{o/w}$. The latter observation has been reported by other workers, and, as noted earlier, it has resulted in the development of the lipid-sieve membrane concept whereby one envisions aqueous pores in the membrane surface. The authors postulate that these small, polar, relatively lipid-insoluble compounds penetrate the membrane by following a route lined by the polar groupings of membrane constituents (i.e., localized polar regions). This concept is an attractive structural explanation of what have been referred to as pores. The accessibility of this route would be limited primarily by the molecular size of the compound as a result of steric hindrance. In fact, it is the first one or two members of a homologous series of compounds that are readily permeable, but beyond these members, it is primarily $K_{o/w}$ that dictates permeability. Table 3 illustrates this effect for several members of various

Table 3 Influence of Chain Length on Membrane Permeability Within Several Homologous Series

Compound	Reflection coefficient, σ
Urea	0.29 ↑
Methyl urea	0.54
Ethyl urea	0.92
Propyl urea	0.93 -
Butyl urea	0.70 ↓
Malononitrile	0.09 ↑
Succinonitrile	0.30 -
Glutaronitrile	0.21 ↓
Methylformamide	0.28 ↑
Methylacetamide	0.51 -
Methylproprionamide	0.22 ↓

The reflection coefficient σ is defined in the text. The direction of the arrows indicates an increase in permeability from the least permeable member of the series.

homologous series. Recall that the smaller the σ, the more permeable the compound. In each instance, permeability decreases after the first member, reaches a minimum, and then increases again.

The other anomalous behavior was the smaller-than-expected permeability of highly branched compounds. This deviation has been explained on the basis that membrane lipids are subject to a more highly constrained orientation (probably a parallel configuration of hydrocarbon chains of fatty acids) than are those in a bulk lipid solvent. As a result, branched compounds must disrupt this local lipid structure of the membrane and will encounter greater steric hindrance than will a straight-chain molecule. This effect with branched compounds is not adequately reflected in simple aqueous lipid-partitioning studies (i.e., in the $K_{o/w}$ value).

With the exception of rather small polar molecules, the majority of compounds, including drugs, appear to penetrate biological membranes via a lipid route. As a result the membrane permeability of most compounds is dependent on $K_{o/w}$. The physicochemical interpretation of this general relationship is based on the atomic and molecular forces to which the solute molecules are exposed in the aqueous and lipid phases. Thus, the ability of a compound to partition from an aqueous to a lipid phase of a membrane involves the balance between solute-water and solute-membrane intermolecular forces. If the attractive forces of the solute-water interaction are greater than those of the solute-membrane interaction, membrane permeability will be relatively poor and vice versa. In examining the permeability of a homologous series of compounds and, therefore, the influence of substitution or chain length on permeability, one must recognize the influence of the substituted group on the intermolecular forces in aqueous and membrane phases (e.g., dipole-dipole, dipole-induced dipole, or van der Waals forces). The membrane permeabilities of the nonelectrolytes studied appear to be largely determined by the number and strength of hydrogen bonds the solute can form with water. Thus, nonelectrolyte permeation is largely a question of physical organic chemistry in aqueous solution. Table 4 summarizes some of the interesting findings of Diamond and Wright with respect to the influence of substituent groups on membrane permeation. These data have been interpreted on the basis of the solutes' ability to form hydrogen bonds with water.

Table 4 Influence of Chemical Substitution on the Membrane Permeability of Several Series of Nonelectrolytes

Substituent group	Influence on membrane permeability	Compound	Example	σ^a
Oxygen and nitrogen functional groups				
Alcoholic hydroxyl group (—OH)	(a) At any given chain length, permeability decreases as the number of —OH groups increases	n-Propanol	$CH_3CH_2CH_2OH$	0.02
		1,2-Propanediol	$CH_3CHOHCH_2OH$	0.84
		Glycerol	$CH_2OHCHOHCH_2OH$	0.95
	(b) Intramolecular H-bonds formed between adjacent —OH groups result in greater permeability compared with the same compound with nonadjacent —OH groups because of decreased H-bond formation with water	2,3-Butanediol	$CH_3CHOHCHOHCH_3$	0.74
		1,3-Butanediol	$CH_3CHOHCH_2CH_2OH$	0.77
		1,4-Butanediol	$CH_2OHCH_2CH_2CH_2OH$	0.86
Ether group (—O—)	Has less of an influence than an —OH group in decreasing permeability	n-Propanol	$CH_3CH_2CH_2OH$	0.02
		Ethyleneglycol-methyl ether	$CH_3-O-CH_2CH_2OH$	0.15
		1,2-Propanediol	$CH_3CHOHCH_2OH$	0.84
Carbonyl group Ketone (—C=O)	Has less of an influence than an —OH group in decreasing permeability; difficulty in measuring permeability of these compounds per se as many are unstable in solution-forming diols and enolic tautomers	Acetone	$\underset{\displaystyle CH_3CCH_3}{O\atop\|}$	0.01
		2-Propanol	$CH_3CHOHCH_3$	0.10
Aldehyde (—HC=O)		2-5-Hexanedione	$\underset{\displaystyle CH_3CCH_2CH_2CCH_3}{O\qquad O\atop\|\qquad\|}$	0.00
		2,5-Hexanediol	$CH_3CHOHCH_2CH_2CHOHCH_3$	0.59
Ester group $\underset{\displaystyle (-C-O-)}{O\atop\|}$	Has less of an influence than an —OH group in decreasing permeability	1,2-Propanediol-1-acetate	$\underset{\displaystyle CH_3C-O-CH_2CHOHCH_3}{O\atop\|}$	0.31
		1,5-Pentanediol	$CH_2OH(CH_2)_3CH_2OH$	0.71

(Continued)

Table 4 Influence of Chemical Substitution on the Membrane Permeability of Several Series of Nonelectrolytes (*Continued*)

Substituent group	Influence on membrane permeability	Compound	Example	σ^a
Oxygen and nitrogen functional groups				
Amide group $O=C-NH_2$	Causes a greater decrease in permeability than any of the above groups	*n*-Propanol	$CH_3CH_2CH_2OH$	0.02
		Acetone	CH_3CCH_3, O	0.08
		Ethyleneglycol-methyl ether	$CH_3-O-CH_2CH_2OH$	0.15
		Proprionamide	$CH_3CH_2CNH_2$, O	0.66
Urea derivatives $R-NH-C-NH_2$, O	These compounds have lower permeability than amides with the same number of carbons and are about as impermeable as the corresponding dihydroxyl alcohols	*n*-Butanl	$CH_3CH_2CH_2CH_2OH$	0.01
		n-Butryamide	$CH_3CH_2CH_2C-NH_2$, O	0.42
		1,4-Butanediol	$CH_2OHCH_2CH_2CH_2OH$	0.86
		n-Propyl urea	$CH_3CH_2CH_2NHCNH_2$, O	0.89
α-Amino acids $R-CHCOOH$, NH_2	These compounds have the lowest $K_{o/w}$ values of all organic molecules and are essentially impermeable due to large dipole-dipole interactions with water	Proprionamide	$CH_3CH_2CNH_2$, O	0.66
		1-Amino-2-propanol	$CH_3CHOHCH_2NH_2$	0.89
		1,3-Propanediol	$CH_2OHCH_2CH_2OH$	0.92
		Alanine	H_2N, $CH_3CHC-OH$, O	0.06

Sulfur functional groups

Sulfur replacement of oxygen	(a) Sulfur compounds have greater $K_{o/w}$ values and permeate membranes more readily than the corresponding oxygen compound; this is a result of poor H-bond formation between sulfur and water compared with the oxygen analog	1-Thioglycerol	$CH_2OHCHOHCH_2SH$	0.69	
		Glycerol	$CH_2OHCHOHCH_2OH$	0.95	←
		Thiodiglycol	$(OHCH_2CH_2)_2S$	0.71	
	(b) Sulfoxides ($R_2S{=}O$) are less permeable than the corresponding ketone ($R_2C{=}O$) due to stronger H-bond formation with water	Diethylene glycol	$(OHCH_2CH_2)_2O$	0.92	
		Acetone	$CH_3\overset{\displaystyle O}{\overset{\|}{C}}CH_3$	0.01	←
		Dimethyl sulfoxide	$CH_3\overset{\displaystyle O}{\overset{\|}{S}}CH_3$	0.92	

[a] The reflection coefficient σ is defined in the text. The direction of the arrows indicates an increase in permeability.
Source: From Refs. 17–19.

Within a homologous series of compounds, the first few small members are readily permeable because of the polar route of membrane penetration. Permeability decreases for the next several members (i.e., σ increases), and then increases as the carbon chain length increases. The regular influence of chain length on permeability is a result not of increased solubility in the lipid phase of the membrane but of the unique interaction of hydrocarbon chains with water. The nonpolar hydrocarbon molecules are surrounded by a local region of water that has a more highly ordered structure than bulk water. This "iceberg" structure of water results in increased $K_{o/w}$, and membrane permeability as the carbon chain length is increased because of the compound being "pushed out" of the aqueous phase by the resulting gain in entropy.

There has been great interest in developing quantitative, structure=activity relationships to predict drug absorption (19). Such relationships could prove extremely useful in the early stages of drug design and in conjunction with high-throughput screening of hundreds of new molecules during early drug discovery to produce optimum absorption characteristics. Another very practical approach involves "data mining," whereby large databases are examined to characterize the properties of those compounds exhibiting good absorption and, perhaps more importantly, the reason for poor absorption.

On the basis of a review of the physical chemical properties of marketed drugs, Lipinski and coworkers have proposed an empirical "rule of 5" (20). This rule may help pharmaceutical scientists in reaching an early decision about the potential candidacy for further development of a new chemical entity. The rule states that a chemical candidate is likely to display poor absorption or poor membrane permeability if two or more of the following criteria are met (and assuming passive membrane transport):

1. There are more than five hydrogen bond donors.
2. There are more than 10 hydrogen bond acceptors.
3. The molecular weight is greater than 500.
4. Log $K_{o/w}$ is greater than 5.

pK_a and pH

Most drug molecules are either weak acids or bases that will be ionized to an extent determined by the compound's pK_a and the pH of the biological fluid in which it is dissolved. The importance of ionization in drug absorption is based on the observation that the nonionized form of the drug has a greater $K_{o/w}$ than the ionized form and, since $K_{o/w}$ is a prime determinant of membrane penetration, ionization would be expected to influence absorption. The observation that pH influences the membrane penetration of ionizable drugs is not a recent finding. At the turn of the previous century, Overton was able to relate pH to the rate of penetration of various alkaloids into cells, and he noted the resulting influence in toxicity. Other investigators have made similar observations with respect to the influence of pH on the penetration of alkaloids through the conjunctival and mammalian skin (21). The rate of penetration of these weak bases is enhanced by alkalinization because of a greater fraction of the nonionized species being present. Travell (22) examined the influence of pH on the absorption of several alkaloids from the stomach and intestine of a cat. Following ligation of the proximal and distal ends of the stomach of the anesthetized cat, a 5-mg/kg solution of strychnine at pH 8.5 caused death within 24 minutes; however, the same dose at pH 1.2 produced no toxic response. Identical results were found with nicotine, atropine, and cocaine. The same trend was also seen when the drug solution was instilled into ligated intestinal segments and after oral administration (via stomach tube) to ambulatory animals. These results indicated that

Table 5 Influence of pH on Drug Absorption from the Small Intestine of a Rat

Drug	pK_a	Percentage absorbed			
		pH 4	pH 5	pH 7	pH 8
Acids					
5-Nitrosalicylic acid	2.3	40	27	<2	<2
Salicylic acid	3.0	64	35	30	10
Acetylsalicylic acid	3.5	41	27	-	-
Benzoic acid	4.2	62	36	35	5
Bases					
Aniline	4.6	40	48	58	61
Aminopyrine	5.0	21	35	48	52
p-Toluidine	5.3	30	42	65	64
Quinine	8.4	9	11	41	54

Drug buffer solutions were perfused through the in situ rat intestine for 30 min, and percentage of drug absorbed was determined from 4 subsequent 10-min samples of the buffer solution.

alkaloids, which are weak bases, will be more rapidly absorbed in the nonionized form (i.e., at high fluid pH) than in the ionized form (low pH). This fundamental observation has sometimes been overlooked in oral acute drug toxicity studies.

In 1940, Jacobs (23) made use of the Henderson–Hasselbalch equation to relate pH and pK_a to membrane transport of ionizable compounds. Extensive experimentation by a group of investigators in the early 1950s (14,24–28) quantitated many of the aforementioned observations concerning the influence of pH and pK_a on drug absorption from the GIT. These studies have resulted in the so-called pH-partition hypothesis. In essence, this hypothesis states that ionizable compounds penetrate biological membranes primarily in the nonionized form (i.e., nonionic diffusion). As a result, acidic drugs should best be absorbed from acidic solutions where pH < pK_a, while basic compounds would best be absorbed from alkaline solutions where pH > pK_a. The data in Table 5 illustrate this principle (29).

The investigators noted some inconsistencies in their data, however, as some compounds (e.g., salicylic acid), which were essentially completely ionized in the buffer solution, were nevertheless rapidly absorbed. To explain these exceptions it was suggested that there was a "virtual membrane pH" (~pH 5.3), different from the bulk pH of the buffer solution, which was the actual pH determining the fraction of drug nonionized and hence dictating the absorption pattern. Although there may indeed be an effective pH at the immediate surface of the intestinal membrane, different from the pH of solutions bathing the lumen, there is overwhelming experimental evidence indicating that many drugs in the ionic form may be well absorbed.

Over the years, there has been an unqualified acceptance of the pH-partition hypothesis, and as a result, many texts and considerable literature on drug absorption indicate that acidic drugs are best absorbed from the acidic gastric fluids of the stomach and basic drugs best absorbed from the relatively more alkaline intestinal fluids. If all other conditions were the same, the nonionized form of the drug would be more rapidly absorbed than the ionized form. However, conditions along the GIT are not uniform, and hence, most drugs, whether ionized or nonionized, acid, or base (i.e., regardless of pH), are best absorbed from the small intestine as a result of the large absorbing surface area of this region.

A good example to illustrate this point is presented in Table 6. The values shown in this table are apparent first-order absorption rate constants (units of reciprocal time,

Table 6 Influence of pH on Drug Absorption from the Stomach and Intestine of a Rat

Drug	Apparent first-order absorption rate constant (1/min)		
	Stomach pH 3	pH 6	Intestine pH 6
Acids			
Salicylic acid	0.015	0.0053	0.085
Barbital	0.0029	0.0026	0.037
Sulfaethidole	0.004	0.0023	0.022
Bases			
Prochlorperazine	<0.002	0.0062	0.030
Haloperidol	0.0028	0.0041	0.028
Aminopyrine	<0.002	0.0046	0.022

Drug buffer solutions were placed into the GIT of an in situ rat preparation. The apparent first-order absorption rate constants are based upon drug disappearance from the buffer solution.

1/time). More rapid absorption rate is indicated by a numerically larger rate constant. There are three important comparisons that should be made in examining these data:

1. By comparing gastric absorption at pH 3 and pH 6, where surface area and factors other than pH are constant, one sees that the general principle is supported; acid drugs are more rapidly absorbed from acidic solution, whereas basic drugs are more rapidly absorbed from relatively alkaline solution.
2. At the same pH (i.e., pH 6), acidic and basic drugs are more rapidly absorbed from the intestine than from the stomach, by virtue of the larger intestinal surface area.
3. Acidic drugs are more rapidly absorbed from the intestine (pH 6), although there is substantial ionization, compared with the rate of gastric absorption, even at a pH where the drug is in a far more acidic solution (pH 3). Again, this is primarily a result of surface area differences.

The pH-partition hypothesis provides a useful guide in predicting general trends in drug movement across biological membranes and it remains a useful concept. There are numerous examples illustrating the general relationship among pH, pK_a, and drug absorption developed in that hypothesis. The primary limitation of this concept is the assumption that only nonionized drug is absorbed, when in fact the ionized species of some compounds can be absorbed, albeit at a slower rate. There is also the presence of unstirred water layers at the epithelial membrane surface, which can alter the rate of drug diffusion. Furthermore, the hypothesis is based on data obtained from drug in solution. In a practical sense, other considerations may also govern the pattern of drug absorption, and these include dissolution rate from solid dosage forms, the large intestinal surface area, and the relative residence times of the drug in different parts of the GIT. These factors are discussed below. In general then, drug absorption in humans takes place primarily from the small intestine regardless of whether the drug is a weak acid or base; gastric absorption, even for acidic drugs, is minimal.

Mechanisms of Drug Absorption

Water-soluble vitamins (B_2, B_{12}, and C) and other nutrients (e.g., monosaccharides, amino acids) are absorbed by specialized mechanisms, which implies membrane participation in transport and the need for energy expenditure. With the exception of a number of antimetabolites used in cancer chemotherapy, L-dihydroxyphenylalanine (L-dopa) and certain antibiotics (e.g., aminopenicillins, aminocephalosporins), the majority of drugs are absorbed in humans by a passive diffusion mechanism. Passive diffusion indicates that the transfer of a compound from an aqueous phase through a membrane may be described by physical chemical laws and by the properties of the membrane; no energy is required. The membrane itself is passive in that it does not partake in the transfer process but acts as a simple barrier to diffusion. The driving force for diffusion across the membrane is the concentration gradient (more correctly, the activity gradient) of the compound across that membrane. This mechanism of membrane penetration may be described mathematically by Fick's first law of diffusion, which has been simplified by Riggs and discussed by Benet (30,31).

$$\left(\frac{dQ_b}{dt}\right)_{g \to b} = D_m \cdot A_m \cdot R_{m/aq}\left(\frac{C_g - C_b}{\Delta X_m}\right) \tag{1}$$

The derivative on the left side of the equation represents the rate of appearance of drug in the blood (amount/time) when the drug diffuses from the gut fluids (g) to the blood (b). The expression reads, the rate of change of the quantity (Q) entering the blood stream. The other symbols have the following meanings (and units): D_m, the diffusion coefficient of the drug through the membrane (area/time); A_m, the surface area of the absorbing membrane available for drug diffusion (area); $R_{m/aq}$, the partition coefficient of the drug between the membrane and aqueous gut fluids (unitless); $C_g - C_b$, the concentration gradient across the membrane, representing the difference in the effective drug concentration (i.e., activity) in the gut fluids (C_g) at the site of absorption and the drug concentration in the blood (C_b) at the site of absorption (amount/volume); and ΔX_m, the thickness of the membrane (length). This equation nicely explains several of the observations discussed previously. Thus, rate of drug absorption is directly dependent on the membrane surface area available for diffusion, indicating that one would expect more rapid absorption from the small intestine compared with that from the stomach. Furthermore, the greater the membrane aqueous fluid partition coefficient ($R_{m/aq}$), the more rapid the rate of absorption, supporting the previous discussion indicating the dependence of absorption rate on $K_{o/w}$. We know that pH will produce a net effect on absorption rate by altering several of the parameters in equation (1). As the pH for a given drug will determine the fraction nonionized, the value of $R_{m/aq}$ will change with pH, generally increasing as the fraction nonionized increases. Depending on the relative ability of the membrane to permit the diffusion of the nonionized and ionized forms, C_g will be altered appropriately. Finally, the value of D_m may be different for the ionized and nonionized forms of the compound. For a given drug and membrane and under specified conditions, equation (1) is made up of a number of constants that may be incorporated into a large constant (P) referred to as the permeability coefficient:

$$\left(\frac{dQ_b}{dt}\right)_{g \to b} = P(C_g - C_b) \tag{2}$$

where P incorporates D_m, A_m, $R_{m/aq}$, and ΔX_m and has units of volume/time, which is analogous to a flow or clearance term. Since the volume into which the drug may distribute from the blood is large compared with the gut fluid volume, and since the rapid circulation of blood through the GIT continually moves absorbed drug away from the site of absorption, $C_g \gg C_b$. This is often referred to as a "sink condition," indicating a

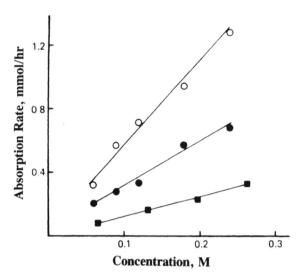

Figure 8 Influence of concentration on the rate of absorption from the in situ rat intestine. The linear dependence of absorption rate on concentration suggests an apparent first-order absorption process over the range studied. Absorption rates have been calculated from the data in reference (14), and the straight lines are from linear regression of the data. Key: (o) erythritol; (●) urea; (■) malonamide.

relatively small drug concentration in the bloodstream at the absorption site (a virtual "sink" exists). As a result, equation (2) may be simplified:

$$\left(\frac{dQ_b}{dt}\right)_{g\to b} \cong P \cdot C_g \tag{3}$$

Equation (3) is in the form of a differential equation describing a first-order kinetic process, and as a result, drug absorption is generally consistent with first-order kinetics. The rate of absorption should increase directly with an increase in drug concentration in the GI fluids.

Figure 8 illustrates the linear dependence of absorption rate on concentration for several compounds placed into the in situ rat intestine. The slopes of these lines represent the constant (P) for absorption in equation (3). Alternatively, one may express these data as the percentage drug absorbed per unit of time as a function of concentration or amount. Several examples illustrating such an analysis are listed in Table 7. The percentage absorbed in any given period is independent of concentration. This constant fractional or percentage absorbed is characteristic of a passive diffusion or first-order kinetic process over the concentration ranges studied. Similar studies by other investigators employing an in situ rat intestine preparation indicate that several other drugs (those listed in Table 6) are absorbed in a first-order kinetic fashion.

It is far more difficult to establish the mechanism(s) of drug absorption in humans. Most investigators analyze drug absorption data in humans (from blood or urine data) by assuming first-order absorption kinetics. For the most part this assumption seems quite valid, and the results of such analyses are consistent with that assumption. One method used to assess the mechanism of drug absorption in humans is based on a pharmacokinetic treatment of blood or urine data and the preparation of log percentage unabsorbed versus time plots. If a straight-line relationship is found, this is indicative of an apparent first-order absorption process, where the slope of that line represents the apparent first-order

Table 7 Influence of Concentration on the Absorption of Various Solutes from the In Situ Rat Intestine

Compound	Concentration (mM)	Percentage absorbed
Urea[a]	60	20.9
	90	19.0
	120	17.0
	180	20.0
	240	17.8
Erythritol[a]	60	54.1
	90	65.0
	120	62.2
	180	54.4
	240	55.5
Malonamide[a]	66	16.9
	132	16.8
	198	16.5
	264	18.4
Salicylic acid[b]	1	12
	2	12
	10	13
Aniline[b]	1	44
	10	43
Benzoic acid[b]	1	12
	2	12
	10	13
Quinine[b]	1	20
	10	20
	0.1	58
Aniline[c]	1	54
	10	59
	20	54

[a] Based on data in Ref. 14.
[b] Based on data in Ref. 15.
[c] Based on data in Ref. 27.

absorption rate constant. Some cautions must be taken in the application of this method. Although the overall absorption process in humans for many drugs appears consistent with the characteristics of a first-order kinetic process, there are some questions regarding which of the sequential steps in the absorption process is rate-limiting. As discussed in a thorough review of mass transport phenomena (32), the $K_{o/w}$ of a solute will govern its movement across a lipid-like membrane as long as the membrane is the predominant barrier to diffusion. However, for such membranes, when the $K_{o/w}$ becomes very large, the barrier controlling diffusion may no longer be the membrane but rather an aqueous diffusion layer surrounding the membrane. Thus, for some molecules, depending on their physicochemical characteristics, the rate-limiting step in membrane transport will be movement through or out of the membrane, while for other compounds the rate-limiting step will be diffusion through an aqueous layer. Our incomplete understanding of drug transport across biological membranes is not that surprising, given the complexity of the system and the experimental requirements needed to make unequivocal statements about this process on a molecular level.

The analysis of absorption data in humans includes traditional modeling and data-fitting techniques as well as so-called moment analysis, in addition to a process referred to as deconvolution (33). Absorption processes are now often characterized by a mean

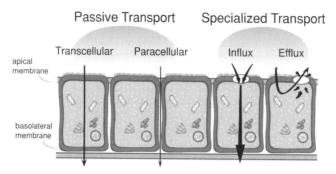

Figure 9 Schematic representation depicting the movement of drug molecules from the absorbing (mucosal or apical) surface of the GIT to the basolateral membrane and from there to blood. (*Left*) Passive, non-energy-dependent processes of transcellular movement through the epithelial cell and paracellular transport via movement between epithelial cells. (*Right*) Specialized carrier-mediated (influx) transport into the epithelial cell and carrier-mediated efflux transport of drug out of the epithelial cell. *Source*: Courtesy of Saguaro Press.

absorption (or input) time (i.e., the average amount of time that the drug molecules spend at the absorption site) or by a process called deconvolution. The former analyses result in a single value (such as absorption half-life or mean absorption time) and the latter analysis results in a profile of the absorption process as a function of time (e.g., absorption rate or cumulative amount absorbed vs. time). These approaches offer alternative ways of interpreting the absorption process.

Most drugs appear to be absorbed in humans by passive diffusion (linear or first-order kinetics) over the therapeutic dose range. The predominant pathway taken by most drugs is through the epithelial cell, the *transcellular* route. It is this route that requires the compound to have a reasonable $K_{o/w}$ (greater than 1 and less than about 10^5). This route is indicated in Figure 9 as the arrow moving through the cell from the mucosal (or apical) absorbing surface to the basolateral membrane. In contrast, small polar molecules ($K_{o/w} < 1$) may have access to a convoluted route that exists between adjacent epithelial cells. This pathway has a tight junction at the apical surface as well as other junctions along the pathway (apical junction complex). This route is referred to as being *paracellular* (Fig. 9). The molecular size cutoff for this route is about 500 Da (34). It remains unclear the extent to which this pathway may be practically affected to increase absorption by so-called tight junction modulators (35).

Since many essential nutrients (e.g., monosaccharides, amino acids, and vitamins) are water soluble, they have low $K_{o/w}$s, which should result in poor absorption from the GIT. However, to ensure adequate uptake of these materials from food, the intestine has developed specialized absorption mechanisms that depend on membrane participation (energy expenditure) and require the compound to have a specific chemical structure. This uptake carrier transport mechanism is illustrated in Figure 9. Absorption by a specialized carrier mechanism has been shown to exist for several agents used in cancer chemotherapy (5-fluorouracil and 5-bromouracil) (36), which may be considered "false" nutrients in that their chemical structures are very similar to essential nutrients for which the intestine has a specialized transport mechanism. These specialized mechanisms are generally found in only a limited section of the small intestine that is sometimes referred to as an "absorption window."

It would be instructive to examine some studies concerned with riboflavin and ascorbic acid absorption in humans, as these illustrate how one may treat urine data to

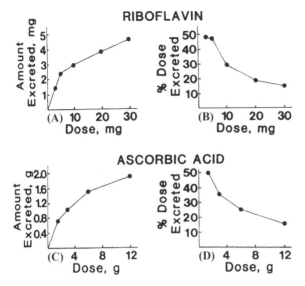

Figure 10 Urinary excretion of riboflavin (**A,B**) and ascorbic acid (**C,D**) in humans as a function of oral dose. Graphs **A** and **C** illustrate the nonlinear dependence of absorption on dose, which is suggestive of a saturable specialized absorption process. Graphs **B** and **D** represent an alternative graph of the same data and illustrate the reduced absorption efficiency as the dose increases. *Source*: Graphs A and C based on the data in Ref. 37 and graphs B and D based on the data in Ref. 38.

explore the mechanism of absorption. If a compound is absorbed by a passive mechanism, a plot of amount absorbed (or amount recovered in the urine) versus dose ingested will provide a straight-line relationship. In contrast, a plot of percentage of dose absorbed (or percentage of dose recovered in the urine) versus dose ingested will provide a line of slope zero (i.e., a constant fraction of the dose is absorbed at all doses). If the absorption process requires membrane involvement, the absorption process may be saturated as the oral dose increases, making the process less efficient at larger doses (i.e., there are more drug molecules than sites on the transporter). As a result, a plot of amount absorbed versus dose ingested will be linear at low doses, curvilinear at larger doses, and approach an asymptotic value at even larger doses. One sees this type of relationship for riboflavin and ascorbic acid in Figure 10A and C, suggesting nonpassive absorption mechanisms in humans (37,38). This nonlinear relationship is reminiscent of Michaelis—Menten saturable enzyme kinetics from which one may estimate the kinetic parameters (K_m and V_{max}) associated with the absorption of these vitamins. Figure 10B and D illustrates an alternative plot, percentage absorbed versus dose ingested. For a nonpassive absorption process, the percentage dose absorbed will decrease as the dose increases as a result of saturation of the transport mechanism, resulting in a reduction in absorption efficiency. It has been suggested (38) that one means of overcoming the decrease in absorption efficiency is to administer small divided doses rather than large single doses, as illustrated later for ascorbic acid.

L-Dopa absorption may be impaired if the drug is ingested with meals containing proteins (39). Amino acids formed from the digestion of protein meals, which are absorbed by a specialized mechanism, may competitively inhibit L-dopa absorption if the drug is also transported by the same transport carrier. There is evidence (in animals) indicating a specialized absorption mechanism for phenylalanine and L-dopa, and there are data illustrating L-dopa inhibition of phenylalanine and tyrosine absorption in humans (40,41). L-Dopa appears to be absorbed by the same specialized transport mechanism responsible for the absorption of other amino acids (42). In a latter section, several of the complicating factors in L-dopa absorption that influence therapy are discussed.

In addition to some anticancer agents being absorbed by a specialized process in humans (e.g., methotrexate) (43), there is evidence to suggest that a similar mechanism exists for the absorption of aminopenicillins (e.g., amoxicillin) (44) and amino-cephalosporins (e.g., cefixime) (45). Absorption of these compounds appears to be linked to cellular amino acid or peptide transporters. Other compounds that have the requisite structural properties may also benefit from those transporting systems (e.g., gabapentin) (46). This behavior may represent an important observation for the new generation of drugs being developed through the application of biotechnology (e.g., peptides), assuming such compounds are sufficiently stable in the GIT. Calcium channel blockers, such as nifedipine, have been shown to increase the absorption of amoxicillin and cefixime (44,45). This may result from the role of calcium in the transport process, the inhibition of which (i.e., calcium channel blockers) enhances absorption.

In direct contrast with specialized uptake transport of a drug into the epithelial cell, is a process referred to as "efflux transport," the facilitated movement of a drug out of the cell. This phenomenon explains the resistance of cancerous cells to some chemo-therapeutic agents (47). It is now apparent that this mechanism exists in epithelial cells of numerous organ systems, including the GIT, liver, lung, kidney, and brain (48). There is a cell surface glycoprotein (P-glycoprotein, P-gp), a multidrug-resistance protein (MDR), which is responsible for the efflux mechanism. This protein belongs to a large family of glycosylated membrane proteins referred to as ATP-binding cassette (ABC) transporters. As depicted in Figure 9, the cell surface glycoprotein will attach to the drug molecule and escort it out of the cell and back into the gut lumen, hence the term, efflux transporter. The presence of this protein in the GIT has significant implications for drug absorption, bioavailability, and drug-drug (and drug-nutrient) interactions (49–54). Substrates for this transporter have a diverse range of structures and include compounds such as (49) anticancer agents (e.g., anthracyclines, taxol, and vinblastine), cardioactive drugs (e.g., digoxin, phenytoin, quinidine, and verapamil), immunosuppressants (e.g., cyclosporine and tacrolimus), erythromycin, and quinine. The P-gp may be inhibited or induced and the efflux transport process may be saturated. The former is the basis for many potential drug-drug and nutrient-drug interactions and the latter limits the efficacy of the transporter.

It is difficult to unequivocally implicate P-gp as the mechanism of an interaction resulting in altered absorption since the absorbing intestinal cells are rich in metabolizing enzymes, especially those responsible for phase I oxidative metabolism, the cytochrome P450 family (CYP450). Within that family the most significant isozyme is CYP3A4, since it is less selective of substrates (a "promiscuous" enzyme), and as a result, it accounts for about 50% of all drug-drug and nutrient-drug interactions. Both P-gp and CYP3A4 are present in the same locations and appear to share the same substrates. As a consequence, it is difficult to unequivocally ascribe alterations in absorption to be the exclusive result of either the efflux transporter or the enzyme. This is the case, for example, for cyclosporine whose absorption is enhanced in the presence of several drugs (e.g., ketoconazole), which may be due to inhibition of P-gp efflux or inhibition of CYP3A4 metabolic activity or both (55). A further complication is the need to consider the systemic effect of altered P-gp activity on drug clearance, an effect that is independent of the absorption process.

Efflux transport and gut wall metabolism tend to decrease systemic drug exposure and thereby reduce systemic bioavailability. It appears that the efflux transporter may act in concert with metabolizing enzymes in the enterocytes by limiting exposure of the enzyme to drug by "pumping" the drug out of the enterocyte and back into the gut. This action reduces the potential for enzyme saturation, which, in turn, minimizes drug from "swamping" the enzyme and being systemically absorbed. These mechanisms are consistent with the protective barrier function of the GIT.

The significance of P-gp in affecting absorption and bioavailability of P-gp substrate drugs can be seen in studies in "knockout" mice that do not have intestinal P-gp. The gene responsible for producing that protein has been "knocked out" of the genetic repertoire. Those animals evidenced a sixfold increase in plasma concentrations (and AUC, area under the plasma concentration-time curve) following oral dosing of the anticancer drug, paclitaxel (Taxol), compared with the control animals (56). Another line of evidence is the recent report of an interaction between the β-adrenergic blocking agents, talinolol and digoxin (57). Talinolol coadministration resulted in a significant increase in digoxin plasma concentrations (and AUC), and since talinolol and digoxin are not substrates for CYP3A3, the effect on absorption may be attributed to inhibition of P-gp, which modulates digoxin absorption.

PHYSIOLOGICAL FACTORS GOVERNING DRUG ABSORPTION

Components and Properties of Gastrointestinal Fluids

The characteristics of aqueous GI fluids to which a drug product is exposed will exert an important influence on what happens to that dosage form in the tract and on the pattern of drug absorption. To appreciate clearly how physiological factors influence drug absorption, one must consider the influence of these variables on the dosage form per se, that is, how these variables influence drug dissolution in the aqueous GI fluids, and finally what influence these variables exert on absorption once the drug is in solution.

One important property of GI fluids is pH, which varies considerably along the length of the tract. The gastric fluids are highly acidic, usually ranging from pH 1 to pH 3.5. There appears to be a diurnal cycle of gastric acidity, the fluids being more acidic at night and pH fluctuating during the day, primarily in response to food ingestion. Gastric fluid pH generally increases when food is ingested and then slowly decreases over the next several hours, fluctuating from pH 1 to about pH 5 (58). There is considerable intersubject variation, however, in GI fluid pH, depending on the general health of the subject, the presence of local disease conditions along the tract, types of food ingested, and drug therapy. Upper GI fluid pH appears to be independent of gender.

An abrupt change in pH is encountered when moving from the stomach to the small intestine. Pancreatic secretions (200–800 mL/day) have a high concentration of bicarbonate, which neutralizes gastric fluid entering the duodenum and thus helps regulate the pH of fluids in the upper intestinal region. Neutralization of acidic gastric fluids in the duodenum is important to avoid damage to the intestinal epithelium, prevent inactivation of pancreatic enzymes, and prevent precipitation of bile acids, which are poorly soluble at acid pH. The pH of intestinal fluids gradually increases when moving in the distal direction, ranging from approximately 5.7 in the pylorus to 7.7 in the proximal jejunum. The fluids in the large intestine are generally considered to have a pH of between 7 and 8.

GI fluid pH may influence drug absorption in a variety of ways. Since most drugs are weak acids or bases, and since the aqueous solubility of such compounds is influenced by pH, the rate of dissolution from a dosage form, particularly tablets and capsules, is dependent on pH. This is a result of the direct dependence of dissolution rate on solubility, as discussed in chapter 4. Acidic drugs dissolve most readily in alkaline media and, therefore, will have a greater rate of dissolution in intestinal fluids compared with gastric fluids. Basic drugs will dissolve most readily in acidic solutions and, thus, the dissolution rate will be greater in gastric fluids compared with intestinal fluids. Since dissolution is a prerequisite step to absorption and often the slowest process, especially for poorly water-soluble drugs, pH will exert a major influence on the overall absorption process. Furthermore, since the major site of drug absorption is the small intestine, it would seem that poorly soluble basic drugs (e.g., dipyridamole, ketaconazole, and diazepam) must first dissolve in the acidic gastric fluids to be well absorbed from the intestine, as the dissolution rate in intestinal fluids will be low. In addition, the disintegration of some dosage forms, depending on their formulation, will be influenced by pH if they contain certain components (e.g., binding agents or disintegrants) whose solubility is pH-sensitive. Several studies (59) have indicated that if the specific products being examined were not first exposed to an acidic solution, the dosage form would not disintegrate and thus dissolution could not proceed.

A complication here, however, is noted with those drugs that exhibit a limited chemical stability in either acidic or alkaline fluids. Since the rate and extent of degradation is directly dependent on the concentration of drug in solution, an attempt is often made to retard dissolution in the fluid where degradation is seen. There are preparations of various salts or esters of drugs (e.g., erythromycin) that do not dissolve in gastric fluid and thus are not degraded there, but they dissolve in intestinal fluid prior to absorption. A wide variety of chemical derivatives or salt forms are used for such purposes. In addition, there are numerous polymers that may be used to coat granules or tablets and that only dissolve at the desired pH, offering protection from degradation at other pHs (e.g., enteric-coated products).

As mentioned previously, pH will also influence the absorption of an ionizable drug once it is in solution, as outlined in the pH-partition hypothesis. All drugs, however, are best absorbed from the small intestine regardless of pK_a and pH. In some instances, especially lower down in the GIT, there is the possibility of insoluble hydroxide formation of a drug or insoluble film formation with components of a dosage form that reduces the extent of absorption of, for example, aluminum aspirin (in chewable tablets) (60,61) and iron (62). The coadministration of acidic or alkaline fluids with certain drugs may exert an effect on the overall drug absorption process for any of the foregoing reasons.

Moreover, in addition to pH considerations, the GI fluids contain various materials which have been shown to influence absorption, particularly bile salts, enzymes, and mucin. Bile salts, which are highly surface active, may enhance the rate and/or extent of absorption of poorly water-soluble drugs by increasing the rate of dissolution in the GI fluids. This effect has been noted in in vitro experiments and has also been seen with other natural surface-active agents (e.g., lysolecithin). Increased absorption of the poorly water-soluble drug griseofulvin after a fatty meal (63,64) reflects the fact that bile is secreted into the gut in response to the presence of fats, and the bile salts that are secreted increase the dissolution rate and absorption of the drug.

Since intestinal fluids contain large concentrations of various enzymes needed for digestion of food, it is reasonable to expect certain of these enzymes to act on a number of drugs. Pancreatic enzymes hydrolyze chloramphenicol palmitate. Pancreatin and trypsin are able to deacetylate N-acetylated drugs, and mucosal esterases appear to attack various esters of penicillin. Oral cocaine ingestion is generally ineffective in producing a pharmacological response because of efficient hydrolysis by esterase enzymes in the gut. This is not true at very large doses, however, such as those resulting from the rupture of bags containing the drug, which are ingested to avoid detection at international borders (severe toxicity and death are often observed).

Mucin, a viscous mucopolysaccharide that lines and protects the intestinal epithelium, has been thought to bind certain drugs nonspecifically (e.g., quarternary ammonium compounds) and thereby prevent or reduce absorption. This behavior may partially account for the erratic and incomplete absorption of such charged compounds. Mucin may also represent a barrier to drug diffusion prior to reaching the intestinal membrane.

Gastric Emptying

Physiologists have for many years been interested in factors that influence gastric emptying and the regulatory mechanisms controlling this process. Our interest in gastric emptying is based on the fact that, since most drugs are best absorbed from the small intestine, any factor that delays movement of drug from the stomach to the small intestine will influence the rate (and possibly the extent) of absorption and therefore the time needed to achieve maximal plasma concentrations and pharmacological response. As a result, and in addition to rate of dissolution or inherent absorbability, gastric emptying may represent a limiting factor in drug absorption. Only in those rare instances where a drug is absorbed by a specialized process in the intestine will the amount of drug leaving the stomach exceed the capacity of the gut to absorb it.

Gastric emptying is determined with a variety of techniques using liquid or solid meals or other markers. Gastric emptying is quantitated by one of several measurements, including emptying time, emptying half-time ($t_{50\%}$), and emptying rate. Emptying time is the time needed for the stomach to empty the total initial stomach contents. Emptying half-time is the time it takes for the stomach to empty one-half of its initial contents. Emptying rate is a measure of the speed of emptying. Note that the last two measures are inversely related (i.e., the greater the rate, the smaller the value for emptying half-time).

Gastric emptying and factors that affect that process need to be understood because of the implications for drug absorption and with regard to optimal dosage form design (65). Gastric-emptying patterns are distinctly different depending upon the absence or presence of food. In the absence of food, the empty stomach and the intestinal tract undergo a sequence of repetitious events referred to as the interdigestive migrating motor (or myoelectric complex, MMC) (66). This complex results in the generation of contractions beginning with the proximal stomach and ending with the ileum. The first of four stages is one of minimal activity that lasts for about one hour. Stage 2, which lasts 30 to 45 minutes, is characterized by irregular contractions that gradually increase in strength leading to the next phase. The third phase, while only lasting 5 to 15 minutes, consists of intense peristaltic waves, which results in the emptying of all remaining gastric contents into the pylorus. The latter phase is sometimes referred to as the "housekeeper" wave. The fourth stage represents a transition of decreasing activity, leading to the beginning of the next cycle (i.e., stage 1). The entire cycle lasts for about two hours. Thus, a solid dosage form ingested on an empty stomach will remain in it for a period dependent on time of dosing relative to the occurrence of the housekeeper. The gastric residence time of a solid dosage form will vary from perhaps 5 to 15 minutes (if ingested at the beginning of the housekeeper) to about two hours or longer (if ingested at the end of the house-keeper wave). It would not be surprising, however, for gastric residence time to be substantially longer. This variability in gastric residence time may explain some of the intersubject variation in rate of absorption, and it raises some question concerning the term, "ingested on an empty stomach." While it is quite common in clinical research studies for a panel of subjects to ingest a solid test dosage form following an overnight fast and, therefore, on an "empty stomach," it is unlikely that all subjects will be in the same phase of the migrating motor complex. It is the latter point, rather than an empty stomach per se, which will determine when emptying occurs and, consequently, when drug absorption is initiated.

The above considerations will not apply to liquid dosage forms, however, which are generally able to empty during all phases of the migrating motor complex.

Various techniques have been used to visualize the gastric emptying of dosage forms. Radiopaque tablets were found to undergo relatively mild agitation in the stomach, a point that needs to be considered in the design and interpretation of disintegration and dissolution tests. While single large solid dosage forms (e.g., tablets and capsules) rely on the housekeeper wave for entry into the small intestine, some controversy remains about the influence of particle (or pellet) size (diameter and volume), shape, and density on gastric emptying. There has been a great deal of recent interest in this issue, which has been investigated primarily with use of γ-scintigraphy (a γ-emitting material is ingested and externally monitored with a γ-camera). These studies are generally performed with the use of nondisintegrating pellets so that movement throughout the tract may be estimated. Particles as large as 5 to 7 mm may leave the stomach. It is likely that a range of particle sizes will empty from the stomach, rather than there being an abrupt cutoff value. The range of values among individuals will be affected by the size of the pylorus diameter and the relative force of propulsive contractions generated by the stomach. The interest in this issue stems from the desire to develop sustained-release dosage forms that would have sufficient residence time in the GIT to provide constant drug release over an extended time. Experimental dosage forms that have been investigated include floating tablets, bioadhesives (that attach to the gastric mucosa), dense pellets, and large dimension forms.

Eating interrupts the interdigestive migrating motor complex. Gastric emptying in the presence of solid or liquid food is controlled by a complex variety of mechanical, hormonal, and neural mechanisms. Receptors lining the stomach, duodenum, and jejunum, which assist in controlling gastric emptying, include mechanical receptors in the stomach, which respond to distension; acid receptors in the stomach and duodenum; osmotic receptors in the duodenum, which respond to electrolytes, carbohydrates and amino acids; fat receptors in the jejunum; and L-tryptophan receptors. Neural control appears to be through the inhibitory vagal system. Hormones involved in controlling emptying include cholecystokinin and gastrin, among others.

As food enters the stomach the fundus and body regions relax to accommodate the meal. Upon reaching the stomach, food tends to form layers that are stratified in the order in which the food was swallowed, and this material is mixed with gastric secretions in the antrum. Nonviscous fluid moves into the antrum, passing around any solid mass. Gastric emptying will begin once a considerable portion of the gastric contents becomes liquid enough to pass the pylorus. Peristaltic waves begin in the fundus region, travel to the pre-pyloric area, and become more intense in the pylorus. The antrum and pyloric sphincter contract, and the proximal duodenum relaxes. A moment later the antrum relaxes and the duodenum regains its tone. The pyloric sphincter will remain contracted momentarily to prevent regurgitation, and the contents in the duodenum are then propelled forward. Emptying is accomplished by the antral and pyloric waves, and the rate of emptying is regulated by factors controlling the strength of antral contraction. Gastric emptying is influenced primarily by meal volume, the presence of acids, certain nutrients, and osmotic pressure. Distension of the stomach is the only natural stimulus known to increase the emptying rate. Fat in any form in the presence of bile and pancreatic juice produces the greatest inhibition of gastric emptying. This strong inhibitory influence of fats permits time for their digestion, as they are the slowest of all foods to be digested. Meals containing substantial amounts of fat can delay gastric emptying for three to six hours or more. These various factors appear to alter gastric emptying by interacting with the receptors noted earlier.

Other than meal volume per se, all the other factors noted earlier result in a slowing of gastric emptying (e.g., nutrients, osmotic pressure, and acidity). It is important to recognize that there are a host of other factors, which are known to influence emptying rate. Thus, a variety of drugs can alter absorption of other drugs via their effect on emptying. For example, anticholinergics and narcotic analgesics reduce gastric-emptying rate, while metoclopramide increases that rate. A reduced rate of drug absorption is expected in the former instance and an increased rate in the latter. The following factors should also be recognized: body position (reduced rate lying on left side), viscosity (rate decreases with increased viscosity), and emotional state (reduced rate during depression, increased rate during stress). As an illustration, one report indicates that absorption rate (and potentially, completeness of absorption) may be altered when comparing posture, lying on the left or right side (67). Acetaminophen and nifedipine absorption rates were faster when the subjects were lying on the right compared with the left side, suggesting more rapid gastric emptying. In the case of nifedipine, the extent of absorption was greater when the subjects were lying on the right side, which may be due to transient saturation of a presystemic metabolic process (see "Metabolism and Transporters" section). Miscellaneous factors, whose exact effect on emptying may vary, include gut disease, exercise, obesity, gastric surgery, and bulimia.

Many investigators have suggested that gastric emptying takes place by an exponential (i.e., first-order kinetic) process. As a result, plots of log volume remaining in the stomach versus time will provide a straight-line relationship. The slope of this line will represent a rate constant associated with emptying. This relationship is not strictly log linear, however, especially at early and later times, but the approximation is useful in that one can express a half-time for emptying ($t_{50\%}$). Hopkins (68) has suggested a linear relationship between the square root of the volume remaining in the stomach and time. There may be a physical basis for this relationship, since the radius of a cylinder varies with the square root of the volume and the circumferential tension is proportional to the radius. Methods for analyzing gastric-emptying data have been reviewed (69).

Gastric-emptying rate is influenced by a large number of factors, as noted earlier. Many of these factors account for the large variation in emptying among different individuals and variation within an individual on different occasions. Undoubtedly, much of this variation in emptying is reflected in variable drug absorption. Although gastric emptying probably has little major influence on drug absorption from solution, emptying of solid dosage forms does exert an important influence on drug dissolution and absorption. A prime example is enteric-coated tablets, which are designed to prevent drug release in the stomach. Any delay in the gastric emptying of these forms will delay dissolution, absorption, and the onset time for producing a response. Since these dosage forms must empty as discrete units, the drug is either in the stomach or the intestine. The performance of this dosage form can be seriously hampered if it is taken with or after a meal, as emptying is considerably delayed. Furthermore, if the drug is to be taken in a multiple-dosing fashion, there is a possibility that the first dose will not leave the stomach until the next dose is taken, resulting in twice the desired dose getting into the intestine at one time. Blythe et al. (70) administered several enteric-coated aspirin tablets containing $BaSO_4$ and radiologically examined emptying of these tablets. The tablets emptied in these subjects anywhere from 0.5 to 7 hours after ingestion. Tablets will empty more rapidly when given prior to a meal compared with administration after a meal. One potential way of minimizing the impact of gastric emptying and release pattern of enteric-coated products is to use capsules containing enteric-coated microgranules. The median time for 50% and 90% emptying of such a dosage form has been shown to be 1 and 3 to 3.5 hours, respectively (71).

Several publications have reviewed the effects of food on drug absorption in humans (72–74) and have offered approaches to predicting food effects (75,76). The effect of food on the GI absorption of drugs is complex and multidimensional, and we are only now beginning to unravel the interplay of numerous variables. The physical presence of food in the GIT may play a significant role in affecting the efficient absorption of a drug from an oral dosage form. The ultimate effect of food on the rate and/or extent of GI absorption is a function of numerous interacting variables. While some general rules may be postulated, the effect of food on a given drug and its dosage form will require, in general, individual investigation. The Food and Drug Administration (FDA) has recognized this complexity and requires that all dosage forms that do not immediately release drug (e.g., controlled-release formulations) undergo a food effects study in humans, for which a "Guidance" has been written (these are available on the FDA Web page, http://www.fda.gov/). The precedence for this requirement is the observation that a sustained-release formulation may "dose dump" its entire contents of drug in the presence of food, and, since the dose is several times the usual single dose, this may lead to toxicity (77,78). The reason for this effect is related to a failure in the controlled-release mechanism (e.g., a film coating dissolves too rapidly in response to the presence of food).

The extent to which food will alter absorption depends upon factors such as physical and chemical characteristics of the drug (e.g., aqueous solubility, $K_{o/w}$, and stability in gut fluids), role of transporters and gut wall enzymes, dose of the drug, characteristics of the dosage form, time of drug administration relative to food ingestion, amount of food, and type of food. When food affects drug absorption, it most often does so by affecting the factors influencing drug dissolution or membrane transport. Other mechanisms may also apply depending on the specific drug (e.g., instability and complexation). It is useful to consider the most important rate-limiting steps in drug absorption in conjunction with what has become known as the "Biopharmaceutical Classification System" (BCS). The latter, illustrated in Figure 11, attempts to classify drugs in terms of their aqueous solubility and membrane permeability and, from that classification, predict the most likely behavior of the drug with regard to absorption following oral administration. The FDA is now using this approach in establishing regulatory standards for new drug entities and for

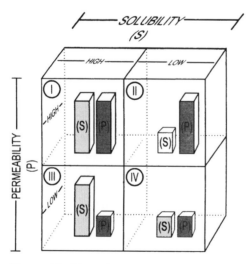

Figure 11 Illustration of the "Biopharmaceutical Classification System" (BCS), which classifies drug absorption potential on the basis of aqueous solubility or membrane permeability. *Source*: Courtesy of Saguaro Press.

generic versions of marketed drugs. The BCS can be easily understood from the simple 2 × 2 matrix illustrated in Figure 11. Drug behavior with respect to aqueous solubility and membrane permeability may be described by one of four possible conditions noted as I to IV. The effects of food on the absorption behavior of compounds classified according to the BCS has been discussed thoroughly (73,76), and they will be highlighted below.

More recently the BCS approach has been modified and expanded to include consideration of the disposition properties of drugs. This new paradigm, referred to as the "Biopharmaceutical Drug Disposition Classification System" (BDDCS), expands considerably the overall usefulness of attempts to classify drugs to better explain and predict their behavior (79,80). The BDDCS is shown in pictorial form in Figure 12. Notice that the system fits into the same basic 2 × 2 BCS matrix, which considers the primary limiting steps in drug absorption, aqueous solubility and membrane permeability. However, the BDDCS also offers information about the elimination mechanism, the presence and type of gut transporters, and the anticipated effect of food on drug absorption. This classification system will undoubtedly find many useful applications as it is further developed and fine-tuned.

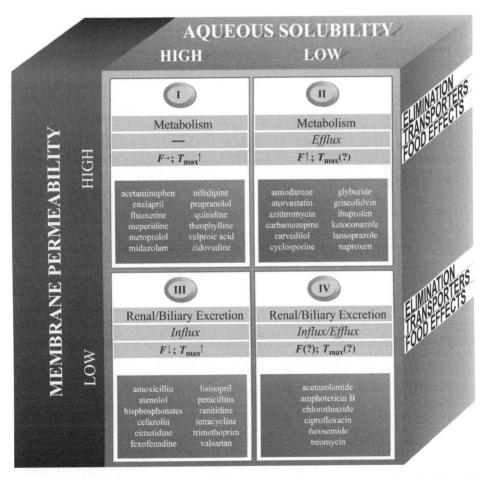

Figure 12 Illustration of the "Biopharmaceutical Drug Disposition Classification System" (BDDCS), which classifies drug absorption potential identically to the BCS (Fig. 11) and incorporates the expected route of elimination and the anticipated role of transporters and food on the absorption process. *Source*: Based on information in Ref. 79. Courtesy of Saguaro Press.

Class I compounds have both good solubility and permeability and generally offer no problems with regard to having a good absorption profile (e.g., acetaminophen, disopyramide, ketoprofen, metoprolol, nonsteroidal anti-inflammatory agents, valproic acid, verapamil). In general, one would not expect the presence of food to influence the absorption of this class of drug. The onset or rate of absorption may be delayed by the presence of food as a consequence of reduced gastric-emptying rate (T_{max}, the time to maximal plasma concentrations, is increased), but the completeness of absorption should not be compromised (fraction of dose absorbed, F, is unchanged).

Drugs in class II have low aqueous solubility (but high membrane permeability), and any factor affecting dissolution rate would be expected to have an impact on the absorption of such compounds. Factors such as fluid pH, volume and viscosity, and bile secretion (especially in response to fatty foods) might be expected to play a role in dissolution rate and thereby affect absorption. Compounds that fall into this class include carbamazepine, cyclosporin, digoxin, griseofulvin, and spironolactone. Food would be expected to exert a potentially significant effect on the absorption of the drugs in this class. The absorption of many compounds in this class is improved in the presence of a fatty meal (F increases). Improved absorption occurs because of the secretion of bile in response to fat and the surfactant and solubilizing properties that bile salts exert on poorly water-soluble compounds (griseofulvin is a classic example). The presence of food, especially fatty foods, will delay gastric emptying and intestinal transit, which in turn allow for more time for drug dissolution and absorption (T_{max} is likely to increase). Many drugs in this class, however, are substrates for gut wall metabolism (especially CYP3A4) and efflux transporters. To the extent that food components may affect those functions, the effective mechanism(s) of any food effect will need to include consideration of those factors.

Drugs in class III have good aqueous solubility but poor membrane permeability (e.g., bidisomide, bisphosphonates, captopril, and furosemide). Food and food components would only be expected to influence absorption of drugs in this class if they affected some aspect of membrane permeability or function or if the permeable form of the molecule was altered (e.g., through ionization). Many of these compounds tend to be absorbed in relatively well-defined and limited areas of the upper small intestine. As a consequence, the physical presence of food may affect the time during which the drug resides at sites of maximal absorption. Food and the viscous milieu that it creates in gut fluids may also create a significant physical barrier to the diffusion of the drug to sites of absorption along the GIT membrane. Several compounds that fall into this class illustrate reduced absorption in the presence of food (F decreases, T_{max} increases), which may also reflect food component effects on any influx transporter.

Class IV drugs have low aqueous solubility and poor membrane permeability and as such are often considered as poor drug candidates for oral administration. Other routes of administration may need to be considered. For example, neomycin falls into this category, and its oral use is to achieve sterilization of the gut. There is too little information about these compounds and the effect of food to offer general observations; however, solubilization and/or involvement of transporters are likely to explain any food effects.

In examining factors that might offer quantitative, predictive rules for the effect of food (especially fatty meals) on drug absorption, several groups have reached some tentative conclusions. On the basis of a chemically diverse group of about 100 drugs (81), the investigators determined that the exposure ratio (AUC_{food}/AUC_{fast}) was inversely related to (log) aqueous solubility and directly related to a (log) solubility ratio (dose/aqueous solubility) and to (log) $K_{o/w}$. As others have observed, food effects are most pronounced for poorly water-soluble, lipophilic compounds. Another group, using regression analysis applied to a more comprehensive set of chemical variables (92 drugs), concluded that those variables permitted a correct categorization of a positive, negative, or no food effect 97%, 79%, and 68% of the time, respectively (76). In those instances associated with a positive food effect (i.e., increased F), solubilization appeared to be the primary factor (class II and perhaps class IV). A negative food effect (decreased F) appeared to be most associated with hydrophilic compounds that are absorbed over a defined length of the GIT (class III).

A drug should always be ingested with a cup of water (ca., 8 oz) to insure easy transit down the esophagus and to provide fluid for disintegration and dissolution. Whether or not the drug should be taken on an empty stomach (e.g., enteric-coated tablets) or with food will depend on the specific drug.

Drugs that should be taken with food include those compounds that are irritating to the tract (e.g., nitrofurantoin), those absorbed high in the tract by a specialized mechanism (e.g., riboflavin and ascorbic acid), and possibly those where the presence of certain food constituents are known to enhance absorption (e.g., griseofulvin). The absorption of griseofulvin (class II), which is a very poorly water-soluble drug, is enhanced when it is coadministered with a fatty meal as discussed previously (63,64). For those compounds that irritate the tract, perhaps the best recommendation is to ingest the drug with or after a light meal that does not contain fatty foods or constituents known to interact with the drug. Nitrofurantoin absorption is improved in the presence of food (82,83). Riboflavin and ascorbic acid, which are absorbed by a specialized process high in the small intestine, are best absorbed when gastric emptying is delayed by the presence of food (37,84). As the residence time of the vitamins in the upper portion of the intestine is prolonged, contact with absorption sites is increased and absorption becomes more efficient (i.e., saturation of transporters is avoided). The influence of food on the absorption of those vitamins is illustrated in Figure 13 along with improved efficacy of ascorbic acid absorption achieved by administering divided doses.

The importance of gastric emptying can probably be most readily appreciated by those investigators who have examined drug absorption in patients after a partial or total

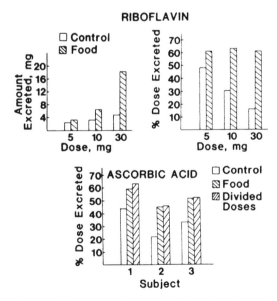

Figure 13 (*Top*) Influence of food on the absorption of different doses of riboflavin. (*Bottom*) Influence of food and divided doses on ascorbic acid absorption in three subjects. *Source*: Based on data from Refs. 37 and 84.

gastrectomy. Muehlberger (85) noted that, following a near-total gastrectomy, patients often complain of "sensitivity" to alcohol. This is probably best explained by ethanol moving rapidly from the poorly absorbing surface of the stomach to the small intestine, where absorption is rapid. Food slows gastric emptying of ethanol, resulting in a slowed absorption, a greater first-pass effect, and lower plasma concentrations (86,87). Gastric emptying has been shown to be important in oral L-dopa therapy, and it has been noted (88) that patients with a partial gastrectomy or gastrojejunostomy exhibit a prompt response with less than average doses of the drug. This observation is consistent with rapid absorption from the small intestine in such patients and is essentially equivalent to introduction of the drug into the duodenum.

For many drugs, as has been shown for acetaminophen, there will be a direct relationship between gastric-emptying rate and maximal plasma concentration (C_{max}) and an inverse relationship between gastric-emptying rate and the time required to attain maximal plasma concentrations (T_{max}). Those relationships are illustrated in Figure 14A and B (89). Also shown in Figure 14 is the influence of a narcotic (heroin) on the gastric emptying and absorption of acetaminophen (Fig. 14C, D) (90). In attempting to predict such relationships, however, it is essential that one consider the physicochemical characteristics of the drug. While increased gastric-emptying rate will probably increase the rate (and possibly the extent) of absorption for drugs best absorbed from the small intestine from rapidly dissolving dosage forms, the converse may be true in other circumstances. For example, if the dosage form must first be exposed to the acidic gastric fluids to initiate disintegration or dissolution, rapid emptying may reduce the rate and extent of absorption (e.g., ketoconazole, a basic compound). Similarly, if the drug dissolves slowly from the dosage form, a shortened residence time in the gut may reduce the extent of dissolution and absorption. One needs a good deal of fundamental understanding of the chemistry of the drug, its dosage form, and the absorption mechanism before being able to anticipate or rationalize the influence of these various factors on the efficacy of absorption.

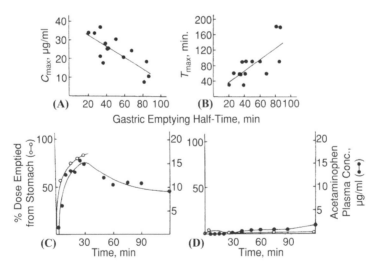

Figure 14 (**A,B**) Maximum acetaminophen plasma concentration (C_{max}) and time to achieve that concentration (T_{max}) as a function of gastric-emptying half-time. (**C**) Percentage of an acetaminophen dose emptied from the stomach (○–○) and acetaminophen plasma concentrations (•–•) as a function of time in one subject. (**D**) The same plot and for the same subject as in (**C**) after a 10-mg intramuscular dose of heroin. *Source*: Parts A and B from Ref. 89 and parts C and D from Ref. 90.

A final point that should be mentioned here, although it has received relatively little attention, is that of esophageal transit. Delay in movement down the esophagus will delay absorption and, in addition, for certain drugs, may also cause local mucosal damage. Capsule disintegration has been observed to occur in the esophagus within three to five minutes. Esophageal transit is delayed when solid dosage forms are swallowed with little fluid or when the subject is supine (91,92). Antipyrine absorption from capsules (93) has been shown to be delayed when esophageal transit was prolonged. To avoid this delay the dosage form should be swallowed with water or other fluids, and the subject should be in a standing or sitting position. This appears to be especially true for the drug class used for treating osteoporosis, bisphosphonates, which must be ingested with adequate fluids while the patient sits in a chair to avoid potentially serious esophageal erosion.

Intestinal Transit

Once a dosage form empties from the stomach and enters the small intestine, it will be exposed to an environment totally different from that in the stomach, as discussed previously. Since the small intestine is the primary site of drug absorption, the longer the residence time in this region, the greater the potential for complete absorption, assuming chemical stability in the intestinal fluids and no formation of water-insoluble derivatives.

There are primarily two types of intestinal movements: propulsive and mixing. Propulsive movements, generally synonymous with peristalsis, will determine intestinal transit rate and therefore the residence time of a drug in the intestine. This time of residence is important since it will dictate the amount of time the dosage form has in which to release the drug, permit dissolution, and allow for absorption. Obviously, the greater the intestinal motility, the shorter the residence time and the less time there is for those processes to proceed. Intestinal motility will be most important for those dosage forms that release drug slowly (e.g., sustained-release products) or require time to initiate release (e.g., enteric-coated products) as well as those drugs that dissolve slowly or where absorption is maximal only in certain regions of the intestine. Peristaltic waves propel intestinal contents down the tract at about 1 to 2 cm/sec. Peristaltic activity is increased after a meal as a result of the gastroenteric reflex initiated by distension of the stomach and results in increased motility and secretion.

Mixing movements of the small intestine are a result of contractions dividing a given region of the intestine into segments, producing an appearance similar to a chain of sausages. These contractions result in the mixing of the intestinal contents with secretions several times a minute. These movements bring the gut contents into optimal contact with the surface epithelium and thereby provide a larger effective area for absorption. In addition, the muscularis mucosa produces folds in the surface epithelium, resulting in an increased surface area and rate of absorption. The villi contract during this process, which results in a "milking" action so that lymph flows from the central lacteal into the lymphatic system.

These mixing motions will tend to improve drug absorption for two reasons. Any factor that increases rate of dissolution will increase the rate (and possibly the extent) of absorption, especially for poorly water-soluble drugs (BCS classes III and IV). Since rate of dissolution depends on agitation intensity, mixing movements will tend to increase dissolution rate and thereby influence absorption. As rate of absorption depends directly on membrane surface area and since mixing increases the contact area between drug and membrane, these motions are expected to increase rate of absorption.

Metoclopramide will increase the rate of gastric emptying, which will often, but not always, increase the rate of drug absorption. However, metoclopramide will also increase the rate of intestinal transit and thus reduce the residence time in the intestine. These two effects may have an opposing influence on absorption. The net effect on absorption depends on the characteristics of the drug and its dosage form as well as the mechanism of absorption. Metoclopramide or similar-acting drugs will probably have little, if any, effect on absorption of a drug given orally in solution, unless the compound (e.g., riboflavin) is absorbed by a specialized process high in the small intestine, in which case there is likely to be a reduction in the amount absorbed. Metoclopramide will probably increase the rate of absorption of a drug from a solid dosage form because of its effect on gastric emptying if the drug is rapidly released and readily dissolved. On the other hand, if the drug dissolves slowly from the dosage form, the extent of absorption may be reduced as a consequence of shortened residence time in the intestine, even though gastric-emptying rate is increased. Similar reasoning may be applied to the influence on drug absorption of various anticholinergics (e.g., atropine and propantheline) and narcotic analgesics, which reduce gastric-emptying and intestinal transit rates. While there will be a reduction in gastric-emptying rate and thus a delay in absorption, these compounds will increase intestinal transit time and possibly increase the extent of absorption, particularly for slowly dissolving drugs or dosage forms that release drug slowly.

Transit through the small intestine appears to be quite different in a variety of ways from movement through the stomach. Once emptied from the stomach, material (such as pellets and tablets) will move along the small intestine and reach the ileocecal valve in about four hours. While this value may range from about one to six hours, intestinal residence time appears to be relatively consistent among normal subjects (94). Values similar to this have been found for food and water movement along the small intestine. Transit appears to be less dependent on the physical nature of the material (liquid vs. solid and size of solids) compared with the response of the stomach. Furthermore, food appears not to influence intestinal transit as it does gastric emptying.

Four hours in the small intestine is a relatively short time for a dosage form to completely dissolve or release drug and then be absorbed. This time would be even more critical to the performance of poorly water-soluble drugs, slowly dissolving coated dosage forms (enteric or polymer coated), and sustained-release forms. Assuming less efficient absorption from the colon (discussed later in the chapter), gastric residence time may prove a critical issue to the performance of certain drugs and drug dosage forms (especially those in the latter categories) as a result of the relatively short intestinal residence time.

There is less information available concerning the factors that may influence intestinal transit time compared with what we know about gastric residence time. Although based upon small populations, there appear to be no gender-related differences in intestinal transit time (95); however, vegetarians appear to have longer intestinal transit times compared with nonvegetarians (96). The latter point may have implications for drug therapy in the third world where the diet is primarily vegetarian. Other factors that result in an increased transit time include reduced digestive fluid secretion, reduced thyroxin secretion, and pregnancy (97–99).

The distal portion of the GIT, the colon (Fig. 1), has as its primary function water and electrolyte absorption and the storage of fecal matter prior to its being expelled. The proximal half of the colon is concerned with absorption and the distal half with storage. Although there are mixing and propulsive movements in the colon, they tend to be rather sluggish. Large circular constrictions occur in the colon, which are similar to the segmenting contractions seen in the small intestine. The longitudinal muscles lining the colon also contract, producing a bulging similar in appearance to sacs and referred to as haustrations. These movements increase the surface area of the colon and result in efficient water absorption.

Contents within the colon are propelled down the tract not by peristaltic waves but by a "mass movement" that occurs only several times a day, being most abundant the first hour after breakfast as a result of a duodenocolonic reflex. The greatest proportion of time moving down the GIT is spent by a meal moving through the colon. In the presence of a diarrheal condition, fluid absorption is incomplete, which results in a watery stool.

Colonic residence time is considerably longer than in other parts of the GIT, and it is also more variable. The transit time can be as short as several hours to as long as 50 to 60 hours. Transit along the colon is characterized by abrupt movement and long periods of stasis. In one study of 49 healthy subjects, the average colonic residence time was 35 hours, with the following times associated with different regions: 11 hours in the right (ascending) colon, 11 hours in the left (descending) colon, and 12 hours in the rectosigmoid colon (100). The latter values do not appear to be influenced by particle size (i.e., pellets vs. tablets), but these times are highly variable and are shortened in response to ingestion of a laxative (average time for a 5-mm tablet in the ascending colon is 8.7 vs. 13.7 hours) (101,102). Furthermore, the ingestion of food, which is known to increase colonic activity, does not appear to have a dramatic effect on the movement of dosage forms from the ileum into the colon nor on the movement within the colon (103). Any differences in colonic transit times as a function of age and gender are not clear at this time due to conflicting reports and investigation in small populations of subjects.

The colonic mucosal pH varies along the length of the colon: right colon, pH 7.1; transverse colon, pH 7.4; left colon, pH 7.5; sigmoid colon, pH, 7.4; and rectum, pH 7.2. These values were determined in a group of 21 subjects (mean age 54 years), and they are somewhat higher than previous estimates (ca., pH 6.7 in the right colon) (104). Those values contrast with the proximal small intestine with a pH of about 6.6 and the terminal ileum with a pH of about 7.4. This near-neutral pH in conjunction with low enzymatic activity has made the colon an interesting potential site for drug absorption. Indeed, there is active interest in delivery of drug dosage forms to the colon for site-specific absorption, especially for peptides (105,106). The characteristics of the colon that are thought to provide a good environment for drug absorption include mild pH, little enzyme activity, and long residence time. The disadvantages of the colon, however, include several considerations that substantially limit this area for providing efficient absorption: small surface area, relatively viscous fluid-like environment (which varies along the length of the colon), and the large colonies of bacteria. The latter factors would limit dissolution and contact with the absorbing surface membrane and may result in presystemic drug metabolism.

The intention of colon-specific drug delivery is to prevent the drug from being released from the dosage form (by coating or other release-controlling mechanism) until it reaches the distal end of the large intestine (i.e., the ileocecal valve). Drug release needs to be delayed for about five hours, but clearly, this delay time will vary from patient to patient and will depend upon a host of factors that may affect gastric emptying and intestinal transit (e.g., food and drugs). The dosage form should then release the drug over the next 10 to 15 hours while in the colon. The results of studies that have examined colonic absorption are not that encouraging, although they do indicate that absorption does occur but to a variable extent (depending on the drug). The hormone, calcitonin, provided an absolute bioavailability from the colon of less than 1%; however, no comparison to oral dosing was made (107). The relative bioavailability of ranitidine solution from the cecum was about 15% of that following gastric or jejunal administration (108). Benazepril-relative bioavailability following a colonic infusion was about 23% that of an oral solution (109). Figure 15 illustrates the plasma concentration-time profiles for

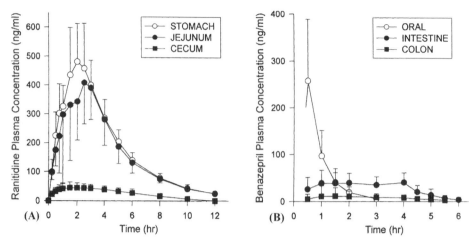

Figure 15 (**A**) Ranitidine plasma concentrations as a function of time following administration of a solution into the stomach, jejunum, or cecum. Each value is the mean of eight subjects (*the cross-hatched vertical bars* are standard deviations). (**B**) Benazepril plasma concentrations as a function of time following a solution dose taken orally or administered as a four-hour intestinal or four-hour colonic infusion. Each value is the mean of 7 to 13 subjects. *Source*: Part A based on data from Ref. 108 and part B based on data from Ref. 109.

those two drugs. The long-lasting analog of vasopressin, dDAVP, a nonapeptide, had a relative bioavailability of about 17% and 21% compared with duodenal and gastric (and jejunal) solution administration, respectively. Rectal administration provided absorption comparable to that from the colon (110). Sumatriptan solution was absorbed from the cecum to an extent of about 23% compared to an oral (and jejunal) dose (111). In all cases, rate of absorption is substantially slower than that from the upper regions of the GIT. Furthermore, in some instances, the metabolite to parent drug concentration ratios change depending on the site of administration, which may reflect a number of causes (e.g., different extent of presystemic metabolism and differences in metabolite absorption). The latter needs to be a consideration for those compounds whose metabolites are either pharmacologically active or toxic.

Although the epithelial surface membrane of the colon may not permit efficient drug absorption (compared with the small intestine), it nonetheless can be an effective site for the absorption of some drugs. The latter is evidenced by continued absorption from controlled-release dosage forms many hours after reaching the colon.

A relevant consideration of absorption from the colonic area is with regard to rectal drug administration. While this is not a frequently used route (at least in the United States), it is employed to some extent, especially in infants, children, and those unable to swallow medication. Absorption from the rectum is generally considered to be relatively poor, at least in comparison to absorption from regions of the upper GIT (112). The reasons for this are essentially those outlined earlier for the colon: small absorbing surface area, little fluid content, and poor mixing movements. There are, in addition, two other considerations. First, the presence of fecal material may result in drug attachment (adsorption) and offer a barrier to diffusion to the absorbing membrane. Second, the extent of absorption will be dependent on the retention time of the dosage form in the rectum. This may be a critical issue for infants who often have irregular bowel movements.

Blood Flow

The entire GIT is highly vascularized and therefore well perfused by the bloodstream. The splanchnic circulation, which perfuses the GIT, receives about 28% of cardiac output, and this flow drains into the portal vein and then goes to the liver prior to reaching the systemic circulation. An absorbed drug will first go to the liver, which is the primary site of drug metabolism in the body; the drug may be metabolized extensively prior to systemic distribution. This has been referred to as the hepatic "first-pass" effect, or presystemic hepatic elimination, and it has important implications in bioavailability and drug therapy.

The fact that the GIT is so well perfused by the bloodstream permits efficient delivery of absorbed materials to the body. As a result of this rapid blood perfusion, the blood at the site of absorption represents a virtual sink for absorbed material. Under normal conditions, then, there is never a buildup in drug concentration in the blood at the site of absorption. Therefore, the concentration gradient will favor further unidirectional transfer of drug from the gut to the blood. Usually, then, blood flow is not an important consideration in drug absorption. Generally, the properties of the dosage form (especially dissolution rate) or the compound's inherent membrane permeability will be the limiting factors in absorption.

There are circumstances, however, where blood flow to the GIT may influence drug absorption. Those compounds absorbed by active or specialized mechanisms require membrane participation in transport, which in turn depends on the expenditure of metabolic energy by intestinal cells. If blood flow and therefore oxygen delivery is reduced, there may be a reduction in absorption of those compounds.

The rate-limiting step in the absorption of those compounds that readily penetrate the intestinal membrane (i.e., have a large permeability coefficient) may be the rate at which blood perfuses the intestine. However, absorption will be independent of blood flow for those compounds that are poorly permeable. Extensive studies have illustrated this concept in animals (113–115). The absorption rate of tritiated water, which is rapidly absorbed in the intestine, is dependent on intestinal blood flow; but a poorly absorbed compound, such as ribitol, penetrates the intestine at a rate independent of blood flow. In between these two extremes are a variety of intermediate compounds whose absorption rate is dependent on blood flow at low flow rates but independent of blood flow at higher flow rates. By altering blood flow to the intestine of the dog, as blood flow decreased the rate of sulfaethidole absorption also decreased. These relationships are illustrated in Figure 16.

An interesting clinical example of the influence of blood flow on drug absorption is that provided by Rowland et al. (116). After oral ingestion of aspirin, one subject fainted while blood samples were being taken. Absorption ceased at the time of fainting, but continued when the subject recovered. Interestingly, there was no reduction in the total amount of aspirin absorbed compared with another occasion when the subject did not faint. Another investigator observed a three-hour delay in the absorption of sulfamethoxypyridazine in a patient who fainted (117). The most reasonable explanation for these observations is the fact that in a fainting episode blood is preferentially shunted away from the extremities and other body organs, including the GIT, thereby reducing blood perfusion of the tract and resulting in a decreased rate of absorption (sink conditions no longer apply). It is possible that generalized hypotensive conditions may be associated with altered drug absorption. In that regard, the influence of congestive heart failure and other disease conditions that will alter GIT blood flow as well as the presence of other drugs that may alter flow need to be considered. For

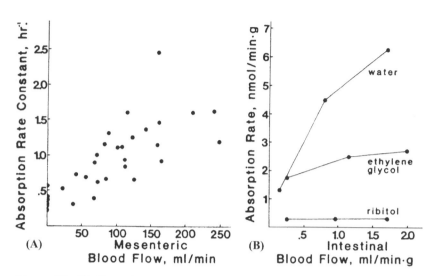

Figure 16 (**A**) Absorption rate constant of sulfaethidole in dogs as a function of mesenteric blood flow. (**B**) Absorption rate of several compounds in rats as a function of intestinal blood flow. *Source*: Part A based on data from Ref. 115 and part B based on data from Ref. 114.

example, it has been suggested that digoxin absorption is impaired in congestive heart failure but improves after compensation (118). The influence of such conditions on absorption has been reviewed elsewhere (119), but there is relatively little information available.

Blood flow to the GIT increases shortly after a meal and may last for several hours. Digestive processes in general seem to enhance blood flow to the tract. For reasons discussed previously, however, coadministration of a drug with a meal would normally not be expected to improve drug absorption on the basis of increased blood flow. Strenuous physical exercise appears to reduce blood flow to the tract and may reduce absorption rate.

COMPLICATING FACTORS IN DRUG ABSORPTION

Drug Interactions: Physical-Chemical Factors

A variety of factors may affect the rate or extent of absorption. Interactions in absorption are mediated by physical-chemical, physiological, or biochemical factors. Physical-chemical considerations include the characteristics of the dosage form and altered solubility, dissolution, and chemical stability within the GIT. Physiological factors include residence time in the tract (i.e., gastric-emptying and intestinal transit rates) and blood flow to the absorbing membrane as well as its characteristics. Biochemical factors would include enzymatic activity in the GIT. Drug-food and drug-drug interactions may alter absorption by one or more of the foregoing mechanisms.

As discussed previously, drug absorption may be impaired or improved when food is present in the GIT. Food may reduce the rate or extent of absorption by virtue of reduced gastric-emptying rate, which is particularly important for compounds unstable in

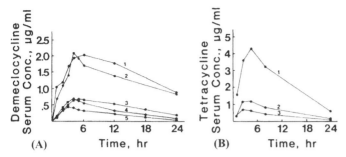

Figure 17 (A) Demeclocycline serum concentrations as a function of time in four to six subjects after oral ingestion of demeclocycline in the absence or presence of dairy meals. Key: 1, meal (no dairy products); 2, water; 3, 110 g cottage cheese; 4, 240 mL buttermilk; 5, 240 mL whole milk. (B) Tetracycline serum concentrations as a function of time in six subjects after oral ingestion of tetracycline in the absence or presence of iron salts (equivalent to 40 mg elemental iron). Key: 1, control; 2, ferrous gluconate; 3, ferrous sulfate. *Source*: Part A based on data from Ref. 122 and part B based on data from Ref. 123.

gastric fluids and for dosage forms designed to release drug slowly. Food provides a rather viscous environment that will reduce the rate of drug dissolution and drug diffusion to the absorbing membrane. Drugs may also bind to food particles or react with GI fluids secreted in response to the presence of food.

The absorption of tetracycline is reduced by calcium salts present in dairy foods and by several other cations, including magnesium and aluminum (120–122), which are often present in antacid preparations. In addition, iron and zinc have been shown to reduce tetracycline absorption (123). Figure 17 illustrates several of these interactions. These cations react with tetracycline to form a water-insoluble and nonabsorbable complex. Obviously, these offending materials should not be coadministered with tetracycline antibiotics. Heavy metals, in general, may create this type of problem, and it is a good precaution to separate in time the administration of those metals from drug ingestion.

The tetracycline example cited above is one type of physical-chemical interaction that may alter absorption. The relative influence of complexation on drug absorption will depend on the water solubility of the drug, the water solubility of the complex, and the magnitude of the interaction (i.e., the complexation stability constant). If the drug itself is poorly water soluble, the absorption pattern will be governed by rate of dissolution. Often such compounds are incompletely and erratically absorbed. As a result, complexation will probably exert more of an influence on the absorption of such a compound than on one that is normally well absorbed, although this will depend on the nature of the complex. If the complex is water insoluble, as in the case of tetracycline interactions with various metal cations, the fraction complexed will be unavailable for absorption. Although most complexation interactions are reversible, the greater the stability constant of the complex, the greater the relative influence on absorption. Generally, however, because the interaction is reversible, complexation is more likely to influence the rate rather than the extent of absorption.

Surface-active agents, because they are able to form micelles above the critical micelle concentration, may bind drugs either by inclusion within the micelle (solubilization) or by attachment to its surface. Below the critical micelle concentration, surfactant monomers have a membrane-disrupting effect, which can enhance drug penetration across a membrane. The latter influence has been seen in drug absorption studies in animals. The influence of surface-active agents on drug absorption will depend on the surfactant concentration and the physicochemical characteristics of the drug. If the drug is capable of partitioning from the aqueous to the micellar phase, and if the micelle is not absorbed, which is usually the case, there may be a reduction in rate of absorption. Micellar concentrations of sodium lauryl sulfate or polysorbate 80 (Tween 80) increase the rectal absorption rate of potassium iodide in the rat but reduce the absorption rate of iodoform and triiodophenol (124,125). Since potassium iodide is not solubilized by the micelle, the enhanced rate of absorption is attributed to the influence of the surfactant on the mucosal membrane. The other compounds, which partition into the micelle, exhibit a reduced rate of absorption since there is a decrease in their effective (i.e., unbound) concentration. Similar observations, using pharmacological response data in goldfish, have been made for several barbiturates in the presence of varying surfactant concentrations.

In addition to the aforementioned effects of surfactants, one must consider their influence on drug dissolution from pharmaceutical dosage forms. If the drug is poorly water soluble, enhanced dissolution rate in the presence of a surface-active agent, even if part of the drug is solubilized, will result in increased drug absorption. The absorption rate of sulfisoxazole suspensions given rectally to rats increased with increasing polysorbate 80 concentration. At surfactant concentrations in excess of that needed to solubilize the drug completely, there was a reduced rate of absorption; however, the rate was greater than that from the control suspension (i.e., without surfactant) (126).

Another important type of physical-chemical interaction, which may alter absorption, is that of drug binding or adsorption onto the surface of another material. As with complexation and micellarization, adsorption will reduce the effective concentration gradient between gut fluids and the bloodstream, which is the driving force for passive absorption. While adsorption frequently reduces the rate of absorption, the interaction is often readily reversible and will not affect the extent of absorption. A major exception is adsorption onto charcoal, which in many cases appears to be irreversible, at least during the time of residence within the GIT. As a result, charcoal often reduces the extent of drug absorption. Indeed, this fact along with the innocuous nature of charcoal is what makes it an ideal antidote for oral drug overdose. The effectiveness of that form of therapy will depend on the amount of charcoal administered and the time delay between overdose and charcoal dosing. Another interesting aspect of charcoal dosing is its influence on shortening the elimination half-life of certain drugs. This is a particularly attractive noninvasive means of enhancing drug elimination from the body for drugs that undergo enterohepatic recycling (phenobarbital is a good example).

In addition to charcoal, adsorption is often seen with pharmaceutical preparations that contain large quantities of relatively water-insoluble components. A good example is antidiarrheal products and perhaps antacids. The importance of the strength of binding as it influences absorption has been illustrated by Sorby (127), who showed that both attapulgite and charcoal reduce the rate of drug absorption but only charcoal reduced the extent of absorption. Lincomycin is an example of a drug whose absorption in impaired by an antidiarrheal preparation (128). Another type of compound that has been shown to alter drug absorption due to binding is the anion-exchange resins, cholestyramine and colestipol. The foregoing physical-chemical interactions, which may alter drug therapy, may be minimized by not coadministering the interacting compounds simultaneously but separating their ingestion by several hours.

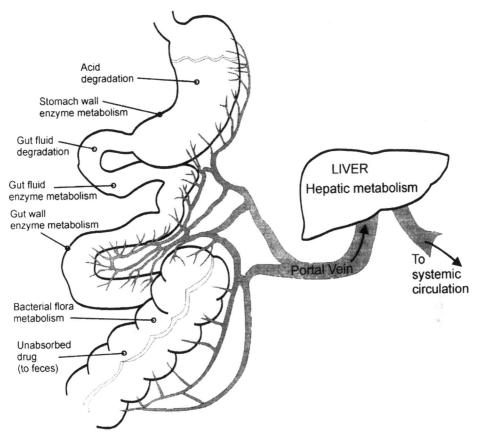

Figure 18 Diagrammatic sketch indicating sites along the GIT where drug may be chemically altered or enzymatically metabolized. *Source*: Courtesy of Saguaro Press.

Metabolism and Transporters: Drug-Drug and Drug-Nutrient Interactions

Drug molecules may be chemically or metabolically altered at various sites along the GIT, including within gut fluids, within the gut wall, and by microorganisms present in the low end of the tract. These sites are noted in Figure 18. Several examples of enzymatic alteration of certain drugs in gut fluids have been noted previously. Gut fluids contain appreciable quantities of various enzymes, which are needed to accomplish digestion of food. An additional consideration in that regard is that of acid- or base-mediated drug breakdown. Numerous drugs are unstable in acidic media (e.g., erythromycin, penicillin) and will therefore degrade and provide lower effective doses depending on the pH of the gastric fluid, solubility of the drug, and the residence time of the dosage form in the stomach. Chemical modification of the drug by, for example, salt or ester formation may provide a more stable derivative whose absorption will be influenced to a smaller degree by the factors noted above. An interesting example of a prodrug that must first be acid-hydrolyzed to produce the active chemical form is clorazepate. Upon hydrolysis in the gut fluids, the active form, *N*-desmethyldiazepam, is produced. In this instance, unlike the examples cited above, acid hydrolysis is a prerequisite for absorption of the pharmacologically active form. As a result, pH of gastric fluids and gastric-emptying time and variables that influence those factors are expected to affect the absorption profile of clorazapate. Greater concentrations of *N*-desmethyldiazepam are achieved at the lower gastric pH, which is consistent with the more rapid acid hydrolysis at acidic pH (129).

As noted in a preceding section, mucosal cells lining the gut wall represent a significant potential site for drug metabolism. The metabolic activity of this region has been studied by a variety of techniques, ranging from subcellular fractions to tissue homogenates to methods involving the whole living animal. Metabolic reactions include both phase I and phase II processes. It appears that the entire small intestine, especially the jejunum and ileum, have the greatest enzymatic activity, although most regions of the GIT can partake in metabolism. It is not a simple matter, especially in the whole animal, to distinguish among the several sites of metabolism responsible for "presystemic elimination." The latter refers to all processes of chemical or metabolic alteration prior to the drug reaching the systemic circulation, which take place primarily in the gut and liver (first-pass effects). It is this presystemic elimination that contributes to differences in drug effects as a function of route of administration, and which may seriously compromise the clinical efficiency of certain drugs given orally. There are many drugs that have been shown to undergo extensive metabolism in the gut wall, including, among others, atorvastatin, simvastatin, felodipine, buspirone, midazolam, cyclosporine, and tacrolimus (130). L-Dopa appears to be metabolized by decarboxylase enzymes present in the gastric mucosa, which, as discussed previously, suggests the importance of rapid gastric emptying to achieve maximal absorption of the unchanged compound (131).

Salicylamide and *p*-aminobenzoic acid are interesting examples because they illustrate another aspect of gut metabolism, which is that of saturation. In addition, factors affecting absorption rate, such as the presence of food, will influence the fraction of the dose reaching the systemic circulation in the form of intact drug. Figure 19 illustrates the relationship between the area under the salicylamide plasma concentration-time curve as a function of the oral dose of sodium salicylamide (132). Normally, that relationship is expected to be linear, and the line should go through the origin. The curvilinearity, especially at low doses, suggests some form of presystemic elimination, which becomes

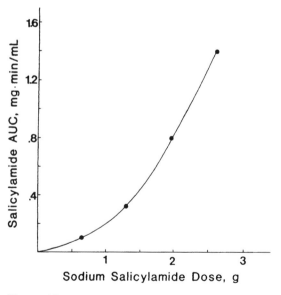

Figure 19 Area under the salicylamide plasma concentration-time curve (AUC) as a function of the oral dose of sodium salicylamide. Each point is the average of five subjects. *Source*: Based on data from Ref. 132.

saturated above a certain ("breakthrough") dose. The drug is metabolized in the gut wall to sulfate and glucuronide conjugates, although metabolism in the liver also occurs on the first pass. Extrapolation of the straight-line segment to the x-axis, in Figure 19 gives an intercept that has been referred to as the breakthrough dose, which approximates the dose needed to saturate the enzyme system (~ 1–1.5 g for salicylamide). Doses less than that value produce only small plasma concentrations of the unchanged drug. Another interesting aspect of this phenomenon is that the rate of drug presentation to the enzyme system will influence the fraction of the dose reaching the systemic circulation unchanged and will alter the metabolic pattern. The latter factors, therefore, will be influenced by the dosage form characteristics and the rate of gastric emptying. The more rapid the rate of absorption, the more likely the enzyme system will become saturated. The latter will result in greater plasma concentrations of unchanged drug and a metabolic pattern with a lower percentage of the drug recovered as the saturable metabolite. At any given dose, the more rapidly soluble sodium salicylamide produces greater plasma concentrations of unchanged drug compared with salicylamide. The more rapidly soluble dosage forms of salicylamide (solution and suspension) produce smaller fractions of the dose in the form of the saturable metabolite (sulfate conjugate) compared with a slowly dissolving tablet (133).

Observations similar to that above have been made for p-aminobenzoic acid, and these illustrate the influence of food. In that instance it was shown that a delay in gastric emptying, produced by the presence of food (fat or glucose), resulted in a greater percentage of the dose being metabolized to the saturable metabolite (acetyl derivative), which is consistent with a reduced rate of absorption and a slowing of presentation of the drug to the site of metabolism. Similar findings would also apply to ethanol absorption; a reduced gastric emptying will maximize metabolic first-pass effects and lower plasma concentrations of intact ethanol.

An interesting example of gut metabolism and gender-dependent differences is that of ethanol. Females appear to have greater blood ethanol concentrations following an oral dose compared with males given the same dose. The latter is true even if the data are corrected for differences in body weight and lean body mass. Ethanol is metabolized by alcohol dehydrogenase present in the gastric mucosa, and it appears that this enzyme is present in smaller quantities in females. The lower enzyme concentration results in a greater fraction of the dose not being metabolized compared with males and a subsequent higher blood ethanol concentration. Estimates of absorption suggest that females absorb about 91% of the dose as ethanol compared with about 61% in males (134). Evidence suggests that alcohol deydrogenase activity is lower in young women (younger than ~ 50 years), elderly males, and alcoholics (135).

The impact of presystemic elimination may be clearly understood by considering the following relationships among the several steps involved in making the drug available to the systemic circulation. The significance of this relationship is its multiplicative nature, since most of the processes are sequential. These relationships assume linear or first-order kinetics (i.e., there is no nonlinearity or saturation effects).

$$F_{\text{systemic}} = f_{\text{released}} \cdot f_{\text{absorbed}} \cdot f_{\text{hepatic}} \qquad (4)$$

The fraction of the orally administered dose that is bioavailable to the systemic circulation (F_{systemic}) is dependent on the fraction of the dose that is released from the dosage form (f_{released}) multiplied by the fraction that is absorbed into the portal circulation on its way to the liver (f_{absorbed}; this is the fraction that escapes GIT metabolism) multiplied by the fraction of the dose that escapes the hepatic first-pass effect (f_{hepatic}). Since this is a multiplicative process, if, for example, f_{released} is 1.0, f_{absorbed} is 0.5 and f_{hepatic} is 0.5, then the overall F_{systemic} is 0.25 (i.e., 25% of the dose reaches the systemic circulation). The absorption process can be broken down further into its component parts.

$$F_{\text{systemic}} = f_{\text{released}} \cdot \left(f_{\text{gut fluid}} \cdot f_{\text{gut wall}} \cdot f_{\text{gut flora}} \right) \cdot f_{\text{hepatic}} \tag{5}$$

The fractions of the dose of drug that escape metabolism in the gut fluid, gut wall, and gut flora are $f_{\text{gut fluid}}$, $f_{\text{gut wall}}$, and $f_{\text{gut flora}}$, respectively. In the above example, an f_{absorbed} of 0.5 represents the product of the three processes that affect absorption. It is often common to express the fraction surviving a specific process as $1 - \text{ER}$ (extraction ratio) for that process. Thus, the above relationship may be written as,

$$F_{\text{systemic}} = f_{\text{released}} \cdot \left(1 - \text{ER}_{\text{gut fluid}} \right) \cdot \left(1 - \text{ER}_{\text{gut wall}} \right) \tag{6}$$
$$\cdot \left(1 - \text{ER}_{\text{gut flora}} \right) \cdot \left(1 - \text{ER}_{\text{hepatic}} \right)$$

A change in the ER value for any of the above processes will have an effect on the systemically available dose of the orally administered drug.

An especially interesting and extensively researched drug-food (or drug-nutrient) interaction is that between grapefruit juice (as well as other fruit juices) and certain drugs, especially those with a high metabolic clearance that undergo substantial presystemic (first-pass) metabolism. The discovery of this interaction is an excellent example of serendipity and an illustration of Pasteur's famous statement, "In the field of experimentation, chance favors only the prepared mind." In their original study (136), the experimenters were attempting to examine the influence of ethanol on the pharmacokinetics of coadministered drugs. The ethanol was mixed (serendipitously) with grapefruit juice to mask the taste of the ethanol. A substantial interaction was noted with felodipine, an approximate threefold increase in bioavailability. Since that initial observation, numerous studies have indicated that many other drugs with diverse chemical structures having a high metabolic clearance participate in this interaction with grapefruit juice (not ethanol!). Many studies have been devoted to determining the mechanism(s) of this interaction, and the readers are referred to a recent symposium and book chapter that cover this topic (137,138). While we have a better understanding of the nature of the interaction, it now appears that there may be several processes going on.

The drugs that undergo this interaction are substrates for one of the major drug-metabolizing isozymes in the body, cytochrome P450 3A4 (CYP3A4). This enzyme has been referred to as being promiscuous (in a biochemical sense) in that it will accommodate and metabolize a very wide range of drug molecules, most of which are lipid soluble. Since this isozyme is responsible for the metabolism of many drugs, it is also involved in many drug-drug and, in this case, nutrient-drug interactions. This enzyme and many other isozymes are present in the mucosal surface cells (enterocytes) of the GIT. Therefore, the gut surface represents a potential site for drug metabolism. Phytochemicals present in grapefruit juice (furanocoumarins) are able to inhibit the CYP3A4 enzyme, resulting in less than usual presystemic GI metabolism of the drug (139). Since more of the dose of drug survives this metabolic step, there is a greater oral bioavailability of the drug. Enzyme inhibition could also be expressed in liver enzyme activity (resulting in increased bioavailability); however, liver enzymes appear to play a less significant role in this interaction than those in the GIT. The latter, however, may be more or less true depending upon the drug whose interaction is under investigation. For example, in the metabolic interaction between saquinavir and midazolam, saquinavir more than doubled the systemic oral bioavailability (F_{systemic}) of midazolam (0.41–0.90). It was determined that the hepatic ER decreased from 0.39 to 0.17; however, the GIT ER decreased from 0.33 to 0 (50). The latter change had the greatest impact on the increased

Table 8 Drugs Known to Interact with Grapefruit Juice

Anti-infectives: artemether, saquinavir
Anti-lipemic: atorvastatin, lovastatin, simvastatin
Cardiovascular: carvedilol, nicardipine, cilostazole, nitrendipine, felodipine, nimodipine, nifedipine, verapamil, nisoldipine
CNS: buspirone, carbamazepine, diazepam, midazolam, trizolam
Other:
Antihistamine: astemizole, terfenadine
Estrogen: ethinyl estradiol
GI: cisapride
Immunosuppressants: cyclosporine, tacrolimus

Source: From Ref. 140.

value for $F_{systemic}$. It is also important to note that these values are associated with large intersubject variability.

A complicating factor, however, in this interaction is that many compounds that are substrates for CYP3A4 are also substrates for P-gp, the efflux transporter protein that resides in the membrane surface of the GIT enterocyte. This transporter was noted in a previous section that discussed the transport process. There is evidence to suggest that the drug interaction with grapefruit juice also involves inhibition of this efflux transporter (137). Both CYP3A4 metabolic inhibition and P-gp efflux transport inhibition will result in increased drug bioavailability. It is possible that these two mechanisms are acting in tandem in an attempt to limit foreign compounds (such as drugs) from entering the systemic circulation.

A recent study (140) has also indicated that these interactions occur in elderly patients. This is especially important since most interaction studies are typically performed in young subjects, yet the elderly are more likely to be taking the drugs that undergo these interactions. Table 8 lists drug examples in different therapeutic categories that are known to participate in this grapefruit juice interaction (140). It should be recognized too that these compounds will also interact with any other drug (e.g., ketoconazole) capable of inhibiting CYP3A4 and/or P-gp.

The illustration mentioned earlier should offer a clear caution that components of food may interact with drugs, resulting in substantial positive or negative therapeutic effects. As will be noted below, this principle also applies to so-called dietary supplements, including botanicals used for the treatment of numerous medical conditions.

In addition to food- or nutrient-based interactions in the metabolism of drugs, it has become quite clear in recent years that so-called dietary supplements, including botanicals have the potential to participate in drug interactions. The latter observation has special relevance because of the extensive use of such products worldwide (ca., $15 billion/yr in the United States alone), their easy commercial availability (no prescription required), and their common use with prescribed drugs. Furthermore, many people consider such "natural" products to be safe and free of any adverse effects (it should be pretty easy to recall many poisons that occur in nature and are, therefore, natural). There are several recent examples of botanical drug interactions, which should serve as a warning that we have just begun to see the tip of the iceberg. This should not be at all surprising when one considers the large number and variety of chemicals (phytochemicals) present in botanicals that are ingested for medicinal value.

St. John's wort, which is extensively used for the treatment of mild depression, has been shown to induce intestinal P-gp and intestinal and hepatic CYP3A4 in humans (141).

That mechanism explains the significant reduction in cyclosporin and anti-AIDS (e.g., indinavir) plasma concentrations. It is likely that similar effects will be noted with the compounds listed in Table 8 (however, the effects noted in Table 8 are in the opposite direction of those seen in the presence of St. John's wort).

The GI microflora provides another potential site for drug metabolism within the GIT, and it has received some attention. In normal subjects, the stomach and proximal small intestine contain small numbers of microorganisms. The concentrations of these organisms increase toward the distal end of the intestine. A wide variety of aerobic and anaerobic organisms are present in the gut. The microflora, derived primarily from the environment, tend to adhere to the luminal surface of the intestine. Within an individual, the microflora tends to remain rather stable over long periods of time. The primary factors governing the numbers and kinds of microorganisms present in the tract include the activity of gastric and bile secretions, which tend to limit the growth of these organisms in the stomach and upper part of the GIT, and the propulsive motility of the intestine, which is responsible for continually cleansing the tract, thereby limiting the proliferation of microorganisms. Gastric atrophy permits increased numbers of microorganisms to pass into the small intestine, and reduced intestinal motility results in overgrowth.

Studies conducted mostly in animals, indicate a wide range of primarily phase I metabolic pathways. Various drugs that are glucuronidated in the body are secreted into the intestine via the bile, and these are subject to cleavage by bacterial glucuronidase enzymes. The cleavage product may then be in a form available for absorption. Various drug conjugates may be similarly deconjugated by other bacterial enzymes (e.g., the glycine conjugate of isonicotinic acid). Although some drugs may be rendered inactive, bacterial metabolism of other drugs may give rise to more active or toxic products. The formation of the toxic compound cyclohexylamine from cyclamate is an example (142).

Salicylazosulfapyridine (sulfasalazine), which is used in treating ulcerative colitis, provides an interesting example of a drug whose metabolites represent the active pharmacological species. The parent drug is metabolized to 5-aminosalicylate and sulfapyridine. In conventional rats, both metabolites and their conjugates appear in urine and feces. In germ-free rats, however, the metabolites are not excreted. This suggests that the intestinal flora plays a role in reducing the parent compound and formation of the two metabolites. If this is the case, factors influencing the population and types of intestinal microorganisms may in turn influence the absorption and effectiveness of the drug. For example, concomitant antibiotic therapy, by reducing the population of microorganisms, may prevent the parent drug from being metabolized.

Disease States

GI disorders and disease states have the potential to influence drug absorption. Although this important area has not been explored thoroughly, numerous studies have addressed this issue. Unfortunately, many of these studies have not been correctly designed, and this has resulted in conflicting reports and our inability to reach generally valid conclusions. The majority of these studies are conducted by administration of an oral dose and measurement of the AUC. The latter parameter is frequently used in assessing bioavailability. The resulting AUC is compared to that from a control group of different subjects or within the same subject during the time the disorder is present and compared to the value prior to or after the disorder is resolved. The problem here is that a value for AUC depends as much on the body's ability to clear or eliminate the drug as it does on absorption (i.e., AUC = dose absorbed/clearance). Differences in the former parameter are likely to be present between subjects as well as within a subject from time to time (especially in the presence of a disease). Therefore, values of AUCs after oral dosing may lead to incorrect conclusions. To use such a value properly, one must be certain that drug clearance is not different between or within a subject. In the ideal situation an intravenous dose would be given to establish the correctness of that assumption. Unfortunately, this is an approach that is not generally used.

Elevated gastric pH is seen in subjects with achlorhydria, as a result of reduced acid secretion. The absorption of tetracycline, which is most soluble at acidic pH, appears to be unaffected by achlorhydria and after surgery where the acid-secreting portion of the stomach was removed (143,144). The absorption of clorazepate is expected to be reduced in achlorhydria (for the reasons discussed earlier), but as yet the data are not conclusive. The clinical significance of altered gut pH with regard to drug absorption is not clearly established. Alterations in drug absorption due to changes in gut pH will most likely be mediated by its influence on dissolution rate.

Changes in gastric emptying are expected to influence the rate and possibly the extent of absorption, for the reasons discussed previously. Emptying may be severely hampered and absorption altered soon after gastric surgery as a result of pyloric stenosis and in the presence of various disease states. Riboflavin absorption is increased in hypothyroidism and reduced in hyperthyroidism, conditions that alter gastric-emptying and intestinal transit rates (145).

Diarrheal conditions may decrease drug absorption as a result of reduced intestinal residence time. The absorption of several drugs was decreased in response to lactose- and saline-induced diarrhea (146). Digoxin absorption from tablets was impaired in one subject who developed chronic diarrhea as a result of X-ray treatment (147). Abdominal radiation or the underlying disease has been shown to reduce digoxin and clorazepate absorption (148). A dosage form that provides rapid drug dissolution (e.g., solution) may partially resolve this problem.

Various malabsorption syndromes are known to influence the absorption of certain nutrients. Although not thoroughly investigated, such syndromes may exert an influence on the efficacy of drug absorption. Heizer et al. (149) have noted reduced absorption of digoxin in patients with sprue, malabsorption syndrome, and pancreatic insufficiency. The dosage form of digoxin, especially dissolution rate from tablets, will partially determine the influence of malabsorption states on absorption, the problem being compounded by poorly dissolving tablets. Phenoxymethyl penicillin absorption is reduced in patients with steatorrhea (150), and ampicillin and nalidixic acid absorption appears to be impaired in children with shigellosis (151).

There are a variety of other disease states whose influence on drug absorption has been reported, including cystic fibrosis, villous atrophy, celiac disease, diverticulosis, and Crohn's disease. The results of these studies are frequently divergent, and therefore general statements cannot be made. A thorough discussion of these findings is beyond the scope of this chapter.

As most drugs are best absorbed from the small intestine, any surgical procedure that removes a substantial portion of the small intestine is likely to influence absorption; however, and as discussed previously, the characteristics of the dosage form may affect the findings. Although the procedure has fallen out of favor, intestinal bypass surgery has been used in treatment of the morbidly obese. A number of studies have been conducted to examine absorption prior to and after surgery. As noted in the introduction to this section, care must be exercised in study design and evaluation of data, as large weight loss may alter drug elimination from the body compared with the presurgery condition. Further complications include the time that the study is conducted relative to the time of surgery, and the length and sections of the intestine removed. Reduced efficiency of drug absorption, however, is a likely outcome of surgical shortening of the GIT (152). One excellent study (153) employed intravenous and oral dosing at each of several times postsurgery (1–2 weeks, 6 and 12 months). This design permits valid conclusions about the absorption process. There was a significant reduction after surgery in ampicillin absorption but no change in propylthiouracil absorption.

In those instances where a patient's response to a drug is less than expected and there is reason to believe that this is a result of impaired absorption due to any of the pathological conditions or disease states cited earlier, a first attempt in seeking to improve drug therapy is to optimize absorption from the GIT. To do this, a practical approach might well be to administer the drug in a form readily available for absorption. In most cases, if such a form is marketed or easily prepared, administration of a drug in solution will represent the best way to achieve maximal absorption, as this will eliminate the time for drug dissolution in the gut needed by solid oral dosage forms. When absorption cannot be sufficiently improved by use of a drug solution, alternative routes of administration must be considered (e.g., intramuscular).

Age

The majority of the information discussed to this point and most of the literature concerned with drug absorption involve studies performed in young, healthy (usually male) adults. In contrast, there is considerably less information concerning absorption in subjects at either end of the age spectrum (i.e., pediatric and geriatric populations). For a variety of reasons, one would expect the absorption process in the latter groups to be different from that in young adults; unfortunately, at this time there is little information to present valid general statements.

The pediatric population (neonates, infants, and children) presents a particularly difficult group in which to conduct clinical experimentation because of ethical considerations. A further complication is the rapid development of organ function, which is likely to influence results even over a relatively short experimental period (e.g., 2–4 weeks), especially in neonates and infants. An additional consideration in the latter groups is whether the neonate is premature or full-term. Most often, plasma concentration-time data are obtained after an oral dose for the purpose of estimating elimination half-life or to provide a basis for the development of a multiple-dosing regimen. Such data provide very limited information about the rate or extent of absorption. Indeed, most reviews of drug disposition in the pediatric population indicate the lack of rigorous information about absorption. There are initiatives to encourage the study of drugs in the pediatric population, and this will undoubtedly result in useful new information.

Gastric fluid is less acidic in the newborn than in adults since acid secretion is related to the development of the gastric mucosa. This condition appears to last for some time, as pH values similar to the adult are not reached until after about two years. The higher gastric fluid pH along with smaller gut fluid volume may influence dissolution rate and the stability of acid-unstable drugs. The gastric-emptying rate appears to be slow, approaching adult values after about six months. An interesting example in support of that suggestion is a study that examined riboflavin absorption in a 5-day-old and a 10-month-old infant (154). The maximum urinary excretion rate was considerably greater in the infant, while excretion rate in the neonate was constant and prolonged. These data suggest more rapid absorption in the infant, while absorption in the neonate proceeds for a longer time. For the reasons discussed previously, these data suggest slower emptying and/or intestinal transit rates in the neonate (recall that riboflavin is absorbed by a specialized process high in the small intestine). Intestinal transit tends to be irregular and may be modified by the type of food ingested and the feeding pattern.

Intestinal surface area and total blood flow to the GIT in the neonates and infants are smaller than that in adults and may influence the efficiency of absorption. With regard to the use of rectal suppositories, one must keep in mind that the completeness of absorption will be a function of retention time in the rectum. Since bowel movements in the neonates and infants are likely to be irregular, the retention time may limit the efficiency of absorption by that route. In light of the little information available about absorption in the young, it would seem reasonable to attempt to optimize absorption by using solution or suspensions rather than solid dosage forms.

Only in recent years has there been any substantial progress made in better understanding drug disposition in the elderly. Active research programs in gerontology have begun to provide more information about rational drug dosing in the elderly. There are a number of important and unique characteristics of the elderly, which make a compelling argument for the need for such information (e.g., they ingest more drugs per capita, their percentage of the population is increasing, and they suffer from more disease and physical impairments). As noted for the pediatric population, a variety of complex issues are associated with the conduct of research in the elderly. Careful consideration must be given to experimental design and data analysis. Some considerations include the appropriate definition of age, cross-sectional versus longitudinal study design, and health status of the subject (155,156).

There have been numerous statements in the literature to the effect that GI absorption in the elderly is impaired and less efficient than in young adults. Although there have been few data to support the suggestion, one basis for that statement has been the results obtained from the application of the so-called xylose tolerance test, which is often used in assessing malabsorption. This conclusion of impaired absorption in the elderly presents a good example of the need for careful study design and appropriate pharmacokinetic analysis of data. Figure 20 illustrates the results of several studies that

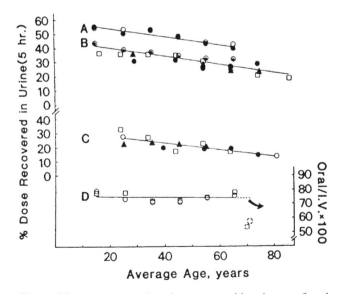

Figure 20 Percentage xylose dose recovered in urine as a function of age after a 5-g intravenous dose (**A**), 5-g oral dose (**B**), and 25-g oral dose (**C**). Line D is the ratio of urinary recoveries (oral to intravenous) after 5-g doses (y-axis *on right*). Symbols represent data obtained from different studies. *Source*: From Ref. 157.

have examined xylose absorption (157). Most studies indicate an inverse relationship between urinary xylose recovery and age after an oral dose (lines B and C). It is this observation that has suggested reduced absorption with age. However, the same inverse relationship is found after an intravenous dose (line A), an observation that cannot be explained by impaired absorption but, rather, by reduced renal clearance of xylose. Line D shows the ratio of urinary recovery (oral to intravenous), which suggests that absorption is not altered with age. A more complete study in which each subject (age range 32–85 years) received both an oral and an intravenous dose indicates no relationship between xylose bioavailability and age (158).

There are substantial changes in a variety of physiological functions in the elderly, which may influence drug absorption (155), including a greater incidence of achlorhydria, altered gastric emptying, reduced gut blood flow, and smaller intestinal surface area. One recent example indicates that gastric pH may be an important determinant of drug absorption in the elderly (159). Dipyridamole is a poorly water-soluble weak base whose dissolution would be optimal in an acidic environment. Elevated gastric pH due to achlorhydria (a condition that is more prevalent in the elderly than in the young) results in impaired absorption of dipyridamole. The ingestion of glutamic acid by achlorhydric subjects improves absorption. There are, in addition, other factors that may influence absorption such as a greater incidence of GI disease, altered nutritional intake and eating habits, and ingestion of drugs, which may affect the absorption of other drugs. Although data are still somewhat limited, the general impression is that the rate of absorption is frequently reduced, while there is little, if any, change in the extent of absorption (155). This is a tentative statement that needs to be qualified for the specific drug and for the health status of the subject. For example, the absorption of drugs that undergo hepatic first-pass metabolism may be greater in the elderly (e.g., propranolol) as a consequence of reduced hepatic clearance with age.

REFERENCES

1. Hamman JH, Enslin GM, Kotze AF. Oral delivery of peptide drugs-barriers and developments. Drug Deliv 2005; 19:165–177.
2. Wender PA, Mitchell DJ, Pattabiraman K, et al. The design, synthesis, and evaluation of molecules that enable or enhance cellular uptake: peptoid molecular transporters. Proc Natl Acad Sci U S A 2000; 97:13003–13008.
3. Rothbard JB, Garlington S, Lin Q, et al. Conjugation of arginine digomers to cyclosporin A facilitates topical delivery and inhibition of inflammation. Nat Med 2000; 6:1253–1257.
4. Hole JW. Human Anatomy and Physiology. 2nd ed. Dubuque, Iowa: Wm. C. Brown Company, 1981:414, 439.
5. Leonhardt H. Color Atlas/Text of Human Anatomy. Vol 2. 4th ed. New York: Thieme Medical Publishers, 1993:213.
6. Fujita T, Tanaka K, Tokunaga J. SEM Atlas of Cells and Tissues. New York: Igaku-Shoin, 1981:122, 123, 129, 135.
7. Trier JS. Morphology of the epithelium of the small intestine. In: Code CF, ed. Handbook of Physiology, Section 6, Alimentary Canal, Vol 3, Intestinal Absorption. Washington, D.C: American Physiological Society, 1968:1133.
8. Tortora GJ, Anagnostakos NP. Principles of Anatomy and Physiology. 6th ed. New York: Harper and Row, 1990:770.
9. Gershkovich P, Qadri B, Yacovan A, et al. Different impacts of intestinal lymphatic transport on the oral bioavailability of structurally similar synthetic lipophilic cannabinoids: dexanabinol and PRS-2111,120. Eur J Pharm Sci 2007; 31:298–305.
10. Fordtran JS, Rector FC Jr., Ewton MF, et al. Permeability characteristics of the human small intestine. J Clin Invest 1965; 44:1935–1944.

11. Danielli JF, Davson H. A contribution to the theory of permeability of thin films. J Cell Comp Physiol 1935; 5:495–508.
12. Davson H, Danieli JF. The Permeability of Natural Membranes. 2nd ed. New York: Cambridge University Press, 1952.
13. Junqueira LC, Carneiro J, Kelley RO. Basic Histology. 6th ed. East Norwalk, CT: Appleton and Lange, 1989:32.
14. Hober R, Hober J. Experiments on the absorption of organic solutes in the small intestine of rats. J Cell Comp Physiol 1937; 10:401–422.
15. Schanker LS. Absorption of drugs from the rat colon. J Pharmacol Exp Ther 1959; 126:283–290.
16. Wright EM, Diamond JM. Patterns of non-electrolyte permeability. Proc R Soc Lond B Biol Sci 1969; 172:203–225.
17. Wright EM, Diamond JM. Patterns of non-electrolyte permeability. Proc R Soc Lond B Biol Sci 1969; 172:227–271.
18. Diamond JM, Wright EM. Molecular forces governing nonelectrolyte permeation through cell membranes. Proc R Soc Lond B Biol Sci 1969; 172:273–316.
19. vande Waterbeemd H, Lennernas H, Artursson P, eds. Drug Bioavailability—Estimation of Solubility, Permeability, Absorption and Bioavailability, Weinheim, Germany: Wiley-VCH, 2003.
20. Lipinski CA, Lombardo F, Dominy BW, et al. Experimental and computational approaches to estimate solubility and permeability in drug discovery and development settings. Adv Drug Deliv Rev 1997; 23:3–25.
21. Faulkner JM. Nicotine posioning by absorption through the skin. J Am Med Assoc 1933; 100:1664–1665.
22. Travell J. The influence of the hydrogen ion concentration on the absorption of alkaloids from the stomach. J Pharmacol Exp Ther 1940; 69:21–33.
23. Jacobs MH. Some aspects of cell permeability to weak electrolytes. Cold Spring Harbor Symp Quant Biol 1940; 8:30–399.
24. Shore PA, Brodie BB, Hogben CAM. The gastric secretion of drugs: a pH partition hypothesis. J Pharmacol Exp Ther 1957; 119:361–369.
25. Schanker LS, Shore PA, Brodie BB, et al. Absorption of drugs from the stomach. I. The rat. J Pharmacol Exp Ther 1957; 120:528–539.
26. Hogben CAM, Schanker LA, Tocco DJ, et al. Absorption of drugs from the stomach. II. The human. J Pharmacol Exp Ther 1957; 120:540–545.
27. Schanker LS, Tocco DJ, Brodie BB, et al. Absorption of drugs from the rat small intestine. J Pharmacol Exp Ther 1958; 123:81–87.
28. Hogben CAM, Tocco DJ, Brodie BB, et al. On the mechanism of intestinal absorption of drugs. J Pharmacol Exp Ther 1959; 125:275–282.
29. Doluisio JT, Billups NF, Dittert LW, et al. Drug absorption. I. An in situ rat gut technique yielding realistic absorption rates. J Pharm Sci 1969; 58:1196–1200.
30. Benet LZ. Biopharmaceutics as a basis fro the design of drug products. In: Ariens EJ, ed., Drug Design. Vol 4. New York: Academic Press, 1973:26–28.
31. Riggs DS. The Mathematical Approach to Physiological Problems. Baltimore: Williams & Wilkins, 1963:181–185.
32. Flynn GL, Yalkowsky SK, Roseman TJ. Mass transport phenomena and models: theoretical concepts. J Pharm Sci 1974; 63:479–510.
33. Mayersohn M. Drug absorption. J Clin Pharmacol 1987; 27:634–638.
34. He Y-L, Murby S, Warhurst G, et al. Species differences in size discrimination in the paracellular pathway reflected by oral bioavailability of poly (ethylene glycol) and D-peptides. J Pharm Sci 1998; 87:626–633.
35. Johnson PH, Frank D, Costantino HR. Discovery of tight junction modulators: significance fro drug development and delivery. Drug Discov Today 2008; 13:261–267.
36. Evered DF, Randall HG. The absorption of amino acid derivatives of nitrogen mustard from rat intestine in vitro. Biochem Pharmacol 1962; 11:371–376.

37. Levy G, Jusko WJ. Factors affecting the absorption of riboflavin in man. J Pharm Sci 1966; 55: 285–289.

38. Mayersohn M. Ascorbic acid absorption in man-pharmacokinetic implications. Eur J Pharmacol 1972; 19:140–142.

39. Gillespie NG, Mena I, Cotzias GC, et al. Diets affecting treatment of Parkinsonism with levodopa. J Am Diet Assoc 1973; 62:525–528.

40. Wade DN, Mearrick PT, Morris JL. Active transport of L-dopa in the intestine. Nature 1973; 242: 463–465.

41. van Woert MH. Phenylalanine and tyrosine metabolism in Parkinson's disease treated with levodopa. Clin Pharmacol Ther 1971; 12:368–375.

42. Lennernas H, Nilsson D, Aquilonius S-M, et al. The effect of L-leucine on the absorption of levodopa, studied by regional jejunal perfusion in man. Br J Clin Pharmacol 1993; 35: 343–250.

43. Zimmerman J. Methotrexate transport in the human intestine. Biochem Pharmacol 1992; 43: 2377–2383.

44. Westphal J-F, Trouvin J-H, Deslandes A, et al. Nifedipine enhances amoxicillin absorption kinetics and bioavailability in human. J Pharmacol Exp Ther 1990; 255:312–317.

45. Duverne C, Bouten A, Deslandes A, et al. Modification of cifixime bioavailability by nifedipine in humans: involvement of the dipeptide carrier system. Antimirob Agents Chemother 1992; 36:2462–2467.

46. Stewart BH, Kugler AR, Thompson PR, et al. A saturable transport mechanism in the intestinal absorption of gabapentin is the underlying cause of the lack of proportionality between increasing dose and drug levels in plasma. Pharm Res 1993; 10:276–281.

47. Gottesman II, Pastan I. Biochemistry of multidrug resistance mediated by the multidrug transporter. Annu Rev Biochem 1993; 62:385–427.

48. Tanigawara Y. Role of p-glycoprotein in drug disposition. Ther Drug Monit 2000; 22: 137–140.

49. Asperen JV, Tellingen OV, Beijnen JH. The pharmacological role of p-glycoprotein in the intestinal epithelium. Pharmacol Res 1998; 37:429–435.

50. Zhang Y, Benet LZ. The gut as a barrier to drug absorption-combined role of cytochrome P450 3A and P-glycoprotein. Clin Pharmacokin 2001; 40:159–168.

51. Mizuno N, Niwa T, Yotsumoto Y, et al. Impact of drug transporter studies on drug discovery and development. Pharmacol Rev 2003; 55:425–461.

52. Aszalos A. Drug-drug interactions affected by the transporter protein P-glycoprotein (ABCB1, MDR1). I. Preclinical aspects. Drug Discov Today 2007; 12:833–837.

53. Aszalos A. Drug-drug interactions affected by the transporter protein P-glycoprotein (ABCB1, MDR1). II.Clinical aspects. Drug Discov Today 2007; 12:838–843.

54. Szakacs G, Varadi A, Ozvegy-Laczka C, et al. The role of ABC transporters in drug absorption, distribution, metabolism, excretion and toxicity (ADME-Tox). Drug Discov Today 2008; 13:379–393.

55. Wacher J, Salphati L, Benet LZ. Active secretion and enterocyte drug metabolism barriers to drug absorption. Adv Drug Deliv Rev 1996; 20:99–112.

56. Sparreboom A, van Asperen J, Mayer U, et al. Limited oral bioavailability of taxol and active epithelial secretion of paclitaxel (Taxol) caused by p-glycoprotein in the intestine. Proc Natl Acad Sci U S A 1997; 94:2031–2035.

57. Westphal K, Weinbrenner A, Giessmann T, et al. Oral bioavailability of digoxin is enhanced by talinolol: evidence for involvement of intestinal p-glycoprotein. Clin Pharmacol Ther 2000; 68: 6–12.

58. Dressman JB, Amidon GL, Reppas C, et al. Dissolution testing as a prognostic tool for oral drug absorption: immediate release dosage forms. Pharm Res 1998; 15:11–22.

59. Bates TR, Young JM, Wu CM, et al. pH-dependent dissolution rate of nitrofurantoin from commercial suspensions, tablets and capsules. J Pharm Sci 1974; 63:643–645.

60. Levy G, Sahli BA. Comparison of the gastrointestinal absorption of aluminum acetylsalicylate and acetylsalicylic acid in man. J Pharm Sci 1962; 51:58–62.

61. Levy G, Procknal JA. Unusual dissolution behavior due to film formation. J Pharm Sci 1962; 51:294.
62. Blezek CE, Lach JL, Guillory JK. Some dissolution aspects of ferrous sulfate tablets. Am J Hosp Pharm 1970; 27:533–539.
63. Crounse RG. Human Pharmacology of griseofulvin. The effect of fat intake on gastrointestinal absorption. J Invest Dermatol 1961; 37:529–533.
64. Kraml M, Dubuc J, Beall D. Gastrointestinal absorption of griseofulvin. I. Effect of particle size, addition of surfactants and corn oil on the level of griseofulvin in the serum of rats. Can J Biochem Physiol 1962; 40:1449–1451.
65. Moes AJ. Gastroretentive dosage forms. Crit Rev Ther Drug Carrier Syst 1993; 10:143–195.
66. Minami H, McCallum RW. The physiology and pathophysiology of gastric emptying in humans. Gastroenterol 1984; 86:1592–1610.
67. Renwick AG, Ahsan CH, Challenor VF, et al. The influence of posture on the pharmacokinetics of orally administered nifedipine. Br J Clin Pharmacol 1992; 34:332–336.
68. Hopkins A. The pattern of gastric emptying: a new view of old results J Physiol 1966; 182: 144–149.
69. Elashoff JD, Reedy TJ, Meyer JH. Analysis of gastric emptying data. Gastroenterol 1982; 83: 1306–1312.
70. Blythe RH, Grass GM, MacDonnell DR. The formulation and evaluation of enteric coated aspirin tablets. Am J Pharm 1959; 131:206–216.
71. Alpsten M, Bogentoft C, Ekenved G, et al. Gastric emptying and absorption of acetylsalicylic acid administered as enteric-coated micro-granules. Eur J Clin Pharmacol 1982; 22:57–61.
72. Welling P. Effects of food on drug absorption. Annu Rev Nutr 1996; 16:383–415.
73. Fleisher D, Li C, Zhou Y, et al. Drug, meal and formulation interactions influencing drug absorption after oral administration. Clin Pharmacokinet 1999; 36:233–254.
74. Charman WN, Porter CJH, Mithani S, et al. Physicochemical and physiological mechanisms for the effects of food on drug absorption: the role of lipids and pH. J Pharm Sci 1997; 86:269–282.
75. Jones HM, Parrott N, Ohlenbusch G, et al. Predicting pharmacokinetic food effects using biorelevant solubility media and physiologically based modeling. Clin Pharmacokinet 2006; 45: 1213–1226.
76. Gu C-H, Li H, Levons J, et al. Predicting effect of food on extent of drug absorption based on physicochemical properties. Pharm Res 2007; 24:1118–1130.
77. Hendeles L, Weinberger M, Milavetz G, et al. Food-induced 'dose-dumping' from a once-a-day theophylline product as a cause of theophylline toxicity. Chest 1985; 87:758–765.
78. Gai MN, Isla A, Andonaegui MT, et al. Evaluation of the effect of 3 different diets on the bioavailability of 2 sustained release theophylline matrix tablets. Int J Clin Pharmacol Ther 1997; 35:565–571.
79. Wu C-Y, Benet LZ. Predicting drug disposition *via* application of BCS: transport/absorption/ elimination interplay and development of a biopharmaceutical drug disposition classification system. Pharm Res 2005; 22:11–23.
80. Custodio JM, Wu C-Y, Benet LZ. Predicting drug disposition, absorption/elimination/ transporter interplay and the role of food on drug absorption. Adv Drug Deliv Rev 2008; 60: 717–733.
81. Singh BN. A quantitative approach to probe the dependence and correlation of food-effect with aqueous solubility, dose/solubility ratio, and partition coefficient (log D) for orally active drugs administered as immediate-release formulations. Drug Dev Res 2005; 65:55–75.
82. Bates TR, Sequeira JA, Tembo AV. Effect of food on nitrofurantoin absorption. Clin Pharmacol Ther 1974; 16:63–68.
83. Rosenberg HA, Bates TR. The influence of food on nitrofurantoin bioavailability. Clin Pharmacol Ther 1976; 20:227–232.
84. Yung S, Mayersohn M, Robinson JB. Ascorbic acid absorption in man: influence of divided dose and food. Life Sci 1981; 28:2505–2511.
85. Meuhlberger CW. The physiological action of alcohol. J Am Med Assoc 1958; 167: 1842–1845.

86. Horowitz M, Maddox A, Bochner M, et al. Relationships between gastric emptying of solid and caloric liquid meals and alcohol absorption. Am J Physiol 1989; 257:G291–G298.
87. Jones AW, Jonsson KA, Kechagias S. Effect of high-fat, high-protein, and high-carbohydrate meals on the pharmacokinetics of a small dose of ethanol. Br J Clin Pharmacol 1997; 44: 521–526.
88. Fermaglich J, O'Doherty S. Effect of gastric motility on levodopa. Dis Nerv Syst 1972; 33:624–625.
89. Heading RC, Nimmo J, Prescott LF, et al. The dependence of paracetamol absorption on the rate of gastric emptying. Br J Pharmacol 1973; 47:415–421.
90. Prescott LF, Nimmo WS, Heading RC. Drug absorption interactions. In: Grahame-Smith DG, ed. Drug Interactions. Baltimore: Macmillan, 1977:45.
91. Channer KS, Virjee J. Effect of posture and drink volume on the swallowing of capsules. Br Med J 1982; 285:1702.
92. Hey H, Jorgenson F, Sorensen K, et al. Oesophageal transit of six commonly used tablets and capsules. Br Med J 1982; 285:171–179.
93. Channer KS, Roberts CJC. Effect of delayed esophageal transit on acetaminophen absorption. Clin Pharmacol Ther 1985; 37:72–76.
94. Davis SS, Hardy JG, Fara JW. Transit of pharmaceutical dosage forms through the small intestine. Gut 1986; 27:886–892.
95. Madsen JL. Effects of gender, age, and body mass index on gastrointestinal transit times. Dig Dis Sci 1992; 37:1548–1553.
96. Price JMC, Davis SS, Wilding IR. The effect of fibre on gastrointestinal transit times in vegetarians and omnivores. Int J Pharm 1991; 76:123–141.
97. Pirk F. Changes in the motility of the small intestine in digestive disorders. Gut 1967; 8: 486–490.
98. Guyton AC. Basic Human Physiology: Normal Functions and Mechanisms of Disease. Philadelphia: W B Saunders, 1971:428.
99. Parry E, Shields R, Turnbull AC. Transit time in the small intestine in pregnancy. J Obstet Gynaecol 1970; 77:900–901.
100. Metcalf AM, Phillips SF, Zinsmeister AR, et al. Simplified assessment of segmental colonic transit. Gastroenterology 1987; 92:40–47.
101. Watts PJ, Barrow L, Steed KP, et al. The transit rate of different sized model dosage forms through the human colon and the effects of a lactulose-induced catharsis. Int J Pharm 1992; 87: 215–221.
102. Akin DA, Davis SS, Sparrow RA, et al. Colonic transit of different sized tablets in healthy subjects. J Control Release 1993; 23:147–156.
103. Price JMC, Davis SS, Sparrow RA, et al. The effect of meal composition on the gastrocolonic response: implications for drug delivery to the colon. Pharm Res 1993; 10:722–726.
104. McDougall CJ, Wong R, Scudera P, et al. Colonic mucosal pH in humans. Dig Dis Sci 1993; 38: 542–545.
105. Friend DR. Colon-specific drug delivery. Adv Drug Deliv Rev 1991; 7:149–199.
106. Wilding I. Site-specific drug delivery in the gastrointestinal tract. Crit Rev Ther Drug Carrier Syst 2000; 17:557–620.
107. Antonin KH, Saano V, Bleck P, et al. Colonic absorption of human calcitonin in man. Clin Sci 1992; 83:627–631.
108. Williams MF, Dukes GF, Heizer W, et al. Influence of gastrointestinal site of drug delivery on the absorption characteristics of ranitidine. Pharm Res 1992; 9:1190–1194.
109. Chan KKH, Buch A, Glazer RD, et al. Site-differential gastrointestinal absorption of benazepril hydrochloride in health volunteers. Pharm Res 1994; 11:432–437.
110. d'Agay-Abensour L, Fjellestad-Paulsen A, Hoglund P, et al. Absolute bioavailability of an aqueous solution of 1-deamino-8-D-arginine vasopressin from different regions of the gastrointestinal tract in man. Eur J Clin Pharmacol 1993; 44:473–476.
111. Warner PE, Brouwer KLR, Hussey EK, et al. Sumatriptan absorption from different regions of the human gastrointestinal tract. Pharm Res 1995; 12:138–143.

112. De Boer AG, Moolenaar F, de Leede LGJ, et al. Rectal drug administration: clinical pharmacokinetic considerations. Clin Pharmacokinet 1982; 7:285–311.
113. Winne D. Formal kinetics of water and solute absorption with regard to intestinal blood flow. J Theor Biol 1970; 2:1–18.
114. Winne D, Remischovsky J. Intestinal blood flow and absorption of nondissociable substances. J Pharm Pharmacol 1970; 22:640–641.
115. Crouthamel WG, Diamond L, Dittert LW, et al. Drug absorption. VII. Influence of mesenteric blood flow on intestinal drug absorption in dogs. J Pharm Sci 1975; 64:664–671.
116. Rowland M, Riegelman S, Harris PA, et al. Absorption kinetics of aspirin in man following oral administration of an aqueous solution. J Pharm Sci 1972; 61:379–385.
117. Kruger-Thiemer E. Pharmacokinetics and dose-concentration relationships. In: Ariens EJ, ed. Physico-Chemical Aspects of Drug Action. Elmsford, NY: Pergamon Press, 1968:63–113.
118. Oliver GC, Tazman R, Frederickson R. Influence of congestive heart failure on digoxin level. In: Storstein O, ed. Symposium on Digitalis. Oslo: Gyldendal Norsk Forlag, 1973:336–347.
119. Benowitz NL. Effects of cardiac disease on pharmacokinetics: pathophysiologic considerations. In: Benet LZ, Massoud N, Gainbertoglio JG, eds. Pharmacokinetics Basis for Drug Treatment. New York: Raven Press, 1984:89–103.
120. Price KE, Zolli Z Jr., Atkinson JC, et al. Antibiotic inhibitors. I. The effect of certain milk constituents. Antibiot Chemother 1957; 7:672–688.
121. Price KE, Zolli Z Jr., Atkinson JC, et al. Antibiotic inhibitors. II. Studies on the inhibitory action of selected divalent cations for oxytetracyctine. Antibiot Chemother 1957; 7:689–701.
122. Scheiner J, Altemeier WA. Experimental study of factors inhibiting absorption and effective therapeutic levels of declomycin. Surg Gynecol Obstet 1962; 114:9–14.
123. Neuvonen PJ, Turakka H. Inhibitory effect of various iron salts on the absorption of tetracycline in man. Eur J Clin Pharmacol 1974; 7:357–360.
124. Riegelman S, Crowell WJ. The kinetics of rectal absorption. II. The absorption of anions. J Am Pharm Assoc (Scientific Edition) 1958; 47:123–127.
125. Riegelman S, Crowell WJ. The kinetics of rectal absorption. III. The absorption of undissociated molecules. J Am Pharm Assoc (Scientific Edition) 1958; 47:127–133.
126. Kakemi K, Arita T, Muranishi S. Absorption and excretion of drugs. XXVII. Effect of nonionic surface-active agents on rectal absorption of sulfonamides. Chem Pharm Bull (Tokyo) 1965; 13:976–985.
127. Sorby DL. Effect of adsorbents on drug absorption. I. Modification of promazine absorption by activated attapulgite and activated charcoal. J Pharm Sci 1965; 54:677–683.
128. Wagner JG. Design and data analysis of biopharmaceutical studies in man. Can J Pharm Sci 1966; 1:55–68.
129. Abruzzo CW, Macasieb T, Weinfeld R, et al. Changes in the oral absorption characteristics in man of dipotassium clorasepate at normal and elevated gastric pH. J Pharmacokinet Biopharm 1977; 5:377–390.
130. Galetin A, Hinton LK, Burt H, et al. Maximal inhibition of intestinal first-pass metabolism as a pragmatic indicator of intestinal contribution to the drug-drug interactions for CYP3A4 cleared drugs. Curr Drug Metab 2007; 8:685–693.
131. Rivera-Calimlim L, Dujovne CA, Morgan JP, et al. Absorption and metabolism of L-dopa by the human stomach. Eur J Clin Invest 1971; 1:313–320.
132. Fleckenstein L, Mundy GR, Horovitz RA, et al. Sodium salicylamide: relative bioavailability and sujective effects. Clin Pharmacol Ther 1976; 19:451–458.
133. Levy G, Matsuzawa T. Pharmacokinetics of salicylamide in man. J Pharmacol Ther 1967; 156: 285–293.
134. Frezza M, Di Padova C, Pozzato G, et al. High blood alcohol levels in women: the rold of decreased gastric alcohol dehydrogenase and first-pass metabolism. N Engl J Med 1990; 322: 95–99.
135. Seitz HK, Egerer G, Simanowski UA, et al. Human gastric alcohol dehydrogenase activity: effect of age, sex and alcoholism. Gut 1993; 34:1433–1437.

136. Bailey DG, Spence JD, Munoz C, et al. Interaction of citrus juices with felodipine and nifedipine. Lancet 1991; 337:268–269.
137. Hall SD, Thummel KE, Watkins PB, et al. Molecular and physical mechanisms of first-pass extraction. Drug Metab Dispos 1999; 27:161–166.
138. Bailey DG, Arnold JMO, Spence JD. Inhibitors in the diet: grapefruit juice-drug interactions. In: Levy RH, Thummel KE, Trager WE, et al., eds Metabolic Drug Interactions: New York: Lippincott Williams & Wilkins, 2000:661–667.
139. Schmeidlin-Ren P, Edwards DJ, Fitzsimmons ME, et al. Mechanisms of enhanced oral availability of CYP3A4 substrates by grapefruit constituents: decreased enterocyte CYP3A4 concentration and mechanism-based inactivation by furanocoumarins. Drug Metab Dispos 1997; 25:1228–1233.
140. Dresser GK, Bailey DG, Carruthers SG. Grapefruit juice-felodipine interaction in the elderly. Clin Pharmacol Ther 2000; 68:28–34.
141. Durr D, Stieger B, Kullak-Ublick GA, et al. St. John's wort induces intestinal p-glycoprotein/ MDR1 and intestinal and hepatic CYP3A45. Clin Pharmacol Ther 2000; 68:598–604.
142. Smith RL. The role of the gut flora in the conversion of inactive compounds to active metabolites. In: Aldridge WN, ed. A Symposium on Mechanisms of Toxicity. New York: Macmillan, 1971:228–244.
143. Kramer PA, Chapron DJ, Benson J, et al. Tetracycline absorption in elderly patients with achlorhydria. Clin Pharmacol Ther 1978; 23:467–472.
144. Ochs HR, Greenblatt DJ, Dengler HJ. Absorption of oral tetracycline in patients with Billroth-II gastrectomy. J Pharmacokinet Biopharm 1978; 6:295–303.
145. Levy G, MacGillivray MH, Procknal JA. Riboflavin absorption in children with thyroid disorders. Pediatrics 1972; 50:896–900.
146. Prescott LF. Gastrointestinal absorption of drugs. Med Clin N Am 1974; 58:907–916.
147. Jusko WJ, Conti DR, Molson A, et al. Digoxin absorption from tablets and elixir: the effect of radiation-induced malabsorption. JAMA 1974; 230:1554–1555.
148. Sokol GH, Greenblatt DJ, Lloyd BL, et al. Effect of abdominal radiation therapy on drug absorption in humans. J Clin Pharmacol 1978; 18: 388–396.
149. Heizer WD, Smith TW, Goldfinger SE. Absorption of digoxin in patients with malabsorption syndromes. N Engl J Med 1971; 285:257–259.
150. Davis AE, Pirola RC. Absorption of phenoxymethyl penicillin in patients with steatorrhea. Austrelas Ann Med 1968; 17:63–65.
151. Nelson JD, Shelton S, Kusmiesz HT, et al. Absorption of ampicillin and nalidixic acid in infants and children with acute shigellosis. Clin Pharmacol Ther 1972; 13:879–886.
152. Severijnen R, Bayat N, Bakker H, et al. Enteral drug absorption in patients with short small bowel. Clin Pharmcokinet 2004; 43:951–962.
153. Kampmann JP, Klein H, Lumholtz B, et al. Ampicillin and propylthiouracil pharmacokinetics in intestinal bypass patients followed up to a year after operation. Clin Pharmacokinet 1984; 9: 168–176.
154. Jusko WJ, Khanna N, Levy G, et al. Riboflavin absorption and excretion in the neonate. Pediatrics 1970; 45:945–949.
155. Mayersohn M. Special pharmacokinetic considerations in the elderly. In: Evans WE, Schentag JJ, Jusko WJ, eds. Applied Pharmacokinetics: Principles of Therapeutic Drug Monitoring. 3rd ed. Vancouver, WA: Applied Therapeutics, 1992:9.1–9.43.
156. Mayersohn M. Pharmacokinetics in the elderly. Environ Health Perspect 1994; 102(suppl 11): 119–124.
157. Mayersohn M. The "xylose test" to assess gastrointestinal absorption in the elderly: a pharmacokinetic evaluation of the literature. J Gerontol 1982; 37:300–305.
158. Johnson SL, Mayersohn M, Conrad KA. Gastrointestinal absorption as a function of age: xylose absorption in healthy adult subjects. Clin Pharmacol Ther 1985; 38:331–335.
159. Russell TL, Berardi RR, Barnett JL, et al. pH-related changes in the absorption of dipyridamole in the elderly. Pharm Res 1994; 11:136–143.

3
Pharmacokinetics

David W. A. Bourne
College of Pharmacy, University of Oklahoma, Oklahoma City, Oklahoma, U.S.A.

INTRODUCTION

Drug therapy is a dynamic process. When a drug product is administered, absorption usually proceeds over a finite time interval; and distribution, metabolism, and excretion (ADME) of the drug and its metabolites proceed continuously at various rates. The relative rates of these "ADME processes" determine the time course of the drug in the body, most importantly at the receptor sites that are responsible for the pharmacologic action of the drug.

The usual aim of drug therapy is to achieve and maintain effective concentrations of drug at the receptor site. However, the body is constantly trying to eliminate the drug and, therefore, it is necessary to balance absorption against elimination so as to maintain the desired concentration. Often the receptor sites are tucked away in a specific organ or tissue of the body, such as the central nervous system, and it is necessary to depend on the blood supply to distribute the drug from the site of administration, such as the gastrointestinal tract, to the site of action.

Since the body may be viewed as a very complex system of compartments, at first, it might appear to be hopeless to try to describe the time course of the drug at the receptor sites in any mathematically rigorous way. The picture is further complicated by the fact that, for many drugs, the locations of the receptor sites are unknown. Fortunately, body compartments are connected by the blood system, and distribution of drugs among the compartments usually occurs much more rapidly than absorption or elimination of the drug. The net result is that the body behaves as a single homogeneous compartment with respect to many drugs, and the concentration of the drug in the blood directly reflects or is proportional to the concentration of the drug in all organs and tissues. Thus, it may never be possible to isolate a receptor site and determine the concentration of drug around it, but the concentration at the receptor site usually can be controlled if the blood concentration can be controlled.

The objective of pharmacokinetics is to describe the time course of drug concentrations in blood in mathematical terms so that (*i*) the performance of pharmaceutical dosage forms can be evaluated in terms of the rate and amount of drug they deliver to the blood, and (*ii*) the dosage regimen of a drug can be adjusted to produce and maintain therapeutically effective blood concentrations with little or no toxicity. The primary objective of this chapter will be to describe the graph paper and calculator level, mathematical tools needed to accomplish these aims when the body behaves as a single homogeneous compartment and when all pharmacokinetic processes obey first-order kinetics.

On some occasions, the body does not behave as a single homogeneous compartment, and multicompartment pharmacokinetics is required to describe the time course of drug concentrations. In other instances certain pharmacokinetic processes may not obey first-order kinetics, and saturable or nonlinear models may be required. More information about these complexities may be found on the Web site http://www.boomer.org/c/p4/. Additionally advanced pharmacokinetic analyses require the use of various computer programs, such as those listed on the Web site http://www.boomer.org/pkin/soft.html. Readers interested in such advanced topics are referred to a number of texts that describe these more complex pharmacokinetic models in detail (1–5) and to the Web site http://www.boomer.org/pkin/.

PRINCIPLES OF FIRST-ORDER KINETICS

Definition and Characteristics of First-Order Processes

The science of kinetics deals with the mathematical description of the rate of the appearance or disappearance of a substance. One of the most common types of rate processes observed in nature is the first-order process in which the rate is dependent on the concentration or amount of only one component. An example of such a process is radioactive decay in which the rate of decay (i.e., the number of radioactive decompositions per minute) is directly proportional to the amount of undecayed substance remaining. This may be written mathematically as follows:

$$\text{Rate of radioactivity decay} \propto [\text{undecayed substance}] \qquad (1)$$

or

$$\text{Rate of radioactive decay} = k(\text{undecayed substance}) \qquad (2)$$

where k is a proportionality constant called the first-order rate constant.

Chemical reactions usually occur through collision of at least two molecules, very often in a solution, and the rate of the chemical reaction is proportional to the concentrations of all reacting molecules. For example, the rate of hydrolysis of an ester in an alkaline-buffered solution depends on the concentration of both the ester and hydroxide ion:

$$\text{Ester} + \text{OH}^- \rightarrow \text{Acid}^- + \text{Alcohol} \qquad (3)$$

The rate of hydrolysis may be expressed as follows:

$$\text{Rate of hydrolysis} \propto [\text{Ester}] \cdot [\text{OH}^-] \qquad (4)$$

or

$$\text{Rate of hydrolysis} = k[\text{Ester}] \cdot [\text{OH}^-] \qquad (5)$$

where k is the proportionality constant called the second-order rate constant.

But, in a buffered system, $[\text{OH}^-]$ is constant. Therefore, at a given pH, the rate of hydrolysis is dependent only on the concentration of the ester and may be written:

$$\text{Rate of hydrolysis}_{(\text{pH})} = k^* \cdot [\text{Ester}] \qquad (6)$$

where k^* is the pseudo-first-order rate constant at the pH in question. (The pseudo-first-order rate constant, k^*, is the product of the second-order rate constant and the hydroxide ion concentration:

$$k^* = k \cdot [\text{OH}^-].)$$

Fortunately, most ADME processes behave as pseudo-first-order processes—not because they are so simple, but because everything except the drug concentration is constant. For example, the elimination of a drug from the body may be written as follows:

$$\begin{bmatrix} \text{Drug} \\ \text{in} \\ \text{body} \end{bmatrix} + \begin{bmatrix} \text{Enzymes;} \\ \text{membranes;} \\ \text{pH; protein} \\ \text{binding; etc.} \end{bmatrix} \rightarrow \begin{array}{c} \text{Metabolized or} \\ \text{excreted drug} \end{array} \qquad (7)$$

If everything except the concentration of drug in the body is constant, the elimination of the drug will be a pseudo-first-order process. This may seem to be a drastic oversimplification, but most in vivo drug processes, in fact, behave as pseudo-first-order processes.

Differential Rate Expressions

In the previous discussion of radioactive decay it was noted that the rate of decay is directly proportional to the amount of undecayed substance remaining. In a solution of a radioactive substance, a similar relationship would hold for the concentration of undecayed substance remaining. If a solution of a radioactive substance were allowed to decay and a plot were constructed of the concentration remaining versus time, the plot would be a curve such as that shown in Figure 1.

In this system, the rate of decay might be expressed as a change in concentration per unit time, $\Delta C/\Delta t$, which corresponds to the slope of the line. But the line in Figure 1 is

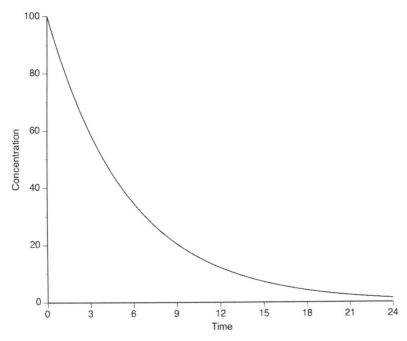

Figure 1 Plot of concentration remaining versus time for a first-order process (e.g., radioactive decay).

curved, which means that the rate is constantly changing and therefore cannot be expressed in terms of a finite time interval. By resorting to differential calculus, it is possible to express the rate of decay in terms of an infinitesimally small change in concentration (dC) over an infinitesimally small time interval (dt). The resulting function, dC/dt, is the slope of the line, and it is this function that is proportional to concentration in a first-order process.

Thus,

$$\text{Rate} = \frac{dC}{dt} = -kC \tag{8}$$

The negative sign is introduced because the concentration is falling as time progresses.

Equation (8) is the differential rate expression for a first-order reaction. The value of the rate constant, k, could be calculated by determining the slope of the concentration versus time curve at any point and dividing by the concentration at that point. However, the slope of a curved line is difficult to measure accurately, and k can be determined much more easily using an integrated rate expression.

Integrated Rate Expressions and Working Equations

Equation (8) can be rearranged and integrated as follows:

$$\frac{dC}{C} = -k \, dt \tag{9}$$

$$\int \frac{dC}{C} = -k \int dt \tag{10}$$

$$\ln C = -kt + \text{constant}$$

where $\ln C$ is the natural logarithm (base e) of the concentration.

The constant in equation (10) can be evaluated at zero time when $kt = 0$ and $C = C_0$, the initial concentration. Thus,

$$\ln C_0 = \text{constant}$$

and

$$\log C = -kt + \ln C_0 \tag{11}$$

Equation (11) is the integrated rate expression for a first-order process and can serve as a working equation for solving problems. It is also in the form of the equation of a straight line:

$$y = mx + b$$

Therefore, if $\ln C$ is plotted against t, as shown in Figure 2, the plot will be a straight line with an intercept (at $t = 0$) of $\ln C_0$, and the slope of the line (m) will be $-k$. Such plots are commonly used to determine the order of a reaction; that is, if a plot of $\ln C$ versus time is a straight line, the reaction is assumed to be a first-order or pseudo-first-order process.

The slope of the line and the corresponding value of k for a plot such as that shown in Figure 2 may be calculated using the following equation:

$$\text{slope } (m) = \frac{\ln C_1 - \ln C_2}{t_1 - t_2} = -k \tag{12}$$

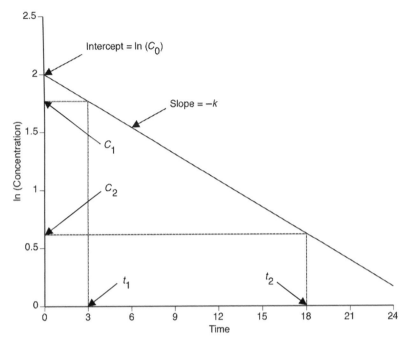

Figure 2 Plot of ln (concentration remaining) versus time for a first-order process.

Example. A solution of an ester in pH 10.0 buffer (25°C) one hour after preparation was found to contain 3 mg/mL. Two hours after preparation, the solution contained 2 mg/mL. Calculate the psuedo-first-order rate constant for hydrolysis of the ester at pH 10.0 (25°C).

$$\text{slope}(m) = \frac{\ln 3 - \ln 2}{(1-2)\,\text{hr}} = -k$$

$$= \frac{1.099 - 0.693}{-1}$$

$$= -0.406/\text{hr} = -k$$

$$k = 0.406/\text{hr}$$

Note that since $\ln C$ is dimensionless, the rate constant, k, has the dimensions of reciprocal time (i.e., day^{-1}, hr^{-1}, min^{-1}, sec^{-1}).

Another useful working equation can be obtained by rearranging equation (11) as follows:

$$\ln C - \ln C_0 = -kt$$

$$\ln C_0 - \ln C = kt \tag{13}$$

$$\ln \frac{C_0}{C} = kt$$

Equation (13) shows that since k is a constant for a given process, the value of t is determined solely by the ratio C_0/C. For example, when C_0/C is equal to 2 the value t will be the same, no matter what the value of the initial concentration (C_0) was.

Example. For the ester hydrolysis above ($k = 0.406$/hr), if $C_0 = 3$ mg/mL, when would $C = 1.5$ mg/mL?

$$\ln \frac{C_0}{C} = kt$$

$$\ln \frac{3}{1.5} = 0.406 \times t$$

$$\ln 2 = 0.406 \times t$$

$$0.693 = 0.406 \times t$$

$$t = 1.71 \text{ hr}$$

If $C_0 = 1.5$ mg/mL, when would $C = 0.75$ mg/mL?

$$\ln \frac{C_0}{C} = kt$$

$$\ln \frac{1.5}{0.75} = 0.406 \times t$$

$$\log 2 = 0.406 \times t$$

$$t = 1.71 \text{ hr}$$

The time required for the concentration to fall to $C_0/2$ is called the half-life, and the foregoing example shows that the half-life for a first-order or pseudo-first-order process is a constant throughout the process; it also demonstrates that a first-order process theoretically never reaches completion, since even the lowest concentration would only fall to half its value in one half-life.

For most practical purposes, a first-order process may be deemed "complete" if it is 95% or more complete. Table 1 shows that five half-lives must elapse to reach this point. Thus the elimination of a drug from the body may be considered to be complete after five half-lives have elapsed (i.e., 97% completion). This principle becomes important, for example, in crossover bioavailability studies in which the subjects must be rested for sufficient time between each drug administration to ensure that "washout" is complete.

The half-life of a first-order process is very important. Since it is often desirable to convert a half-life to a rate constant, and vice versa, a simple relationship between the two is very useful. The relationship may be derived as follows:

$$\ln \frac{C_0}{C} = kt$$

Table 1 Approach to Completeness with Increasing Half-Lives

Number of half-lives elapsed	Initial concentration remaining (%)	"Completeness" of process (%)
0	100.0	0.0
1	50.0	50.0
2	25.0	75.0
3	12.5	87.5
4	6.25	93.75
5	3.13	96.87
6	1.56	98.44
7	0.78	99.22

when $C_0/C = 2$ and $t = t_{1/2}$. Thus,

$$\ln 2 = kt_{1/2}$$
$$0.693 = kt_{1/2}$$

$$k = \frac{0.693}{t_{1/2}} \tag{14}$$

$$t_{1/2} = \frac{0.693}{k} \tag{15}$$

Examples of Calculations

Equations (13) to (15) can be used to solve three types of problems involving first-order processes. These types of problems are illustrated in the following examples:

TYPE 1: Given the rate constant or half-life and the initial concentration, calculate the concentration at some time in the future.

Example. A drug solution containing 500 units/mL has a half-life of 10 days. What will the concentration be in seven days?

$$k = \frac{0.693}{t_{1/2}} = \frac{0.693}{10 \text{ day}} = 0.069/\text{day}$$

$$\ln \frac{C_0}{C} = kt$$

$$\ln \frac{500 \text{ units/mL}}{C} = 0.069/\text{day} \times 7 \text{ day} = 0.483$$

$$\frac{500}{C} = \text{anti ln}(0.483) = e^{0.483} = 1.62$$

$$C = 308 \text{ units/mL}$$

TYPE 2: Given the half-life or rate constant and the initial concentration, calculate the time required to reach a specified lower concentration.

Example. A drug solution has a half-life of 21 days. How long will it take for the potency to drop to 90% of the initial potency?

$$k = \frac{0.693}{21 \text{ day}} = 0.033/\text{day}$$

$$\ln \frac{C_0}{C} = kt$$

$$\ln \frac{100\%}{90\%} = 0.033 \times t$$

$$t = 3.2 \text{ day}$$

TYPE 3: Given an initial concentration and the concentration after a specified elapsed time, calculate the rate constant or half-life.

Example. A drug solution has an initial potency of 125 mg/5 mL. After one month in a refrigerator, the potency is found to be 100 mg/5 mL. What is the half-life of the drug solution under these storage conditions?

$$\ln \frac{C_0}{C} = kt$$

$$\ln \frac{125 \text{ mg}/5 \text{ mL}}{100 \text{ mg}/5 \text{ mL}} = k \times 30 \text{ day}$$

$$k = 0.0074/\text{day}$$

$$t_{1/2} = \frac{0.693}{0.0074/\text{day}} = 94 \text{ day}$$

For each type of problem the following assumptions are made: (*i*) The process follows first-order kinetics, at least over the time interval and concentration range involved in the calculations and (*ii*) all time and concentration values are accurate.

The latter assumption is particularly critical in solving problems such as type 3, where a rate constant is being calculated. It would be unwise to rely on only two time points to calculate such an important value. Normally, duplicate or triplicate assays would be performed at six or more time points throughout as much of the reaction as possible. The resulting mean assay values and standard deviation values would be plotted on semilogarithmic graph paper and a straight line carefully fitted to the data points. The half-life could then be determined using equation (14).

Example. A solution of an ester in pH 9.5 buffer (25°C) was assayed in triplicate several times over a 20-hour period. The data obtained are presented in Table 2. The results were plotted on semilogarithmic graph paper as shown in Figure 3. Calculate the pseudo-first-order rate constant for the hydrolysis of the ester at pH 9.5 (25°C).

By fitting a straight line ("best-fit" line) through the data points in Figure 3 (this can be done by eye using a transparent straight edge) and extrapolating to $t = 0$, the intercept C_0 is found to be 3.13 mg/mL. The half-life is the time at which the concentration equals 1.57 mg/mL ($C_0/2$), and this is found by interpolation to be 2.4 hours. The value of k can be given by

$$k = \frac{0.693}{t_{1/2}} = \frac{0.693}{2.4 \text{ hr}} = 0.289/\text{hr}$$

Table 2   Concentration of an Ester Vs. Time

Time (hr)	Concentration (mg/mL) $\pm$ SD
2	1.83 $\pm$ 0.15
4	1.01 $\pm$ 0.09
6	0.58 $\pm$ 0.07
8	0.33 $\pm$ 0.06
10	0.18 $\pm$ 0.04
12	0.10 $\pm$ 0.02
16	0.031 $\pm$ 0.006
20	0.012 $\pm$ 0.002

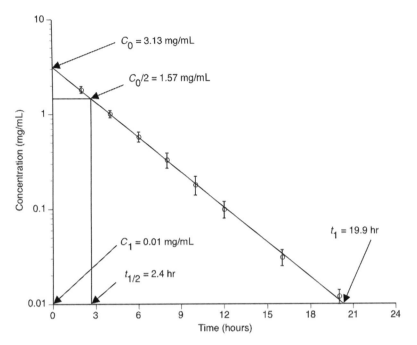

Figure 3 Semilogarithmic plot of concentration versus time for the hydrolysis of an ester. (Data shown in Table 2. One standard deviation is indicated by error bars.)

A value for k can also be determined directly from points on the line using equation (12). In Figure 3 values for C_0, C_1, t_0, and t_1 can be read from the "best-fit" line as 3.13 mg/mL, 0.01 mg/mL, 0 hour, and 19.9 hours, respectively. Thus:

$$k = -\text{slope} = \frac{\ln C_0 - \ln C_1}{t_1 - t_0}$$

$$k = \frac{\ln 3.13 - \ln 0.01}{19.9 - 0.0} = 0.289/\text{hr}$$

Semilogarithmic graph paper is readily available from many graph paper manufacturers. It consists of a logarithmic scale on the y-axis and a Cartesian scale on the x-axis (Fig. 3). On the logarithmic scale, the spatial distribution of lines is such that the position of each line is proportional to the logarithm of the value represented by the line. For example, plotting a concentration of 1.83 mg/mL on semilogarithmic paper is equivalent to looking up the logarithm of 1.83 and plotting it on a Cartesian scale. This type of graph paper is extremely useful for kinetic calculations because raw concentration data can be plotted directly without converting to logarithms, and concentration values can be extrapolated and interpolated from the plot without converting logs to numbers.

For example, to determine the half-life in the preceding example, the C_0 value and the time at which $C = C_0/2$ were both read directly from the graph. If Figure 3 had been a plot of ln C (on a Cartesian scale) versus time, it would have been necessary to read ln C_0 from the graph, convert it to C_0, divide by 2, convert back to ln $(C_0/2)$, then read the half-life of the graph. If the rate constant is determined for this example using equation (12), the slope must be calculated. To calculate the slope of the line it is necessary to first read two concentrations from the graph and then take the logarithm of each concentration as described in equation (12).

FIRST-ORDER PHARMACOKINETICS: DRUG ELIMINATION FOLLOWING RAPID INTRAVENOUS INJECTION

It was mentioned previously that drug elimination from the body most often displays the characteristics of a first-order process. Thus, if a drug is administered by rapid intravenous (IV) injection, after mixing with the body fluids its rate of elimination from the body is proportional to the amount remaining in the body.

Normally, the plasma concentration is used as a measure of the amount of drug in the body, and a plot of plasma concentration versus time has the same characteristics as the plot in Figure 1. A semilogarithmic plot of plasma concentration versus time is a straight line and allows the calculation of k_{el} from the slope, where k_{el} is the overall elimination rate constant. The intercept at $t = 0$ is C_p^0, the hypothetical plasma concentration after the drug is completely mixed with body fluids but before any elimination has occurred.

A typical semilogarithmic plasma concentration versus time plot is shown in Figure 4. This figure shows that pharmacokinetic data can also be expressed in terms of a half-life, called the biologic half-life, which bears the same relationship to k_{el} as that shown in equations (14) and (15).

Since all the kinetic characteristics of the disappearance of a drug from plasma are the same as those for the pseudo-first-order disappearance of a substance from a solution by hydrolysis, the same working equations (equations 11 and 13) and the same approach to solving problems can be used.

Example. A 250 mg dose of a drug was administered to a patient by rapid IV injection. The initial plasma concentration (C_p^0) was 2.50 µg/mL. After four hours the

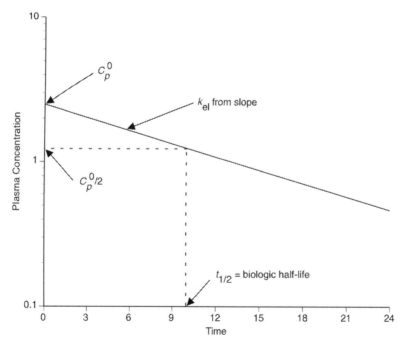

Figure 4 Semilogarithmic plot of plasma concentration versus time for a drug administered by rapid IV injection. *Abbreviation*: IV, intravenous.

plasma concentration was 1.89 μg/mL. What is the biologic half-life ($t_{1/2}$) of the drug in this patient?

$$\ln\frac{C_p^0}{C_p} = k_{el}t$$

$$\ln\frac{2.50}{1.89} = k_{el} \times 4$$

$$k_{el} = \frac{0.280}{4} = 0.0699/\text{hr}$$

$$t_{1/2} = \frac{0.693}{0.0699/\text{hr}} = 9.91 \text{ hr}$$

Note that this approach involves the following assumptions: (*i*) the drug was eliminated by a psuedo-first-order process, (*ii*) there was rapid mixing of the drug in blood, and (*iii*) the drug was rapidly distributed so that an "initial plasma concentration" could be measured before any drug began to leave the body. The latter assumption implies that the body behaves as a single homogeneous compartment throughout which the drug distributes instantaneously following IV injection. In pharmacokinetic terms, this is referred to as the one-compartment model. Although most drugs do not, in fact, distribute instantaneously, they do distribute very rapidly, and the one-compartment model can be used for many clinically important pharmacokinetic calculations.

An important parameter of the one-compartment model is the apparent volume of this one compartment, because it directly determines the relationship between the plasma concentration and the amount of drug in the body. This volume is called the apparent volume of distribution, V_d, and it may be calculated using the relationship:

$$\text{Volume} = \frac{\text{Amount}}{\text{Concentration}}$$

The easiest way to calculate V_d is to use C_p^0, the plasma concentration when distribution is complete (assumed to be instantaneous for a one-compartment model) and the entire dose is still in the body. Thus,

$$V_d = \frac{\text{Dose}}{C_p^0} \tag{16}$$

Example. Calculate V_d for the patient in the previous example.

$$V_d = \frac{250 \text{ mg}}{2.50 \text{ μg/mL}}$$

$$V_d = 100 \text{ L}$$

Note: Since 1 μg/mL = 1 mg/L, dividing the dose in milligrams by the plasma concentration in micrograms per milliliter will give V_d in liters.

The apparent volume of distribution of a drug very rarely corresponds to any physiologic volume and, even in cases where it does, it must never be construed as showing that the drug enters or does not enter various body spaces.

Example. For example, the 100 L volume calculated in the foregoing example is much greater than either plasma volume (about 3 L) or whole blood volume (about 6 L) in a standard (70 kg) man; it is even greater than the extracellular fluid volume (19 L) and total body water (42 L) in the same average man (4). On the basis of calculated value of V_d it cannot be said that the drug is restricted to the plasma, or that it enters or does not enter red blood cells, or that it enters or does not enter any or all extracellular fluids.

A discussion of all the reasons for this phenomenon is beyond the scope of this chapter, but a simple example will illustrate the concept. Highly lipid soluble drugs are preferentially distributed into adipose tissue. The result is that plasma concentrations are extremely low after distribution is complete. When the apparent volumes of distribution are calculated, they are frequently found to exceed total body volume, occasionally by a factor of two or more. This would be impossible if the concentration in the entire body compartment were equal to the plasma concentration. Thus, V_d is an empirically fabricated number relating the concentration of drug in plasma (or blood) with the amount of drug in the body. For drugs such as pentobarbital, the ratio of the concentration in adipose tissue to the concentration in plasma is much greater than unity, resulting in a large value for V_d.

PHARMACOKINETIC ANALYSIS OF URINE DATA

Occasionally, it is inconvenient or impossible to assay the drug in plasma, but it may be possible to follow the appearance of the drug in urine. If the drug is not metabolized to any appreciable degree, the pharmacokinetic model may be written as shown in Scheme 1.

$$D_B \xrightarrow{k_{el}} D_U$$

Scheme 1

A plot of cumulative amount of drug appearing in urine (D_U) versus time will be the mirror image of a plot of amount of drug remaining in the body (D_B) versus time. This is illustrated in Figure 5, which shows that the total amount of drug recovered in urine throughout the entire study (D_U^∞) is equal to the dose (D_B^0) and, at any time, the sum of drug in the body (D_B) plus drug in urine (D_U) equals the dose (D_B^0).

A kinetic equation describing urine data can be developed as follows. If

$$\frac{dD_B}{dt} = -k_{el}D_B$$

then,

$$\frac{dD_U}{dt} = +k_{el}D_B$$

But

$$D_B + D_U = D_U^\infty$$
$$= \text{Amount recovered in urine}$$

Then,

$$D_B = D_U^\infty - D_U$$

Therefore,

$$\frac{dD_U}{dt} = k_{el}(D_U^\infty - D_U)$$

or

$$\frac{dD_U}{D_U^\infty - D_U} = k_{el}\,dt$$

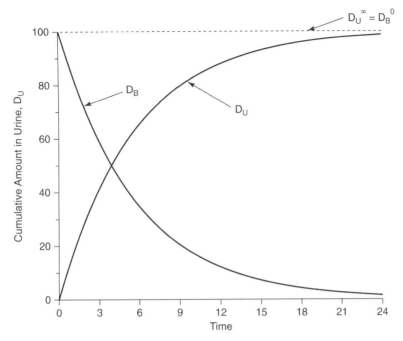

Figure 5 Plot of cumulative amount of drug in urine, D_U (*solid line*), and amount of drug in body, D_B (*dashed line*), versus time according to Scheme 1.

Integration gives

$$\int \frac{dD_U}{D_U^\infty - D_U} = k_{el} \int dt$$

$$-\ln(D_U^\infty - D_U) + \ln(D_U^\infty - D_U^0) = k_{el}t$$

Since $D_U^\infty = 0$ (there is no drug in urine when $t = 0$),

$$\ln(D_U^\infty - D_U) - \ln D_U^\infty = -k_{el}t$$

$$\ln(D_U^\infty - D_U) = -k_{el}t + \ln D_U^\infty \qquad (17)$$

Equation (17) is in the form of an equation for a straight line ($y = mx + b$), where t is one variable (x), $-k_{el}$ is determined from the slope (m), $\ln D_U^\infty$ is the constant (b), and $\ln (D_U^\infty - D_U)$ the other variable (y). Thus a plot of $\ln (D_U^\infty - D_U)$ versus time is a straight line with a slope providing a value of k_{el} and an intercept of $\ln D_U^\infty$. Since D_U^∞ is the total amount excreted and D_U is the amount excreted up to time t, $D_U^\infty - D_U$ is the amount remaining to be excreted (ARE). A typical ARE plot is shown in Figure 6.

Example. The plot in Figure 6 was constructed using the data shown in Table 3. Note that the concentration of the drug in each urine specimen is not the information analyzed. The total amount excreted over each time interval and throughout the entire study must be determined. As a result, the experimental details of a urinary excretion study must be very carefully chosen, and strict adherence to the protocol is required. Loss of a single urine specimen, or even an unknown part of a urine specimen, makes construction of an ARE plot impossible.

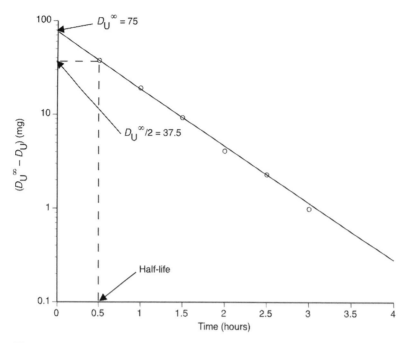

Figure 6 Semilogarithmic plot of drug ARE into urine, $D_U^\infty - D_U$, versus time. *Abbreviation*: ARE, amount remaining to be excreted.

Table 3 Drug Excreted into the Urine Vs. Time

Time interval (hr)	Amount excreted (mg)	Cumulative amount excreted, D_U[a] (mg)	$D_U^\infty - D_U$ (mg)
0.0–0.5	37.5	37.5	37.8
0.5–1.0	18.5	56.0	19.3
1.0–1.5	10.0	66.0	9.3
1.5–2.0	5.2	71.2	4.1
2.0–2.5	1.8	73.0	2.3
2.5–3.0	1.3	74.3	1.0
3.0–6.0	1.0	75.3	0.0
6.0–12.0	0.0	75.3	0.0

[a]$D_U^\infty = 75.3$ mg.

CLEARANCE RATE AS AN EXPRESSION OF DRUG ELIMINATION RATE

A clearance rate is defined as the volume of blood or plasma completely cleared of drug per unit time. It is a useful way to describe drug elimination because it is related to blood or plasma perfusion of various organs of elimination, and it can be directly related to the physiologic function of these organs. For example, the renal clearance rate (RCR) of a drug can be calculated using the following equation:

$$RCR = \frac{\text{Amount excreted in urine per unit time}}{\text{Plasma concentration}} \qquad (18)$$

Example. In the example plotted in Figure 6, the amount of drug excreted over the 0- to 0.5-hour interval was 37.5 mg. If the plasma concentration at 0.25 hour (the middle of the interval) was 10 µg/mL, what was the RCR? From equation (18),

$$RCR = \frac{37.5 \, mg/0.5 \, hr}{100 \, \mu g/mL}$$
$$= 7.5 \, L/hr$$
$$= 125 \, mL/min$$

The glomerular filtration rate (GFR) in normal males is estimated to be 125 mL/min, and the results of the example calculation suggest that the drug is cleared by GFR. If the RCR had been less than 125 mL/min, tubular reabsorption of the drug would have been suspected. Had it been greater than 125 mL/min, tubular secretion would have been involved in the drug elimination.

Drugs can be cleared from the body by metabolism as well as renal excretion, and when this occurs, it is not possible to measure directly the amount cleared by metabolism. However, the total clearance rate (TCR), or total body clearance, of the drug can be calculated from the total amount administered (dose) and "total" concentration, area under the plasma concentration versus time curve (AUC) (see sect. "Area under the Plasma Concentration versus Time Curve") using the following equation.

$$TCR = \frac{Dose}{AUC} \tag{19}$$

Example. One hundred milligram of drug was given IV to a patient, and plasma concentrations were measured. The AUC was determined to be 87 mg.min/L. Calculate the TCR of the drug.

$$TCR = \frac{100 \, mg}{87 \, mg \cdot min/L} = 1.15 \, L/min$$

When a drug is eliminated by both metabolism and urinary excretion, it is possible to calculate the metabolic clearance rate (MCR) by the difference between TCR and RCR:

$$MCR = TCR - RCR \tag{20}$$

The RCR can be determined from urine and plasma data using equation (18), and the TCR can be determined using equation (19). Alternately, the RCR can be calculated by multiplying the TCR by the fraction of the dose excreted unchanged into urine, f_e:

$$RCR = f_e \, TCR \tag{21}$$

If it is assumed that the fraction of the dose not appearing as unchanged drug in urine has been metabolized, the MCR can be calculated as follows:

$$MCR = (1 - f_e)TCR \tag{22}$$

Example. An IV dose of 250-mg was given to a normal volunteer. The measured AUC was 289 mg.hr/L, and 60% of the dose was recovered as unchanged drug in urine. Calculate TCR, RCR, and MCR for the drug in this person.

$$AUC = \frac{250 \, mg}{289 \, mg.hr/L} = 0.865 \, L/hr$$
$$= 14.4 \, mL/min$$

$$\text{RCR} = f_e \, \text{TCR}$$
$$= 0.6 \times 14.4 \; \text{mL/min}$$
$$= 8.64 \; \text{mL/min}$$

$$\text{MCR} = (1 - f_e) \, \text{TCR}$$
$$= (1 - 0.6) \times 14.4 \; \text{mL/min}$$
$$= 5.76 \; \text{mL/min}$$

It should be emphasized that the assumption that any drug not appearing as unchanged drug in urine has been metabolized may introduce a great amount of error into the values of the clearance rates estimated using equations (21) and (22). By this assumption, unchanged drug eliminated in the feces would be included with metabolized drug, as would any orally administered drug that was unabsorbed.

PHARMACOKINETICS OF DRUG ELIMINATED BY SIMULTANEOUS METABOLISM AND EXCRETION

Although some drugs are excreted unchanged in urine, most are partially eliminated by metabolism. Usually both the urinary excretion of unchanged drug and the metabolism are first-order processes, with the rate of excretion and metabolism dependent on the amount of unchanged drug in the body. This results in a "branch" in the kinetic chain, representing exit of drug in the body as depicted in the accompanying pharmacokinetic model (Scheme 2).

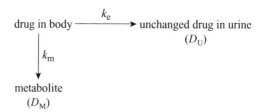

Scheme 2

In this scheme, the rate of loss of drug from the body is determined by both k_e and k_m, and this can be written in differential form as follows:

$$\frac{dD_B}{dt} = -k_e D_B - k_m D_B$$
$$= -(k_e + k_m) D_B \tag{23}$$

Thus, the overall elimination rate constant (k_{el}) here is the sum of the urinary excretion rate constant (k_e) and the metabolism rate constant (k_m):

$$k_{el} = k_e + k_m \tag{24}$$

For drugs that are both metabolized and excreted unchanged, semilogarithmic plots of plasma concentrations versus time will provide values of k_{el}.

Urine data are required to determine the individual values of k_e and k_m. The required equations are derived next.

Derivation. From Scheme 2, the differential equation describing overall rate of disappearance of drug from the body may be written:

$$\frac{dD_B}{dt} = -k_{el}D_B$$

and the following integrated equation can be written as (see also equation 10):

$$\ln D_B = \ln D_B^0 - k_{el}t$$

Taking antilogs yields

$$D_B = D_B^0 \exp(-k_{el}t) \tag{25}$$

It should be noted that equation (25) is another form of an integrated rate equation. This form makes use of an exp $(-x)$ term and may be referred to as an exponential rate expression. These expressions are useful for visualizing the characteristics of a first-order process. For example, when $t = 0$, exp $(-k_{el}t) = 1$, and $D_B = D_B^0$. When $t = t_{1/2}$, exp $(-k_{el}t_{1/2}) = 0.5$, and $D_B = 0.5 \times D_B^0$. When $t = \infty$, exp $(-k_{el}t) = 0$, and $D_B = 0$. Thus, the value of exp $(-k_{el}t)$ varies from 1 to 0 as time varies from 0 to ∞. At any time between 0 and ∞, the fraction of the dose remaining in the body is equal to exp $(-k_{el}t)$.

Exponential rate expressions are also useful in deriving kinetic equations because they can be substituted into differential equations that can then be integrated. For example, from Scheme 2 the differential equation describing the rate of appearance of unchanged drug in urine may be written as:

$$\frac{dD_U}{dt} = +k_e D_B \tag{25a}$$

Substituting equation (25) into equation (25a) gives:

$$\frac{dD_U}{dt} = +k_e[D_B^0 \exp(-k_{el}t)]$$

$$dD_U = +ke[D_B^0 \exp(-k_{el}t)]dt$$

Integration yields:

$$D_U = -\frac{k_e}{k_{el}} D_B^0 \exp(-k_{el}t) + \text{constant}$$

at $t = 0$, $D_U = 0$, and exp $(-k_{el}t) = 1$; therefore, the constant equals $(k_e/k_{el}) D_B^0$, and

$$D_U = \frac{k_e}{k_{el}} D_B^0 [1 - \exp(-k_{el}t)] \tag{26}$$

At $t = \infty$ after elimination is complete, the total amount of drug excreted unchanged in urine (D_U^∞) can be calculated using equation (26) as follows:

$$D_U^\infty = \frac{k_e}{k_{el}} D_B^0 (1 - 0)$$

$$\frac{D_U^\infty}{D_B^0} = \frac{k_e}{k_{el}} = f_e \tag{27}$$

Equation (27) shows that the fraction of the dose appearing as unchanged drug in urine (f_e) is equal to the fraction of k_{el} attributable to k_e. (An equation analogous to equation 27 for D_M^∞ and k_m could be derived in much the same way.)

Table 4 Drug Recovered in Urine Vs. Time

Time interval (hr)	Amount excreted unchanged (mg)	Cumulative amount excreted unchanged, D_U^a (mg)	$D_U^\infty - D_U$ (mg)
0.0–0.5	75	75	215
0.5–1.0	55	130	160
1.0–1.5	40	170	120
1.5–2.0	30	200	90
2.0–3.0	40	240	50
3.0–6.0	40	280	10
6.0–12.0	10	290	0
12.0–24.0	0	290	0

[a]$D_U^\infty = 290$ mg.

Substituting equation (27) into equation (26) and rearranging gives:

$$D_U^\infty - D_U = D_U^\infty \cdot \exp(-k_{el})$$

Taking logarithm's yields

$$\ln(D_U^\infty - D_U) = -k_{el}t + \ln D_U^\infty \qquad (28)$$

Equation (28) is identical to equation (17), for the case in which all eliminated drug was excreted unchanged in urine. $(D_U^\infty - D_U)$ is the ARE, and equation (28) shows that an ARE plot of unchanged drug in urine versus time will be a straight line with a slope providing a value of k_{el} even when the drug is partially eliminated by metabolism (Figs. 6 and 7). Using equation (27) and the total amount of unchanged drug excreted in urine (D_U^∞), it is possible to calculate k_e. Also, k_m can be calculated from equation (24). Thus, all the rate constants in Scheme 2 can be calculated solely on the basis of urinary excretion of unchanged drug.

Example. Five hundred milligrams of a drug was administered IV to a normal healthy volunteer, and various amounts of unchanged drug were recovered from the urine over the 24-hour postdrug period (Table 4). Calculate k_{el}, k_e, and k_m for this drug. A plot of $(D_U^\infty - D_U)$ on a log scale versus time is shown in Figure 7. A half-life of 1.2 hours can be estimated from the line in Figure 7.

$$k_{el} = \frac{0.693}{1.2\text{hr}} = 0.578/\text{hr}$$

From equation (27):

$$\frac{D_U^\infty}{D_B^0} = \frac{k_e}{k_{el}}$$

$$\frac{290 \text{ mg}}{500 \text{ mg}} = \frac{k_e}{0.578/\text{hr}}$$

$$k_e = 0.335/\text{hr}$$

From equation (24),

$$k_{el} = k_e + k_m$$

$$k_m = 0.578 - 0.335 = 0.243/\text{hr}$$

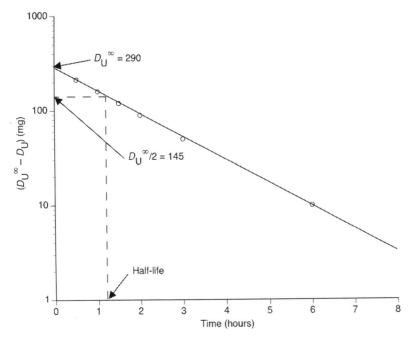

Figure 7 Semilogarithmic plot of amount of unchanged drug remaining to be excreted into urine, $D_U^\infty - D_U$, versus time according to Scheme 2.

It is important to reemphasize the following assumptions inherent in this type of calculation:

1. It must be assumed that urine collections were accurately timed and that complete urine specimens were obtained at each collection time. It is also assumed that the assay procedure is accurate and reproducible.
2. It is assumed that all processes of elimination obey first-order kinetics.
3. It is assumed that any drug not appearing unchanged in urine has been metabolized. Furthermore, if the drug is not administered by IV injection, it must also be assumed that the dose is completely absorbed. (The IV route was chosen for the preceding example specifically to avoid the need to introduce this assumption.)

Significance of k_e and k_m in Patients with Kidney or Liver Disease

In the foregoing example, the drug was administered to a healthy subject who had normal kidney and liver function. The estimated biologic half-life in this person was 1.2 hours. If the same drug were administered to a person with no kidney function but with a normal liver, it would be impossible for this individual to excrete unchanged drug. They would, however, be able to metabolize the drug at the same rate as a normal individual. The net result would be that the overall k_{el} would be reduced to the value of k_m, and the biologic half-life would increase to

$$\frac{0.693}{k_m} = \frac{0.693}{0.243/hr} = 2.85 \text{ hr}$$

Thus, the biologic half-life of a drug can increase dramatically when the organs of elimination are diseased or nonfunctional; it may increase to varying degrees if these organs are partially impaired.

At the present time, no simple relationship exists between clinical measurements of liver function and the value of k_m. Fortunately, kidney function can be measured quantitatively using standard clinical tests, and it is directly related to k_e for a number of drugs. Great success has been achieved in using kidney clearance measurements to predict the biologic half-lives of a number of drugs.

KINETICS OF DRUG ABSORPTION

For all commonly used routes of administration except IV, the drug must dissolve in body fluids and diffuse through one or more membranes to enter the blood or plasma. Thus, all routes except IV are classed as extravascular routes, and absorption is defined as appearance of the drug in blood or plasma.

The most common extravascular route is oral. When a solution or a rapidly dissolving solid dosage form is given orally, the absorption process often obeys first-order kinetics. In these cases, absorption can be characterized by evaluating the absorption rate constant, k_a, using plasma concentration versus time data.

The Method of "Residuals" ("Feathering" the Curve)

When absorption is first-order, the kinetic model may be written as shown in Scheme 3:

$$D_G \xrightarrow{\ k_a\ } D_B \xrightarrow{\ k_{el}\ } D_E$$

Scheme 3

where D_G = drug at the absorption site (gut); D_B = drug in the body; D_E = eliminated drug; k_a = first-order absorption rate constant, and k_{el} = overall elimination rate constant.

The differential equations describing the rates of change of the three components of Scheme 3 are

$$\frac{dD_G}{dt} = -k_a D_G \tag{29}$$

$$\frac{dD_B}{dt} = k_a D_G - k_{el} D_B \tag{30}$$

$$\frac{dD_E}{dt} = +k_{el} D_B \tag{31}$$

To determine k_a from plasma concentration versus time data, it is necessary to integrate equation (30). This is best achieved through exponential expressions. First, integration of equation (29) gives

$$D_G = D_G^0 \exp(-k_a t) \tag{32}$$

where D_G^0 is the initial amount of drug presented to the absorbing region of the gut. (D_G^0 = dose, if absorption is complete.)

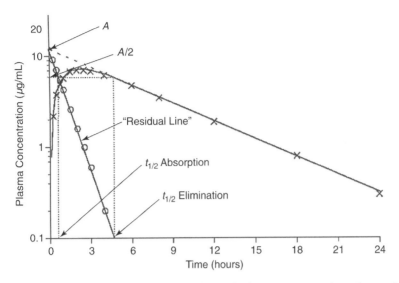

Figure 8 Semilogarithmic plot of observed plasma concentrations (*crosses*) and "residuals" (*circles*) versus time for an orally administered drug absorbed by a first-order process.

Substituting equation (32) into equation (30) gives

$$\frac{dD_B}{dt} = +k_a D_G^0 \exp(-k_a t) - k_{el} D_B \tag{33}$$

Integration of equation (33) may be accomplished with Laplace transforms (6,7). The result is

$$D_B = \frac{D_G^0 k_a}{k_a - k_{el}} [\exp(-k_{el}t) - \exp(-k_a t)] \tag{34}$$

Thus, the amount of drug in the body following administration of an extravascular dose is a constant $[(D_G^0 k_a)/(k_a - k_{el})]$ multiplied by the difference between two exponential terms—one representing elimination $[\exp(-k_{el}t)]$ and the other representing absorption $[\exp(-k_a t)]$.

Dividing both sides of equation (34) by V_d yields an equation for plasma concentration versus time:

$$C_p = \frac{D_G^0 k_a}{V_d(k_a - k_{el})} [\exp(-k_{el}t) - \exp(-k_a t)] \tag{35}$$

Equation (35) describes the line in Figure 8, which is a semilogarithmic plot of C_p versus time for an orally administered drug absorbed by a first-order process. The plot begins as a rising curve and becomes a straight line with a negative slope after six hours. This behavior is the result of the biexponential nature of equation (35). Up to six hours, both the absorption process $[\exp(-k_a t)]$ and the elimination process $[\exp(-k_{el}t)]$ influence the plasma concentration. After six hours, only the elimination process influences the plasma concentration.

This separation of the processes of absorption and elimination is the result of the difference in the values of k_a and k_{el}. If k_a is much larger than k_{el} (a good rule is that it must be at least five times larger), the second exponential term in equation (35) will approach zero much more rapidly than the first exponential term. And at large values of t, equation (35) will reduce to

$$C_p = \frac{D_G^0\, k_a}{V_d(k_a - k_{el})} [\exp(-k_{el}t)] \tag{36}$$

or

$$C_p = A \cdot \exp(-k_{el}t)$$

where A is a constant term.

Converting to logarithms we obtain

$$\ln C_p = -k_{el}t + \ln A \tag{37}$$

Thus after six hours the semilogarithmic plot of C_p versus time shown in Figure 8 becomes a straight line, and k_{el} can be determined from the slope. Therefore, the overall elimination rate constant for a drug may be accurately determined from the "tail" of a semilogarithmic plot of plasma concentration versus time following extravascular administration if k_a is at least five times larger than k_{el}.

The value of k_a can also be determined from plots like Figure 8 using the following logic: In Figure 8 the curved line up to six hours is given by

$$C_{p1} = A \cdot \exp(-k_{el}t) - A \cdot \exp(-k_a t)$$

The straight line after six hours and the extrapolated (dashed) line before six hours are given by

$$C_{p2} = A \cdot \exp(-k_{el}t)$$

The difference (residual) between the curved line and the extrapolated (dashed) line up to six hours is given by

$$\text{Residual} = C_{p2} - C_{p1}$$
$$= A \cdot \exp(-k_a t)$$

Converting to logs:

$$\ln(\text{residual}) = -k_a t + \ln A \tag{38}$$

As shown in Figure 8, a semilogarithmic plot of residuals versus time is a straight line with a slope of $-k_a$.

It should be noted that the intercepts (A) for both the extrapolated (dashed) line (equation 37) and the residuals line (equation 38) are the same and are equal to the constant in equation (35):

$$A = \frac{D_G^0\, k_a}{V_d(k_a - k_{el})} \tag{39}$$

A is a function of the two rate constants (k_a and k_{el}), the apparent volume of distribution (V_d), and the amount of drug absorbed (D_G^0). After k_a and k_{el} have been evaluated and A has been determined by extrapolation, a value for V_d can be calculated if it is assumed that D_G^0 is equal to the dose administered, i.e., absorption is 100% complete.

Example. Figure 8 is a plot of the data shown in Table 5. The extrapolated value of A is 11.8 µg/mL.

Table 5 Plasma Concentrations and "Residuals" Vs. Time

Time (hr)	Observed C_p (µg/mL)	Extrapolated C_p (µg/mL)	Residuals (µg/mL)
0.0	0.0	11.8	11.8
0.25	2.2	11.4	9.2
0.5	3.8	10.9	7.1
0.75	5.0	10.6	5.6
1.0	5.8	10.1	4.3
1.5	6.8	9.4	2.6
2.0	7.1	8.7	1.6
2.5	7.1	8.1	1.0
3.0	6.9	7.5	0.6
4.0	6.2	6.4	0.2
6.0	4.8	4.8	–
8.0	3.5	3.5	–
12.0	1.9	1.9	–
18.0	0.8	0.8	–
24.0	0.3	0.3	–

The $t_{1/2}$ (elimination) is the time at which the elimination line crosses $A/2 = 4.5$ hour:

$$k_{el} = \frac{0.693}{t_{1/2}(\text{elimination})} = 0.154/\text{hr}$$

The $t_{1/2}$ (absorption) is the time at which the residuals line crosses $A/2 = 0.7$ hour:

$$k_a = \frac{0.693}{t_{1/2}(\text{absorption})} = 0.990/\text{hr}$$

Assuming that the 100-mg dose of drug was completely absorbed, the V_d can be calculated from equation (39):

$$A = 11.8\mu\text{g/mL} = \frac{100\,\text{mg} \times 0.990/\text{hr}}{V_d(0.990 - 0.154)/\text{hr}}$$

$$V_d = 10.0\,\text{L}$$

This method of calculation is often referred to as the "method of residuals" or "feathering the curve." It is important to remember that the following assumptions were made:

1. It is assumed that k_a is at least five times larger than k_{el}; if not, neither constant can be determined accurately.
2. It is assumed that the absorption and elimination processes are both strictly first order; if not, the residuals line and, perhaps, the elimination line will not be straight.
3. It is assumed that absorption is complete; if not, the estimate of V_d will be erroneously high.

The Wagner–Nelson Method (8)

A major shortcoming of the method of residuals for determining the absorption rate constant from plasma concentration versus time data following administration of oral solid dosage forms is the necessity to assume that the absorption process obeys first-order kinetics. Although this assumption is often valid for solutions and rapidly dissolving dosage forms for which the absorption process itself is rate determining, if release of drug from the dosage form is rate determining, the kinetics are often zero-order, mixed zero- and first-order, or even more complex processes.

The Wagner–Nelson method of calculation does not require a model assumption concerning the absorption process. It does require the assumption that (*i*) the body behaves as a single homogeneous compartment and (*ii*) drug elimination obeys first-order kinetics. The working equations for this calculation are developed next.

Derivation. For any extravascular drug administration, the mass balance equation can be written as amount absorbed (*A*) equals amount in body (*W*) plus amount eliminated (*E*), or

$$A = W + E$$

Taking the derivative with respect to time yields

$$\frac{dA}{dt} = \frac{dW}{dt} + \frac{dE}{dt}$$

But

$$W = V_d C_p$$

or

$$\frac{dW}{dt} = V_d \frac{dC_p}{dt}$$

and

$$\frac{dE}{dt} = k_{el} W$$
$$= k_{el} V_d C_p$$

Therefore,

$$\frac{dA}{dt} = V_d \frac{dC_p}{dt} + k_{el} V_d C_p$$

$$dA = V_d dC_p + k_{el} V_d C_p \, dt$$

Integrating from $t = 0$ to $t = t$

$$\int_0^t dA = V_d \int_0^t dC_p + k_{el} V_d \int_0^t C_p \, dt$$

$$A_t = V_d C_p^t + k_{el} V_d \int_0^t C_p \, dt$$

On rearranging we have

$$\frac{A_t}{V_d} = C_p^t + k_{el} \int_0^t C_p \, dt \tag{40}$$

where A_t/V_d is the amount of drug absorbed up to time t divided by the volume of distribution, C_p^t is plasma (serum or blood) concentration at time t, and $\int_0^t C_p \, dt$ is the area under the plasma (serum or blood) concentration versus time curve up to time t (see sect. "Area under the Plasma Concentration versus Time Curve"). An equation similar to equation

(40) can be derived by integration from $t = 0$ to $t = \infty$. Since $C_p = 0$ at $t = \infty$, the equation becomes

$$\frac{A_{max}}{V_d} = k_{el} \int_0^\infty C_p \, dt \qquad (41)$$

where A_{max} is the total amount of drug absorbed from the dosage form divided by the volume of distribution; and $\int_0^\infty C_p \, dt$ is the area under the entire plasma (serum or blood) concentration versus time curve (see sect. "Area under the Plasma Concentration versus Time Curve").

Equation (41) is useful for comparing the bioavailabilities of two dosage forms of the same drug administered to the same group of subjects. If it is assumed that k_{el} and V_d are the same for both administrations, it can be seen that the relative availabilities of the dosage forms is given by the ratio of the areas under the plasma concentration versus time curves:

$$\frac{A_{max_1}}{A_{max_2}} = \frac{\int_0^\infty (C_p \, dt)_1}{\int_0^\infty (C_p \, dt)_2} \qquad (42)$$

Other methods of comparing bioavailabilities will be discussed in a later section.

A great deal can be learned about the absorption process by applying equations (40) and (41) to plasma concentration versus time data. Since there is no model assumption with regard to the absorption process, the calculated values of A_t/V_d can often be manipulated to determine the kinetic mechanism that controls absorption. This is best illustrated by an example.

Example. A tablet containing 100 mg of a drug was administered to a healthy volunteer and the plasma concentration (C_p) versus time data shown in Table 6 were obtained. Figure 9 shows a semilogarithmic plot of these C_p versus time data. The half-life for elimination of the drug can be estimated from the straight line "tail" of the plot to be 4.7 hours. The overall elimination rate constant is then

$$k_{el} = \frac{0.693}{4.7 \text{ hr}} = 0.147/\text{hr}$$

Table 6 An Example of Wagner–Nelson Calculation

Time (hr)	C_p (μg/mL)	$\int_0^t C_p \, dt$	$k_{el} \int_0^t C_p \, dt$	$\frac{A_t}{V_d}$	$\frac{A_{max}}{V_d} - \frac{A_t}{V_d}$
0.25	0.6	0.1	0.0	0.6	9.4
0.50	1.2	0.3	0.1	1.3	8.7
0.75	1.8	0.7	0.1	1.9	8.1
1.0	2.3	1.2	0.2	2.5	7.5
1.5	3.4	2.6	0.4	3.8	6.2
2.0	4.3	4.5	0.7	5.0	5.0
3.0	6.0	9.7	1.5	7.5	2.5
6.0	5.6	27.1	4.1	9.7	0.3
12.0	2.3	50.8	7.6	9.9	0.1
18.0	0.9	60.4	9.1	10.0	–
24.0	0.4	64.3	9.6	10.0	–

Note $A_{max}/V_d = 10.0$.

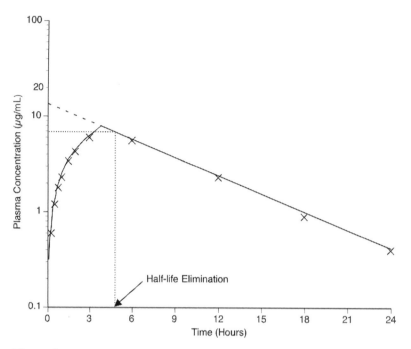

Figure 9 Semilogarithmic plot of observed plasma concentrations (*crosses*) versus time for an orally administered drug absorbed by a zero-order process (data shown in Table 6).

Table 6 illustrates the steps involved in carrying out the Wagner–Nelson calculation. The third column ($\int_0^t C_p\,dt$) shows the area under the C_p versus time curve calculated sequentially from $t = 0$ to each of the time points using the trapezoidal rule (see sect. "Area under the Plasma Concentration versus Time Curve"). The fourth column ($k_{el} \int_0^t C_p\,dt$) shows each of the preceding areas multiplied by k_{el} (as estimated from the tail) constituting the second term of the Wagner–Nelson equation (see equation 40). The fifth column (A_t/V_d) shows the sums of the values indicated in the second and fourth columns according to equation (40). A_{max}/V_d is the maximum value in the fifth column (i.e., 10.0), and the sixth column shows the residual between A_{max}/V_d and each sequential value of A_t/V_d in the fifth column.

If the absorption process obeyed first-order kinetics, a semilogarithmic plot of the residuals in the sixth column would be a straight line, and k_a could be determined from the slope. However, the regular Cartesian plot of the residuals shown in Figure 10 is a straight line showing that the absorption process obeys zero-order kinetics; that is, the process proceeds at a constant rate (25 mg/hr), stopping abruptly when the dose has been completely absorbed.

This example illustrates the usefulness of the Wagner–Nelson calculation for studying the mechanism of release of drugs from dosage forms in vivo. Whereas the absorption process itself usually obeys first-order kinetics, dissolution of capsules, tablets, and especially sustained-release dosage forms often must be described by more complex kinetic mechanisms. Although pure zero-order absorption, such as that just illustrated, is almost never observed in practice, many sustained-release dosage forms are designed to produce as close to zero-order release as possible since constant absorption produces constant plasma levels.

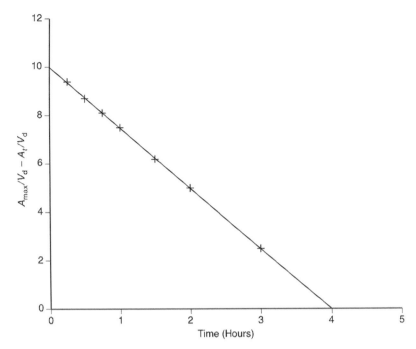

Figure 10 Plot of the residuals (*crosses*) between A_{max}/V_d and A_t/V_d versus time (last column of Table 6).

The Method of "Inspection"

Often, it is unnecessary to calculate an exact value for an absorption rate constant. For example, when several oral tablets containing the same drug substance are all found to be completely absorbed, it may be sufficient to merely determine if the absorption rates are similar. In another instance, it would be possible to choose between an elixir and a sustained-release tablet without assigning accurate numbers to the absorption rate constant for the two dosage forms.

In these instances, the *time of the peak* in the plasma concentration versus time curve provides a convenient measure of the absorption rate. For example, if three tablets of the same drug are found to be completely absorbed and all give plasma peaks at one hour, it could be concluded that all three tablets are absorbed at essentially the same rate. (In fact, if all tablets are completely absorbed and all peak at the same time, it would be expected that all three plasma concentration versus time curves would be identical, within experimental error.)

The time of the peak can also be used to roughly estimate the absorption rate constant. If it is assumed that k_a is at least $5 \times k_{el}$, then it can be assumed that absorption is at least 95% complete at the peak time; that is, the peak time represents approximately five absorption half-lives (Table 1). The absorption half-life can then be calculated by dividing the time of the peak by 5, and the absorption rate constant can be calculated by dividing the absorption half-life by 0.693.

Example. Inspection of Figure 8 gives a peak time of about 2.5 hours. The absorption half-life can be estimated to be 0.5 hour and the absorption rate constant to be 1.4/hr.

BIOAVAILABILITY (EXTENT OF ABSORPTION)

If a drug is administered by an extravascular route and acts systemically, its potency will be directly related to the amount of drug the dosage form delivers to the blood. Also, if the pharmacologic effects of the drug are related directly and instantaneously to its plasma concentration, the rate of absorption will be important because the rate will influence the height of the plasma concentration peak (response) and the time at which the peak occurs (onset). Thus, the *bioavailability of a drug product is defined in terms of the amount of active drug delivered to the blood and the rate at which it is delivered.*

Whenever a drug is administered through an extravascular route, there is a danger that part of the dose may not reach the blood (i.e., absorption may not be complete). When the IV route is used, the drug is placed directly in the blood; therefore an IV injection is, by definition, 100% absorbed. The absolute bioavailability of an extravascular dosage form is defined relative to an IV injection. If IV data are not available, the relative bioavailability may be defined relative to a standard dosage form. For example, the bioavailability of a tablet may be defined relative to an oral solution of the drug.

In the section "Kinetics Of Drug Absorption" we dealt with methods of determining the rate (and mechanism) of absorption. In this section we will deal with methods of determining the extent of absorption. In every example, the calculation will involve a comparison between two studies carried out in the same group of volunteers on different occasions. Usually, it will be necessary to assume that the volunteers behaved identically on both occasions, especially with regard to their pharmacokinetic parameters.

Area Under the Plasma Concentration Vs. Time Curve

In the development of equations for the Wagner–Nelson method of calculation, the following equation was derived (see equation 42):

$$\frac{A_{\max_1}}{A_{\max_2}} = \frac{\int_0^\infty (C_p\,dt)_1}{\int_0^\infty (C_p\,dt)_2}$$

This equation shows that the amounts of drug absorbed from two drug products (i.e., the relative bioavailability of product 1 compared with product 2) can be calculated as the ratio of the AUCs, assuming k_{el} and V_d were the same in both studies.

If dosage form 2 (equation 42) is an IV dosage form, the *absolute bioavailability* of the extravascular dosage form (dosage form 1) is given by:

$$\text{Absolute bioavailability} \atop \text{(extravascular dosage form)} = \frac{\text{AUC}_{\text{extravascular}}}{\text{AUC}_{\text{IV}}} \tag{43}$$

The AUC for a plasma concentration versus time curve can be determined using the trapezoidal rule. For this calculation, the curve is divided into vertical segments, as shown in Figure 11. The top line of each segment is assumed to be straight rather than slightly curved, and the area of the segment is calculated as though it were a trapezoid; for example, the area of segment 10 is

$$\text{Area}_{10} = \frac{C_{p9} + C_{p10}}{2} \times (t_{10} - t_9) \tag{44}$$

The total AUC is then obtained by summing the areas of the individual segments.

It should be readily apparent that the trapezoidal rule does not measure AUC exactly. However, it is accurate enough for most bioavailability calculations, and the segments are chosen on the basis of the time intervals at which plasma was collected.

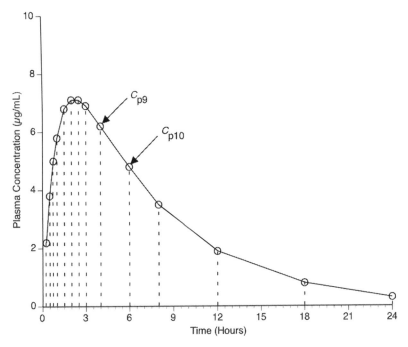

Figure 11 Plot of plasma concentrations (*circles*) versus time with the curve divided into vertical segments (data shown in Table 7).

Example. The AUC for Figure 11 can be calculated from the data given in Table 7.

Assuming that the AUC for a 100-mg IV dose given to the same group of volunteers was 86.7 hr.μg/mL, the absolute bioavailability of the extravascular dosage form is

$$\text{Absolute bioavailability} = \frac{\text{AUC}_\infty}{\text{AUC}_{\text{IV}}} \times 100 = \frac{67.2}{86.7} \times 100 = 77.5\%$$

It is not necessary to apply the trapezoidal rule to the entire plasma concentration versus time curve to calculate the total AUC. After the semilogarithmic plot becomes a straight line, the remaining area out to $t = \infty$ can be calculated using the following equation:

$$\text{AUC}_{(t \text{ to } \infty)} = \frac{C_p^t}{k_{\text{el}}} \tag{45}$$

Once a semilogarithmic plasma concentration versus time plot begins to follow simple first-order elimination kinetics, the remaining AUC can be calculated in one step using equation (45).

Example. In the previous problem, the AUC from 24 hours to infinity is given by

$$\text{AUC}_{(24 \text{ hr to } \infty)} = \frac{0.3 \ \mu g/mL}{0.15/hr} = 2.0 \ hr.\mu g/mL$$

It follows that if the entire semilogarithmic plot were straight, as would be the case for a one-compartment drug following IV administration, the total AUC would be given by

$$\text{AUC}_{\text{IV}} = \frac{C_p^0}{k_{\text{el}}} \tag{45(a)}$$

Table 7 Calculation of AUC using the Trapezoidal Rule

Time (hr)	C_p (µg/mL)	Area of segment (hr.µg/mL)	Cumulative area up to time = t (hr.µg/mL)
0.0	0.0		
		0.275	0.275
0.25	2.2		
		0.75	1.025
0.5	3.8		
		1.1	2.125
0.75	5.0		
		1.35	3.475
1.0	5.8		
		3.15	6.625
1.5	6.8		
		3.475	10.10
2.0	7.1		
		3.55	13.65
2.5	7.1		
		3.50	17.15
3.0	6.9		
		6.55	23.70
4.0	6.2		
		11.0	34.70
6.0	4.8		
		8.3	43.0
8.0	3.5		
		10.8	53.8
12.0	1.9		
		8.1	61.9
18.0	0.8		
		3.3	65.2
24.0	0.3		
		2.0	67.2[a]
∞	–		

[a]$\text{AUC}_\infty = 67.2$ hr.µg/mL.
Abbreviation: AUC, area under the plasma concentration versus time curve.

Example. For IV administration in the foregoing problem, the AUC was calculated as follows:

$$\text{AUC}_{\text{IV}} = \frac{13.0\,\mu\text{g/mL}}{0.15/\text{hr}} = 86.7\,\text{hr.}\mu\text{g/mL}$$

Cumulative Urinary Excretion

In the development of equations for calculating urine data when the drug is partially metabolized and partially excreted unchanged in urine, the following equation was derived (see equation 27):

$$\frac{D_{\text{U}}^{\infty}}{D_{\text{B}}^{0}} = f_e$$

where D_U^∞ is the amount of drug recovered from urine, D_B^0 is the amount of drug absorbed, and f_e is the fraction of the absorbed amount recovered as unchanged drug in urine. Equation (27) may be rearranged and written for two dosage forms as follows:

$$D_{U_1}^\infty = D_{B_1}^0 \times f_{e_1}$$

and

$$D_{U_2}^\infty = D_{B_2}^0 \times f_{e_2}$$

Dividing the first equation by the second gives:

$$\frac{D_{U_1}^\infty}{D_{U_2}^\infty} = \frac{D_{B_1}^0 \times f_{e_1}}{D_{B_2}^0 \times f_{e_2}}$$

Assuming that $f_{e_1} = f_{e_2}$, we have

$$\frac{D_{U_1}^\infty}{D_{U_2}^\infty} = \frac{D_{B_1}^0}{D_{B_2}^0} = \text{Relative bioavailability} \qquad (46)$$

Similarly,

$$\frac{D_{U(\text{extravascular})}^\infty}{D_{U(IV)}^\infty} = \text{Absolute bioavailability} \qquad (47)$$

Thus, if it is assumed that the same fraction of absorbed drug always reaches the urine unchanged, the bioavailability can be calculated as the ratio of total amounts of unchanged drug recovered in urine.

Example. When a drug was administered IV to a group of volunteers, 80% of the 500-mg dose (i.e., 400 mg) was recovered unchanged in urine. When the same drug was administered orally to the same volunteers, 280 mg was recovered unchanged in urine. What is the absolute bioavailability of the drug following oral administration? From equation (47),

$$\text{Absolute bioavailability} = \frac{280}{400} \times 100 = 70\%$$

For this calculation, it is unnecessary to assume that V_d and/or k_{el} is the same for the two studies. It is only necessary that f_e be the same in both studies. This is usually a valid assumption unless the drug undergoes a significant amount of "first-pass" metabolism in the gut wall or liver following oral administration or a significant amount of decomposition at an intramuscular (IM) injection site. When this occurs, the availability of the extravascular dosage form may appear to be low, but the fault will not lie with the formulation. The bioavailability will be a true reflection of the therapeutic efficacy of the drug product, and reformulation may not increase bioavailability.

The Method of "Inspection"

Bioavailability studies are frequently carried out for the sole purpose of comparing one drug product with another with the full expectation that the two products will have identical bioavailabilities; that is, their rates and extents of absorption will be identical. Such studies are called *bioequivalence studies* and are often employed when a manufacturer wishes to market a "generic equivalent" of a product already on the market. To take advantage of the safety and efficacy data the product's originator has filed with the FDA, the second manufacturer must show that his/her product gives an *identical plasma concentration versus time curve.*

In these cases it is not necessary to determine the absolute bioavailability or the absorption rate constant for the product under study. It is only necessary to prove that the plasma concentration versus time curve is not significantly different from the reference product's curve. This is done by comparing the means and standard deviations of the plasma concentrations for the two products at each sampling time using an appropriate statistical test.

A discussion of the statistical methods used in analyzing the data from bioequivalence studies is beyond the scope of this chapter. For a discussion of these considerations, the reader is referred to a description by Westlake (9).

MULTIPLE-DOSING REGIMENS (REPETITIVE DOSING)

Drugs are infrequently used in single doses to produce an acute effect; the way aspirin is used to relieve a headache. More often, drugs are administered in successive doses to produce a repeated or prolonged effect, the way aspirin is used to relieve the pain and inflammation of arthritis. A properly designed multiple-dosing regimen will maintain therapeutically effective plasma concentrations of the drug while avoiding toxic concentrations. Such regimens are easily designed if the pharmacokinetic parameters of the drug are known.

When drugs are administered on a multiple-dosing regimen, each dose (after the first) is administered before the preceding doses are completely eliminated. This results in a phenomenon known as *accumulation*, during which the amount of drug in the body (represented by plasma concentration) builds up as successive doses are administered. The phenomenon of accumulation for a drug administered IV is shown in Figure 12.

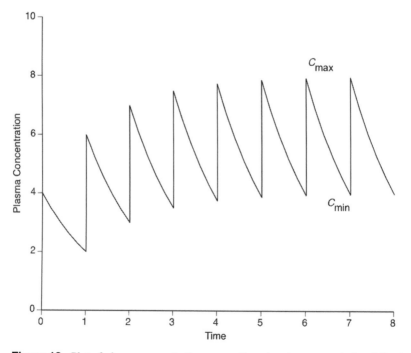

Figure 12 Plot of plasma concentration versus time showing accumulation following multiple IV injections.

Figure 12 shows that the plasma concentrations do not continue to build forever but reach a plateau where the same maximum (C_{max}) and minimum (C_{min}) concentrations are reproduced over and over. The objectives of designing a dosing regimen are to keep C_{min} above the *minimum effective concentration* (MEC) and to keep C_{max} below the *minimum toxic concentration* (MTC).

Repetitive IV Dosing

The plasma concentrations in Figure 12 can be calculated as follows: From equation (25) the plasma concentration at the *end of the first dosing interval* (*T*) is given by:

$$C_{p_1}^T = C_{p_1}^0 \exp(-k_{el}T) \tag{48}$$

Immediately after the second dose is given, the plasma concentration will be:

$$C_{p_2}^0 = C_{p_1}^T + C_{p_1}^0 = C_{p_1}^0 \exp(-k_{el}T) + C_{p_1}^0 \tag{49}$$

and so on.

It is now helpful to define the parameter *R* as the *fraction of the initial plasma concentration that remains at the end of any dosing interval*; *R* is given by the following equation:

$$R = \exp(-k_{el}T) \tag{50}$$

As was pointed out in section "Pharmacokinetics of Drug Eliminated by Simultaneous Metabolism and Excretion", when $T = t_{1/2}$, $R = 0.5$. The plot in Figure 12 was constructed using these conditions; therefore, the plasma concentration at the end of each dosing interval is half the concentration at the beginning of the dosing interval.

Equations (48) and (49) can be simplified to

$$C_{p_1}^T = C_{p_1}^0 R$$

for the *plasma concentration at the end of the first dosing interval*, and

$$C_{p_2}^0 = C_{p_1}^0 R + C_{p_1}^0$$

for the *plasma concentration at the beginning of the second dosing interval*.

The series can be carried further for more doses:

$$C_{p_2}^T = \left(C_{p_1}^0 R + C_{p_1}^0 \right) R$$

$$C_{p_3}^0 = \left(C_{p_1}^0 R + C_{p_1}^0 \right) R + C_{p_1}^0$$

$$C_{p_3}^T = \left[\left(C_{p_1}^0 R + C_{p_1}^0 \right) R + C_{p_1}^0 \right] R \text{, etc.}$$

The plasma concentrations at the beginning and end of the *n*th dosing interval are given by the following power series:

$$\text{Beginning} = C_{p_1}^0 + C_{p_1}^0 R + C_{p_1}^0 R^2 + \cdots + C_{p_1}^0 R^{n-1} \tag{51}$$

$$\text{End} = C_{p_1}^0 R + C_{p_1}^0 R^2 + C_{p_1}^0 R^3 + \cdots + C_{p_1}^0 R^n \tag{52}$$

Since R is always smaller than 1, R^n becomes smaller as n increases. For example, if $R = 0.5$, $R^{10} = 0.001$. Therefore, the high-power terms in equations (51) and (52) become negligible as n increases, and additional doses do not change the value of $C_{p_n}^0$ or $C_{p_n}^T$ significantly. This explains why the plasma concentrations reach a plateau instead of continuing to rise as more doses are given.

Hence, C_{max} and C_{min} (see Figure 12) are defined as the plasma concentrations at the beginning and end, respectively, of the nth dosing interval after the *plateau* has been reached (i.e., n approaches ∞). When $n = \infty$, equations (51) and (52) become

$$C_{max} = \frac{C_{p_1}^0}{1 - R} \tag{53}$$

$$C_{min} = C_{max}\,R = \frac{C_{p_1}^0\,R}{1 - R} \tag{54}$$

Thus, the maximum and minimum plasma concentrations on the plateau of a repetitive IV dosing regimen can be calculated if the dosing interval (T), the overall elimination rate constant (k_{el}), and the initial plasma concentration (C_p^0) are known.

Example. A drug has a biologic half-life of four hours. Following an IV injection of 100 mg, C_p^0 is found to be 10 μg/mL. Calculate C_{max} and C_{min} if the 100-mg IV dose is repeated every six hours until a plasma concentration plateau is reached.

$$k_{el} = \frac{0.693}{4\,\text{hr}} = 0.173/\text{hr}$$

$$\begin{aligned} R &= \exp(-k_{el} \cdot T) \\ &= \exp(-0.173 \times 6) = \exp(-1.038) \\ &= 0.354 \end{aligned}$$

$$C_{max} = \frac{10\,\mu\text{g/mL}}{1 - 0.354} = 15.5\,\mu\text{g/mL}$$

$$C_{min} = 15.5\,\mu\text{g/mL} \times 0.354 = 5.49\,\mu\text{g/mL}$$

Example. As indicated earlier, when $T = t_{1/2}$, $R = 0.5$. As a result, on the plateau in Figure 12,

$$C_{max} = \frac{C_p^0}{1 - 0.5} = 2 \times C_p^0$$

$$C_{min} = \frac{C_p^0 \times 0.5}{1 - 0.5} = C_p^0$$

Thus, when a dose is administered every half-life, C_{max} will be twice C_p^0, and C_{min} will be half C_{max} or equal to C_p^0.

The second example illustrates a very simple and often-used dosage regimen; that is, administration of a *maintenance dose every half-life*. The calculations indicate that on this regimen, C_{min} will be $C_{max}/2$ and C_{max} will be $2 \times C_p^0$. Figure 12 indicates that approximately *five half-lives will be required to reach the plasma concentration plateau*. If the drug has a relatively long half-life, many hours, perhaps days, may be required for the plasma concentrations to reach the ideal range. If the patient's condition is serious, the physician may not want to wait for this to happen. It is under these circumstances that a *loading dose* is indicated. The loading dose immediately puts the plasma concentrations in the plateau range, and the maintenance dose maintains that condition.

For IV administration, the easiest way to determine the loading dose is in terms of C_p^0 and C_{max}. For example, if the desired C_{max} is 20 µg/mL, and a dose of 100 mg gives a C_p^0 of 10 µg/mL, a loading dose of 200 mg should give a C_p^0 of 20 µg/mL, which is the desired C_{max}. If this loading dose is followed by maintenance doses of 100 mg every half-life, the plasma concentrations can be maintained at the plateau from the very beginning and throughout the entire dosing regimen. Thus, *for the maintenance dose of every half-life regimen, the ideal loading dose is twice the maintenance dose.*

Example. Consider another drug that is toxic if plasma concentrations are allowed to remain above 35 µg/mL (MTC) and the MEC in plasma is about 10 µg/mL. Thus, this drug has a *narrow therapeutic index* and the calculation of a precise dosing regimen is very important. When administered IV in a dose of 7.5 mg/kg to adults, the C_p^0 is about 25 µg/mL with a half-life of about of three hours. What would be a good dosing regimen for this drug?

Since 25 µg/mL is well above the MEC but below the MTC, a loading dose of 7.5 mg/kg might be given initially. After one half-life (3 hours), the plasma concentration should be 12.5 µg/mL. Since this is just above the MEC and corresponds to half the initial 25 µg/mL, a maintenance dose of 3.75 mg/kg could be administered. With repeated 3.75 mg/kg maintenance doses every three hours, C_{max} should be 25 µg/mL and C_{min} should be 12.5 µg/mL, which would allow some margin for error on either side.

Repetitive Extravascular Dosing

Although the equations become considerably more complex than those for the IV case, C_{max} and C_{min} can be calculated when the drug is administered by an extravascular route. The required equations may be developed as follows: The equation describing the plasma concentration versus time curve following one extravascular administration was discussed previously. Equation (35) may be written as follows:

$$C_p = \frac{FD}{V_d} \times \frac{k_a}{k_a - k_{el}} [\exp(-k_{el}t) - \exp(-k_a t)] \tag{55}$$

where D is the dose administered and F is the fraction of the administered dose absorbed (FD = D_G^0 in equation 35).

If n doses of the drug are administered at fixed time intervals (T), the plasma concentrations following the nth dose are given by

$$C_p = \frac{FD}{V_d} \times \frac{k_a}{k_a - k_{el}} \left[\frac{1 - \exp(-nk_{el}T)}{1 - \exp(-k_{el}T)} \exp(-k_{el}t') - \frac{1 - \exp(-nk_a T)}{1 - \exp(-k_a T)} \exp(-k_a t') \right] \tag{56}$$

where t' is the time elapsed after the nth dose. When n is large (i.e., when the plasma concentrations reach a plateau), the terms "exp $(-nk_{el}T)$" and "exp $(-nk_a T)$" become negligibly small, and equation (56) simplifies to

$$C_p = \frac{FD}{V_d} \times \frac{k_a}{k_a - k_{el}} \left[\frac{\exp(-k_{el}t')}{1 - \exp(-k_{el}T)} - \frac{\exp(-k_a t')}{1 - \exp(-k_a T)} \right] \tag{57}$$

Equation (57) can be used to calculate the C_{max} and C_{min} values on the plasma concentration plateau by substituting values for t' that correspond to the "peaks" and "valleys" in the C_p versus time curve. Thus, if $t' = t_{max}$ (the time of the peak), equation (57) gives C_{max}:

$$C_{max} = \frac{FD}{V_d} \times \frac{k_a}{k_a - k_{el}} \left[\frac{\exp(-k_{el}t_{max})}{1 - \exp(-k_{el}T)} - \frac{\exp(-k_a t_{max})}{1 - \exp(-k_a T)} \right] \tag{58}$$

If $t' = 0$ (the time at which another dose is to be given), equation (57) gives C_{min}:

$$C_{min} = \frac{FD}{V_d} \times \frac{k_a}{k_a - k_{el}} \left[\frac{1}{1 - \exp(-k_{el}T)} - \frac{1}{1 - \exp(-k_a T)} \right] \tag{59}$$

Example. The results of a single IM dose show that the dose is completely absorbed ($F = 1.0$), $V_d = 20$ L, $k_{el} = 0.3$/hr, and the time of the peak is about one hour ($k_a = 3.47$/hr). If 800 mg doses are administered IM every six hour, what will C_{max} and C_{min} be when the plasma concentration plateau is reached?

$$C_{max} = \frac{1.0 \times 800\,\text{mg}}{20\,\text{L}} \times \frac{3.47/\text{hr}}{(3.47 - 0.3)/\text{hr}} \left[\frac{\exp(-0.3 \times 1)}{1 - \exp(-0.3 \times 6)} - \frac{\exp(-3.47 \times 1)}{1 - \exp(-3.47 \times 6)} \right]$$
$$= 37.5\,\mu\text{g/mL}$$

From equation (59),

$$C_{min} = \frac{1.0 \times 800\,\text{mg}}{20\,\text{L}} \times \frac{3.47/\text{hr}}{(3.47 - 0.3)/\text{hr}} \left[\frac{1}{1 - \exp(-0.3 \times 6)} - \frac{1}{1 - \exp(-3.47 \times 6)} \right]$$
$$= 8.67\,\mu\text{g/mL}$$

The foregoing example shows the calculation of the two most important features of a repetitive dosing regimen, the maximum and minimum plasma concentrations on the plateau. But if equation (56) had been used, it would have been possible to calculate the plasma concentration at any time throughout an entire dosing regimen. Although these calculations are complex and laborious when done by hand, relatively inexpensive programmable calculators and now personal computers can solve equation (56) in seconds. As a result, a plasma concentration versus time plot can be generated for an entire dosing regimen in a very short time.

REFERENCES

1. DWA Bourne. Mathematical Modeling of Pharmacokinetic Data. Lancaster, PA: Technomic Publishing Company, 1995.
2. Bauer L. Applied Clinical Pharmacokinetics. 2nd ed. New York: McGraw-Hill Medical, 2008.
3. Rowland M, Tozer TN. Clinical Pharmacokinetics. 3rd ed. Media, PA: Lippincott Williams & Wilkins, 1995.
4. Shargel L, Wu-Pong S, Yu ABC. Applied Biopharmaceutics and Pharmacokinetics. 5th ed. New York: McGraw-Hill Medical, 2005.
5. Winter ME. Basic Clinical Pharmacokinetics. 4th ed. Baltimore, MD: Lippincott Williams & Wilkins, 2004.
6. Mayersohn M, Gibaldi M. Mathematical methods in pharmacokinetics. I. Use of the Laplace transform for solving differential rate equations. Am J Pharm Educ 1970; 34(4):608–614.
7. Web site http://www.boomer.org/c/p3/c02/c0208.html. Accessed on February 24, 2009.
8. Wagner JG, Nelson E. Kinetic analysis of blood levels and urinary excretion in the absorptive phase after single doses of drug. J Pharm Sci 1964; 53(11):1392–1403.
9. Westlake WJ. The design and analysis of comparative blood-level trials. In: Swarbrick J, ed. Current Concepts in the Pharmaceutical Sciences: Dosage Form Design and Bioavailability. Philadelphia, PA: Lea & Febiger, 1973.

4

Factors Influencing Oral Drug Absorption and Drug Availability

Juergen Siepmann and Florence Siepmann
Department of Pharmaceutical Technology, College of Pharmacy, Université Lille Nord de France, Lille, France

Alexander T. Florence
Centre for Drug Delivery Research, The School of Pharmacy, University of London, London, U.K.

INTRODUCTION

The scope of this chapter[a] is limited largely to considering factors affecting the absorption of drugs from solid oral delivery systems, as the basic principles of drug absorption have been discussed in chapter 2 of this volume. The discussion is restricted to drugs absorbed by passive diffusion that therefore can appear to obey first- or zero-order absorption kinetics (depending on the drug concentration within the contents of the gastrointestinal tract, GIT). Absorption of a drug after administration of an oral delivery system involves at least four steps: first and ideally, delivery of the drug to the site from which it will be optimally absorbed; second, the release and dissolution of the drug from the dose form; third, passage of the molecularly dispersed drug through the barrier membranes of the GIT; and finally, movement of the drug away from the site of absorption into the general circulation. Each of these steps is considered in turn. The order of the first two steps is not absolute; the drug may dissolve either before or after reaching its absorption site, the difference clearly affecting outcomes. It is imperative that the drug be in solution before it can be absorbed. The slowest of the four steps mentioned earlier determines the rate of availability of the drug from an oral dosage form. Those factors related to the physicochemical properties of the drug and the design and production of the dosage form, the pharmaceutical variables, can be closely controlled. Those variables resulting from the anatomical, physiological, and pathological characteristics of the patient, the biological or patient variables, are almost by definition more difficult to minimize. However, dosage forms should be designed with the physiological constraints in mind. This will be even

---

[a]Based on the chapter by Betty-Ann Hoener and Leslie Z. Benet, published in the 4th edition.

more important in the future with the increased emphasis on personalized medicines, addressed briefly in the last chapter in volume 2.

GETTING THE DRUG TO ITS SITE OF ABSORPTION

When an oral dosage form is swallowed by a patient, it travels through the GIT (Fig. 1). During its passage the dosage form encounters great anatomical and physiological variations. These patient variables have been discussed in chapter 2 of this volume. Two of these variables are most important in affecting the delivery of the drug from its dosage form. The first variable, hydrogen ion concentration, exhibits a 10^7-fold difference between the mucosal fluids of the stomach and the intestine. The second variable, the available surface area of the absorbing membranes, changes dramatically between different regions of the GIT (chap. 2), but one variable frequently defines inter- and intrapatient variability, namely GIT transit time. The transit times of nondisintegrating dose forms is determined largely by gastric-emptying rates.

Gastric Emptying

Since increased membrane surface area and decreased thickness of the absorbing membrane favor the small intestine rather than the stomach as the primary site for drug

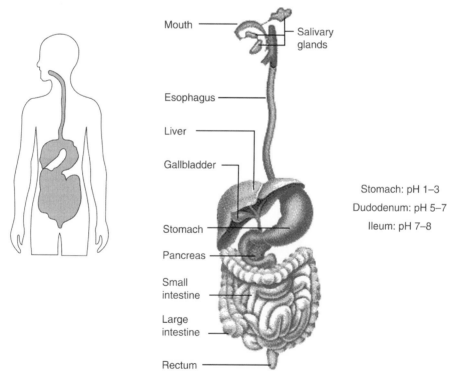

Figure 1 Diagrammatic representation of the complexity of the gastro-intestinal tract, with an impression (*left*) of the size of the GI tract in an adult. The average pH values of the stomach, duodenum, and ileum are shown. The small intestine contains bile salts and other agents, which can affect drug solubility and absorption. The large intestine presents another complexity in the form of the ascending, transverse, and descending colon, so nondisintegrating dosage forms have complex terrains to traverse.

absorption, the rate at which the drug reaches the small intestine can significantly affect its rate of absorption. Hence, gastric-emptying rate may often be the rate-determining step in the absorption of a drug. Light physical activity stimulates stomach emptying, but strenuous exercise delays emptying (1,2). If a patient is lying on his or her left side, the stomach contents have to move uphill to get into the intestine. The emotional state of the patient can either reduce or speed up the stomach-emptying rate (1,2). Numerous pathological conditions may alter gastric-emptying rate (3). Furthermore, drugs administered concomitantly may affect the stomach-emptying rate by themselves influencing GI motility. Any substance in the stomach delays emptying and, therefore, can delay the absorption of some drugs. If the stomach contents differ appreciably in pH, temperature, osmolarity, or viscosity from those conditions normally expected in the intestine, the stomach delays emptying until those conditions approach normal. Food, by altering many of these equilibrium conditions, can affect the rate of stomach emptying. In addition, the volume, composition, and caloric content of a meal can alter the stomach-emptying rate (1,2). Figure 2 illustrates the relationship between the position of a coated controlled-release capsule in the GI tract and plasma concentrations of 4-aminosalicylic acid. This emphasizes the points made earlier. In one case, drug is released in the colon as

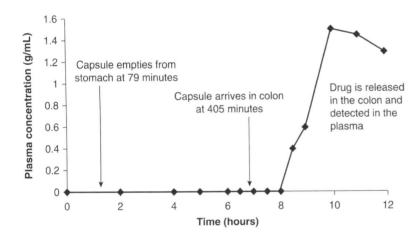

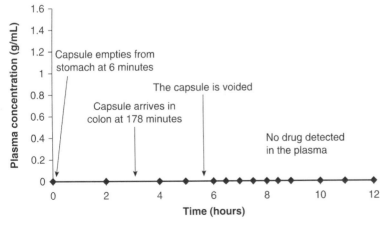

Figure 2 Plasma profiles for 4-ASA delivered from a coated capsule designed to target the colon for two different volunteers with different GI transit times. *Source*: From Refs. 4 and 5.

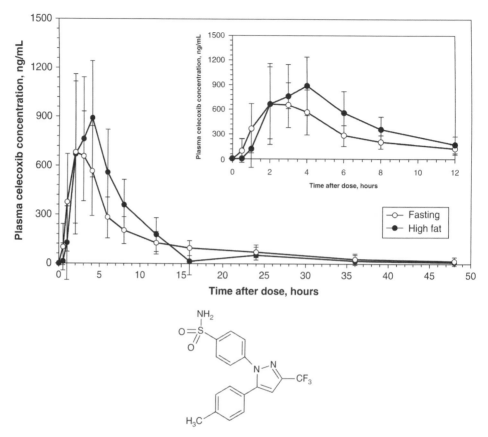

Figure 3 The effect of fasting and a high fat intake on the plasma concentrations of celcoxib (*structure shown*) as a function of time. *Source*: From Ref. 8.

intended, while in the other, the capsule is voided and zero plasma levels are detected (4). Prediction of the rate of absorption in an individual can be difficult, thus it is a problem to predict the range of pharmacokinetic factors that pertains to a large population.

The timing of meals relative to the timing of the oral dosing of a drug can influence the rate, and possibly the extent, of drug availability. It can be anticipated that taking a drug shortly before, after, or with a meal may delay the rate of drug availability as a function of decreased-emptying rate. However, the effect of food on the *extent* of availability cannot be so readily predicted (6). Food does not always affect drug absorption, one case being that of telbivudine (7). And in the case of celcoxib (Fig. 3), a high fat meal *increases* the peak plasma levels of the drug and the overall bioavailability.

To understand food effects such as the prolonged retention of the dose form or released drug in the stomach, one must be aware of the acid stability of the drug itself. Erythromycin, for example, is acid labile. Figure 4 illustrates the decreased *extent* of availability of erythromycin when two 250 mg tablets of erythromycin were taken on a fasting stomach with 20 or 250 mL of water or with 250 mL of water immediately after high-fat, high-protein, and high-carbohydrate meals (9). However, the *rate* of availability of this poorly absorbed water-soluble, acid-labile antibiotic was not affected by food (i.e., peak time was approximately the same for all dosings), indicating that stomach emptying is not the rate-determining step in the absorption of erythromycin from this drug delivery system. The *extent* of availability was, however, markedly decreased. This decrease might

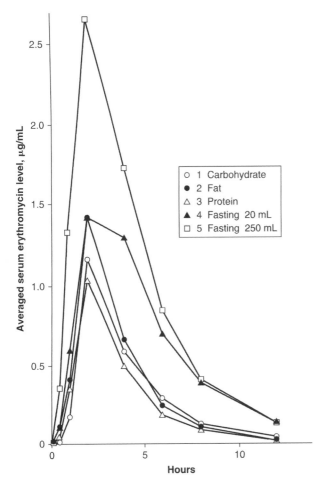

Figure 4 Mean serum erythromycin levels in healthy volunteers given 500 mg of erythromycin stearate with 20 mL of water (▲), 250 mL of water (□), or 250 mL of water immediately after a high-carbohydrate meal (○), 250 mL of water immediately after a high-fat meal (●), and 250 mL of water immediately after a high-protein meal (△). *Source*: From Ref. 9.

be due to complexation between drug and food or, more likely, due to degradation of the antibiotic when it is retained in the acid environment of the stomach for longer periods.

A further example of an *increase* in the extent of availability of a drug taken with food is illustrated in Figure 5. Here the cumulative amount of unmetabolized nitrofurantoin excreted in the urine is plotted against time. Healthy male volunteers took nitrofurantoin as a capsule containing 100 mg of the drug in a *macrocrystalline* form (circles) and as a tablet containing 100 mg of the drug in the *microcrystalline* form (squares) (the significance of the *macro-* and *microcrystalline* forms are discussed later in this chapter). The dosage forms were taken with 240 mL of water, either on an empty stomach (open symbols) or immediately after a standard breakfast (solid symbols).

It can be seen that food delays the absorption of nitrofurantoin from both the tablet and the capsule dosage forms, as indicated by the initial phase of each plot. However, food enhanced the *extent* of availability of the drug from both dosage forms, as indicated by the cumulative amount of drug excreted at 24 hours. It appears that delaying the rate of transit of nitrofurantoin through the GIT gives this poorly soluble drug more time to

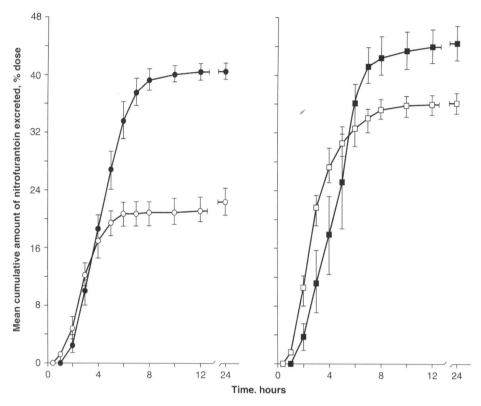

Figure 5 Mean cumulative urinary excretion of nitrofurantoin after oral administration of a 100-mg *macro*crystalline capsule to fasting (○) and nonfasting (●) subjects and a 100-mg *micro*crystalline tablet to fasting (□) and nonfasting (■) subjects. Vertical bars represent standard errors of the mean. The *macro*crystalline nitrofurantoin (Macrodantin™) was introduced to modify the absorption rate of nitrofurantoin to prevent side effects from high plasma levels. *Source*: from Ref. 10.

dissolve in the GI fluids. Thus, more nitrofurantoin gets into solution and, therefore, more is absorbed.

Hence, food delays stomach emptying and, as a result, may decrease the *rate* of availability of a drug from its oral dosage form (Fig. 6). The *extent* of availability of that drug, however, may be increased, decreased, or unaffected by meals. Thus, it is important for patients to be counseled on the importance of the timing of their medications relative to their mealtimes.

A good summary of food effects is given by Schmidt and Dalhoff (11). The most important interactions are those associated with a high risk of treatment failure arising from a significantly *reduced bioavailability* in the fed state. Such interactions are frequently caused by the following:

1. Chelation with components in food (e.g., alendronic acid, clodronic acid, didanosine, etidronic acid, penicillamine, and tetracycline)
2. Chelation with dairy products (e.g., ciprofloxacin and norfloxacin)
3. Other direct interactions between the drug and certain food components (e.g., avitriptan, indinavir, itraconazole solution, levodopa, melphalan, mercaptopurine, and perindopril)

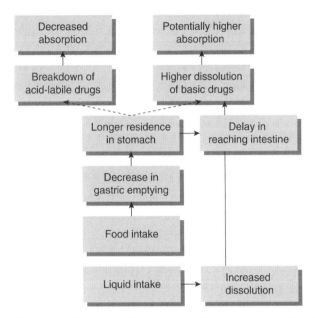

Figure 6 Schematic of some of the effects of food and liquid intake on drug absorption.

4. Physiological responses to food intake, in particular gastric acid secretion, which may reduce the bioavailability of certain drugs (e.g., ampicillin, azithromycin capsules, didanosine, erythromycin stearate or enteric coated, and isoniazid)

On the other hand, drug *bioavailability* may be *increased* because of the following:

1. A food-induced increase in drug solubility (e.g., albendazole, atovaquone, griseofulvin, isotretinoin, lovastatin, mefloquine, saquinavir, and tacrolimus)
2. The secretion of gastric acid (e.g., itraconazole capsules) or bile (e.g., griseofulvin and halofantrine) in response to food intake

For most drugs, such an increase results in a desired increase in drug effect, but in others it may result in serious toxicity (e.g., halofantrine).

The listing of drugs under the categories mentioned earlier can only be understood with reference to the chemical structures of the molecules concerned. Some drugs (such as the tetracyclines) are well known to chelate with divalent ions in particular, such as calcium in dairy products. Chelation often occurs between a keto group and an adjacent hydroxyl, but clearly will depend on the state of ionization of the molecule, hence will be pH dependent. With the tetracyclines there are several opportunities for chelation because of the potential – C=O and C–OH adjacent binding sites. Some other examples are discussed in the following sections. Chelation usually involves the formation of dimers or trimers such that the complex is larger and less well absorbed. There are cases, however, when the chelate is more lipophilic and can enhance absorption.

Chelation with Components in Food

Alendronic acid, clodronic acid, etidronic acid, and other bisphosphonates are implicated in binding to components, for example calcium in food. Their mode of therapeutic action is to bind to hydroxyapatite, which depends on the P-C-P group and the R_1 side chain

Table 1 Chemical Structure of Bisphosphonates

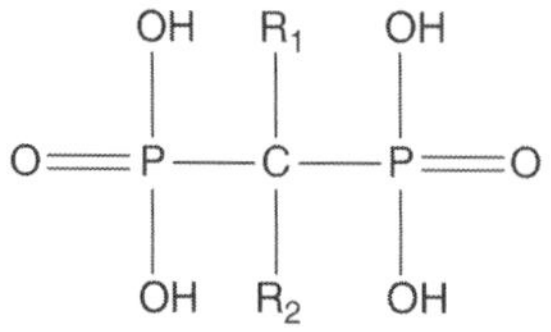

$$O = \overset{\overset{\displaystyle OH}{|}}{\underset{\underset{\displaystyle OH}{|}}{P}} - \overset{\overset{\displaystyle R_1}{|}}{\underset{\underset{\displaystyle R_2}{|}}{C}} - \overset{\overset{\displaystyle OH}{|}}{\underset{\underset{\displaystyle OH}{|}}{P}} = O$$

Bisphosphonate	R1 side chain	R2 side chain
Etidronate[a]	OH	CH_3
Clodronate[a]	Cl	Cl
Pamidronate[b]	OH	$CH_2CH_2NH_2$
Alendronate[a]	OH	$(CH_2)_3NH_2$
Risedronate[a]	OH	CH_2-3-pyridine
Tiludronate[a]	H	CH_2-S-phenyl-Cl
Ibandronate[b]	OH	$CH_2CH_2N(CH_3)$(pentyl)
Zoledronate[b]	OH	CH_2-imidazole
YH 529	OH	CH_2-2-imidazo-pyridinyl
Incadronate	H	N-(cyclo-heptyl)
Olpadronate	OH	$CH_2CH_2N(CH_3)_2$
Neridronate	OH	$(CH_2)_5NH_2$
EB-1053	OH	CH_2-1-pyrrolidinyl

[a]Bisphosphonates approved for use in nonmalignant conditions.
[b]Bisphosphonates approved for use in malignancy for one or more indications.
Other agents are only available for experimental purposes.

(Table 1). The biological activity is dependent on the R_2 side chain. The various structures in this class are given in Table 1. Being very hydrophilic they have poor and variable bioavailability, hence binding to food components is important clinically.

With penicillamine whose structure is shown in the following figure, there should be no surprise at chelation with components in food, as its primary mode of action is through chelation of copper in Wilson's disease. Iron is among the metals thus affected. When iron and penicillamine are taken together, chelation of penicillamine by iron in the gut reduces its absorption and activity.

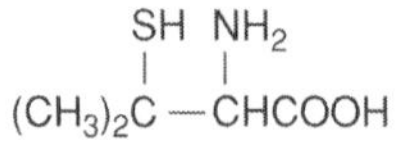

$$(CH_3)_2\overset{\overset{\displaystyle SH}{|}}{C} - \overset{\overset{\displaystyle NH_2}{|}}{C}HCOOH$$

Penicillamine

Orally administered iron has been shown to reduce the effects of penicillamine. A period of at least two hours, or preferably eight hours, should elapse between administration of penicillamine and iron supplements or other iron-containing products. Penicillamine can also bind zinc, and this interferes with the absorption of both the drug and the metal.

Normal dietary intake can significantly interfere with penicillamine absorption. In one study penicillamine levels were reduced to 52% of those from the fasting dose after food (12,13).

Chelation with Dairy Products

The quinolones have the requisite binding structures as can be seen in the following diagrams of ciprofloxacin and norfloxacin, namely the adjacent C=O and -OH groups.

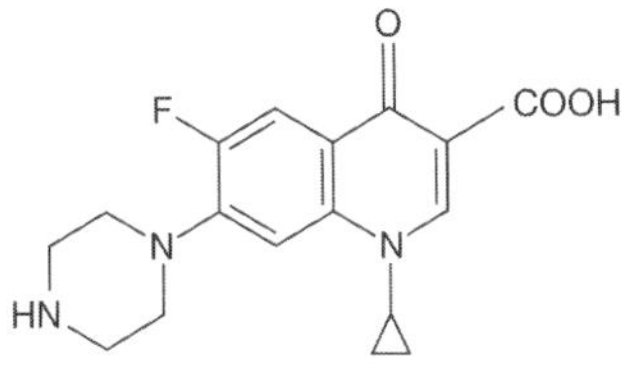

Ciprofloxacin

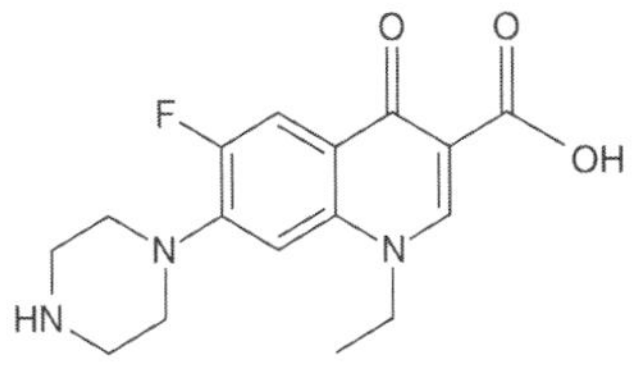

Norfloxacin

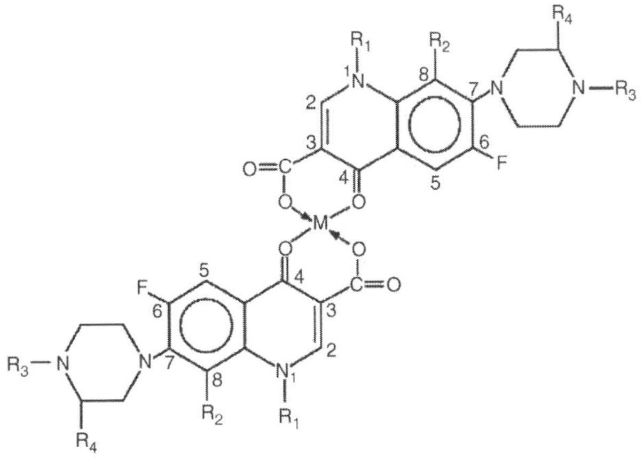

Quinolone dimer-metal ion chelate

The presumed structure of a dimer–metal ion chelate is shown above (14). This effective size increase through the linking of two quinolones molecules is one reason for reduced absorption.

Large Objects

Large objects, such as nondisintegrating dosage forms, are handled by the stomach quite differently from liquids and particles smaller than about 2 mm in diameter (15). These larger devices can remain in the stomach pouch until they are swept out by a series of contractions called a migrating motor complex (MMC). This MMC occurs about every three hours in the fasted stomach (16). However, when a patient has eaten a meal, the MMC does not occur until after most of the food has left the stomach (15). Thus, there can be a considerable delay in the absorption of drugs from solid dosage forms that do not disintegrate or release their contents by some other mechanism while in the stomach. The effect of size and the rate of delivery of the drug from its dosage form, frustratingly, *may* or *may not* affect the extent of availability.

GI Motility

Other patient variables may affect GI motility and, thereby, the extent and/or rate of availability of a drug from a delivery system. As illustrated in chapter 2 of this volume, the degree of physical activity, age, disease state, and emotional condition of a patient may increase or decrease GI motility. Other drugs taken concurrently may affect GI motility and, thus, indirectly affect the rate and extent of availability of a particular drug. This concurrent therapy may increase or decrease GI motility, thereby increasing or decreasing the *rate* at which a drug reaches its absorption site. Such changes in GI motility may increase, decrease, or have no effect on the *extent* of availability of a drug from an oral dosage form.

Average serum digoxin levels in an elderly female patient taking 0.375 mg of digoxin daily in a tablet dosage form are shown in Figure 7. When the patient was also given three

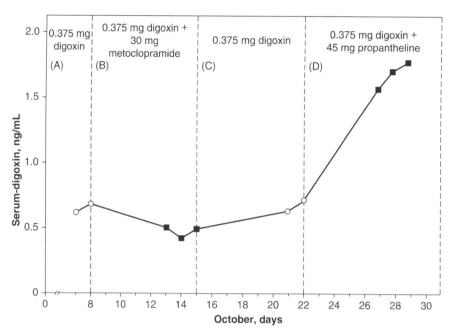

Figure 7 Variations in serum digoxin concentration in an elderly female patient during treatment with digoxin and metoclopramide or propantheline. *Source*: From Ref. 17.

daily 10 mg oral doses of metoclopramide, a drug that increases GI motility, the serum digoxin levels dropped, indicating a decrease in the extent of digoxin bioavailability. It is possible that this decreased extent of availability occurred because there was insufficient time for the digoxin to be released from its dosage form, or to dissolve in the fluids of the stomach or small intestine, before it moved completely through the GI tract.

An increase in GI motility does not, however, always decrease the extent of availability of a drug. Figure 8 illustrates the plasma level versus time curves obtained after oral administration of a 100-mg tablet of atenolol to six healthy male volunteers. When the atenolol was given one hour after a 25-mg dose of metoclopramide, a slight increase in the rate of availability was observed (e.g., decreased t_{max}), but the extent of availability of the atenolol was not significantly different from when atenolol was administered alone. Therefore it appears that, under these study conditions, stomach emptying is neither the rate-determining step in absorption nor does an increase in gastrointestinal motility significantly affect the amount of drug available to the general circulation (18).

Concurrent drug therapy may also *decrease* the motility of the GIT. Figure 7 shows average digoxin serum levels in an elderly female patient receiving 0.375 mg of digoxin daily in tablet form. After receiving three daily doses of a 15-mg tablet of propantheline, a drug that slows GI motility, the patient's serum digoxin level increased significantly. Since the digoxin tablet was moving more slowly through its principal site of absorption, the small intestine, it is probable that there was more time for the tablet to disintegrate and/or for the digoxin to dissolve, thereby increasing the extent of availability.

Returning to Figure 8, it can be seen that the oral administration of two 15 mg tablets of propantheline 1.5 hours before atenolol delayed the rate of availability of this β-blocker, while increasing its extent of availability (18). This increased extent might be due to more complete dissolution of the drug, resulting from its increased time in the GIT.

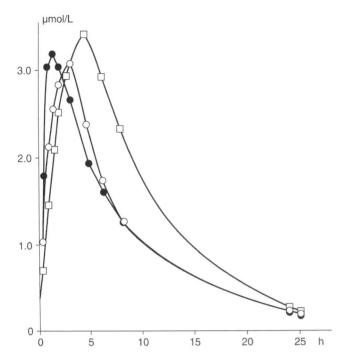

Figure 8 Mean plasma levels of atenolol in six male volunteers after a 100-mg tablet alone (○), with 25 mg of metoclopramide (●), or with 30 mg of propantheline (□). *Source*: From Ref. 18.

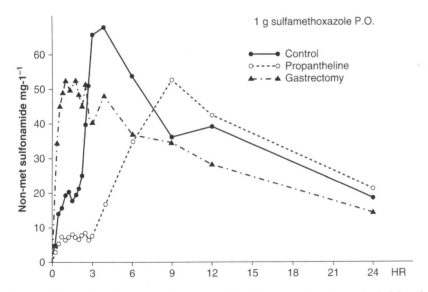

Figure 9 Blood levels of nonmetabolized sulfamethoxazole following oral administration of 1.0 g, as two 0.5 g tablets, under three different conditions. *Source*: From Ref. 19.

Blood levels versus the time curves obtained after oral administration of two 0.5 g tablets of sulfamethoxazole to male patients are pictured in Figure 9 (each subject took the drug with 300 mL of lightly sugared tea). When a 15-mg tablet of propantheline was taken 30 minutes before the sulfamethoxazole was given and a second propantheline tablet taken with it, both the rate and extent of availability of the drug from the tablet dosage form decreased (see dotted line in Fig. 9). Here, it is possible that slowing the passage of a drug through the GIT increased the opportunity for drug degradation to take place.

Thus, drugs that alter GI motility may increase or decrease the *rate* of availability of another drug. In addition, concurrent therapy may increase, decrease, or not affect the *extent* of availability of a drug. It should be noted that knowledge of the effect of a drug on GI motility can usually lead to an accurate prediction of its potential effect on the *rate* of availability of a second drug if, and only if, this is the rate-determining step in absorption, but this knowledge usually does not allow the pharmacist to predict how changes in motility may affect the *extent* of availability of the second drug. To make such a prediction, additional information, such as degradation and drug-binding mechanisms along the GI tract, must be known.

Since gastric emptying can significantly affect the availability of a drug, it might be suspected that patients who have undergone partial or total gastrectomies exhibit abnormal rates or extents of availability. Figure 9 also illustrates the increased *rate* of availability of sulfamethoxazole in a patient who had previously undergone a partial gastrectomy. Since the patient had most of his stomach removed, the drug could reach its principal site of absorption, the small intestine, without delay. Some pathological conditions are also accompanied by altered gastrointestinal motility, which may affect availability (3).

Understanding one of the key conditions in the GI tract, namely pH, can be enhanced by direct measurement of the pH values, which can be achieved by using telemetric devices (Fig. 10) (4). Concomitant measurement of plasma levels as a function of time can pinpoint the key elements in determining bioavailability. Such studies are especially valuable in examining outliers in clinical trials, such as those exhibiting very low bioavailability or indeed enhanced levels of drug.

Degradation in the GIT

Absorption is not the only process that can occur along the GIT. A drug may be degraded or metabolized before it can be absorbed. Chemical degradation, especially pH-dependent

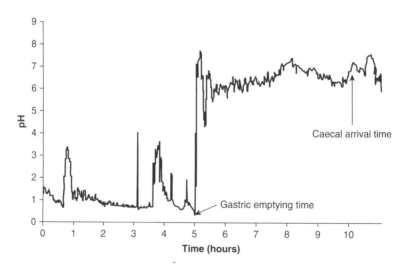

Figure 10 pH profile from one subject using the Bravo® pH capsule. The capsule was given 30 minutes before food (standard breakfast), and a standard lunch was administered at 4 hours. *Source*: From Ref. 4.

reactions, can occur in the solubilizing fluids of the GIT. Drugs that structurally resemble nutrients, such as polypeptides, nucleotides, or fatty acids, may be especially susceptible to enzymatic degradation (1,2). Digestion of these molecules can result as a consequence of the normal functions of the GIT. Moreover, the GIT is rich in microflora. These resident microorganisms can metabolize drug molecules before absorption. The variety of degradations attributable to bacteria has been reviewed (20). In various disease states both the fluids and the microflora of the GIT may be altered, and drug therapy may need to be modified if the rate and extent of availability are affected by these changes (3).

It would seem that metabolism and degradation of a drug within the GIT would serve primarily to reduce its extent of availability. In some instances, however, these processes may enhance availability. For example, clindamycin palmitate is less soluble than clindamycin HCl. A suspension of the palmitate ester is a more stable, better-tasting dosage form than a solution of clindamycin HCl. The palmitate ester is rapidly hydrolyzed in the GIT to free the more soluble active parent antibiotic drug, which becomes rapidly available to the systemic circulation. Molecules such as clindamycin palmitate are prodrugs, synthesized to enhance the pharmaceutical properties of the parent molecule. These may depend on degradation in the GIT to release the active parent molecule. Consequently, although metabolism or degradation in the GIT decreases the extent of availability for most drugs, with some prodrugs the degradative processes may be essential for complete bioavailability.

GETTING THE DRUG INTO SOLUTION: FACTORS AFFECTING THE RATE OF DISSOLUTION

Once the dosage form reaches the absorption site, it must release its therapeutic agent. Figure 11A depicts the disintegration and dissolution processes involved in the gastrointestinal absorption of a drug administered in a tablet dosage form. Figure 11B indicates more comprehensively the various solubility problems that may be encountered after the administration of a drug in an oral dosage form.

The dissolution process is primarily dependent on pharmaceutical variables, with possible exceptions such as pH dependency, which may be a patient variable. The relative importance of the various processes in Figure 11 may be explained in terms of the equation proposed by Noyes and Whitney in 1897 (21), which was further detailed by Nernst and Brunner (22) in 1904.

The Noyes–Whitney equation states:

$$\frac{dc}{dt} = K(c_s - c_t) \tag{1}$$

where dc/dt denotes the dissolution rate of a particle in its own solution, K is a constant, c_s represents the drug solubility in the liquid unstirred boundary layer surrounding the drug particle, and c_t the drug concentration in the well-stirred bulk fluid. Thus, the dissolution rate of a drug particle in its own solution is proportional to the difference in concentration between its saturation concentration and the concentration in the bulk fluid.

This equation was derived on the basic assumption that the diffusion of the dissolved species through the liquid unstirred layer surrounding the particle is the rate-limiting step in the dissolution process (Fig. 12). Three major processes can be distinguished during the dissolution of a solid particle (e.g., drug crystal): (*i*) the breakdown of the solid-state bonds, (*ii*) the diffusion of the individualized species

(A)

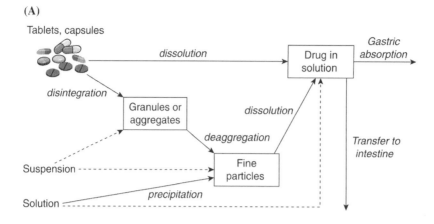

(B)

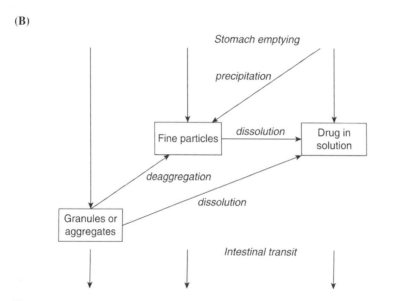

Figure 11 Schematic of events that occur in the GI tract after administration of different dose forms. (**A**) Events in the stomach and (**B**) in the intestine. Arrows drawn with continuous lines indicate primary pathways that most drugs administered in a particular dosage form undergo. Arrows drawn with dashed lines indicate that the drug is administered in this state in the dosage form, for example, as a suspension or solution. Arrows labeled "precipitation" indicate situations in which a drug is already in solution, but which then precipitates as fine particles, usually due to a change in pH of the aqueous environment. Other arrows indicate secondary pathways usually inconsequential in achieving therapeutic efficacy.

(e.g., molecules or ions) through the liquid unstirred boundary layer surrounding the particle, and (*iii*) convection within the stirred bulk fluid.

Often, the breakdown of the solid-state bonds as well as convection within the stirred bulk fluid are much more rapid than the diffusion through the liquid unstirred boundary layer ("diffusion layer" in Fig. 12). As these three processes take place sequentially, the much slower diffusion step is rate limiting for the overall dissolution rate. Thus, to quantify the rate at which a solid particle dissolves in its own solution,

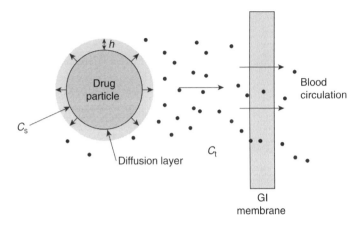

• Drug molecule

Figure 12 Diagrammatic representation of a dissolving drug particle, showing the liquid unstirred boundary layer of thickness, h, the saturation concentration of the drug in the liquid unstirred boundary layer at the particle surface, c_s, and the drug concentration at time t in the well-stirred bulk fluid, c_t. Once dissolved drug molecules/ions reach the GI membrane, they can be absorbed. It should be remembered that the process is a *dynamic* one: As long as solid drug excess exists, a continuous supply of molecularly dispersed drug available for absorption is provided.

Fick's first law of diffusion can be used (23):

$$\frac{dM}{dt} = -SD\frac{dc}{dx} \tag{2}$$

where dM represents the mass that is transported in the time interval dt, S denotes the surface area available for diffusion, D is the diffusion coefficient, dc represents the difference in concentration, and dx the distance to be overcome.

Applying this equation to the diffusion step through the liquid unstirred layer surrounding the drug particle (illustrated in Fig. 12) and considering that

(i) dc can be substituted by "$c_s - c_t$" (drug solubility–drug concentration in the bulk fluid at time t), because the breakdown of the solid-state bonds is rapid compared to drug diffusion (thus, the concentration directly at the particle's surface is the maximum possible concentration)

(ii) dx can be substituted by "h" (the thickness of the unstirred boundary layer)

(iii) the view point here is that the (positive) change in concentration in the bulk fluid allows deriving the Nernst–Brunner equation (22):

$$\frac{dM}{dt} = SD\frac{c_s - c_t}{h} \tag{3}$$

To calculate with *concentrations* instead of *amounts*, both sides of this equation can be divided by volume of the bulk fluid V, resulting in

$$\frac{dc}{dt} = \frac{SD}{Vh}(c_s - c_t) \tag{4}$$

where dc is the amount of drug dissolved in the time interval dt, D the diffusion coefficient of the drug in the liquid unstirred boundary layer surrounding the drug particle, S

the effective surface area of the drug particle, h the thickness of the unstirred liquid boundary layer surrounding the drug particle, c_s the solubility of the drug in the liquid unstirred boundary layer, and c_t the concentration of the drug in the well-stirred bulk fluid.

The following subsections will consider the pharmaceutical implications of the terms given in equation (4).

Effective Surface Area of the Drug Particles

Particle Size

The smaller the drug particles, the greater the surface area for a given mass of drug. Thus equation (4) predicts that dissolution rate increases as particle size decreases. Experiments confirm this expectation both with drug powders and with drug granules. Smaller granules dissolve more quickly than larger ones, and there has been shown to be a graded response in the case of phenacetin, a hydrophobic drug. That is, for the investigated five size ranges an increasing amount of drug dissolves over a specified time as the particle size decreases and surface area increases. However, in this example the drug was granulated (see chap. 14, for further discussion) whereby the hydrophilic diluent gelatin was incorporated into the particle. When phenacetin particles themselves were dissolved in 0.1 N HCl, there was a paradoxical finding: the dissolution rate increased with increasing particle size and decreasing particle surface area. A clue to the cause was given by the effect of the surface-active agent, polysorbate (Tween) 80, which when added to the 0.1 N HCl medium, resulted in the dissolution rate obeying equation (4). It is probable that decreasing the particle size of a hydrophobic drug may at times actually decrease its *effective* surface area, such as was proposed for phenacetin. Smaller phenacetin particles had more air adsorbed on their surfaces and these thus floated on the surface of the dissolution medium. A surfactant allows the particles to be readily wetted, thus their absolute surface area virtually equals effective surface area (24). Gastric juice has a relatively low surface tension (42.7 mN/m) compared with water, which has a surface tension of approximately 70 mN/m. The low surface tension of the gastric juice aids in the wetting of both the hydrophobic particles and the hydrophilic granules.

It is possible that large tablets do not rapidly disintegrate into smaller granules, but when they do disintegrate, the hydrophilicity of some granule formulations enables them to be more readily wetted than the powdered form. There are several instruments now available to allow ready understanding of the processes occurring during disintegration, one being the Mettler Toledo Lasentec™ D600L[a]. In particular, the size distribution of different materials present in the formulation can be measured.

The effect of particle size reduction on the bioavailability of nitrofurantoin was shown in Figure 5. The *microcrystalline* form (<10 μm) is more rapidly and completely absorbed from the tablet dosage form than is the *macro*crystalline form (74–177 μm) from the capsule dosage form. This is not a completely satisfactory illustration of the effect of particle size on the rate and extent of availability, since other manufacturing variables have not been held constant. Nevertheless, it does demonstrate some correlation between particle size, dissolution rate, and rate of availability.

In summary, the effective surface area of a drug particle plays a major role for the resulting dissolution rate. The effective surface area may be increased by physically reducing the particle size, by adding hydrophilic diluents to the final dosage form, or by adding surface-active agents to the dissolution medium or to the dosage form.

---

[a]www.mt.com/lasentec.

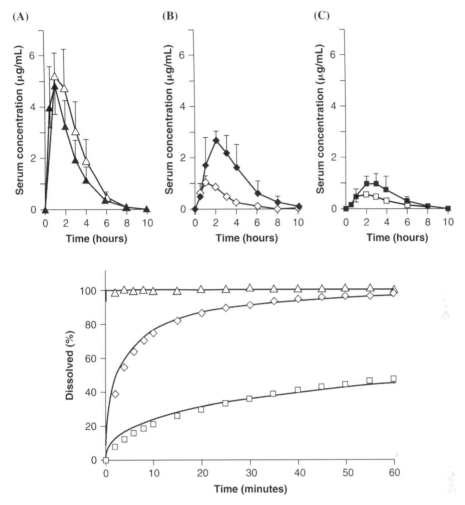

Figure 13 (*Upper figure*) Serum concentration–time profiles of cilostazol after oral administration of the suspensions at a dose of 100 mg/body in beagle dogs. Results are expressed as the mean with the bar showing SD values of four experiments. (**A**) △, NanoCrystal® suspension (fasted); ▲, NanoCrystal suspension (fed); (**B**) ◇, jet-milled suspension (fasted); ◆, jet-milled suspension (fed); (**C**) □, hammer-milled suspension (fasted); ■, hammer-milled suspension (fed). (*Lower figure*) Dissolution of the different batches of the drug in 900 mL water. △ NanoCrystal form, □ hammer-milled suspension, ◇ jet-milled suspension. *Source*: From Ref. 25.

Nanocrystals

Aspects of pharmaceutical nanotechnology are discussed in volume 2, chapter 12, but it is appropriate here to refer to the newer technologies that can achieve particle sizes within the nanotechnology domain. Reduction of particle size below the 300-nm diameter range vastly increases the surface area of the drug, although the additional surface area can lead to the problems as experienced with phenacetin (as described earlier). Figure 13 shows the effect of particle size reduction in the nanosize range of cilostazol, both on the serum concentrations of drug and on the dissolution behavior in vitro. To achieve greater intrinsic solubility (rather than greater dissolution rate through increased area), particle diameters must be below about 150 nm depending on the surface energy of the crystals.

Disintegration and Deaggregation

The rate of disintegration of the dosage form and the size of the resulting aggregates can be the rate-limiting step in the dissolution process. Disintegration is a particularly important step in the dissolution of drugs from *coated* dosage forms. Tablets, pellets, or capsules are coated for several reasons, as will be discussed in chapter 10 of this volume. Rationales for the use of coating include, for instance, the need to protect a drug during storage or from the very low pH in the stomach. Dosage forms may be coated so that they release their active ingredients slowly for prolonged action. Some drugs are coated to protect the patient's GIT from local irritation. Whatever the reason, these coatings are made from materials having various degrees of hydrophilicity that may or may not break down and allow their active ingredients to dissolve. Some coated tablets do not break down at all, and these dosage forms can be recovered intact in the feces.

As illustrated in Figure 11, after a dosage form disintegrates into large particles, these large particles must deaggregate to yield fine particles. Hence, deaggregation may be a rate-limiting step in the dissolution process as well.

Effects of Manufacturing Processes

Lubricating agents are often added to capsule or tablet dosage forms so that the powder mass or the finished dosage forms will not stick to the processing machinery. When the hydrophilic lubricating agent sodium lauryl sulfate (SLS) was added, 325 mg salicylic acid tablets dissolved in 0.1 N HCl more rapidly than did control tablets containing no lubricant. If, however, the *hydrophobic* lubricant magnesium stearate was added, the dissolution rate decreased. Most lubricants (and all the effective ones) are very hydrophobic. They act by particle coating. Thus, they must be properly formulated to avoid reducing dissolution rate and bioavailability. Once again, increasing hydrophilicity of a dosage form enhances its dissolution rate in an aqueous medium, but increasing its hydrophobicity decreases its dissolution rate.

Disintegrating agents, such as starch, tend to swell with wetting. In swelling the starch can break apart the dosage form. As more starch is added, the drug generally dissolves more quickly because the dosage form itself disintegrates more rapidly. The effect of micronization, cogrinding, and spray-drying on fenofibrate can be seen from the in vitro data in Figure 14 (26).

Clearly, unprocessed fenofibrate dissolved very slowly. Micronization led to a significant reduction in the drug particle size and, thus, to an increase in the surface area available for diffusion and to accelerated drug dissolution (Fig. 14A), as discussed earlier. Importantly, cogrinding with lactose resulted in a steep increase in the dissolution rate, which cannot be explained by changes in the particle size (Fig. 14B). Instead, the presence of hydrophilic lactose was likely to allow for a facilitated wetting of the drug particles and, thus, accelerated drug dissolution. The fact that the addition of the surfactant SLS further increased the release rate confirms this hypothesis. Interestingly, spray-drying allowed transforming the initially crystalline drug almost completely into the amorphous state. Thus, the apparent drug solubility significantly increased, resulting in a high drug dissolution rate (Fig. 14C). However, the obtained solution was not stable, and recrystallization occurred rapidly.

The possible effects on dissolution rate of the force used in compressing the drug-diluent mixture into a tablet dosage form can be summarized as follows: as compression force is increased, the particles may be more tightly bound to one another. On the other hand, it is also possible that higher pressures may fracture the particles so that they break into yet smaller particles. Depending on which of these two extremes is dominant for a given formulation, any of the combinations is possible. The effect of the compression force on the dissolution rate of a tablet dosage form would appear to be unpredictable.

(A)

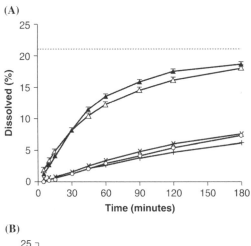

(B)

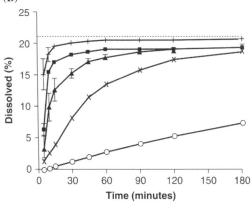

(C)

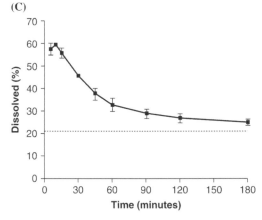

Figure 14 Dissolution profiles of 60 mg fenofibrate in FaSSIF ($n = 3$, ±SD). (**A**) Comparison of commercial preparations: (▲) indicates micronized active in physical mixture with lactose. (○) indicates unprocessed drug substance in physical mixture with lactose. (△) indicates Lipidil® powder; (+) indicates Lipanthyl® powder; (×) indicates Secalip® powder. (**B**) Coground mixtures: (○) indicates unprocessed drug substance in physical mixture with lactose; (×) indicates micronized active in physical mixture with lactose; (■) indicates a binary coground mixture with lactose; (▲) indicates a binary coground mixture with PVP (1:1), physically blended with lactose; (+) indicates a tertiary coground mixture with SLS/lactose (1:44). (**C**) Spray-dried formulation with lactose and SLS. Dotted lines indicate the fenofibrate solubility limit in the medium. *Abbreviations*: FaSSIF, fasted-state simulated intestinal fluid; SLS, sodium lauryl sulfate. *Source*: From Ref. 26.

From the few studies discussed here it can be seen that manufacturing processes can determine the dissolution rate of a drug from its final dosage form. Whether changes in these manufacturing variables are beneficial or detrimental to the ultimate bioavailability of a drug depends on the physicochemical properties of the drug and its dosage form. So-called inert ingredients and manufacturing methods, which are usually carefully guarded trade secrets, may exert subtle effects on bioavailability of the drug products that are selected. It is clear that the observation and, if possible, measurement of the parameters, both macroscopic and microscopic, which can affect drug release and absorption, should be studied in preformulation. Chapter 11 of this volume is devoted to preformulation studies.

Saturation Solubility of the Drug

The next term in equation (4) that can be manipulated is c_s, the saturation solubility of the drug. This variable can be influenced by both patient and pharmaceutical variables. The patient variables include the changes in pH as well as the amounts and types of secretions along the GIT. Additionally, both the physical and chemical properties of a drug molecule can be modified to increase or decrease its saturation solubility.

Salt Form of the Drug

Table 2 lists the large variety of salt forms of drugs approved by the FDA in the period 1995 to 2005, as collated by Serajuddin (27). Salt forms can be chosen to optimize the

Table 2 Salt Forms of NCEs Approved by the FDA from 1995 to 2006

Salts of basic drugs	Total number
Hydrochloride	54
Methanesulfonate (mesylate)	10
Hydrobromide/bromide	8
Acetate	5
Fumarate	5
Sulfate/bisulfate	3
Succinate	3
Citrate	2
Phosphate	2
Maleate	2
Nitrate	2
Tartrate	2
Benzoate	1
Carbonate	1
Pamoate	1
Total of all salts of basic drugs	101

Salts of acidic drugs	**Total number**
Sodium	12
Calcium	4
Potassium	2
Tromethamine	1
Total of all salts of acidic drugs	19

Abbreviation: NCEs, new chemical entities.
Source: Adapted from Refs. 27–39.

Table 3 Aqueous Solubility of Monosalts of Avitriptan Containing Various Counterions

Acid used	pK_a of acid	Solubility (mg/mL at 25°C)
HCl	−6.1	3.4 (9.0)[a]
Methanesulfonic acid	−1.2	16.3
Tartaric acid	3.0, 4.4	14.7
Lactic acid	3.9	15.2
Succinic acid	4.2, 5.6	16.1
Acetic acid	4.8	16.5

[a]Value in parentheses is for the dihydrochloride salt.
Source: Adapted from Ref. 27.

stability of the drug substance or, as it is often the case, to enhance the physical properties such as solubility (Table 3). The preparation of more soluble forms of drugs by salt formation is discussed in reference (40).

Since the salt form of a drug is more soluble in an aqueous medium, the dissolution rate for the salt form of a drug should be greater than the dissolution rate of the nonionized form of the drug. However, the solubility of the salt depends on the counterion; generally, the smaller the counterion, the more soluble the salt.

If dissolution is the rate-determining step in absorption, then, for a series of salts and the nonionized form of a drug, it can be anticipated that the rate of availability of the drug will increase as solubility increases. The weakly acidic drug *p*-aminosalicylic acid (PAS) is available as the potassium, calcium, or sodium salt. The solubility of nonionized PAS is 1 g/600 mL of water, that of KPAS is 1 g/10 mL, of CaPAS is 1 g/7 mL, and of NaPAS is 1 g/2 mL. Healthy adult volunteers took, on a fasting stomach with 250 mL of water, tablets containing either 4 g of PAS or tablets containing 4 g of one of the salts (containing 2.6–2.8 g of PAS) (40). Mean plasma concentrations (corrected to a 4-g dose of PAS) versus time curves are shown in Figure 15.

Although the rates of availability of the salts are not significantly different, their rank order does correlate with solubility. All the salt forms were more rapidly available than the nonionized PAS to a significant extent. Furthermore, the extent of availability of the acid form is only about 77% of that of the salt forms, indicating that the drug may not have completely dissolved before the dosage form moved through the GIT. Since commercial tablets were used, it is probable that other dosage form variables were not held constant. Thus, the decrease in rate and extent of availability of the PAS may not be exclusively due to differences in solubility.

pH Effects

As indicated, the ionized form of a drug will be more soluble than the nonionized form in the aqueous fluids of the GIT. The now classic studies on the beneficial effects of changing nonionized drugs into salt forms were reported by Nelson for tetracycline in 1959 (41), and Nelson and coworkers for tolbutamide in 1962 (42). Table 4 shows portions of the data of these studies.

Urinary excretion of the drugs or of their metabolites was taken as the in vivo measure of the relative absorption rate for the salts and the nonionized forms of the drugs. It has to be pointed out that no comparison can be made between tetracycline and tolbutamide. They are combined here only to illustrate that the same principles hold for both: positively and negatively charged drug ions. Note that the salt forms of the drugs dissolve much faster than the nonionized forms (or zwitterion for tetracycline) in all

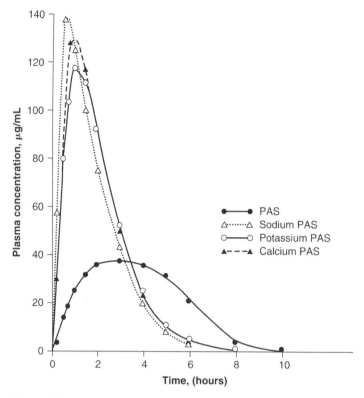

Figure 15 Mean plasma concentrations of unchanged drug from 12 subjects following administration of four different preparations of PAS. Data were corrected to 70 kg of body weight and to a dose equivalent of 4 g of free acid. *Abbreviation*: PAS, *p*-aminosalicylic acid. *Source*: From Ref. 40.

Table 4 Correlation of Dissolution Rates with Biological Measurements for Tolbutamide and Tetracycline Absorption in Humans

Drug as non-disintegrating pellet	In vitro dissolution rate[a] (mg/cm².hr)		Average amount excreted (mg) to time indicated[b]			
	0.1 N HCl[c] or simulated gastric fluid[a]	pH 7.2 buffer[c] or simulated neutral intestinal fluid[d]	1 hr	2 hr	3 hr	Lowering of blood sugar level (mg/100 mL) after 1 hr
Tolbutamide	0.21 (N → N)	3.1 (N → I)	5	7	12	5.2
Sodium tolbutamide	1069 (I → N)	868 (I → I)	21	65	117	9.1
Tetracycline	2.6 (N → I)	0.001 (N → N)	0.2	1.5	3.3	
Tetracycline HCl	4.1 (I → I)	7.8 (I → N)	3.0	12.0	20.4	

[a]The (N → N), etc., designations for the dissolution data are explained in the text.
[b]Tolbutamide excretion measured as the carboxytolbutamine metabolite.
[c]Tolbutamide study.
[d]Tetracycline study.
Source: From Refs. 41 and 42.

media and that more of the salt forms of the drug are absorbed and subsequently excreted in each period. For a dissociable drug, either an acid or a base, such as tolbutamide or tetracycline, the pH of the GI fluids determines whether the drug is ionized or nonionized. The dependence of the dissolution rate of a drug on pH is indirectly considered in the Nernst–Brunner equation (equation 3). That equation may be rewritten as

$$\frac{dM}{dt} = \frac{SD}{h}(c_h - c_t) \tag{5}$$

where dM is the amount of drug dissolved in the time interval dt, S represents the effective surface area of the drug particle, D denotes the diffusion coefficient of the dissolved species through the liquid unstirred layer surrounding the drug particle, h is the thickness of this unstirred liquid layer, c_t is the drug concentration in the bulk fluid at time t, and c_h denotes the saturation solubility of the drug in *the boundary layer* at any particular pH (Fig. 12). Then, for a weakly acidic drug:

$$AH \rightleftarrows A^- + H^+ \tag{6}$$

$$K_a = \frac{[A^-][H^+]}{[AH]} \tag{7}$$

$$c_h = [AH] + [A^-] \tag{8}$$

$$c_h = [AH]\left(1 + \frac{K_a}{[H^+]}\right) \tag{9}$$

so

$$\frac{dM}{dt} = \frac{DS}{h}\left\{[AH]\left(1 + \frac{K_a}{[H^+]}\right) - c_t\right\} \tag{10}$$

Therefore, as pH increases, the dissolution rate of a weak acid increases. Similarly, for a weak base:

$$BH^+ \rightleftarrows B + H^+ \tag{11}$$

$$K_a = \frac{[B][H^+]}{[BH^+]} \tag{12}$$

$$c_h = [BH^+] + [B] \tag{13}$$

$$c_h = [B]\left(1 + \frac{[H^+]}{K_a}\right) \tag{14}$$

so

$$\frac{dM}{dt} = \frac{DS}{h}\left\{[B]\left(1 + \frac{[H^+]}{K_a}\right) - c_t\right\} \tag{15}$$

Referring to Table 4, we can see that the dissolution rate of the weak *acid* tolbutamide *increases* when the pH *increases*, as predicted by equation (10). Additionally, for the weak *base* tetracycline, as predicted by equation (15), the dissolution rate *decreases* when the pH *increases*. Thus far, the more rapid dissolution of the salt forms of these drugs and the direction of change of the dissolution rate with pH have been accounted for with equations (6) to (15). However, there are six possible dissolution rate comparisons that can be made for each set of nonionized drug and its salt in the two buffers. The letters in Table 4 indicate similar measurements in the two studies.

- N → N indicates a nonionized solid drug dissolving in a medium in which the dissolved solute in the bulk solution is nonionized.
- N → I indicates a nonionized solid drug dissolving in a medium in which the dissolved solute in the bulk solution is ionized.
- I → I indicates an ionized solid drug dissolving in a medium in which the dissolved solute is ionized.
- I → N indicates an ionized solid drug becoming nonionized solute after dissolution.

Process I → I should be faster than process N → N, since the solubility of the dissolving substance will be much greater for the salt than for the nonionized molecule in an aqueous medium. A similar explanation can be used for (I → N)>(N → N) and (I → I)>(N → N) and (I → I)>(N → I), but it must be remembered that c_h in equation (5) is the saturation solubility of the drug in the stationary *diffusion layer*, not in the stirred *bulk solution*. Importantly, the dissolving solid might change the pH of the liquid environment immediately surrounding the solid particle; thus, the dissolution rate might be governed by the solubility of the drug in the diffusion layer. The I → N and N → N comparison is especially significant in the oral administration of weakly acidic drugs and their salts, since the acidic region of the stomach is the first solvent medium encountered following normal oral dosing. Frequently, administering the sodium or potassium salt of an acidic drug actually speeds up absorption by increasing the effective surface area of the solid drug according to the following hypothesized process. The salt acts as its own buffer in the diffusion layer and goes into solution in this layer. However, when the salt molecules diffuse out of the layer and encounter the bulk solution, they precipitate out as *very fine* nonionized *prewetted* particles. The large surface area thus favors rapid dissolution when additional fluid becomes available for one of the following reasons: (*i*) dissolved drug is absorbed, (*ii*) more fluid accumulates in the stomach, or (*iii*) the fine particles are emptied into the intestine. The classic study of Lee et al. (43) comparing serum levels of penicillin V following administration of the salt and free acid to dogs is explained by this phenomenon also. However, in at least three cases—aluminum acetylsalicylate (44), sodium warfarin (45), and the pamoate salt of benzphetamine (46)—administration of the salt slowed dissolution of the drug and subsequent absorption as compared with the nonionized form. This decrease appears to be due to precipitation of an insoluble particle or film on the surface of the tablet, rather than in the bulk solution. Precipitation of an insoluble particle or film onto the surface of the tablet decreases the effective surface area by preventing deaggregation of the particles.

The comparison of I → N and N → I may also be explained by the buffered pH in the unstirred diffusion layer and leads to an interesting comparison between a process under *kinetic* control versus one under *thermodynamic* control. Because the bulk solution in process N → I favors formation of the ionized species, a much larger quantity of drug could be dissolved in the N → I solvent if the dissolution process were allowed to reach *equilibrium*. However, the dissolution *rate* will be controlled by the solubility in the unstirred diffusion layer; accordingly, faster dissolution of the salt in the buffered diffusion layer (process I → N) might occur. In comparing N → I and N → N, or I → N and I → I, the pH of the diffusion layer is identical in each set, and the differences in dissolution rate are likely to be explained either by the thickness of the diffusion layer or the concentration gradient of the drug. One might assume that a diffusion layer at a different pH than that of the bulk solution is thinner than a diffusion layer at the same pH because of the acid-base interaction at the interface. In addition, when the bulk solution is at a different pH than that of the diffusion layer, the bulk solution might act as a sink and c_t might be eliminated from equations (1), (3), (4), and (5). A decrease both in the diffusion layer thickness, h, and in the drug concentration in the well-stirred bulk at time t, c_t, favor faster dissolution in processes N → I and I → N as opposed to N → N and I → I, respectively (equations 3–5).

Furthermore, Nelson (47) studied a series of weak organic acids and found (I → I) > (I → N) for the sodium salt of four of these compounds. For example, the dissolution rate of sodium benzoate in pH 6.83 buffer was 1770 mg/100 min.cm^2 versus 980 mg/100 min.cm^2 in a pH 1.5 solution. Corresponding values of I → I and I → N were 820 versus 200 mg/100 min.cm^2 for sodium phenobarbital, 2500 versus 1870 mg/100 min.cm^2 for sodium salicylate, and 810 versus 550 mg/100 min.cm^2 for sodium sulfathiazole. The acid forms of these drugs all showed the expected (N → I) > (N → N) relationship (48).

As stated earlier, the preceding explanation of the data in Table 4 is presented with reference to a specific theory of dissolution. Although this theory may not be fully appropriate for some drug products, it does provide a basis for understanding the general principles that dictate the (I → N) ≈ (I → I) > (N → I) > (N → N) relationship observed in dissolution rate measurements for a nonionized drug and its salt form.

The pH of a solution affects not only the *active* ingredients of a dosage form but also the *inert* ingredients. Three commercial dosage forms of nitrofurantoin are compared in Table 5. Nitrofurantoin is a weak acid with $pK_a = 7.2$. Equation (10) predicts that as the pH of the dissolution medium *increases*, the dissolution half-life of nitrofurantoin should *decrease*. For the suspension of microcrystalline nitrofurantoin and for the capsule containing 100 mg of nitrofurantoin in the macrocrystalline form, the experimental results follow this prediction. In contrast, for the tablet containing 100 mg of nitrofurantoin in the microcrystalline form, the dissolution half-life *increases* with *increasing* pH. This can be explained by the fact that the tablet did not disintegrate at pH 7.2. Thus, for this formulation it appears that the physicochemical properties of the *dosage form* rather than the physicochemical properties of the *drug* determine the resulting drug release rate. Strictly speaking the terms "drug *release* rate" and "drug *dissolution* rate" are not synonymous. Several processes (and not only drug dissolution) can be involved in the release of a drug from a dosage form. However, this distinction is not always made in the literature. Interestingly, both the capsule and tablet formulations, which must both disintegrate, are less rapidly available than the suspension (see the dissolution scheme shown in Fig. 11.).

Table 5 Effect of pH on the Dissolution Half-Life of Nitrofurantoin from Commercial Dosage Forms at 37°C

	Mean dissolution half-time[a] (min)	
Commercial dosage form	pH 1.12	pH 7.20
Aqueous suspension[b]	12.5 (1.2)	2.64 (0.34)
Compressed tablet[c]	77.9 (19.0)	167.0 (35)
Gelatin capsule[d]	212.0 (44)	160.0 (24)

[a]Determined from log-normal probability plots of individual rate data. Mean of five determinations (SD).
[b]Furadantin suspension containing microcrystalline (<10 μm) drug.
[c]Furadantin tablets containing microcrystalline (<10 μm) drug.
[d]Macrodantin capsules containing microcrystalline (74–177 μm) drug.
Source: From Ref. 49.

It has been mentioned that the pH of the bulk fluids may not reflect the pH of the stationary diffusion layer. As the active or inert ingredients of a dosage form dissolve, they may alter the pH of the stagnant diffusion layer, without significantly changing the pH of the bulk fluids. Moreover, it is possible to intentionally add buffering agents to a capsule or tablet dosage form. The small amount of buffer may not alter the pH of the bulk fluids of the GIT, but can buffer the pH in the unstirred diffusion layer to a pH favoring rapid dissolution of the drug. Such an effect was hypothesized when dissolution rates were compared for buffered versus plain (no alkaline additives) tablets of aspirin (48). Later, more extensive studies on the effects of a variety of buffers on the dissolution of aspirin tablets were carried out (50). Hydrophilic buffers and buffers that released carbon dioxide increased the dissolution rate; however, hydrophobic buffers decreased the dissolution rate, possibly by effectively waterproofing the tablets.

In summary, the effects of pH on the dissolution rate of a drug from an oral dosage form depend on (*i*) the pH of the GI fluids, a patient variable, (*ii*) the acid or base strength of the drug, a pharmaceutical variable, as well as (*iii*) the physicochemical properties of the dosage form, another pharmaceutical variable. Furthermore, by intentionally designing the dosage form such that it buffers the unstirred diffusion layer, it is possible to control a patient variable by a pharmaceutical ploy.

Usually, drugs in a salt form are more quickly available and, often, available to a greater extent. However, there are instances when the drug may not be formulated in the salt form, even when a proper, stable formulation of the salt may be produced. Sodium tolbutamide dissolves faster than tolbutamide when both in vitro dissolution data and in vivo urinary excretion measurements are compared. As would be expected, the pharmacological effect (i.e., lowering of the blood sugar level) is also more pronounced after one hour for the salt form. However, the product is actually formulated containing the acidic (nonionized) tolbutamide, because a rapid decrease in blood sugar is not desirable.

The solid state is discussed extensively in chapter 9 of this volume. What follow are summaries to complete the picture of the parameters that can affect drug absorption.

Solvate Formation

One variable that can influence the saturation solubility of a drug is its degree of solvation. Since the anhydrous, hydrated, and alcoholated forms of a drug have slightly different solubilities, they may well have different dissolution rates and, therefore, different rates of absorption. However, these differences may not be clinically significant (51).

Polymorphism

Yet another property of a drug that may affect its saturation solubility and, hence, its dissolution rate is its crystalline state (see chap. 8). Many drugs exhibit polymorphism (52); that is, they are available in several different crystalline states. Chloramphenicol palmitate is available in at least two different forms, A and B. The B form is the more soluble one. Figure 16 shows the mean serum level of chloramphenicol versus time curves obtained after oral administration to male volunteers of chloramphenicol palmitate suspensions containing the equivalent of 1.5 g of chloramphenicol (53). The fraction of the B form of chloramphenicol palmitate ranges from 0% in suspension M to 100% in suspension L. Since the suspensions were identical except for the crystalline form, it appears that the increase in rate and extent of availability with an increasing percentage of the B form is due to the increasing rate of dissolution. A warning, however, is necessary. In general, the more soluble polymorph is the least stable *thermodynamically*. Thus, older

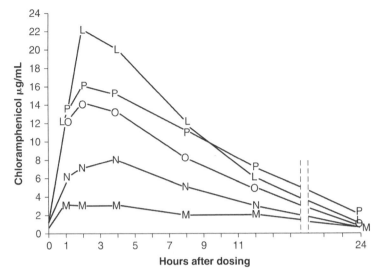

Figure 16 Comparison of mean blood serum levels obtained with chloramphenicol palmitate suspensions containing varying ratios of A and B polymorphs, following a single oral dose equivalent to 1.5 g of chloramphenicol. Percentage of polymorph B in the suspension: M, 0%; N, 25%; O, 50%; P, 75%; L, 100%. *Source*: From Ref. 53.

dosage forms may contain more of the more stable, but less soluble polymorph. Aging may significantly affect the bioavailability of drugs exhibiting polymorphism. Pharmacists must, for this and many other reasons, be aware of the storage requirements of all drugs dispensed. They must also counsel their patients on the proper storage of their medicines and the importance of discarding out-of-date drugs.

Complexation

Several studies have examined the effects of complex formation on the rate and extent of drug availability. A drug may complex with both absorbable and nonabsorbable excipients in a dosage form. This complexation may occur within the dosage form or in the solubilizing fluids, and the resulting complex may be more or less soluble compared with the drug itself. The rate and extent of availability of promazine from a suspension of the drug adsorbed on either activated charcoal or the clay attapulgite were compared with the availability of the drug from an aqueous solution (54). Healthy adults took, on an empty stomach, 45 mL of either the solution or one of the suspensions with 120 mL of water. The *rate* of availability of promazine from the attapulgite suspension was less than from the solution, but the *extent* of absorption was the same. When compared with the solution, the promazine-activated charcoal suspension showed both a decreased rate and extent of availability. However, the association constant for the promazine-attapulgite complex was greater than for the promazine-activated charcoal complex. Thus, it appears that it is not the magnitude of the association constant of the complex, but the *rate* at which the complex dissociates, that determines whether absorption of the drug is as rapid or as complete as in the absence of complex formation.

In addition to possible complexation with other ingredients in the dosage form, a drug may complex with the natural components of the GIT. The mucin, enzymes, bile, and physiological surfactants found in the mucosal fluids may interact with a given drug. The influence of these interactions on the availability of the drug depends on the physicochemical properties of the drug and those of the endogenous compound, as discussed in chapter 2 of this volume. It is possible that both increased and decreased drug solubilities are encountered. Thus, for drugs for which the rate of availability is dissolution rate limited, such interactions may be beneficial or detrimental. Once again, patient variables may control the availability of the drug from its dosage form.

Biorelevant Dissolution Media

The purpose of the study, the results of which are illustrated in Figure 17, was to characterize the dissolution of itraconazole in different dissolution media and to elucidate the effects of various additives to represent the fed and fasted conditions (55). Dissolution studies are important as we have seen. The appropriate choice of dissolution media can assist in obtaining meaningful results especially with very poorly soluble drugs. In Figure 17 albumin in levels up to 4% has been added to study the dissolution of itraconazole, a poorly water-soluble drug whose structure is shown below the figure.

Clearly, the dissolution rate of the poorly water-soluble drug significantly increases with increasing albumin content of the release medium, which can be attributed to protein-drug binding and the increased solubility of itraconazole in the presence of this protein (51).

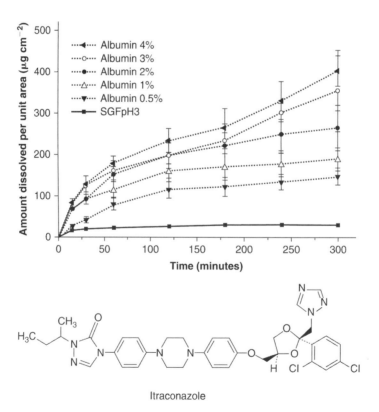

Itraconazole

Figure 17 Effects of albumin presence in simulated gastric fluid (SGF) on the dissolution of itraconazole (*structure shown*). *Source*: Adapted from Ref. 55.

Solid-Solid Interactions

Preparing a solid solution of a drug is one additional way of controlling its dissolution rate. For this chapter, the term "solid solution" will be used to describe any solid system in which one component is dispersed at the *molecular* level within another (56).

Importantly, for extremely small particles the saturation solubility (c_s) of the drug may increase as particle size decreases. This increase in solubility can be described by the Kelvin equation (57):

$$c_s^{\text{micro}} = c_s \exp\left(\frac{2\gamma M}{r\rho RT}\right) \tag{16}$$

where c_s^{micro} is the saturation solubility of the microscopic particle, c_s the saturation solubility of the drug (macroparticles), γ the interfacial tension between drug particles and the solubilizing fluids, M the molecular weight of the drug, r the radius of the microscopic drug particle, R the ideal gas constant, ρ the density of the microscopic drug particle, and T the absolute temperature.

Figure 18 depicts the dissolution rates of griseofulvin, an insoluble antifungal agent, and griseofulvin-succinic acid samples as described by Goldberg et al. (58). Several conclusions can be drawn from these experiments. The first is that physically reducing the particle size of the griseofulvin by micronization increased the rate of dissolution in accordance with equation (3), but did not increase the concentration of drug above its

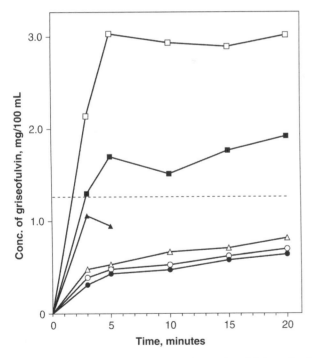

Figure 18 Dissolution rates of various griseofulvin and griseofulvin-succinic acid samples as determined by the oscillating bottle method: griseofulvin, crystalline (●); griseofulvin, micronized (▲); eutectic mixture (■); physical mixture at eutectic composition (○); solid solution (□); physical mixture at solid solution composition (△). The dashed line indicates the equilibrium solubility of griseofulvin in water. *Source*: From Ref. 58.

equilibrium solubility. Second, physical mixtures of griseofulvin and succinic acid, at ratios corresponding to those in the solid solution and eutectic mixture, had dissolution rates similar to griseofulvin alone. Therefore, succinic acid does not itself increase the solubility of griseofulvin (e.g., by a complexation mechanism). Finally, the solid solution and the eutectic mixture were very rapidly soluble. Both gave supersaturated solutions, as predicted by equation (16), because of the extremely small—in the extreme case, molecular—size of the griseofulvin "particles" in these states.

Solid solutions and eutectic mixtures have been used, at least in research laboratories, to increase the rate of dissolution of drugs (59). However, since the drug is in an unstable thermodynamic state, it is critical that the stability of the formulation be maintained. Otherwise, the preparation may revert to a state of having even less favorable dissolution properties than those of a micronized formulation, as shown by the dissolution characteristics of the physical mixtures in Figure 18.

Concentration of the Dissolved Drug in Bulk Solution

In equations (3–5), the saturation solubility of the drug in the diffusion layer is not the only concentration affecting the resulting dissolution rate. The determinant is, rather, the difference between c_s (or more precisely c_h) and c_t, the concentration of dissolved drug in the bulk fluids of the GIT. Thus, the driving force for dissolution is the concentration gradient, "$c_s - c_t$" (or more precisely "$c_h - c_t$"). It is usually assumed that c_t is much smaller than c_s (or c_h), meaning that dissolution occurs under sink conditions. If a drug is absorbed through the GI membrane very slowly, drug concentration in the GIT fluids may build up. This buildup can, by decreasing the gradient, decrease the resulting dissolution rate. Additionally, the bulk fluids may not be identical with the solubilizing fluids of the stationary diffusion layer. A drug may be more soluble in the boundary layer and then precipitate in the bulk fluids, especially if the pH differs between these two sites (as described earlier). However, these precipitated particles are often quite small, and thus may rapidly redissolve (see the dissolution scheme presented in Fig. 11). On the other hand, the drug may be more soluble in the bulk fluids than in the unstirred boundary layer because of a difference in pH or by complexation with other components. Also, the volume of the bulk fluids is much larger than the volume of the boundary layer. Thus, a large absolute amount of drug in the bulk fluids may still give a small value of c_t.

Figure 4 illustrates a situation in which this may not be true. When 250 mL of water was taken with erythromycin tablets, the extent of absorption was much greater than when the tablets were taken with only 20 mL of water. In the latter case, dissolution probably did not occur under sink conditions. Hence, the dissolution rate decreased, and it appears that not all of the erythromycin had a chance to dissolve in the GIT. As a general rule pharmacists should advise patients to take their oral medications with a full glass of water to ensure that dissolution occurs under optimal conditions.

Diffusion Coefficient Divided by the Thickness of the Stationary Diffusion Layer, *D/h*

Although it is possible to control the dissolution rate of a drug by controlling its particle size and solubility, the pharmaceutical manufacturer has very little, if any, control over the *D/h* term in the Nernst–Brunner equation (equation 3). The thickness of the unstirred diffusion layer, *h*, probably increases as particle size increases. Furthermore, *h* decreases when the "stirring rate" increases. In vivo, as GI motility increases or decreases, *h* can be expected to decrease or increase. It has to be pointed out that drug particles in a pharmaceutical formulation are often polydisperse (60). Their size distribution in terms of number of particles tends to be skewed toward the smaller particles. Furthermore, as dissolution proceeds, the particles become smaller. Hence, h can vary considerably both initially and throughout the dissolution process.

The other virtually uncontrollable term in equation (3) is D, the diffusion coefficient of the drug within the liquid unstirred boundary layer surrounding the drug particle. For a spherical, ideal drug molecule in a highly diluted solution, the following equation can be used to calculate D:

$$D = \frac{kT}{6\pi\eta R} \tag{17}$$

where k is the Boltzmann's constant, T the absolute temperature, R the radius of the molecule in solution, and η the viscosity of the solution.

Both, k and π are constants. The radius R is a property of the drug molecule. The viscosity, η, of the GI fluids can vary. An increase in the viscosity decreases the dissolution rate. In addition, increasing the viscosity of the stomach's contents slows gastric emptying, thereby delaying delivery of the drug to the generally most important absorption site (the small intestine). Increasing the temperature of the GI fluids tends to increase the diffusion rate. Patients might be advised to take oral dosage forms with warm liquids. However, extremely hot liquids will delay stomach emptying. In summary, D and h are largely uncontrollable factors, although they may influence drug availability.

GASTROINTESTINAL MEMBRANE TRANSPORT

Once a drug is in solution at the absorption site, it must move through the GIT membrane and then into the general circulation. In chapter 2, Fick's law was used to describe this transport:

$$\frac{dM}{dt} = D_{\text{membrane}}\, S_{\text{membrane}}\, R_{\text{membrane/aqueous}}\, \frac{c_t - c_{\text{blood}}}{L} \tag{18}$$

with dM/dt the amount of drug transported through the membrane in the time interval dt, D_{membrane} the diffusion coefficient of the drug in the membrane, S_{membrane} the surface area of the membrane, $R_{\text{membrane/aqueous}}$ the partition coefficient of the drug between the membrane and the aqueous contents of the GIT, c_t the concentration of dissolved drug in the GIT contents at time t, c_{blood} the drug concentration in the blood, and L the thickness of the membrane.

The larger the value of c_t is, the more quickly the drug moves through the membrane. This c_t is the same concentration of dissolved drug in the bulk fluids that was minimized in equations (3) and (5) to increase the rate of dissolution (Fig. 12). As the bulk fluids of the GIT are aqueous, c_t increases as the water solubility of the drug increases; $R_{\text{membrane/aqueous}}$, however, decreases. Thus, to be absorbed, a drug can neither be so lipophilic that it will not dissolve in the aqueous fluids of the GIT nor so hydrophilic that it will not penetrate into the lipid GI membranes. Lipinski and colleagues empirically derived the "Rule of 5" (Table 6) (61). This rule allows drug developers to select drug candidate molecules with acceptable hydrophilicity and lipophilicity, that is, molecules likely to have good oral availability. Although diffusion across the GI membrane can be one of the major rate-limiting steps in oral absorption, it has been extensively covered in chapter 2 and will not receive further treatment here.

Table 6 The "Rule of 5": Drugs that have More than Two Strikes Are Likely to Be Poorly Absorbed on Oral Administration

1. There are more than 5 H-bond donors (expressed as sum of OHs and NHs)
2. There are more than 10 H-bond acceptors (expressed as the sum of Ns and Os)
3. Molecular weight is > 500
4. $\log P$ is > 5
5. Compounds that are substrates for biological transporters are exceptions to the rule

Source: Ref. 61.

The GI wall is not, however, an *inert* barrier. Some drugs may be actively transported into the enterocytes, as discussed in chapter 2. Additionally, it is known that there are efflux transporters in these cells. The most studied is P-glycoprotein (P-gp), which is a relatively nonselective carrier for a wide variety of drugs (62). In addition, the enterocytes also contain drug-metabolizing enzymes, particularly cytochrome P4503A4 (CYP3A4), which metabolizes a significant number of marketed drugs (63). To further complicate the picture, some drugs are substrates of both P-gp and CYP3A4 (57). Thus, drug molecules that are absorbed from the lumen of the GI tract may be pumped back out and/or metabolized before they reach the blood. This will limit the overall availability of these drugs. As if this were not enough of a challenge, both P-gp and/or CYP3A4 can be upregulated and/or downregulated by other drugs, herbal products, and food (62–65).

REMOVING THE DRUG FROM THE SITE OF ABSORPTION

The fourth basic process that may influence drug absorption is the removal of the drug from the site of absorption. Drugs that have crossed the GI membrane generally are removed in the flowing blood (66). It can be seen in equation (18) that if there were no blood flow, the concentration of drug in the blood, c_{blood}, would quickly approach c_t, and net transfer of drug across the GIT would cease. Thus, a decreased blood flow might decrease the rate or removal of passively absorbed drugs (67,68). Decreased flow could possibly also interfere with active transport systems owing to the reduction of the supply of oxygen to the tissues. Winne and Ochsenfahrt (68) and Winne (69) have developed models and derived equations for GI absorption considering both blood flow and countercurrent exchanges. For the following theoretical discussion, a simplified equation is presented as a modification of equation (18) (66):

$$\frac{dM}{dt} = \frac{c_t - c_{blood}}{1/P_{membrane}S_{membrane} + 1/\alpha\,BF} \tag{19}$$

where $P_{membrane} = D_{membrane}R_{membrance/aqueous}/L$, α is the fraction of blood flowing through the capillaries near the GI membrane, and BF the GI blood flow.

The denominator of equation (19) can be interpreted as the resistance of the region between the GI lumen and the blood pool. Winne and Remischovsky (70) divided this resistance into two parts (first and second terms of the denominator): (*i*) the resistance to transport in the region between the gastrointestinal lumen and the capillary blood (mainly resistance of the membrane) and (*ii*) the resistance to drainage by blood. Figure 19 indicates the influence of blood flow on the rate of intestinal absorption for eight substances from the jejunum of the rat. The absorption of highly permeable materials

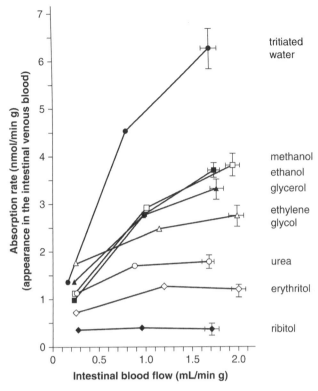

Figure 19 Dependence of intestinal absorption on blood flow as reported by Winne and Remischovsky. All data are corrected to a concentration of 50 nmol/mL in the solution perfusing jejunal loops of rat intestine. Bracketed points indicate the 50% confidence intervals. *Source*: From Ref. 70.

(those with a small first term in the denominator of equation 19), such as very lipid-soluble or pore-diffusable substances, should be blood flow limited. Conversely, the absorption rate of drugs characterized by low membrane permeability (those with a large first term in the denominator of equation 19) may be independent of blood flow. From Figure 19 it may be seen that the absorption of freely permeable tritiated water is very sensitive to blood flow, but that ribitol, a sugar that penetrates the GI membrane with great difficulty, is essentially unaffected by changes in the intestinal blood flow in the range studied. As would be expected from equation (19), the absorption rate of intermediate substances, such as urea, appear to be flow limited at low blood flow rates, but then become insensitive to blood flow at higher rates. Winne and coworkers (67–70) have reported a blood flow dependence for several relatively small drug molecules. Crouthamel et al. (71) also noted a decrease in the absorption rate of sulfaethidole and haloperidol as a function of decreased mesenteric blood flow rates, using an in situ canine intestinal preparation. Haas and coworkers (72), using a guinea pig model, found a strong correlation between spontaneously varying portal blood flow and the amount of digitoxin and digoxin absorbed following intraduodenal infusion of the drug. Digitoxin, the most lipophilic of the cardiac glycosides chosen, shows the most pronounced effects as a function of the blood flow. Digoxin also showed increasing absorption rates as a function of blood flow. Ouabain, the most hydrophilic of the three, showed no such dependence.

These results are consistent with the predictions of equation (19) for the effects of blood flow on the absorption rate of drugs.

These animal studies should indicate to the pharmacist that blood flow can, under certain circumstances, be an important patient variable that may affect the absorption of drugs. Patients in heart failure would generally be expected to have a decreased cardiac output and, therefore, a decreased splanchnic blood flow. This can lead to a decreased rate of absorption for drugs when the blood flow rates in equation (19) become rate limiting. Other disease states and physical activity can also decrease blood flow to the GIT (1–3). Thus, the pharmacist must be aware of the possible effects of the blood flow rate, especially alterations in the rate, on the availability of drugs.

PHYSICOCHEMICAL VERSUS BIOCHEMICAL FACTORS INFLUENCING DRUG ABSORPTION AND DRUG AVAILABILITY

The extent of oral drug availability (F_{oral}) may be described as the product of absorption availability (F_{abs}), the extent of availability through the gastrointestinal membranes (F_G), and the availability through the liver (F_H):

$$F_{oral} = F_{abs}F_G F_H \tag{20}$$

First-pass loss in the GIT will be due to metabolic processes within the intestinal membrane (due primarily to CYP3A and phase 2 enzymes present in the intestine such as glucuronosyltransferases, sulfotransferases, and glutathione S-transferases). First-pass *hepatic* loss will be due to liver metabolism as well as biliary excretion. Although transporters present in the intestinal epithelium can affect F_G, their consequences are probably reflected as a result of changes in intestinal metabolism. Absorption transporters should decrease intestinal metabolism by accelerating the drug transport through the intestinal membrane and allowing less access of drug to intestinal enzymes, while efflux transporters would increase intestinal metabolism since the drug molecule may be repeatedly absorbed by passive processes increasing access to intestinal enzymes (73). While extremely important in determining bioavailability, P-gp efflux transporters are outwith the scope of this text. It is true, however, that excipients in formulations (such as surfactants) (74) can affect P-gp function, and this can change the normal behavior of these influential efflux pump systems (for further reading see Ref. 75).

The physicochemical processes described in detail in this chapter (i.e., disintegration, dissolution, saturation solubility, and diffusion) will primarily affect the F_{abs} term in equation (20). However, these physicochemical processes, together with gastric emptying and gastrointestinal motility, can also affect the *rate* of absorption, as described earlier in this chapter. For a drug susceptible to GI metabolism, F_G could be expected to increase if absorption rate could increase to the point that intestinal metabolism could be saturated, leading to further increases in F_G. In a similar manner a fast absorption rate could also possibly lead to saturation of hepatic enzymes during first pass resulting in an increase in F_H.

SUMMARY

Drug availability following oral dosing may be thought of as the result of four basic steps: (*i*) getting the drug to its absorption site, (*ii*) getting the drug into solution, (*iii*) moving the dissolved drug through the membranes of the GIT, and (*iv*) moving the drug away from the site of absorption into the general circulation. Although steps (*i*), (*iii*), and (*iv*) were discussed briefly, these topics are also found in chapters 2 and 5 of this volume. Step (*ii*) and the combination of factors influencing the dissolution rate of a drug from its dosage form served as the major topic of this chapter. Dissolution rate was discussed in terms of the parameters found in the Nernst–Brunner equation (equation 3). Although this equation is derived in terms of a specific model for dissolution, which, in fact, may not always accurately describe the physical process, we believe that the treatment gives pharmacists a point of reference from which they can predict and interpret availability data that are rate limited by the dissolution step. Two terms in the Nernst–Brunner equation are of major importance and are susceptible to manipulation by the pharmaceutical manufacturer in preparing the dosage form, by the patient in the manner in which he or she takes the drug and stores it between drug dosing, and by the biological system, specifically the GIT of the patient, through interactions with the dosage form and the drug. These two variables are the effective surface area of the drug particles and the saturation solubility of the particular chemical form of the drug. We believe that pharmacists must be aware of these variables and how they can change in each of the three situations listed previously before they can make rational judgments about which of many pharmaceutical alternatives should be dispensed under a specific set of conditions. Knowledge of these variables and their potential for change also allows pharmacists to make rational assumptions about possible drug-related factors that may be responsible for ineffective drug treatment. Under these conditions, pharmacists may be able to recommend an alternative formulation that will prove to be efficacious.

REFERENCES

1. Bachrach WH. Physiology and pathologic physiology of the stomach. Ciba Clin Symp 1959; 11: 1–28.
2. Davenport HW. Gastric digestion and emptying: absorption. In: Davenport HW, ed. Physiology of the Digestive Tract. 3rd ed. Chicago: Year Book Medical Publishers, 1971:163–171.
3. Benet LZ, Hoener B. Pathological limitations in the application of rate control systems. In: Prescott L, ed. Proceedings of the 2nd International Conference on Drug Absorption: Rate Control in Drug Therapy. Edinburgh: Churchill-Livingstone, 1983:155–165.
4. McConnell EL, Fadda HM, Basit AW. Gut instincts: explorations in intestinal physiology and drug delivery. Int J Pharm 2008; 364:213–226.
5. Tuleu C, Basit AW, Waddington WA, et al. Colonic delivery of 4-aminosalicylic acid using amylose-ethylcellulose-coated hydroxypropylmethylcellulose capsules. Aliment Pharmacol Ther 2002; 16:1771–1779.
6. Welling PG. Effect of food on drug absorption. Annu Rev Nutr 1996; 16:383–415.
7. Zhou XJ, Lloyd DM, Chao GC, et al. Absence of food effect on the pharmacokinetics of telbivudine following oral administration in healthy subjects. J Clin Pharmacol 2006; 46:275–281.
8. Paulson, SK, Vaughn MB, Jessen SM, et al. Pharmacokinetics of celecoxib after oral administration in dogs and humans: effect of food and site of absorption. J Pharmacol Exp Ther 2001; 297:638–645.
9. Welling PG, Huang H, Hewitt PF, et al. Bioavailability of erythromycin stearate: influence of food and fluid volume. J Pharm Sci 1978; 67:764–766.
10. Bates TR, Sequeira JA, Tembo AV. Effect of food on nitrofurantoin absorption. Clin Pharmacol Ther 1974; 16:63–68.
11. Schmidt LE, Dalhoff K. Food-drug interactions. Drugs 2002; 62:1481–1502.
12. Osman MA, Ptael RB, Schuna A, et al. Reduction in oral penicillamine absorption by food, antacid, and ferrous sulfate. Clin Pharmacol Ther 1983; 33:465–470.
13. Schuna A, Osman MA, Patel RB, et al. Influence of food on the bioavailability of penicillamine. J Rheumatol 1983; 10:95–97.

14. El-Kommos ME, Saleh GA, El-Gizawi SM, et al. Spectrofluorometric determination of certain quinolone antibacterials using metal chelation. Talanta 2003; 60:1033–1050.
15. Fara JW. Physiological limitations: gastric emptying and transit of dosage forms. In: L. Prescott, ed. Proceedings of the 2nd International Conference on drug Absorption, Rate Control in Drug Therapy, Edinburgh, 1983:144–150.
16. Dooley CP, Di Lorenzo C, Valenzuela JE. Variability of migrating motor complex in humans. Dig Dis Sci 1992; 37:723–728.
17. Manninen V, Apajalahti A, Melin J, et al. Altered absorption of digoxin in patients given propantheline and metoclopramide. Lancet 1973; 1:398–400.
18. Regardh CG, Lundborg P, Persson BA. The effect of antacid, metoclopramide and propantheline on the bioavailability of metoprolol and atenolol. Biopharm Drug Dispos 1981; 2:79–87.
19. Antonioli JA, Schelling JL, Steininger E, et al. Effect of gastrectomy and of an anticholinergic drug on the gastrointestinal absorption of a sulfonamide in man. Int J Clin Pharmacol 1971; 5: 212–215.
20. Sousa T, Paterson R, Moore V, et al. The gastrointestinal microbiota as a site for the biotransformation of drugs. Int J Pharm 2008; 362:1–25.
21. Noyes AA, Whitney WR. Ueber die Aufloesungsgeschwindigkeit von festen Stoffen in ihren eigenen Loesungen. Z Physikal Chem 1897; 23:689–692.
22. Nernst W, Brunner E. Theorie der Reaktionsgeschwindigkeit in heterogenen Systemen. Zeitschrift fuer Physikalische Chemie 1904; 47:52–110.
23. Fick A. Ueber Diffusion. Annalen der Physik 1855; 94:59–86.
24. Prescott LF, Steel RF, Ferrier WR. The effects of particle size on the absorption of phenacetin in man. A correlation between plasma concentration of phenacetin and effects on the central nervous system. Pharmacol Ther 1970; 11:496–504.
25. Jinno JI, Kamada N, Miyake M, et al. Effect of particle size reduction on dissolution and oral absorption of a poorly water soluble drug, cilostazol in beagle dogs. J Control Release 2006; 111: 56–64.
26. Vogt M, Kunath K, Dressman JB. Dissolution enhancement of fenofibrate by micronization, cogrinding and spray drying: comparison with commercial preparations. Eur J Pharm Biopharm 2008; 68:283–288.
27. Serajuddin ATM. Salt formation to improve drug solubility. Adv Drug Deliv Rev 2007; 59: 603–616.
28. Hussar DA. New drugs of 1995. J Am Pharm Assoc 1996; 36:158–188.
29. Hussar DA. New drugs of 1996. J Am Pharm Assoc 1997; 37:192–234.
30. Hussar DA. New drugs of 1997. J Am Pharm Assoc 1998; 38:155–198.
31. Hussar DA. New drugs of 1998. J Am Pharm Assoc 1999; 39:151–206.
32. Hussar DA. New drugs of 1999. J Am Pharm Assoc 2000; 40:181–231.
33. Hussar DA. New drugs of 2000. J Am Pharm Assoc 2001; 41:229–272.
34. Hussar DA. New drugs of 2001. J Am Pharm Assoc 2002; 42:227–266.
35. Hussar DA. New drugs of 2002. J Am Pharm Assoc 2003; 43:207–248.
36. Hussar DA. New drugs of 2003. J Am Pharm Assoc 2004; 44:168–210.
37. Hussar DA. New drugs of 2004. J Am Pharm Assoc 2005; 45:185–217.
38. New drugs and biologic product approval, 2005. AJHP News. February 15, 2006. Available at: www.ashp.org.
39. New drugs and biologic product approval, 2006. AJHP News. February 15, 2007. Available at: www.ashp.org.
40. Stahl PH. Preparation of water-soluble compounds through salt formation. In: Wermuth CG, ed. The Practice of Medicinal Chemistry. 2nd ed. Amsterdam: Elsevier, 2003:601–615.
41. Nelson E. Influence of dissolution rate and surface on tetracycline absorption. J Am Pharm Assoc 1959; 48:96–103.
42. Nelson E, Knoechel EL, Hamlin WE, et al. Influence of the absorption rate of tolbutamide on the rate of decline of blood sugar levels in normal humans. J Pharm Sci 1962; 51:509–514.

43. Lee CC, Froman RO, Anderson RC, et al. Gastric and intestinal absorption of potassium penicillin V and the free acid. Antibiot Chemother 1958; 8:354–360.

44. Levy G, Sanai BA. Comparison of the gastrointestinal absorption of aluminum acetylsalicylic and acetylsalicylic acid in man. J Pharm Sci 1962; 51:58–62.

45. O'Reilly RA, Nelson E, Levy G. Physicochemical and physiologic factors affecting the absorption of warfarin in man. J Pharm Sci 1966; 55:435–437.

46. Higuchi WI, Hamlin WE. Release of drug from a self-coating surface: benzphetamine pamoate pellet. J Pharm Sci 1963; 52:575–579.

47. Nelson E. Comparative dissolution rates of weak acids and their sodium salts. J Am Pharm Assoc 1958; 47:297–299.

48. Levy G, Leonards JR, Procknal JA. Development of in vitro dissolution tests which correlate quantitatively with dissolution rate-limited drug absorption in man. J Pharm Sci 1966; 54: 1719–1722.

49. Bates TR, Young JM, Wu CM, et al. pH-dependent dissolution rate of nitrofurantoin from commercial suspensions, tablets and capsules. J Pharm Sci 1974; 63:643–645.

50. Javaid KA, Cadwallader DE. Dissolution of aspirin from tablets containing various buffering agents. J Pharm Sci 1972; 61:1370–1373.

51. Poole JW, Owen G, Silverio J, et al. Physicochemical factors influencing the absorption of the anhydrous and trihydrate forms of ampicillin. Curr Ther Res 1968; 10:292–303.

52. Hableblian J, McCone W. Pharmaceutical application of polymorphism. J Pharm Sci 1969; 58: 911–929.

53. Aguiar AJ, Krc J, Kinkel AW, et al. Effect of polymorphism on the absorption of chloramphenicol palmitate. J Pharm Sci 1967; 56:847–853.

54. Sorby DL. Effect of adsorbents on drug absorption. I. Modification of promazine absorption by activated attapulgite and activated charcoal. J Pharm Sci 1965; 54:677–683.

55. Ghazal HS, Dyas AM, Ford JL, et al. In vitro evaluation of the dissolution behaviour of itraconazole in bio-relevant media. Int J Pharm 2009; 366(1–2):117–123.

56. Kwan KC, Alien DJ. Determination of the degree of crystallinity in solid-solid equilibria. J Pharm Sci 1969; 58:1190–1193.

57. Hiestand EN, Higuchi WI, Ho NFH. Theories of dispersion techniques. In: Lachman L, Lieberman HA, Kanig JL, eds. Theory and Practice of Industrial Pharmacy. 2nd ed. Philadelphia: Lea & Febiger, 1976:159.

58. Goldberg AH, Gibaldi M, Kanig JL. Increasing dissolution rates and gastrointestinal absorption of drugs via solid solutions and eutectic mixtures. III. Experimental evaluation of griseofulvin-succinic acid solid solution. J Pharm Sci 1966; 55:487–492.

59. Goldberg A. Methods of increasing dissolution rates. In: Leeson IJ, Carstensen JT, eds. Dissolution Technology. Washington, DC: Academy of Pharmaceutical Sciences, American Pharmaceutical Association, 1974:147–162.

60. Benet LZ. Theories of dissolution: Multiparticulate systems. In: Leeson IJ, Carstensen JT, eds. Dissolution Technology. Washington, DC: Academy of Pharmaceutical Sciences, American Pharmaceutical Association, 1974:29–57.

61. Lipinski CA, Lombardo F, Dominy BW, et al. Experimental and computational approaches to estimate solubility and permeability in drug discovery and development settings. Adv Drug Deliv Rev 1997; 23:3–25.

62. Wacher VJ, Salphati L, Benet LZ. Active secretion and enterocytic drug metabolism barriers to drug absorption. Adv Drug Deliv Rev 1996; 20:99–122.

63. Evans WE, Relling MV. Pharmacogenomics: translating functional genomics into rational therapeutics. Science 1999; 286:487–491.

64. Johne A, Brockmoller J, Bauer S, et al. Pharmacokinetic interaction of digoxin with an herbal extract from St. John's wort (Hypericum perforatum). Clin Pharmacol Ther 1999; 66:338–345.

65. Piscitelli SC, Burstein AH, Chaitt D, et al. Indinavir concentrations and St. John's wort. Lancet 2000; 355:547–548.

66. Benet LZ, Greither A, Meister W. Gastrointestinal absorption of drugs in patients with cardiac failure. In: Benet LZ, ed. The Effect of Disease States on Drug Pharmacokinetics. Washington: Academy of Pharmaceutical Association, 1976:33–50.
67. Ther L, Winne D. Drug absorption. Annu Rev Pharmacol 1971; 11:57–70.
68. Winne D, Ochsenfahrt H. Die formale Kinetic der Resorption unter Berucksichtigung der Darmdurchblutung. J Theor Biol 1967; 14:293–315.
69. Winne D. The influence of villous countercurrent exchange on intestinal absorption. J Theor Biol 1976; 53:145–176.
70. Winne D, Remischovsky J. Intestinal blood flow and absorption of nondissociable substances. J Pharm Pharmacol 1970; 22:640–641.
71. Crouthamel WG, Diamond L, Dittert LW, et al. Drug absorption. VII. Influence of mesenteric blood flow on intestinal drug absorption in dogs. J Pharm Sci 1975; 64:661–671.
72. Haas A, Lullman H, Peters T. Absorption rates of some cardiac glycosides and portal blood flow. Eur J Pharmacol 1972; 19:366–370.
73. Wacher VJ, Silverman JA, Zhang Y, et al. Role of P-glycoprotein and cytochrome P450 3A in limiting oral absorption of peptides and peptidomimetics. J Pharm Sci 1998; 11:1322–1330.
74. Doo MH, Li H, Jang HI, et al. Effect of nonylphenol ethoxylates (NPEs) on barrier functions of epithelial cell membranes: opening of tight junctions and competitive inhibition of P-gp-mediated efflux. Int J Pharm 2005; 302:145–153.
75. Takano M, Yumoto R, Murakami T. Expression and function of efflux drug transporters in the intestine. Pharmacol Ther 2006; 109:137–161.

5

Effect of Route of Administration and Distribution on Drug Action

Maureen D. Donovan
Division of Pharmaceutics, University of Iowa, Iowa City, Iowa, U.S.A.

INTRODUCTION

The ultimate goal of drug therapy is to deliver an active pharmaceutical agent to the site(s) within the body where it can exert its desired action. Once a drug is absorbed or delivered to the bloodstream, multiple steps are involved in the process of subsequently delivering the drug to its active site, and the steps involved are commonly referred to as *drug distribution*. These distribution steps rely on the same transfer processes that are involved in drug absorption: dissolution within the body fluids or tissues; partitioning, active or facilitated transport across cell membranes; and bulk flow within the vascular system. The accessibility to each of these processes and the order in which they are encountered play a significant role in determining the final distribution of the drug within the body. As an example, when hydrocortisone, an anti-inflammatory corticosteroid with significant immunosuppressive activity, is administered intravenously (as the water-soluble sodium phosphate or sodium succinate ester), it rapidly reaches many of the tissues within the body and exerts multiple pharmacologic effects. These ester prodrugs can also be injected intramuscularly, and similar systemic effects are observed because of the rapid absorption of the drug into the vascular system. Hydrocortisone can also be administered orally via liquid or solid dosage forms, but since the orally absorbed drug first travels via the bloodstream to the liver before it reaches the rest of the body, some of the drug is metabolized, and not all of the absorbed drug is able (or "available") to reach the other body tissues. The amount of hydrocortisone that can be administered via these systemic delivery routes is limited by the wide variety of pharmacologic effects it exerts throughout the body, so other modes of administration have been developed. To maximize its anti-inflammatory effects while limiting secondary effects at distant body sites, methods to deliver hydrocortisone "locally" have also been developed. Hydrocortisone acetate is injected directly into joint spaces (intra-articular or intrasynovial administration) or into soft tissue spaces. Topical applications of various forms of hydrocortisone (typically ester derivatives) directly to the skin surface in creams, ointments, and lotions; to the eye in combination with antibiotics; or even rectally in suppositories or as a foam have been marketed.

The need to administer this single pharmacologic agent as different chemical analogs and in various dosage forms to achieve the desired effect while limiting secondary effects is driven by the need to control the absorption and subsequent distribution of a drug to maximize its effectiveness while minimizing exposure to other body systems. This balance is achieved (or at least attempted) by knowledge of the factors controlling the absorption and distribution of the drug within the body.

In most cases, it is the goal of *systemic* drug administration to have the drug enter the bloodstream and be carried rapidly throughout the rest of the body. The drug is initially "diluted" by the blood volume, and the resulting concentration in the blood becomes the driving force for passive diffusion of the drug out of the vascular system into the adjacent tissues where the concentration is lower (see chap. 2, equation 2). It does this by leaving the bloodstream and entering the adjacent tissues, either by partitioning, by active transport across the vascular tissues, or by escaping between the vascular endothelial cells in regions where the vasculature might be considered "leaky" (e.g., liver, respiratory tract). Once in the adjacent tissues, further diffusion of the drug to more distant tissues is the result of the concentration gradient then present between these tissues. This process continues as long as the new drug continues to enter the bloodstream and results in the exposure of all of the body tissues to the drug. Because of the varying compositions of the tissues and the resulting partitioning and binding differences, however, vastly different drug concentrations may exist in different regions along with associated differing pharmacologic effects and differing durations of these effects.

At the same time while the bloodstream is delivering the absorbed drug throughout the body, other processes are acting to eliminate the drug from the body or from particular regions of the body through processes generally referred to as "clearance." The major organs for metabolism and excretion in the body are the liver, kidneys, and lungs, yet nearly all of the other tissues also exhibit some ability to metabolize and clear drugs. Transporters present within the cell membranes can also act to escort drugs out of individual cells (see chap. 2). These clearance mechanisms result in the reduction of drug concentrations within cells, organs, and tissues and eventually result in the depletion of the drug from the body.

GENERAL ASPECTS OF DRUG DISTRIBUTION[a]

Figure 1 provides a diagram that summarizes the processes of distribution after the drug reaches the general circulation and demonstrates that drug distribution is critical in designing appropriate drug dosage regimens. This has led to the determination of "apparent" volumes of distribution (as discussed in chap. 3), which can be used to relate the amount of drug in the body (or in a hypothetical compartment of the body) to a measured plasma or blood concentration. The volume of distribution is a function of four major factors: (*i*) the size of the organs into which the drug distributes; (*ii*) the partition coefficient of the drug between the organ and the circulating blood; (*iii*) the blood flow to the distributing organs; and (*iv*) the extent of protein binding of the drug both in the plasma and in various tissues.

Effects of Organ Size, Blood Flow, and Partition Coefficient on Distribution

A particular organ in the body may act as a site of distribution or as a site of both distribution and elimination. The relative importance of the various organs as storage or

---

[a]Excerpted from Oie and Benet, Modern Pharmaceutics, 4th Edition.

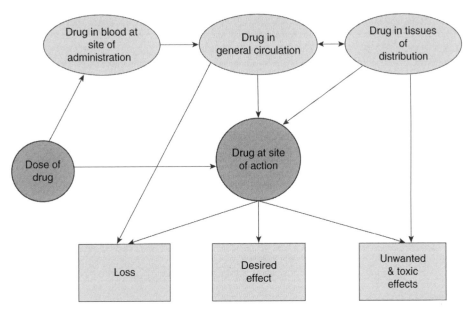

Figure 1   Process of drug absorption and distribution following administration of a single dose. The drug reaches the desired site of action either directly or via the general circulation. The drug may also reach other tissue sites or may be eliminated by physiologic clearance mechanisms. *Source*: Modified from Ref. 1.

elimination sites depends on how fast the drug gets to each organ and how much space or volume is available to hold the drug. Table 1 presents a compilation of the volumes and blood flows of the different regions of the human body for an average adult male, as compiled by Dedrick and Bischoff (2) by using the mean estimates of Mapleson (3).

The various regions of the body are listed in decreasing order relative to blood flow per unit volume of tissue (adrenals highest and bone cortex lowest). This value essentially describes how fast a drug can be delivered to a body region per unit volume of tissue and reflects the relative rates at which tissues may be expected to come to equilibrium with the blood. How much drug can be stored or distributed into a tissue will depend on the size of the tissue (volume) and the ability of the drug to concentrate in the tissue (i.e., the partition coefficient between the organ and blood, $K_{O/B}$). For example, the blood flow per unit volume of thyroid gland (Table 1) is one of the highest in the body, whereas the gland itself is quite small. Thus, if partition of the drug between the thyroid and blood were approximately 1, we would expect to see that the drug in the tissue would rapidly come into equilibrium with that in the blood but that a relatively small total amount of drug would actually be present in the thyroid. In comparison, for certain drugs containing iodine moieties, $K_{O/B}$ for the thyroid is very large, and a significant amount of drug will distribute into this small gland relatively rapidly. In addition, Table 1 lists the volume of blood contained within each tissue and is believed to be in equilibrium with the tissue. Thus, the volume of the thyroid in Table 1 is considered to be 20 mL of tissue and 49 mL of blood. Note that total volume of all tissues in column 3 is 70 L, including the 5.4 L of blood volume. This blood volume can be further categorized into 1.4 L of arterial blood (listed in the last column as being in equilibrium with the air in the lungs) and 4 L of venous blood (in equilibrium with tissues A through O).

When discussing drug distribution, it is often convenient to combine various tissue regions into general categories. For example, following an IV bolus injection, the heart,

Table 1 Volumes and Blood Supplies of Different Body Regions for a Standard Man[a]

Tissue	Reference letters	Volume (L)	Blood flow (mL/min)	Blood flow (mL/100 mL)	Volume of blood in equilibrium with tissue (mL)
Adrenals	A	0.02	100	500	62
Kidneys	B	0.3	1240	410	765
Thyroid	C	0.02	80	400	49
Gray matter	D	0.75	600	80	371
Heart	E	0.3	240	80	148
Other small glands and organs	F	0.16	80	50	50
Liver plus portal system	G	3.9	1580	41	979
White matter	H	0.75	160	21	100
Red marrow	I	1.4	120	9	74
Muscle	J	30	300/600/1500	1/2/5	185/370/925
Skin				1/2/5	18/37/92
Nutritive	K	3	30/60/150		
Shunt	L		1620/1290/300	54/43/10	
Nonfat subcutaneous	M	4.8	70	1.5	43
Fatty marrow	N	2.2	60	2.7	37
Fat	O	10.0	200	2.0	123
Bone cortex	P	6.4	≈ 0	≈ 0	≈ 0
Arterial blood	Q	1.4			
Venous blood	R	4.0			
Lung parenchymal tissue	S	0.6			
Air in lungs	T	2.5 + half Tidal Volume			1400[b] 999/795/185[c]
Total		70.0[d]	6480		5400

[a]Standard man = 70-kg body weight, 1.83-m^2 surface area, 30–39 years old.
[b]Arterial blood.
[c]Skin-shunt venous blood.
[d]Excluding the air in the lung.

brain, liver, and kidneys achieve the highest and earliest drug concentrations, with equilibrium between these tissues and blood being rapidly achieved. Thus, Dedrick and Bischoff (2) combined these tissues and other well-perfused regions (see A through H in Table 1) into a well-perfused compartment that they designate as the viscera. Similarly, regions I, J, K, and M are combined into a "lean tissue" compartment, whereas poorly perfused regions N and O are designated as the adipose compartment. Blood flows and volumes for these compartments can be calculated by summing the appropriate terms in Table 1.

Using a similar perfusion model containing these three lumped compartments and a blood compartment, Bischoff and Dedrick (4) were able to describe thiopental concentrations in various tissues, as shown in Figure 2. Concentrations in the dog liver, representative of the visceral tissues, are already at a maximum by the time the first sample is taken, since very rapid equilibrium is achieved between these tissues and the blood. Drug uptake into the less well-perfused skeletal muscle, representative of the lean tissue, is slower, with a peak concentration occurring at about 20 minutes with an

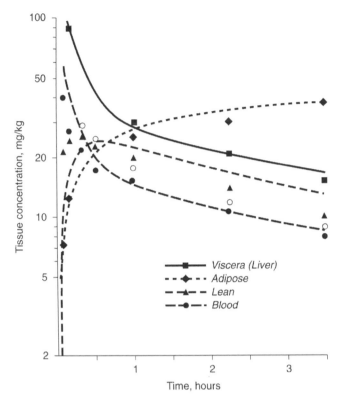

Figure 2 Thiopental concentration in various tissues following 25 mg/kg IV bolus doses. Solid symbols indicate data in dogs; the open circles represent data from humans. Lines correspond to predicted values in various tissues using a perfusion model containing compartments corresponding to the blood, viscera, lean, and adipose tissues. *Source*: From Refs. 1 and 4.

apparent distribution equilibrium occurring between one and two hours. Uptake into the poorly perfused adipose tissue is even slower. In fact, peak levels in this tissue had not been reached by the time the last samples were taken.

Since the site of action for the barbiturates is the brain, we might expect the pharmacologic activity to correspond to the time course of thiopental concentrations in the viscera, which, in turn, would be approximated by blood levels, since a rapid equilibrium is attained between the viscera and the blood. Although the pharmacologic action of thiopental may terminate quickly (within an hour) owing to decreased blood and brain concentrations, traces of the drug may be found in the urine for prolonged periods (days) owing to accumulation in the fatty tissues. At 3½ hours, most of the lipid-soluble thiopental left in the body is in the fat, and at later times, this percentage may even increase before distribution equilibrium is reached. At these later times, the removal rate of the barbiturate from the body will be controlled by the slow movement of drug out of the fatty tissue as a result of the high partition into the fat and the low blood flow to this region.

Protein Binding

The macromolecular protein building blocks present within the body possess a variety of chemical properties. Some contain highly charged regions, and others have tertiary structures that result in regions of significant hydrophobicity or hydrophilicity. Drug molecules that come into contact with these macromolecules may interact with specific regions, and in some cases, this may result in the drug molecule binding with the macromolecule for a considerable period of time, typically via ionic or hydrophobic associations. The interactions can happen in any tissue or compartment within the body, and for the time period that the drug molecule is associated with the macromolecule, it does not contribute to the diffusible concentration of drug molecules. This effectively reduces the concentration of "free" drug and can alter (or determine) the distribution pattern of the drug. While there is still a lack of complete understanding of tissue binding, binding affinities to proteins in the blood are well characterized for a number of drug compounds.

There are two primary proteins within the blood that are involved with most drug binding. They are albumin, which commonly interacts with drugs that have acid properties, and α_1-acid glycoprotein (gp), which binds with a number of basic drug molecules. Some of the lipoproteins present in the blood also interact and bind with certain drug molecules. If a drug has a high binding affinity to one of the plasma proteins, it is likely that most of the drug will remain in the bloodstream rather than penetrate into the body tissues. In such a case, changes in the protein concentration in the blood, specifically a decrease in the concentration, may result in an overall increase in the free concentration of the drug, and more drug will be able to distribute outside of the bloodstream. This may lead to an increase in the pharmacologic effect or in the side effects of the drug. The significance of protein (or other macromolecule) binding cannot be disregarded when determining the distribution pattern of a particular drug substance. In particular, for drugs with significant plasma protein binding, further characterization of the distribution changes in conditions where plasma protein concentrations may be altered are needed to minimize the likelihood of toxic or subtherapeutic concentrations of the drug occurring.

Lymphatic Distribution

The previous discussions focused on the blood as the primary fluid enabling the movement of drug throughout the body. In most parts of the body, the lymph is another fluid that can assist with the bulk transport of drugs and other substances into and out of the tissues. Lymph is initially formed from the interstitial fluid (ISF) present in the tissues of the body. This ISF is originally produced by the pressure-driven flow of fluids across the arterioles. The ISF contains many of the components present within the blood, and substances move from the ISF into cells, and other substances exit the cells and enter the ISF on the basis of the local concentration gradients. Much of the ISF is carried away from the tissues by the venous system, but a significant fraction is also emptied into the lymphatic vessels for clearance. Lymph is moved from the periphery into the larger lymphatic vessels, through the lymph nodes, and is eventually emptied into the venous circulation at the right and left subclavian veins. Thus, all of the materials captured by the lymph eventually become part of the systemic circulation, but the time constant for transport via the lymph is typically much longer than that via the blood circulation since there is no physical pumping mechanism that directly acts on lymph to move it throughout the body. Since the endothelial cells of the lymphatics are not as tightly arranged as those in the arteries and veins, clearance of larger molecules, molecular aggregates, cells, and other particles frequently occurs via the lymph. In many tissues, the ISF and the lymphatics play a major role in the distribution and clearance of drugs, and one should always consider their role when assessing the tissue distribution patterns of drug molecules.

EFFECT OF ROUTE OF ADMINISTRATION

While it would be preferable to deliver a drug only to its target site, this is usually impossible, both because of the inaccessibility of many tissues and because of a lack of information regarding the exact "active site" of many current drug compounds. Thus, systemic administration is typically used to provide a drug throughout the body, which results in its eventual exposure to the pharmacologic target. If, on the other hand, the pharmacologic target can be reached by topical or local administration, far less drug would need to be administered since an effective local concentration could result from drug partitioning from the administration site into and through the local tissues. While it is likely that some drug would eventually reach the vasculature and enter the bloodstream, the amount would be far less than that had the drug originally been delivered via the bloodstream. The barriers encountered, typical absorption and clearance characteristics, and the resulting drug distribution patterns following systemic or local delivery for many of the commonly utilized routes of delivery are the subject of the remainder of this section.

Intravascular Delivery

The most rapid method of delivering a drug to a target organ or to the systemic circulation is to administer it directly into a vein or artery. A key aspect to drug distribution following intravascular delivery is the path of blood flow in the vessel where the drug solution was injected. For intra-arterial administration, the blood will transfer the drug into the tissues being perfused by that specific artery. Unless a large artery is used, this typically results in local exposure to a high concentration of drug. IV administration, in comparison, transfers the drug away from the tissue and into larger and larger veins, thus significantly diluting the drug concentration, which exposes the more distant tissues to safe yet effective concentrations of the drug.

Intra-arterial Administration/Organ Cannulation

Direct organ cannulation involves the placement of a sterile cannula into an artery supplying blood to a specific organ. This is usually accomplished by placing the cannula into one of the major arteries, frequently the femoral artery, and using angiography to direct the cannula to the organ of interest. While invasive, the cannula ensures that high concentrations of drug are presented to the organ while not requiring these same high concentrations throughout the body. This technique is primarily reserved for the administration of chemotherapeutic agents in the localized treatment of cancer and has been used to successfully reduce the tumor burden in organs such as the liver, pancreas, brain, and eye. Because of the blood flow velocity, it is likely that some fraction of the drug administered via the cannula will pass out of the organ without being transferred to the tissues, thus some systemic exposure to the drug will still likely occur.

Accidental intra-arterial administration, when IV access is desired, in comparison, can have significant negative effects, including even death. When an intra-arterial injection is performed, the organ or tissue perfused by the artery is exposed to extremely high concentrations of drug. This frequently results in significant pain and can result in permanent tissue and nerve damage (5).

Intravenous Delivery

The most frequent mode of intravascular drug administration is via a visible or palpable peripheral vein. The drug entering the bloodstream via one of these veins is initially diluted in the regional blood volume and eventually into greater volumes of blood as it is carried away from the injection site toward the superior or inferior vena cava. For drugs or formulations that require rapid dilution or are given in large volumes, administration via a catheter placed in one of the larger veins, frequently the subclavian or femoral vein, can also be used.

Venous blood enters the heart and passes through the lungs where it undergoes reoxygenation. The blood then returns through the heart, passes into the arterial circulation, and is pumped through the rest of the arterial system to perfuse the body tissues. As mentioned previously, the lungs are major metabolic organs, and some of the administered drug may be metabolized during its passage through the lungs prior to reaching the arterial circulation. This "first-pass pulmonary metabolism" may result in a reduction in the drug concentration presented to the peripheral tissues. Additional drug may also be temporarily lost from the blood because of partitioning and binding to the lung tissues. The relative ease and safety of IV administration, as compared with organ cannulation and intra-arterial administration, however, typically far outweigh the slight delay in reaching the desired tissue sites and the potentially reduced drug concentration experienced with this route of delivery.

Nonvascular Parenteral Routes

For medications that do not require an immediate onset of action or would benefit from sustained, constant blood concentrations without requiring constant infusion, administration can be accomplished using superficial, nonvascular injections. Typically, the sites utilized are the large muscles (intramuscular) or subcutaneous tissue spaces. The muscles, and to a somewhat lesser extent, the subcutaneous tissues are well perfused by the vascular system, thus, both of these sites are frequently used for systemic administration. The peritoneal cavity can also be used for the administration of large volumes of drug solution for systemic or local therapies.

Other parenteral delivery sites include the dermis, a region just below the skin (intradermal); the spinal column (intrathecal, intralumbar, or epidural); the joint spaces (intra-articular or intrasynovial); and the eye (intravitreal, subconjunctival).

Intramuscular Administration

The administration of relatively small volumes (<2–5 mL) of concentrated drug solutions or suspensions into large muscles (deltoid, vastus lateralis, gluteus maximus) can result in therapeutic systemic concentrations of drug. The injected volumes spread within the interstitial spaces of the muscle tissue bringing the drug into close proximity with the muscle capillary network. When aqueous drug solutions are administered, absorption into the systemic circulation is quite rapid, and drug distribution patterns are similar to those observed after IV administration of the same drug, often with only a slight delay due to the necessary absorption step. More prolonged action can be obtained using a lipophilic form of drug dissolved in an oil-based vehicle (e.g., sesame oil). Drug absorption is slowed by the necessity for drug partitioning from the oily vehicle into the aqueous-like ISF prior to systemic absorption.

There is the possibility that the drug may not be entirely absorbed from the administration site or it may be metabolized by the enzymes present within the cells or ISF. For example, Doluisio et al. (6) found that only 77% to 78% of an intramuscular injection of ampicillin sodium was absorbed systemically. The remaining ~12% was likely chemically or enzymatically changed to an inactive form.

Drug suspensions, either in oily or in aqueous vehicles, can also be administered intramuscularly, and their absorption is much slower than that of drug solutions. The solid drug must first dissolve in the vehicle and then mix with or partition into the ISF. Since the ISF volume is low, this dissolution step may be quite slow and can result in the continuous absorption of small amounts of drug for extended periods (days, weeks, months) of time. If this small amount of drug results in a therapeutic concentration at the target site, then an intramuscular injection provides an excellent mode of drug delivery. Unfortunately, there are only a limited number of drugs that are suitable for extended delivery following intramuscular injection because of the limited volumes that can be utilized for these injections and the need for a highly potent drug to achieve therapeutic blood levels following the absorption of the small amounts of drug that can be dissolved in the muscle fluids.

Because of the need to accommodate the volume of fluid contained in an intramuscular injection, the large muscles of the upper arm, thigh, abdomen, or buttocks are typically used as sites of administration. While these tissues are quite similar and would be expected to show similar absorption patterns, it has been shown that significant differences in the rate of absorption of lidocaine hydrochloride (7–9) are observed when different muscle sites are utilized, and the absorption differences can be attributed to the differences in regional blood flow to these muscles. Among the deltoid, vastus lateralis, and gluteus maximus muscles, the blood flow is greatest to the deltoid and least to the gluteus maximus; the magnitude of the lidocaine blood concentrations following administration to these muscles was shown to follow the same pattern (Fig. 3). As lidocaine partitions into the blood vessels, the increased perfusion of the deltoid muscle allows the more rapid removal of lidocaine from this muscle, and this results in a higher drug concentration in the blood. If, instead, a slower, more sustained blood concentration is desired, especially for longer-acting dosage forms, it would be best to administer these in the gluteus maximus because of the lower perfusion of this muscle. As one might also expect, the degree of muscle movement may directly impact absorption because of increases or decreases in blood flow. This effect can be directly observed in geriatric patients whose more sedentary nature can lead to poor and erratic absorption of intramuscular dosage forms.

Subcutaneous Administration

The subcutaneous tissues are composed of adipose and connective tissues and are only moderately perfused by the vascular system. As a result, drug absorption following subcutaneous administration is typically slower than that following intramuscular administration, and it may be somewhat erratic, depending on the amount of adipose tissue present at the site. Lipophilic drug compounds, in particular, may partition into the adipose tissue and remain at the delivery site for an extended period of time. The subcutaneous tissues, however, are more loosely arranged than the muscle tissues, and this enables aqueous-based subcutaneous formulations to readily mix with the ISF and allows for rapid systemic absorption of water-soluble compounds. Aqueous-based suspensions can also be administered subcutaneously. Similar to the behavior of suspensions administered intramuscularly, the dissolution step of the solid drug into the ISF can be quite slow, resulting in an extended duration of the effect following administration.

The significant population of lymphatic vessels present within the subcutaneous tissues also influences the resulting systemic distribution pattern of drugs administered subcutaneously. Since systemic bioavailability is typically estimated by measuring the concentration of the drug in the blood following administration, drugs that distribute into

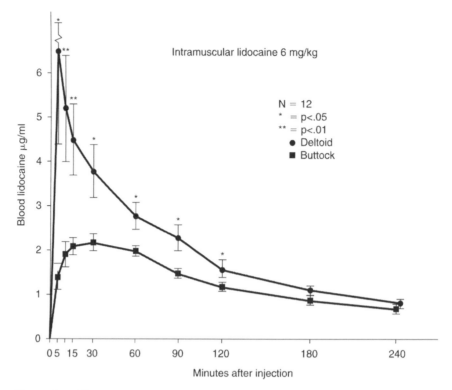

Figure 3 Differences in blood concentration of lidocaine following the intramuscular injection of 6 mg/kg lidocaine (10%) into either the deltoid or the gluteal muscle. Absorption from the deltoid muscle was more rapid than from the gluteus, and higher blood concentrations were obtained from the intradeltoid injection. *Source*: From Ref. 8

the lymph may appear to have lower systemic bioavailabilities while still retaining pharmacologic efficacy. The distribution of drug within the lymph system and its subsequent entry into the vascular system are difficult to precisely control because of the slower flow velocities of the lymph and the dependence of lymphatic clearance on nearby muscle movement. An enhanced effectiveness of a drug whose pharmacologic target is within or associated with the lymphatics may be accomplished using subcutaneous administration.

Intraperitoneal Administration

The peritoneal cavity can accommodate large volumes of fluid and contains a large vascular surface area from the peritoneum, the membrane that defines the cavity. Perhaps the best-known use of the peritoneal cavity is for peritoneal dialysis in the treatment of renal failure. In this case, large volumes of fluids are placed into the peritoneal cavity, and small polar molecules, those typically cleared by the kidneys, equilibrate with the fluids and are thus removed from the body when the peritoneal fluids are evacuated from the cavity. Drugs can also be added to the fluids placed into the peritoneal cavity and can be absorbed into the surrounding vasculature and tissues for systemic delivery. Peritoneal delivery can also be used to administer drugs to the organs of the peritoneal cavity in an effort to limit systemic side effects. A good example of this is the increased survival rate of patients receiving paclitaxel intraperitoneally in addition to IV therapy in the treatment of ovarian cancer (10).

Local Delivery via Injection or Infusion

While limited to highly specialized therapies, the ability to deliver drugs directly via injection to some otherwise poorly perfused or difficult-to-reach tissue sites can enable the local treatment of symptoms or diseases that cannot otherwise be accomplished through systemic administration. Since the drug concentration at any site within the body that is distant from the site of administration is the direct result of the concentration gradient between the blood and adjacent tissue, extremely high blood concentrations are required to reach therapeutic tissue concentrations at many sites. These elevated blood concentrations, however, can lead to numerous unwanted effects of the drug at other sites. Yet, if a tissue site is somewhat isolated or distinct from other nearby structures, it may be possible to inject drug directly into the tissue allowing a local therapeutic concentration to be reached. Since most of these sites receive only a small fraction of the total vascular volume, only small amounts of drug are transferred into the systemic vasculature, and any amounts that are transferred are diluted into the systemic volume of distribution. This typically results in low systemic concentrations of drug and potentially prolonged effective concentrations at the site of administration. Some of the more frequently accessed sites are listed in Table 2.

Mucosal Routes of Drug Administration

While injection of a drug formulation directly into the vascular system or locally at the site of action represents the most reliable method of drug administration, the highly invasive nature of these injections and the risks and discomfort associated with their use

Table 2 Alternative Sites for Direct Injection of Drug Solutions

Site	Characteristics
Cutaneous	
Intradermal	Low volume (<0.1 mL); slow absorption; used for testing allergic response
Intralesional	Used to administer high local drug (e.g., anti-infectives, chemotherapeutics) concentrations
Central nervous system	
Epidural	Local anesthetics; steroids
Intracisternal	Cisterna magna at base of brain; experimental use only
Intrathecal	Into lumbar sac; used for acute and chronic (via pump and catheter) administration
Intraventricular	Requires stereotaxic placement; experimental use
Musculoskeletal	
Intra-articular	Steroids, hyaluronic acid
Intrasynovial	Into soft tissue spaces surrounding joints; steroids, anti-infectives
Ophthalmic	
Anterior chamber	Anti-infectives, anesthetics, viscoelastic agents
Intravitreal	Anti-infectives; placement of drug-eluting implants; gene therapy
Retrobulbar	Behind the eye
Subconjunctival	Used for transscleral delivery
Other accessible organs	
Intracardiac	Infrequently used in emergency medicine; experimental use
Intrapleural	Anti-infectives; anesthetics; chemotherapeutics
Intrauterine	Diagnostics; medical abortion; intrauterine fetal therapy

severely limit their utility in most patient populations. Conveniently, the body possesses several sites containing absorptive epithelia that can be exploited for drug administration. Each of these epithelial surfaces is exposed, either directly or indirectly, to the external environment and is protected by a layer of mucus secreted by cells or glands associated with the tissue. Under normal conditions, the physiologic roles of each of these absorptive sites include nutrient absorption or heat, water, or gas exchange. These sites share common characteristics that enable them to also serve as sites for drug uptake, yet, because of their differing physiologic functions, each of these sites has some unique characteristics that can influence the processes and outcomes of drug absorption.

Mucosal Routes Composed of a Single Epithelial Cell Layer

Gastrointestinal tract The characteristics of the gastrointestinal (GI) tract and the resulting drug absorption from this site are described in detail in chapters 2 and 4, so only a brief description focusing on absorption and subsequent distribution will be provided here. Each segment of the GI tract, stomach, small intestine (duodenum, jejunum, and ileum), and large intestine (colon and rectum), contains a single columnar epithelial layer of cells overlying a submucosal region containing blood and lymph vessels. The primary physiologic function of the GI tract is that of nutrient absorption, thus, the epithelial surfaces have developed a high capacity for the uptake of a variety of chemicals.

Stomach The stomach is responsible for the initial size reduction and chemical breakdown of the ingested foodstuffs. This is accomplished by the contractile activity of the gastric musculature resulting in the mixing and grinding of stomach contents along with the secretion of hydrochloric acid and proteolytic enzymes from the parietal and chief cells, respectively, within the gastric mucosa. Because of the harsh nature of these secretions, the mucus layer overlying the epithelial surface serves to protect the cells from the damaging effects of the secretions. This protective layer can also serve to limit access of other agents, drugs for example, to the cellular surface, thus reducing its absorptive capacity. In addition, the extremely low pH of the secretions limits the absorption of basic compounds at this site because of their highly charged nature under acidic conditions. Any compounds that are absorbed from the stomach and reach the venous blood supply are cleared directly to the liver via the portal vein where they may undergo extensive metabolism prior to reaching the systemic circulation.

Small intestine The epithelial surface of the small intestine, in comparison, is designed for extremely efficient absorption of nutrients. Its total surface area is enhanced by the arrangement of villi on the mucosal surface and by the microvilli present on each epithelial cell. Molecules with good passive permeabilities are well absorbed, and many active and facilitated carrier systems are present within the cells to enhance the absorption of molecules with poor permeabilities. In a protective and clearance function, some of these carrier systems also act to remove molecules from the cell into the intestinal lumen (e.g., P-gp), and high-affinity substrates can see their systemic absorption significantly reduced as a result. The intestinal epithelium, however, has limited capacity to absorb large, macromolecular compounds because of the tight junctional complexes that exist between the epithelial cells, which limit paracellular uptake of these large molecules. This characteristic, combined with the highly proteolytic nature of the luminal contents, limits the utility of the GI tract for the absorption of peptide and protein drug compounds.

The small intestine receives a significant fraction of the total blood volume, and much of the vascular system resides close to the epithelial surface. Each villus on the mucosal surface contains an associated arteriole, venule, and lymphatic vessel, resulting in excellent access to the systemic circulation for drugs absorbed across the intestinal epithelial cells. Drugs taken up by the venous circulation leave the villus, are emptied into the portal vein, and pass through the liver prior to reaching the systemic circulation. As with absorption from the stomach, this passage through the liver can result in significant metabolism of a drug compound, referred to as hepatic first-pass metabolism, and can reduce or nearly eliminate the distribution of the drug outside of the GI tract.

In addition to its role in the absorption of nutrients, the GI tract also plays a role as an immunologic organ. The presence of the lymph system within the entire GI tract facilitates this immunologic role, and in particular, regions of lymphatic tissues organized as nodules referred to as Peyer's patches exist in the lower regions of the small intestine. Drugs can also be taken up by the lymph vessels, and this is a particularly important mechanism for large or extremely lipophilic molecules. Materials transported through the lymph do not enter the portal circulation and thus do not undergo hepatic first-pass metabolism, yet the compounds would still be exposed to metabolic enzymes in the intestinal enterocytes, and even these enzymes can act to significantly reduce the bioavailability of a drug molecule absorbed from the GI tract.

Large intestine   The majority of drug and nutrient absorption takes place in the small intestine, yet the large intestine also contains an epithelial layer capable of absorbing most molecules. While the surface area for absorption is far less than in the small intestine, the epithelial cells still contain microvilli on their luminal surfaces to enhance their absorptive capacity. One of the primary roles of the colon is the reabsorption of water, and this suggests that other small, polar compounds may be reasonably well absorbed in this region. The significance of drug absorption in the colon is demonstrated by the continued drug absorption seen with many extended-release oral dosage forms. Under typical GI transit conditions, well over 50% of the drug release from a 24-hour extended-release dosage form occurs in the large intestine. The continued sustained blood concentrations observed from these dosage forms confirm that good absorption of many compounds also occurs in the large intestine. Improved absorption of many compounds that are subject to proteolytic degradation in the small intestine has also been observed, and this is due, in large part, to the decrease in the population of proteolytic enzymes in the large intestine. The presence of colonic bacteria in the lower large intestine, however, presents a new metabolic barrier, and some drug degradation by these bacteria may occur prior to absorption as a result.

Drugs absorbed from the proximal regions of the large intestine are cleared to the superior and inferior mesenteric veins, which empty into the portal vein, and results in these drugs also being subject to hepatic first-pass metabolism prior to reaching the systemic circulation.

Rectum   The rectum is typically defined to be the distal ∼ 15 cm of the large intestine. It is differentiated from the remainder of the large intestine on the basis of anatomical characteristics and the ability to access this region via the anus rather than needing to rely on transit of material from the upper regions of the GI tract. The mucous membrane in the rectum is somewhat thicker than the tissues in the remainder of the GI tract. While the surface available for absorption is modest in comparison with the other GI segments, both local and systemic effects can be obtained for drugs administered via the rectum. A significant advantage of rectal drug administration is the ability of some of the absorbed drug to bypass first-pass hepatic metabolism. The venous circulation from the rectal tissues involves three primary vessels, the superior, middle, and inferior rectal veins. The superior and middle rectal veins, which drain the upper, approximately, two-thirds of the rectum, empty into the portal vein and expose the drug carried in them to hepatic enzymatic activity. The inferior rectal vein, in comparison, empties into the iliac vein, which eventually empties into the inferior vena cava rather than the portal vein, thus bypassing the liver on first pass. This may lead to an improvement in bioavailability for drugs that have significant hepatic clearance, yet because of the necessity for the drug to be absorbed from the lower rectum, significant variability in bioavailability can be encountered owing to the typical short residence times of dosage forms in this region and to spreading of the drug to other regions of the rectum prior to absorption.

As should be the case for drugs administered for local effect, drug concentrations in the regional tissues are typically much higher than corresponding systemic blood concentrations. An example of this was reported by Ivanov (11) in an investigation of the concentration of hydrocortisone following rectal administration of a foam or suspension containing the drug. A 20-fold increase in tissue concentration, compared with plasma concentration of hydrocortisone, was observed using an optimized foam formulation. These results clearly demonstrate that it is inappropriate to evaluate the effects of a drug administered locally from its systemic concentration.

The rate and extent of rectal absorption is highly dependent on the delivery system used to apply the drug. Various dosage forms, including solutions, suspensions, suppositories, tablets, and foams, have been used to deliver drugs rectally. In an experiment designed to investigate the absorption of metronidazole following rectal administration (Fig. 4), the drug was absorbed most rapidly from a microenema (10 mL volume) and was absorbed most slowly from a fatty base suppository. A PEG base suppository had an absorption rate near that of the microenema, yet the plasma concentration (C_{max}) achieved from the suppository was far greater than that for the enema, likely the result of improved retention of the suppository as compared with the enema. The difference between the two suppository dosage forms was likely due to

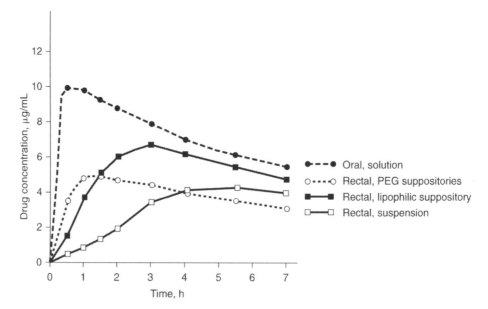

Figure 4 Metronidazole concentrations in the plasma measured after the administration of 500 mg as an oral solution (*filled circles*) or rectally as a suspension (*open circles*) in a PEG base suppository (*filled squares*) or in a fatty base suppository (*open squares*). *Source*: Adapted from Ref. 12.

the more rapid mixing and dissolution of the drug in the rectal fluids from the PEG base than that for the immiscible fatty base formulation, which required an additional partitioning step for the drug to enter the rectal secretions to be available for absorption.

Respiratory tract

Pulmonary region Drug delivery to the lungs is the topic of Chapter 5 in volume 2, thus, only a brief description of drug absorption from this organ will follow to provide a general comparison with other routes of absorption. The lungs receive the entire volume of cardiac output along with a more limited arterial blood supply provided by the bronchial artery. This tremendous volume of blood and the highly permeable epithelium of the lungs suggest that this organ would be an excellent site for drug administration. Indeed, drug absorption from the lungs is extremely rapid and often complete, but the utility of pulmonary delivery is severely limited by the ability to reliably deliver a drug to its intended site of absorption (chap. 5).

The epithelial surfaces in the larger airways (bronchi and bronchioles) are composed of a pseudostratified, ciliated columnar epithelium. Both regions contain goblet cells that secrete mucus over the epithelial surface, and the bronchial epithelium also contains mucus and serous glands. The terminal bronchioles consist primarily of ciliated cuboidal epithelial cells, and the alveoli are comprised of a simple squamous epithelium of two distinct types: alveolar type I and type II cells. The permeability of the alveolar epithelium to gases is well known, but the epithelium has also been shown to be highly permeable to most solutes, including some macromolecules, although absorption of these molecules is somewhat limited because of their size. The bronchial and bronchiolar epithelia are also quite permeable to most small, relatively lipophilic substances, and these regions are frequently the sites for delivery of agents administered for the local treatment of lung disease.

Targeted or local delivery to the bronchial and bronchiolar regions has been effectively used in the treatment of airway diseases such as asthma. Direct inhalation of small (~ 5 μm) drug particles, either in water- or propellant-based aerosols or as dry powders, results in the deposition of these particles along the upper airways, primarily the larger airways. Drug substances dissolve in the mucus layer overlying the epithelial surface and diffuse to the cellular surface where they are absorbed and exert their effects locally. Some of the applied drug may also be absorbed into the systemic circulation, but since these upper airway regions receive only $\sim 2\%$ of total cardiac output, the extent of systemic exposure is somewhat limited. In addition, because of the metabolic capacity of the lung, significant amounts of the drug may be metabolized prior to reaching the systemic vasculature.

An additional factor that acts to reduce the systemic exposure of drugs administered to these airways is the mucociliary clearance system acting at the cellular surface of the larger airways. As previously described, the epithelium in these regions is composed of *ciliated* columnar cells. The cilia on the luminal surfaces act with a coordinated beating pattern to move the overlying mucus layer, along with any entrapped materials, out of the lung and toward the pharynx. The cleared materials are deposited into the esophagus and are transferred to the GI tract for removal. If a significant amount of drug is carried out of the lungs, it is no longer available to exert its local action, and a secondary absorption of the drug can occur in the GI tract, which can result in increased drug concentrations in the systemic circulation.

While the delivery of drugs to the lung for local treatment is important, the large surface area and tremendous blood supply within the lung suggest that this would be an excellent site for systemic drug administration. Unfortunately, from a drug delivery perspective, the pulmonary regions of the lungs are well protected from exposure to nongaseous agents inhaled into the lung. Delivery to this region requires closely controlled, small-sized (~ 2 µm) particles to be carried by the inspired airstream into the alveolar region of the lungs. The drug must then dissolve in or mix with the lung surfactant-containing alveolar fluids, permeate through the alveolar epithelium, and finally reach the associated vascular or lymphatic vessels. While delivery to the alveoli suffers from a lack of efficiency because of losses of drug to the upper airway regions during inhalation, this method has demonstrated its therapeutic and commercial potential by the U.S. FDA approval and marketing of a inhalation device delivering insulin for the treatment of diabetes (Exubera®, codeveloped by Pfizer and Nektar, New York and California, respectively, U.S.). While this product experienced resistance to its adoption by some prescribers and patients, has ongoing issues regarding potential adverse drug effects, and is no longer marketed by the manufacturer, its development and the associated demonstration of efficacy of an inhaled protein-containing drug product validated the potential of this route of delivery for systemically active drug agents.

Because of the dependence of the delivery of drugs to the lungs, either for local or systemic action, on the velocity profile of the inhaled airstream carrying the drug into the lung, significant changes in drug deposition patterns can occur in patients with diseases that increase airway resistance or change airflow patterns. These changes are typically associated with decreased deposition of drug at the intended site and greater losses of drug to the upper airways and associated increases in secondary GI delivery. These deposition changes, along with the subsequent alterations in absorption and distribution patterns, can have significant effects on both the efficacy of the drug and its side effect profile.

Nasal region Similar to the lungs, drug administration to the nasal cavity is most frequently associated with the treatment of local pathologies, including allergies, rhinitis, polyps, etc. Yet, the nasal cavity contains a permeable epithelium that is highly vascularized, as can be attested by anyone who has ever experienced a nosebleed. The nasal mucosa is composed of a single layer of ciliated pseudostratified columnar epithelial cells, and the submucosal region contains a highly responsive vascular system that responds to numerous stimuli with either vasoconstriction or vasodilation and can result in the narrowing of the airways and an associated perception of nasal congestion. The submucosa also contains a significant population of lymphatic vessels, which play important roles in allergic response and immunologic protection. The vascular system empties primarily into the jugular vein and bypasses hepatic first-pass elimination, a significant advantage for this route of delivery.

The primary physiologic roles of the nasal cavity are to cleanse the inspired airstream and warm and humidify the air to near 100% relative humidity and near body temperature. The nasal mucosa also plays an important role in the recovery of water from the exhaled airstream in an attempt to maintain overall physiologic water balance. The short time interval available to accomplish this air conditioning demonstrates that significant heat and water transport can take place across the nasal mucosa in response to the characteristics of the inhaled or exhaled airstream. This is accomplished through the vascular bed acting as a heat sink and supply of water by transudation of its fluid components into the interstitial spaces of the tissue through a highly permeable, fenestrated capillary system. Water is then able to pass rapidly across the leaky epithelium, which possesses fewer tight junctions between the epithelial cells than what is seen in most of the other epithelial tissues. These high permeability and highly vascular properties also make this an excellent site for drug absorption, and this has been exploited both for legitimate and illicit drug therapies.

The leakiness of the nasal mucosa results in high permeabilities of both large molecules and highly polar molecules, most of which typically possess low permeabilities across the tighter epithelia associated with many other delivery sites (13,14). Drugs administered as solutions are typically rapidly absorbed across the nasal mucosa and can enter the systemic circulation within minutes. In many cases, the resulting blood concentrations can mimic those observed following IV administration of an equivalent dose. The small volume of the nasal cavity, however, severely restricts the amount of drug that can be administered via this route, and only a limited number of compounds have sufficiently low doses to achieve therapeutic systemic blood concentrations following nasal administration.

The majority of drugs currently administered via the nasal cavity are intended for local therapy, frequently for the reduction of nasal congestion associated with allergies or colds. These drugs are administered as solutions or suspensions delivered as water-based or propellant-driven aerosols/sprays or drops. Drug administration of dry powders is also under current investigation and is certainly a common mode of cocaine administration for systemic action by illicit drug users. Most of the drugs administered for local effect are also absorbed systemically, but the doses used for local therapy are significantly lower than would be needed for systemic therapeutic effect. The nasal cavity also possesses a considerable population of metabolizing enzymes, both within the mucosal tissues and in the secretions, which serve in a protective role against materials removed from the inspired airstream. Drugs administered to the nasal cavity can undergo significant metabolism prior to their systemic absorption, and this can serve to reduce the systemic exposure for drugs intended for local effect or reduce the bioavailability of drugs intended for systemic effect.

While many drugs are rapidly absorbed from the nasal mucosa, those that have limited permeability may not have a sufficiently long residence time for complete absorption in the nasal cavity because of the mucociliary clearance activity. Just as the ciliated epithelium clears mucus and entrapped materials from the lung, the same mechanisms are operative on the nasal mucosal surface, and unabsorbed substances are efficiently cleared into the nasopharynx, frequently in as little as 15 to 30 minutes. These materials are subsequently swallowed and enter the GI tract where further systemic absorption (or metabolism) may take place. The short and frequently variable residence time for drugs in the nasal cavity has somewhat limited the effective systemic administration of drugs from this site, particularly potent, high molecular weight drugs, such as peptides and proteins.

Numerous reports suggest that a unique distribution pathway exists between the nasal cavity and the brain, which allows drugs administered intranasally to be directly transported into the brain without passing through the systemic vasculature (15). This interesting distribution pattern has been observed for small drug molecules such as dopamine and cocaine (16,17) and for large proteins such interferon β and insulin-like growth factor I (18,19), and can be enhanced for P-gp substrates by the use of P-gp inhibitors (20). The mechanisms responsible for this unique and promising distribution pathway are the subject of current investigation, and most evidence supports that the olfactory region at the uppermost surface of the nasal cavity, along with the trigeminal nerve, plays a role in regulating drug distribution in this pathway.

In addition to the nasal mucosa serving as an administration site for local and systemic drug administration, it has also been successfully utilized for the noninvasive administration of vaccines. As described previously, the nasal mucosa contains a significant population of lymph vessels, all of which eventually empty into the cervical lymph nodes. Macromolecules and particulates can be taken up by the lymphatics, and if antigenic sequences are recognized, a significant immunologic response can be mounted.

The commercialization of intranasally administered vaccines for both human (Flumist®, MedImmune, Maryland, U.S.) and veterinary use (feline upper respiratory infections, Feline UltraNasal® vaccines, Heska, Colorado, U.S.) suggest that this is a promising route for the noninvasive administration of other vaccines currently under development.

Mucosal Routes Composed of Multiple Epithelial Cell Layers

Oral mucosa The tissues within the oral cavity possess varying morphologic characteristics depending on their exact location (Table 3), but, in general, all of the regions are composed of multiple layers of squamous epithelial cells. The number of cell layers differs throughout the oral cavity, but regardless of exact number, these multiple cellular layers represent a greater permeability barrier than for any of the routes described previously containing only a single epithelial layer. Being thinnest, the sublingual region is frequently targeted as the optimal site for drug absorption within the oral cavity. The buccal region is also used frequently because it represents the largest surface area within the mouth. While the gingival region has a keratinized superficial epithelial layer, it is also a common administration site for extended-release dosage forms because of the ability to place a tablet inconspicuously over these surfaces. The vascular system from the oral cavity empties into the internal jugular vein, and unlike most of the rest of the GI tract, drugs absorbed from this site can avoid first-pass hepatic metabolism.

Drugs placed into the oral cavity for either local treatment or systemic absorption must either be in solution as administered or go into solution in the saliva or mucus layers overlying the epithelial cells prior to absorption. Transport across the oral mucosa takes place primarily by passive diffusion across each of the cell layers and thus favors the absorption of relatively lipophilic substances. Unique to the oral mucosa, an additional, noncellular barrier to the absorption of polar molecules also exists several cell layers below the epithelial surface. This barrier is produced by secretions from the prickle cell layer of the mucosa and results in a highly lipophilic intercellular environment that limits the partitioning of hydrophilic substances beyond the barrier. Lipophilic substances, in comparison, can be efficiently absorbed across the mucosal tissue and can yield high systemic bioavailabilities. This rapid and significant systemic absorption is exemplified by the historic use of nitroglycerin in sublingual tablets for the rapid amelioration of angina pain.

The variety of forms of foodstuffs ingested orally have given rise to several nontraditional delivery systems being used for oral mucosal drug administration. These include gums, for example, the nicotine polacrilix gum used as replacement nicotine

Table 3 Regional Differences in Mucosal Tissues in the Oral Cavity

Region	Keratinized surface layer	Approximate thickness (μm)
Buccal	No	500–600
Gingival	Yes	200
Palatal		
Hard	Yes	200
Soft	No	
Sublingual	No	100–200
Tongue		
Dorsal surface	Yes	
Ventral surface	No	

therapy for smoking cessation, and hard candies/lollipops (transmucosal fentanyl citrate). Both of these products were developed to present the incorporated drug in a pleasant, "non-medicinal" form for improved patient acceptance while providing a drug delivery system that could be retained in the oral cavity for a reasonable period of time to increase the amount of drug absorbed into the systemic circulation.

While there can be excellent systemic absorption of drug molecules administered to the oral cavity, in general, the rapid dilution in saliva and the short residence time of the resulting saliva mixture within the oral cavity limit the utility of this route for systemic drug delivery. The subsequent swallowing of the saliva mixture can also result in secondary absorption of the drug agent in the remainder of the GI tract. In addition, any interaction of the drug with the taste receptors on the dorsum of the tongue could elicit a negative response, thus resulting in poor patient utilization of the drug, regardless of its efficacy. Newer delivery systems, including bioadhesive tablets that stick to the mucosal surfaces of the oral cavity and yet can be inconspicuously placed, are being developed to counteract these dilution and residence time effects and have resulted in delivery systems with therapeutically useful bioavailabilities (Striant®, Columbia Laboratories, New Jersey, USA).

Vaginal tissues   Because of the similarities between the dosage forms used both in rectal and vaginal drug administration, the vaginal and rectal mucosa are often believed to behave similarly with regard to their absorption and distribution characteristics. This, however, is an overgeneralization, and closer evaluation shows that the vaginal mucosa has several aspects that affect drug absorption and distribution differently than at other sites of administration.

The vaginal mucosa contains a stratified squamous epithelium composed of five differentiable layers overlying layers of muscle and submucosal tissues containing blood and lymph vessels. The epithelium contains a low population of tight junctions, and instead, cell-cell adhesion is primarily accomplished via desmosomes. The vascular endothelium is also somewhat leaky, which allows for rapid plasma transudation into the vaginal tissues and expedites uptake of macromolecules from the mucosa. The thickness of the vaginal mucosa is estrogen dependent and varies throughout the menstrual cycle, which can lead to intra-patient variability in drug absorption. The blood supply to the vagina originates from multiple nearby regional vessels, including the iliac, uterine, middle rectal, and internal pudendal arteries. The venous return empties directly into the systemic circulation and does not enter the liver directly, thus avoiding first-pass hepatic metabolism. The vaginal mucosa, similar to all of the other epithelia, is a metabolically active tissue, and some local metabolism of vaginally applied drugs can occur.

The vaginal route is typically used for the systemic administration of drugs for female-specific therapies. These include the administration of etonogestrel/ethinyl estradiol as hormonal contraceptives from a controlled-release flexible ring system (NuvaRing®, Organon, New Jersey, U.S.) and progesterone (in various dosage forms) in infertility treatment regimens. In both of these cases, the avoidance of hepatic first-pass metabolism allows lower doses of the drug substances to be administered via the vaginal tract. Recently, reports of increased uterine drug concentrations following vaginal administration compared with systemic administration have been reported (21). This has been coined the "uterine first-pass effect," and it represents a potentially unique distribution pathway that could be exploited for the treatment of uterine-specific pathologies.

A healthy vaginal tract in a woman of child-bearing age contains secretions whose pH is typically in the range of 4 to 5. This low pH is the result of the local conversion of glycogen to lactic acid by the action of the commensal lactobacilli present within the vagina. Prepubescent children and postmenopausal women, however, have vaginal pH values closer to 7. The low pH of the vaginal secretions in adult women can affect drug absorption from the vagina by altering the amount of nonionized drug dissolved in the secretions. Since many drug compounds have a basic character, this will act to reduce the total absorption of these drugs.

The residence time within the vagina can be quite long (at least 24 hours) but is highly variable depending on menstrual cycle and sexual and physical activity. While the extended residence times can be utilized to improve total drug absorption, the intra- and inter-patient variability makes dose reproducibility somewhat difficult for many vaginal delivery systems.

Ocular tissues   Ophthalmic drug delivery systems will be covered in greater detail in Chapter 4 of volume 2, so this short synopsis will only briefly introduce the absorption and resulting distribution properties of drugs administered topically to the eye. Most of the outer surface (80%) of the eye is covered by the conjunctival epithelium; this epithelium is also continuous with the tissues lining the interior surfaces of the eyelids. The conjunctival membrane is composed of a multicellular epithelium and is highly vascularized. The circulatory system within the conjunctiva does not perfuse the remaining ocular tissues and, instead, empties into the systemic circulation.

In general, a significant fraction of a drug solution administered to the eye is lost because of volume overflow from the surface or loss down the nasolacrimal duct. Drug lost to the nasal cavity can subsequently be absorbed or metabolized by the nasal mucosa, potentially resulting in the systemic delivery of the drug. Drugs that come into contact with the conjunctival tissues can be absorbed into the blood vessels associated with this tissue, and this also leads to systemic exposure. Only a small amount of the administered drug is actually absorbed across the ocular tissues, primarily via the cornea. The drug absorbed across the cornea enters the anterior chamber, where it is subsequently diluted and cleared from the eye along with the aqueous humor present in the chamber. Almost no drug is transferred to the posterior chamber following corneal penetration.

Typically, if drug is required in the posterior chamber or at the retina, systemic delivery is used to provide a therapeutic concentration to the retinal or ocular tissues via the arterial circulation. More distant tissues and the vitreous are then reached by the concentration gradient formed at the tissue surface. Alternatively, direct intravitreal injections can be used to place the drug directly into the posterior chamber. The turnover time for the vitreous, however, is rapid, so drug concentrations are not maintained for long periods, and frequent re-administration is necessary. Recently, subconjunctival injections have also been shown to provide drug to the posterior chamber (22). These injections are slightly less invasive than intravitreal injections and may represent a promising technique for drug administration to the posterior chamber. Advances in delivery system development have also brought forth intravitreal implant systems that slowly release drug over many weeks. Obviously, these systems are only suitable for highly potent drug compounds because of size limitations for the implants.

Systemic delivery of peptide and protein compounds following absorption via the conjuctival vasculature has also been attempted in an effort to identify alternatives to injection-based therapy. While this route of administration showed some promise, the limited amount of drug able to be delivered via the eye and the significant degradation of the peptide due to the activity of local proteases demonstrated that this method of delivery required more extensive development to produce an effective delivery system.

Corneal tissues   The cornea is an avascular region of the eye, but nearly all drug penetration from the external surface of the eye into the internal compartment, primarily the anterior chamber, is the result of drug permeation across the cornea. The cornea is a multilayered tissue comprised of a superficial layer of squamous epithelial cells, Bowman's membrane, a collagenous matrix referred to as the stroma, Descemet's membrane, and a single layer of endothelial cells. Compounds that permeate across this tissue must both possess lipophilic character to partition across the epithelium and endothelium and be sufficiently hydrophilic to traverse the stroma. As a result, it is important to optimize the physiochemical properties of drug compounds intended for ophthalmic delivery to assure that they possess the best combination of these characteristics.

Conjunctival scleral tissues   The epithelial layer of the conjuctival tissues is composed of a layer of 5 to 15 stratified squamous epithelial cells. An underlying stromal layer contains blood vessels, lymphatics, and nerves. The epithelial layer represents a significant barrier to the penetration of compounds across the scleral regions of eye, yet the permeability of hydrophilic compounds across the scleral epithelium is significantly greater than that across the cornea. It has been demonstrated that compounds that penetrate the conjuctival tissues can also typically penetrate the underlying sclera and reach the posterior chamber (22).

Non-mucosal Routes of Administration

Skin   Cutaneous and transdermal drug delivery are the topics of Chapter 3 in volume 2, and a more extensive discussion of drug permeation across the skin and its resulting distribution can be found there. As a brief introduction, however, the skin is composed of three anatomical layers, the epidermis, the dermis, and the subcutaneous layer. The epidermis is a multicellular layer containing both metabolically active cells and dead cells. As the cells mature from the basal layer to the external surface, they form an intracellular matrix of crystalline keratin, which plays a major role in the barrier properties of the skin. The dermis contains blood vessels that supply the epidermis with nutrients and oxygen, and it also contains glands that secrete both lipid-like and aqueous-based secretions at the skin surface. The vascular system of the skin bypasses hepatic first-pass metabolism, thus, improved systemic bioavailability of some compounds may be observed following transdermal absorption. Finally, the subcutaneous layer is composed of connective tissue, adipose tissue, and additional blood and lymph vessels.

The physiologic roles of the skin include protection of the body from the elements of the external environment, providing information about the environment (e.g., temperature), and retention of water and other elements within the body. Given that skin primarily serves a physiologic barrier function, it follows that it should also provide a significant barrier to drug absorption. The stratum corneum, the layer of dead, keratinized cells at the external surface of the epidermis, contributes the greatest barrier properties, both to absorption of compounds from the external environment and to loss of substances, particularly water, from the body. The keratinized cells possess a typical cell membrane that excludes all but the most lipophilic substances, and the crystalline intracellular substance contributes an additional, nearly impermeable barrier to these cells. The intercellular spaces of the stratum corneum are filled with a lipid-based material that also provides a significant barrier to the permeation of hydrophilic substances. As a result, the skin is impermeable to nearly all hydrophilic substances, and hydrophobic substances are left to permeate only through the intercellular spaces.

Significant efforts have been devoted to characterizing the optimal properties of compounds for effective permeation across the stratum corneum. In addition, the effects of additional agents that can be combined in topical formulations have been investigated to enhance the delivery of many drugs. In some cases, simply hydrating the stratum corneum can significantly increase the permeability of many substances. This seems to be the result of both hydration of the keratin fibrils within the keratinocytes, improving the permeability of hydrophilic compounds through these cells, and hydration of the polar regions of the lipids within the intercellular spaces, thus making these regions more permeable to a wide variety of compounds.

The hair follicles and sweat glands that penetrate through the skin represent more highly permeable regions on the skin surface, yet, because of their relatively small surface areas, they typically contribute minimally to the total amount of drug absorbed across the skin, except in select cases where the delivery system targets these transport routes (e.g., iontophoretic delivery, nanoparticulate delivery).

The rest of the epidermis is far more permeable to most substances than the stratum corneum, so typically, once a compound has penetrated the stratum corneum, it has ready access to the systemic circulation. For drugs intended for local effect within the skin itself, absorption into the systemic vasculature represents a loss of drug from its primary site of activity. In some cases, topically active drugs are selected or formulated to form depots within the layers of the skin on the basis of their partitioning properties to limit their systemic absorption. In most cases, the amount of drug absorbed, however, is quite small since the local dose of the agent was likely far less than the typical systemic dose. Unfortunately, under some circumstances, excessive transdermal absorption of drugs intended for local therapy can have dangerous and even fatal consequences. This has been recently been demonstrated by the deaths of several women using a topical anesthetic cream prior to laser hair removal (23). In these cases, the women used a lidocaine-containing cream and placed occlusive dressings over the treated regions. This increased the permeability of the lidocaine across the skin because of the hydrating effects of the occlusion, and sufficient lidocaine was absorbed to exert CNS and cardiac effects.

For drugs intended to be administered to the systemic circulation via the skin, a significant amount of drug needs to permeate across the skin and into the vascular system to provide sufficient drug to produce therapeutic blood concentrations. This frequently involves placing a large reservoir of drug on the external surface of the skin and providing a sufficiently large surface area and long-enough time period to transfer the required amount of drug across the skin. Local metabolism of the drug, both prior to absorption by the bacteria present on the skin surface or by the enzymes present within the viable epidermis, can reduce the systemic bioavailability of a drug using the transdermal route for administration.

The number of drugs with optimal permeation characteristics and sufficient potency to be administered via this route is quite limited (24), yet several have been quite successful as commercial products. In addition, considerable effort has also been placed in the development of delivery systems and devices that can enhance the permeability of drugs across the skin. Many of these technologies will be discussed in Chapter 3, volume 2.

EFFECT OF PHYSIOLOGIC CONDITIONS ON DRUG DISTRIBUTION

All of the previous descriptions of drug distribution patterns were based on the physiologic characteristics of a "typical" adult. Yet many adults are not typical, and, as is frequently demonstrated both socially and physically, children are not "mini-adults." In addition, the elderly, while adults, frequently have diminished functionality of many of the key physiologic properties on which we base our generalizations about drug distribution. The remainder of this section will be devoted to a brief introduction regarding some of the major differences among various patient populations that can alter drug distribution patterns and potentially result in ineffective or toxic therapies.

The Pediatric Population (25)

Children have a wide variety of differences in physiology that may affect drug absorption and distribution. Their body masses, body compositions, and surface area/volume ratios change significantly throughout their maturation to adulthood. Infants typically have body water contents of ~80% of total body weight; this fraction decreases by adulthood to ~55%. Similarly, the extracellular water content of an infant is ~40% of total body weight, while in an adult, it is half of this value. These alterations can have dramatic effects on the volumes of distribution of many drugs and will result in significantly different distribution patterns between children and adults of water-soluble drug compounds. Typically, the blood concentration of these drugs will be lower in children, suggesting that an increase in dose is required; yet a significant mass load of drug may actually be located throughout the tissues of the body, and increases in dose may lead to local toxicities or enhanced side effects at many sites.

Plasma protein binding will also influence drug concentrations in the blood, and younger children typically have lower plasma protein concentrations than older children and adults. Binding affinities also seem to be reduced in younger children, and this, along with the presence of additional endogenous substances that act to compete for binding sites, results in total plasma protein binding to be lower in children than in adults. This results in a greater free fraction of a drug for a given total drug concentration and will likely result in higher tissue concentrations of the drug as a result of a steeper concentration gradient between the blood and the tissues.

Many of the tissue barrier functions and metabolic capacities of children are also significantly different from those of adults. Perhaps most critical is the immaturity of the blood-brain barrier in young infants. Until myelination is complete, the barrier properties of the brain are significantly reduced, and this, coupled with the much greater fraction of total body mass that the brain represents in infants compared with adults, results in the possibility for dangerous levels of brain exposure to many drug compounds. A very different barrier, the skin, also shows significant differences between children and adults, a fact that is already appreciated by many health care providers and parents. The skin of children has both a reduced epidermal and a reduced stratum corneum thickness, and the permeation of drugs through children's skin appears to be typically greater than that in adults. This could lead to increased systemic uptake of drugs administered to the skin, whether intended for local or systemic action.

While the absorptive properties of the GI tract appear to be quite similar in children (>6 months in age) and adults, GI motility patterns differ between these two populations. Typically, gastric emptying may be delayed in infants, and the intestinal transit time is shorter in younger children. These differences in motility patterns can result in significantly different absorption patterns for drug compounds and may result in ineffective therapies if the dosing interval is longer than the GI residence time for compounds with short biological half-lives.

The Elderly Population

The aging process causes system-wide changes in body function. Of particular interest regarding drug disposition, alterations in liver and kidney function cause numerous changes in drug metabolism and excretion, which may necessitate decreases in doses, changes in drug therapies to analogs either less susceptible to hepatic extraction or less dependent on renal clearance, or increases in the possibilities that adverse drug reactions will occur (26). With regard to drug absorption and distribution, there are some generalizations that can be made regarding changes in the elderly population compared with younger adults. Typically, there is a reduction in the fraction of total body water and an increase in the proportion of body fat. These changes will affect the volume of distribution of many drugs, as will the observed reduction in plasma protein binding. Other changes are exhibited in GI function, especially in the metabolic and transporter activities in the intestinal tissues, production of gastric acid, and GI motility patterns. Depending on a drug's expected absorption behavior, each of these changes may have a significant effect on the resulting bioavailability from an oral dosage form. The overall reduction in cardiac output and tissue perfusion experienced by the elderly also has a significant effect on drug distribution. Peripheral target sites may have difficulty achieving therapeutic drug concentrations if there is a limited blood supply perfusing the region. Drug absorption from these peripheral sites may also be compromised, thus, drug administration via the skin, or by intramuscular or subcutaneous injection may be more variable and, in general, less efficient than that observed in the younger adult.

Because of the confounding occurrence of multiple physiologic-based pathologies in many elderly adults, it is difficult to define exact cause-and-effect relationships between aging processes and altered drug effects. Regardless of the ability to predict the changes that may occur in the elderly, it is important to identify the changes in individual patients that may alter their individual responses to medications and to modify their therapies accordingly to prevent undesired effects.

SUMMARY

Achievement of a therapeutic concentration of a drug at its site of action within the body involves the interplay of a multitude of complex processes, including those involving the chemistry of the drug and its dosage form and those involving the biochemical and physiologic characteristics of the user. As can be observed from the multitude of routes of delivery and dosage forms available, there is no simple delivery methodology that works best for all drug compounds. Providing optimal drug therapies involves an understanding of the desired pharmacologic target, in particular an estimate of its location within the body; an understanding of the chemical properties of the drug compound; and an understanding of the characteristics of the various body sites at which drugs can be delivered. When the pharmacologic target is localized in a specific region of the body, a targeted local therapy would likely result in the need for a significantly lower dose of the drug with a concomitant reduction in off-target side effects. If systemic therapy is necessary, a coordination of the dynamics of absorption and distribution from the site of administration with those of the desired pharmacologic effect of the drug substance can significantly improve drug therapy. Regardless of whether an individual is the developer of new medications, a prescriber involved in diagnosis and treatment of disease, or a professional involved in medication therapy management, consideration of the role of the route of administration and resulting distribution pattern for a drug product can significantly improve the therapeutic outcome for a patient seeking treatment.

REFERENCES

1. Oie S, Benet LZ. The effect of route of administration and distribution on drug action. In: Banker GS, Rhodes CT, eds. Modern Pharmaceutics. 4th ed. New York: Marcel Dekker, 2002:129–133.
2. Dedrick RL, Bischoff KB. Pharmacokinetics in applications of the artificial kidney. Chem Eng Prog Symp Ser 1968; 64:32–44.

3. Mapleson WW. An electric analogue for uptake and exchange of inert gases and other agents. J Appl Physiol 1963; 18:197–204.

4. Bischoff KB, Dedrick RL. Thiopental pharmacokinetics. J Pharm Sci 1968; 57:1347–1357.

5. Sen S, Nunes Chini E, Brown MJ. Complications after unintentional intra-arterial of drugs: risks, outcomes and management strategies. Mayo Clin Proc 2005; 80:783–795.

6. Doluisio JT, LaPiana JC, Dittert LW. Pharmacokinetics of ampicillin trihydrate, sodium ampicillin, and sodium dicloxacillin following intramuscular injection. J Pharm Sci 1971; 60:715–719.

7. Cohen LS, Rosenthal JE, Horner DW Jr., et al. Plasma levels of lidocaine after intramuscular administration. Am J Cardiol 1972; 29:520–523.

8. Zener JC, Kerber RE, Spivack AP, et al. Blood lidocaine levels and kinetics following high-dose intramuscular administration. Circulation 1973; 47:984–988.

9. Feldman S. Biopharmaceutic factors influencing drug availability. In: Turco S, King RE, eds. Sterile Dosage Forms Their Preparation and Clinical Application. 3rd ed. Philadelphia: Lea & Febiger, 1987:110–113.

10. Almadrones L. Evidence-based research for intraperitoneal chemotherapy in epithelial ovarian cancer. Clin J Oncol Nurs 2007; 11:211–216.

11. Ivanov LV, Lyapunov NA, Orlova IN, et al. Study of bioavailability of hydrocortisone acetate in rectal administration of the foamy preparation to rabbits. Pharm Chem J 1993; 27:846–849.

12. Vromans H, Moolenaar F, Meijer DKF. Rectal absorption of metronidazol from polyethylene glycol suppositories. Pharm Weekbl Sci 1984; 6:18–20.

13. Donovan MD, Flynn GL, Amidon GL. Absorption of polyethylene glycols 600 through 2000: the molecular weight dependence of gastrointestinal and nasal absorption. Pharm Res 2000; 7:863–868.

14. McMartin C, Hutchinson LE, Hyde R, et al. Analysis of structural requirements for the absorption of drugs and macromolecules from the nasal cavity. J Pharm Sci 1987; 76:535–540.

15. Illum L. Is nose-to-brain transport of drugs in man a reality? J Pharm Pharmacol 2004; 56:3–17.

16. Dahlin M, Bergman U, Jansson B, et al. Transfer of dopamine in the olfactory pathway following nasal administration in mice. Pharm Res 2000; 17:737–742.

17. Chow HS, Chen Z, Matsuura GT. Direct transport of cocaine from the nasal cavity to the brain following intranasal cocaine administration in rats. J Pharm Sci 1999; 88:754–758.

18. Ross TM, Martinez PM, Renner JC, et al. Intranasal administration of interferon beta bypasses the blood-brain barrier to target the central nervous system and cervical lymph nodes: a non-invasive treatment strategy for multiple sclerosis. J Neuroimmunol 2004; 151:66–77.

19. Thorne RG, Pronk GJ, Padmanabhan V, et al. Delivery of insulin-like growth factor-1 to the rat brain and spinal cord along olfactory and trigeminal pathways following intranasal administration. Neuroscience 2004; 12:481–496.

20. Graff CL, Pollack GM. Functional evidence for p-glycoprotein at the nose-brain barrier. Pharm Res 2005; 22:86–93.

21. DeZiegler D, Bulletti C, De Monstier B, et al. The first uterine pass effect. Ann N Y Acad Sci 1997; 828:291–299.

22. Hosoya K, Lee VHL, Kim KJ. Roles of the conjunctiva in ocular drug delivery: a review of conjunctival transport mechanisms and their regulation. Eur J Pharm Biopharm 2005; 60: 227–240.

23. Gorgos D. Lidocaine-induced deaths raise questions about medspa management. Dermatology Nursing, October (2005). Available at: http://findarticles.com/p/articles/mi_hb6366/is_/ai_n29215018?tag=artBody;col1. Accessed December 22, 2008.

24. Flynn GL, Stewart B. Percutaneous drug penetration: choosing candidates for transdermal development. Drug Dev Res 1988; 13:169–185.

25. Benedetti MS, Whomsley R, Baltes EL. Differences in absorption, distribution, metabolism, and excretion of xenobiotics between the paediatric and adult populations. Expert Opin Drug Metab Toxicol 2005; 1:447–471.

26. ElDesoky ES. Pharmacokinetic-pharmacodynamic crisis in the elderly. Am J Ther 2007; 14: 488–498.

6

In Vivo Imaging of Dosage Forms

Zheng-Rong Lu
Department of Pharmaceutics and Pharmaceutical Chemistry,
College of Pharmacy, University of Utah, Salt Lake City, Utah, U.S.A.

INTRODUCTION

The preclinical pharmacokinetics and pharmacodynamics of drug formulations are traditionally evaluated in animal models with invasive surgical methods. A large number of experimental animals are sacrificed during the process of preclinical development. The results obtained in the preclinical studies with these invasive methods are often not predictive of the outcome of later clinical studies. Options are very limited for clinical evaluation of the pharmacokinetics and pharmacodynamics of new formulations. The studies with surgery- or biopsy-based tissue sampling often do not accurately reflect the true systemic efficacy of the drug formulations. Many drug compounds have failed to acquire the Food and Drug Administration (FDA) approval for clinical applications after expensive preclinical and clinical studies.

Biomedical imaging, including anatomical, functional, and molecular imaging, provides high-quality and high-resolution tissue images and allows noninvasive visualization and measurement of molecular markers, in vivo interaction of molecular probes, and biological, metabolic, and physiological processes with high sensitivity and specificity (1–4). Recent advancements in biomedical imaging have made it possible to use imaging technologies for noninvasive and longitudinal evaluation of the real-time and whole-body pharmacokinetics and pharmacodynamics of drug formulations in preclinical and clinical development phases and postapproval clinical studies. Biomedical imaging can provide accurate, timely, and quantitative pharmacokinetic and pharmacodynamic information of the drug candidates on the basis of a relatively smaller group of subjects than conventional biopsy- or surgery-based methods. The systemic whole-body information is essential for accurate identification of promising drug dosage forms for further development from the preclinical and early-phase clinical studies. The timely evaluation of pharmacokinetics and pharmacodynamics of a clinical dosage form in patients will also allow the physicians to tailor the best therapies for them.

A variety of currently available biomedical imaging modalities can be used for in vivo studies of drug formulations in the process of preclinical and clinical development. These imaging modalities include computerized tomography (CT), ultrasound, single-photon emission computed tomography (SPECT), positron-emission tomography (PET), magnetic resonance imaging (MRI), and optical imaging. CT and MRI provide high-resolution three-dimensional anatomical images. SPECT, PET, ultrasound, and optical imaging have high sensitivity for functional and molecular imaging. These imaging modalities have complementary properties and can be used independently or collectively for noninvasive in vivo imaging of drug dosage forms. In this chapter, we focus on applications of these imaging modalities in noninvasive in vivo evaluation of the pharmacokinetics and pharmacodynamics of drug dosage forms in preclinical and clinical studies.

IMAGING MODALITIES

Biomedical imaging measures the interactions of electromagnetic waves with the body or the emission of electromagnetic waves from the body. These imaging modalities utilize the physical characteristics of the waves across the electromagnetic spectrum. Covering the range from low-frequency to high-frequency electromagnetic waves, ultrasound imaging, MRI, optical imaging, X-ray radiography, and X-ray CT, γ-scintigraphy, SPECT, and PET are routinely used for preclinical and clinical studies (Table 1).

Ultrasound Imaging

Ultrasound imaging or sonography measures the interaction of high-frequency sound waves (1–10 MHz) with the body (5,6). Sound waves travel fast in solids and liquids, are slow in gas, and have no progression in vacuum. When sound waves are applied to a living subject through a transducer, they are reflected at the interface of tissues or organs of different densities and recorded in the transducer. Stronger signals are generated in the tissues with greater density differences. Images are constructed on the basis of echoes, attenuation of the sound, and sound speed. Advanced ultrasound imaging technologies, for example, Doppler imaging technology, can provide real-time two-dimensional and three-dimensional images. The real-time blood flow can also be visualized with ultrasound in high resolution.

    Microbubbles, microspheres filled with gas or low-density liquid, are used as contrast agents for ultrasound imaging to enhance echo differences between tissue types for more accurate diagnostic imaging (7). These contrast agents are based on the fact

Table 1 Imaging Modalities Available for Preclinical and Clinical Studies

Modality	Energy level	Image generation	Application
Ultrasound	1–10 MHz	Sound echo	Anatomic, functional, and molecular imaging
MRI	42.6/T MHz	Proton relaxation	Anatomic, functional, and molecular imaging
Optical imaging	$3.5–4.5 \times 10^8$ MHz	Fluorescence luminescence	Anatomic, functional, and molecular imaging
X-ray CT	3×10^{11} MHz	X-ray attenuation	Anatomic and functional imaging
SPECT	100–200 keV	γ-Ray emission	Functional and molecular imaging
PET	511 keV	Positron annihilation	Functional and molecular imaging

Abbreviations: MRI, magnetic resonance imaging; CT, computed tomography; SPECT, single-photon emission computed tomography; PET, positron-emission tomography.

that gas is resistant to sound propagation, resulting in strong echoes. The size of the microbubbles is usually smaller than 10 μm. Inert gas with low water solubility, such as air, nitrogen, and SF_6 or C_3F_8, or low-density perfluorocarbon, including C_5F_{12}, and C_6F_{14}, are commonly used for ultrasound contrast agents. Microbubbles are coated with a shell of biocompatible materials, including denatured proteins, lipids, or polymers. These microbubbles are highly echogenic and can directly interact with the incident sound wave. Ultrasound imaging is highly sensitive in detecting the microbubbles. Microbubbles are used as blood pool contrast agents for imaging of the cardiovascular, lymphatic, and reticuloendothelial systems, tumors, gastrointestinal (GI) tract, and tissue perfusion and inflammation. Targeting agents (e.g., antibody, peptide) can be attached to microbubble shell for functional and molecular imaging (8).

Magnetic Resonance Imaging

MRI uses a powerful magnet and radio waves to produce detailed images of the body's organs and structures. MRI measures the longitudinal (T_1) and transverse (T_2) relaxation rates of protons (mainly water protons) in the body (9,10). Water forms more than 50% of the body weight of a normal human adult. Water protons have magnetic moments with random orientations. When placed in a strong magnetic field, the proton magnetic moments align either along or against the static magnetic field (B_0) and create a net magnetization pointing in the direction of the magnetic field. The magnetization magnitude is proportional to the external magnetic field strength. When a radiofrequency (RF) pulse is applied to create an oscillating electromagnetic field (B_1) perpendicular to the main field, the protons absorb energy and the net magnetization is tipped away from the static magnetic field. The second magnetic field oscillates at the Larmor frequency, that is, the proton resonance frequency (42.58 MHz/T). Immediately after the RF pulse, the magnetization returns to its equilibrium state, or ground state, due to longitudinal (T_1) and transverse (T_2) relaxation processes. The longitudinal relaxation, or spin-lattice relaxation, involves the return of protons from the high-energy state to the equilibrium state by dissipating their excess energy to their surroundings. The transverse relaxation, or spin-spin relaxation, involves energy transfer from proton to proton. The decaying magnetization induces a voltage in a tuned detector coil to generate nuclear magnetic resonance (NMR) signal. Three-dimensional images are constructed from the signals of the proton relaxation in different tissues. Image contrast between tissues is the result of differences of proton density, relaxation rates, and flow and diffusion properties.

Paramagnetic materials, including paramagnetic metal ion chelates and nanoparticles, have been developed as contrast agents for MRI to enhance the image contrast in the tissue of interest (11,12). These agents decrease the relaxation rates of water protons, resulting in enhanced MR signals. MRI contrast agents approved for clinical applications are mainly stable paramagnetic chelates, for example, Gadolinium III [Gd(III)] chelates and Mn(II) chelates, and ultrasmall superparamagnetic iron oxide (USPIO). Both Gd(III) and Mn(II) chelates are mainly used as T_1 contrast agents, which produce brighter images. USPIOs are mainly used as T_2 contrast agents, resulting in darker images.

Optical Imaging

Optical microscopy has been broadly used for in vitro study of tissue samples and cells with high spatial resolution. Optical imaging for in vivo studies largely depends on the depth of light penetration into tissues, which is inversely proportional to the light wavelengths. Visible and infrared light can be absorbed by water, proteins, and lipids in the tissues, which limits imaging of deep tissues. Fluorescent and luminescent imaging techniques are the popular optical imaging methods for in vivo imaging (13,14). Fluorescent imaging requires excitation of a fluorochrome with an external light source to emit fluorescence of a longer wavelength. Luminescence imaging measures light emission from a chemical or biochemical reaction without excitation from an external source. Near-infrared (NIR) light (650–900 nm) has relatively low tissue absorption and is commonly used for in vivo imaging. Tissue penetration of NIR can be as deep as a few centimeters. Recently, a new optical imaging technique, fluorescence resonance energy transfer (FRET), using activatable imaging probes has also been developed for in vivo imaging (15).

X-Ray Radiography and Computed Tomography

X rays are a form of electromagnetic radiation of higher energ ($\lambda = \sim 0.01$ nm), which pass through the body and can be recorded in the opposite side of the body. X-ray images are constructed as two-dimensional projection from differential attenuation of X rays by the body tissues through which they pass. Attenuation is a process by which X rays are removed from the beam through absorption and scattering. X-ray attenuation is efficient in dense tissue (such as bone) and less in soft tissues. As a result, bone appears white, air black, and other tissues gray, depending on tissue density in the body. X-ray radiography is commonly used in the imaging of chest, dental structure, bone, neck, skull, abdomen, spine, etc.

X-ray CT provides three-dimensional images of the body with high spatial resolution (16,17,18). In CT imaging, X-ray sources and detectors rotate together around the body, and projections are collected from different angles. The computer processes the data to create two-dimensional and three-dimensional images. X-ray CT gives high-resolution anatomical images of air, soft tissues, and bones in the body but has a low sensitivity for molecular imaging. A major disadvantage of X-ray imaging and CT is the ionization of X rays. It has been reported that exposure to high-dose X rays increases the risk of cancer.

Biologically inert substances containing elements of high atomic weights are effective to attenuate X rays and are used as contrast agents for CT (19). The electrons of these elements have a high probability to interact with incident photons, resulting in substantial attenuation and bright image contrast enhancement. Water-soluble iodinated benzene derivatives are commonly used as CT contrast agents. High doses of these contrast agents are often required to produce good contrast enhancement.

γ-Scintigraphy and Single-Photon Emission Computed Tomography

γ-Scintigraphy detects the γ-rays emitted by the administered radiopharmaceuticals in the body, the derivatives of γ-ray-emitting isotopes (20,21). The radioactive emission is detected by a γ-camera and processed by a computer to generate an image. γ-Scintigraphy gives two-dimensional images of signal intensity distribution. When a rotating camera is used with the same principle of tomography as in X-ray CT, three-dimensional images are produced in a technique called SPECT. Compared with contrast-enhanced MRI and CT, SPECT has a high sensitivity for measuring radiopharmaceuticals in molecular imaging and gives qualitative and quantitative information about the distribution of a γ-emitter in the body. However, it does not provide high-resolution anatomical images of the body.

Radiopharmaceuticals or radiotracers used for γ-scintigraphy and SPECT are composed of the radionuclides decaying by γ-ray emission and with relatively short half-lives (22). The preferable γ-rays are those with energies greater than 30 keV, because γ-rays below 30 keV are not detectable due to the absorption by the body. The commonly used SPECT tracers are the complexes of radioactive transition metal ions (e.g., In-111 and Tc-99m) with short half-lives. Specificity and biodistribution of the tracers can be manipulated by altering the chemical structures of chelating ligands or incorporating tissue-specific agents. Unlike CT and MRI, only picomolar level radiotracer is needed for effective imaging in SPECT.

Positron-Emission Tomography

PET also detects γ-rays from the body after administration of radiopharmaceuticals containing radionuclides that emit positrons (23). The difference between PET and SPECT is that two γ-rays are detected in PET after one decay, compared with one in SPECT. Positrons emitted by PET probes annihilate with electrons in the tissue to give a pair of γ-rays with energy of 511 keV. The γ-rays are emitted at almost $180°$ and are recorded by detectors after escaping from the body. Like SPECT, PET is used for functional imaging and molecular imaging, rather than anatomical imaging. PET provides a much higher signal to noise ratio and spatial resolution than does SPECT.

C-11, N-13, O-15, and F-18 are the commonly used isotopes for PET imaging (24). The major advantage of using these isotopes is that one or more atoms in a biologically active molecule, e.g., a drug compound, can be replaced by a radioactive isotope without changing its chemical structure. This is particularly attractive for in vivo imaging of biological and pharmaceutical properties of a drug or drug candidate. One limitation of using these isotopes is that they have very short half-lives. The half-lives of C-11, N-13, O-15, and F-18 are 20.4, 9.96, 2.07, and 109.7 minutes. Because of the short half-life of the emitters, an on-site cyclotron is required for the production of positron emitters before imaging.

These imaging modalities can be used for noninvasive in vivo evaluation of dosage forms in preclinical and clinical studies. Optical imaging, SPECT, and PET have high sensitivity for functional and molecular imaging. CT and MRI produce high-resolution anatomical images for soft tissues. Ultrasound imaging is the least expensive imaging modality with high sensitivity to microbubbles. Each imaging modality has its own distinct advantages and characteristics. They are complementary to each other and can be used together to obtain more complete in vivo information of dosage forms. Combined imaging modalities, such as PET-CT, SPECT-CT, and PET-MRI, have been developed for preclinical and clinical applications (25,26).

Imaging of Pharmacokinetics and Biodistribution

Therapeutic efficacy of drugs depends to a large extent on the pharmacokinetic properties of drugs delivered in dosage forms. Traditionally, pharmacokinetic data are collected by blood and tissue sampling, followed by quantitative analysis of drugs and metabolites in both preclinical and clinical studies. It is difficult to provide complete in vivo pharmacokinetic data with traditional tissue sampling. Incomplete preclinical data of the kinetics of dosage forms could lead to unpredictable outcome in clinical development. Accurate pharmacokinetic data obtained with specific dose forms are also critical in clinical studies to determine the best dosing strategies to achieve maximum therapeutic efficacy and minimal adverse side effects.

Biomedical imaging provides qualitative and quantitative methods for noninvasive evaluation of real-time and whole-body pharmacokinetics and biodistribution of drugs and their dosage forms. Drugs can be directly labeled with positron-emitting isotopes (e.g., C-11, N-13, O-15, or F-18) without changing their structures. Their pharmacokinetics can be visualized and quantitatively determined by PET. Direct labeling of drug compounds with probes of other imaging modalities, for example, paramagnetic chelates for MRI, fluorescein for optical imaging, and radioactive metal complexes for SPECT, changes their structures and may alter their pharmacokinetic properties. Nevertheless, drug formulations or delivery systems can be labeled with various imaging probes for in vivo imaging.

IN VIVO IMAGING OF LABELED DRUGS

PET Imaging of C-11-Labeled Drugs

A relatively convenient method to prepare C-11-labeled drug compounds is the methylation of drug precursors with C-11 methyl iodide or triflate. Since C-11 has a short half-life, both the synthesis and purification of the labeled drugs have to be performed on site within a short period before injection. In preclinical studies, PET imaging of C-11-labeled drug candidates in animal models can provide whole-body and real-time pharmacokinetic information, including plasma kinetics, and longitudinal normal and diseased tissue biodistribution, in a limited number of experimental animals. The drug concentration can be quantitatively calculated from the radioactivity in the tissues, and pharmacokinetic parameters in the tissues can then be readily calculated from the data. The whole-body pharmacokinetics and biodistribution are critical for selecting the promising drug candidate with favorable pharmacokinetics, uptake, and residence time in the target organ or tissue from preclinical drug screening for further development. For example, PET imaging of C-11-labeled tricyclic carboxamide N-[2-(dimethylamino)ethyl]acridine-4-carboxamide and its analogues, DNA-intercalating agents inhibiting topoisomerases I and II, in an animal tumor model reveals the difference of the analogues in whole-body biodistribution, tumor uptake and retention, metabolism, and renal clearance (27). The comparative imaging with PET allows the identification of promising drug candidates for rapid translation into clinical studies.

Several C-11-labeled imaging agents have been evaluated in nonhuman primates and humans to determine their effective dose with whole-body PET imaging (28–31). PET gives three-dimensional images of the biodistribution of the radiolabeled agents. The PET images can also be reformatted into two-dimensional slice images with thickness as thin as a few millimeters, which allows accurate measurements of the whole-body biodistribution of the labeled agents. Repeated scanning of the same subject measures drug concentration in the major organs and tissues over time. Quantitative determination of concentration-time correlation allows the calculation of the residence time, binding parameters to their targets and elimination rate of the imaging agents. A similar study can also be performed to evaluate whole-body biodistribution and to determine the optimal dose and dosing interval of therapeutics with C-11 whole-body PET in clinical studies. The major limitation of PET is that it cannot differentiate the signal from the drug compounds and their metabolites or catabolites in pharmacokinetic studies.

PET Imaging of F-18-Labeled Drugs

F-18 has a relatively longer half-life and has been commonly used as the positron emitter for PET probes. In the preclinical and clinical development of these probes, PET imaging visualizes the whole-body and dynamic biodistribution of the probes in nonhuman primates and humans, providing accurate dosimetry for clinical use of the F-18-labeled probes (32–35). PET imaging is able to reveal the possible difference in biodistribution of the imaging probes between nonhuman primates and humans, suggesting that PET is effective for accurate measurement of whole-body pharmacokinetics in clinical studies. [F-18]-PET has also been used to study the pharmacokinetics of fluorine-containing therapeutics after one or more fluorine atoms in the drug compounds are replaced with F-18.

5-Fluorouracil (5-FU) is a commonly used anticancer drug for the treatment of GI tumors. However, the response rate to the treatment with 5-FU alone is very low. A recent PET study with F-18-labeled 5-FU in cancer patients has shown that the low efficacy of 5-FU may be caused by the low uptake in tumors and reduced systemic availability through hepatic catabolism (36). Figure 1 shows the transabdominal 5-[^{18}F]FU PET images for a patient with liver metastases before and after treatment with eniluracil. PET image indicates that 5-FU has high accumulation in normal liver because of catabolism and retention of a catabolite α-fluoro-β-alanine (FABL). The treatment with eniluracil inactivates dihydropyrimidine dehydrogenase and blocks the catabolism of 5-FU, resulting in reduced liver exposure to 5-FU. Quantitative analysis of imaging data shows that the initial extraction of 5-[^{18}F]FU from the plasma into the liver is 205-fold higher than the extraction by tumors, and 96% of catabolites are in the liver.

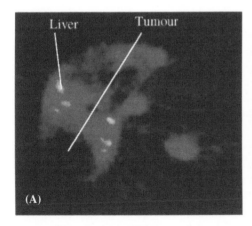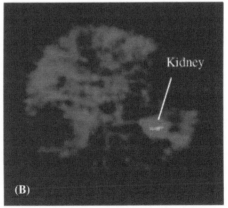

Figure 1 Transabdominal 5-[F-18]FU PET images of a patient with liver metastases before (**A**) and after (**B**) the administration of eniluracil. High signal intensity, the brightness, in the normal liver tissue indicates catabolism and retention of (F-18)FBAL (α-fluoro-β-ananine), a catabolite of 5-FU. Eniluracil inactivates dihydropyrimidine dehydrogenase, blocks 5-FU catabolism, and reduces liver retention of 5-FU and its catabolites (36). *Abbreviation*: 5-FU, 5-fluorouracil.

IN VIVO IMAGING OF LABELED SOLID FORMULATIONS

Solid drug formulations, for example, tablets, microspheres, and capsules, can be labeled with imaging probes to study the in vivo properties of the formulations. Labeling tablets with γ-emitters, In-111 and Tc-99m complexes, allows noninvasive evaluation of GI behavior of tablets in experimental animals and humans with γ-scintigraphy and SPECT. The imaging study can provide accurate information of the GI movement of the tablets and the time and position of the disintegration of tablets (37). Biodistribution of aerosol powder formulations in the lung can be visualized with γ-scintigraphy and SPECT by labeling the formulations with γ-emitters (38). Contrast-enhanced MRI is also effective in the study of in vivo properties of tablets after labeling solid formulations with MRI contrast agents. The incorporation of superparamagnetic iron oxide into tablets enables the localization of tablets by MRI with high spatial resolution due to the magnetic susceptibility of iron oxide particles (39,40). Gd(III) complexes in solid formulations do not generate any enhanced MR signal because water exchange with Gd(III) complexes is necessary for the contrast agents to enhance MR signal. However, the inclusion of Gd(III) chelates in tablets or other solid formulations allows in vivo visualization of drug release from the formulations with MRI (41). Unlike nuclear imaging, the signal in the MR images cannot be linearly correlated with the concentration of MRI contrast agents. Contrast-enhanced MRI can only be used as a qualitative or semiquantitative method for in vivo visualization of the properties of drug formulations.

IN VIVO IMAGING OF POLYMER DRUG CONJUGATES

The conjugation of anticancer drugs to water-soluble biomedical polymers modifies drug pharmacokinetics and improves tumor-targeting efficiency and therapeutic efficacy (41). Imaging probes can be incorporated into polymer drug conjugates for noninvasive study of pharmacokinetics and tumor-targeting efficiency. The chemical modification of the conjugates with imaging probes would not significantly affect the pharmacokinetic properties of the polymers. Effectiveness of the nuclear medicine and MRI for in vivo imaging of labeled polymer conjugates has been demonstrated in preclinical or clinical studies (42–44). In addition to the whole-body biodistribution of the labeled conjugates, the effect of size and structure of the polymers on the pharmacokinetics and tumor-targeting efficiency of the conjugates can be determined by in vivo imaging. For example, size-dependent plasma pharmacokinetics of polyamidoamine (PAMAM) dendrimers are clearly visualized by the contrast-enhanced MRI after the dendrimers are labeled with Gd(III) chelates (45). The dendrimers of higher generations with larger sizes have longer blood circulation than the dendrimers with smaller sizes as shown in the dynamic MR images. MRI studies with paramagnetically labeled polymer conjugates have also revealed the effect of size and structure of polymer conjugates on tumor-targeting efficiency (46–48). Figure 2 shows the two-dimensional coronal dynamic MR images of mice bearing MDA-MB-231 human breast carcinoma xenografts after the intravenous injection of poly[N-(2-hydroxypropyl)methacrylamide]-(Gd-DO3A) conjugate [PHPMA-(Gd-DO3A)] and poly(L-glutamic acid)-(Gd-DO3A) conjugate with similar hydrodynamic sizes (60 kDa). It can be seen in the dynamic MR images that the nondegradable PHPMA-(Gd-DO3A) conjugate circulates in the blood for longer and achieves a higher tumor accumulation than the biodegradable poly(L-glutamic acid)-(Gd-DO3A) conjugate.

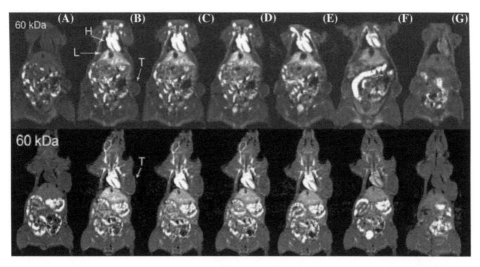

Figure 2 Two-dimensional coronal MR images of mice before (**A**) and at 1 minute (**B**), 10 minutes (**C**), 20 minutes (**D**), 60 minutes (**E**), 4 hours (**F**), and 24 hours (**G**) after intravenous injection of PHPMA-GFLG-(Gd-DO3A) (*top row*) and poly(L-glutamic acid)-(Gd-DO3A) (*bottom row*) conjugates with a molecular weight of 60 kDa at a dose of 0.03 mmol-Gd/kg. The arrows point to the heart (H), liver (L), and tumor (T). Bright signal in the blood in the heart and the liver indicates high concentration of paramagnetically labeled polymer conjugates. Bright signal in the intestines and stomach is from food contents not by the contrast agents.

IN VIVO IMAGING OF LIPOSOMAL DRUG DELIVERY SYSTEMS

Liposomes are commonly used delivery systems for anticancer drugs and therapeutic DNA. Several liposomal drug delivery systems have been approved for cancer treatment. Liposomal drug delivery systems have been investigated by CT, MRI, optical imaging, SPECT, and PET in preclinical or clinical studies (49–52). Imaging probes can be encapsulated inside liposomes or incorporated in the lipid bilayers after the probes are conjugated to lipophilic groups. Different imaging probes can also be incorporated into liposomes for multimodality imaging. For example, coencapsulation of an MRI contrast agent and a CT contrast agent in PEGylated liposomes results in significant signal enhancement for both MRI and CT to effectively visualize the plasma kinetics of liposomes in an animal model (49). Both imaging modalities provide the same kinetic data on the prolonged blood circulation of the PEGylated liposomes. Relatively low liver uptake of the PEGylated liposomes is also shown in both CT and MR images.

PET imaging of 2-[^{18}F]-2-fluoro-2-deoxyglucose [F-18]FDG–encapsulated liposomes in mice reveals some interesting features on how the size and structure of liposomes affect biodistribution and tumor accumulation (50). High tumor accumulation was shown in the PET images with PEGylated liposomes compared with those with the conventional liposomes. Long-circulating liposomes with a size of 100 nm have a lower liver uptake and higher tumor accumulation than those with a size larger than 200 nm. Positively charged liposomes exhibit much higher liver uptake than the negatively charged and neutral liposomes. The neutral liposomes have lower liver uptake than the charged liposomes.

Labeling of PEGylated liposomes with γ-emitters, for example, (In-111)-diethylene-triaminepentaacetate (DTPA) chelates, allows noninvasive study of pharmacokinetics and biodistribution of the liposomal drug delivery systems with SPECT in patients for an

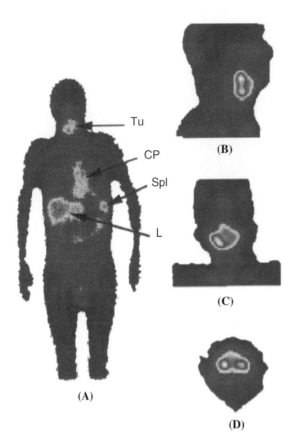

Figure 3 γ-Scintigraphic image (**A**) and sagittal (**B**), coronal (**C**), and axial (**D**) SPECT images showing the biodistribution of the PEGylated liposomes labeled with (In-111)-DTPA in a patient with T3N0M0 squamous cell cancer at the tongue base at 72 hours after administration (52). *Abbreviations*: Tu, tumor; CP, cardiac blood pool; Spl, spleen; L, liver.

extended period (up to 10 days) (52). Figure 3 shows the γ-scintigraphic image and the SPECT images of a patient with T3N0M0 squamous cell cancer at the tongue base 72 hours after administration of the PEGylated liposomes labeled with (In-111)-DTPA. Significant accumulation of the liposomes is shown in the tumor tissue. Substantial liver accumulation is still shown in all tested patients, although the PEGylated liposomes are designed to limit liver accumulation.

IN VIVO IMAGING OF DRUG CONTAINING MICROBUBBLES

In addition to contrast-enhanced ultrasound imaging, coated microbubbles can be used for the delivery of therapeutic agents, including anticancer drugs and plasmid DNA (53,54). Hydrophobic drugs can be loaded in the lipid, surfactant, or polymer shell of the microbubbles. Plasmid DNA can be loaded inside microbubbles. Ultrasound imaging has the sensitivity of visualizing the movement and location of a single microbubble. The combination of ultrasound imaging and drug delivery allows track and localization of the drug loading microbubbles in target tissues. The microbubbles can then be destroyed by high-intensity ultrasound under imaging guidance to release the drug payloads in the target tissues such as tumor tissue. A recent study has demonstrated the feasibility of ultrasound-assisted drug delivery using polymer-coated and doxorubicin-containing microbubbles for cancer treatment in a mouse tumor model (55). Substantial and prolonged tumor accumulation of the microbubbles is shown in ultrasound images. Significant tumor regression is observed after the tumor is treated with ultrasonication.

IN VIVO IMAGING OF GENE DELIVERY SYSTEMS

Nonviral gene delivery systems are promising delivery systems for gene therapy because of the ease of preparation and low immunogenicity. However, currently available nonviral delivery systems suffer from low in vivo delivery efficiency. Noninvasive evaluation of gene delivery systems with biomedical imaging may provide better understanding of the mechanism of in vivo gene delivery, which can help to design safe and efficient nonviral gene delivery systems. Fluorescence imaging and luminescence imaging are commonly used for the study of in vivo gene expression. To study the biodistribution and targeted delivery, gene delivery systems need to be labeled with the imaging probes that can be effectively visualized with suitable imaging modalities. It has been shown that incorporation of Gd(III) chelates into cationic lipids can be used as a tool to study noninvasively the whole-body biodistribution of gene delivery systems with contrast-enhanced MRI in animal models after local injection (56). Incorporation of super-paramagnetic iron oxide nanoparticles and an NIR probe with an siRNA carrier allows noninvasive evaluation of tumor accumulation of the delivery system in a mouse model with both contrast-enhanced MRI and NIR fluorescence imaging (57). It is also feasible to label gene delivery systems with radiotracers to quantitatively visualize the real-time biodistribution of gene delivery systems with SPECT and PET in both preclinical and clinical studies (58). Nuclear imaging provides much higher sensitivity to detect the labeled delivery system than contrast-enhanced MRI.

MULTIMODALITY IMAGING OF PHARMACOKINETICS

Recently, there have been efforts to develop combined imaging modalities with both functional and anatomical imaging for more accurate radiological diagnosis. PET and SPECT have high sensitivity for quantitative measurement of imaging probes in vivo, while CT and MRI provide anatomical images with high spatial resolution. The combined dual imaging modalities include CT-PET, CT-SPECT, MRI-PET, and MRI-SPECT (59–61). CT-PET is now available for both clinical and preclinical applications. Figure 4 shows axial CT, [F-18]FDG-PET and merged CT-PET images of a patient with epithelial malignant pleural mesothelioma and lymph node metastasis (60). The CT image shows the detailed anatomy, and PET image shows the uptake of [F-18]FDG in the tumor. The merged CT–PET image correlates the [F-18]FDG uptake to the anatomy of tumor location. The dual imaging modalities are valuable tools for in vivo imaging of kinetics and biodistribution of dosage forms. Combination of quantitative molecular imaging of nuclear medicine and anatomic imaging of CT or MR can provide quantitative measurement of biodistribution with accurate correlation with anatomy.

IN VIVO IMAGING OF PHARMACODYNAMICS

Biomedical imaging is also effective for noninvasive study of pharmacodynamics of drugs delivered in dosage forms in correlation to their pharmacokinetics in both preclinical and clinical studies. While pharmacokinetics explores what the body does to a

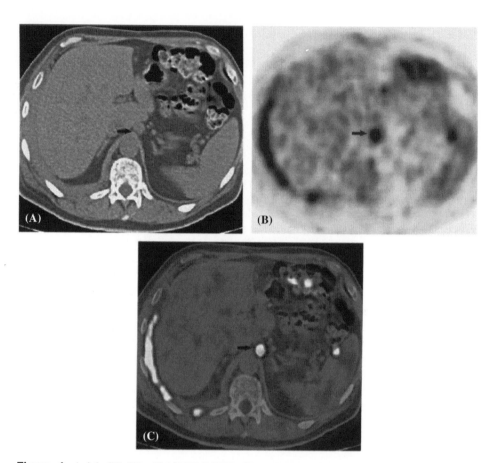

Figure 4 Axial CT (**A**), [F-18]-FDG–PET (**B**) and merged CT–PET images showing the distribution of [F18]-FDG in a patient with epithelial malignant pleural mesothelioma. CT provides high-resolution anatomic image, and PET reveals unusual uptake of [F-18]-FDG in a tumor. The merged image correlates the unusual metabolic activity in the PET image to a metastatic lymph node in the high-resolution CT image. The arrow points to lymph node with metastasis confirmed by biopsy (60). *Abbreviations*: CT, computed tomography; FDG, 2-fluoro-2-deoxyglucose; PET, positron-emission tomography.

drug, pharmacodynamics explores what the drug does to the body. Pharmacodynamics can be determined by imaging as the biochemical or physiological response of target tissues to dosage forms. The biochemical and metabolic responses can be visualized by PET imaging or magnetic resonance spectroscopy (MRS) before any significant morphological change of the target tissues. The physiological response can be imaged by dynamic contrast-enhanced (DCE)-MRI on the basis of vascular and tissue permeability and perfusion. Early and accurate evaluation of pharmacodynamics is essential for both drug development and patient care. Early determination of therapeutic efficacy in drug development allows accurate identification of promising drug candidates or formulations for further development and eliminates nonresponsive drug candidates or formulations before enormous resources are wasted. In patient care, timely recognition of therapeutic response helps the physicians caring the patients to tailor the therapies accordingly to achieve the maximum therapeutic outcome.

PET IMAGING OF THERAPEUTIC RESPONSE

PET with [F-18]FDG is the most commonly used method for noninvasive evaluation of therapeutic response in both preclinical and clinical studies (62,63). [F-18]FDG is a glucose analogue and is taken by cells via glucose membrane transporters. [F-18]FDG is then converted to [F-18]FDG-6-phosphate that cannot be metabolized further in the glycolic pathway. [F-18]FDG remains trapped and preferentially accumulates in the cells with high metabolic activity and high glucose uptake. [F-18]FDG-PET measures metabolic activities of tumor tissue on the basis of accurate quantification of [F-18]FDG uptake. It can differentiate metabolically highly active tumors from less active tumors. Early tumor response to anticancer treatment can be predicted by [F-18]FDG-PET on the basis of the change of tumor metabolism before any significant change of tumor volume can be observed.

In the preclinical evaluation of dosage forms, [F-18]FDG-PET can be used as a measurable biomarker to evaluate therapeutic efficacy of anticancer drugs in animal models. High-resolution small animal PET is available for evaluation of therapeutic efficacy in preclinical studies. The feasibility of using [F-18]FDG-PET to assess therapeutic efficacy in experimental animal models has been demonstrated in numerous preclinical studies. In a study of evaluating the efficacy of photodynamic therapy in a mouse tumor model, tumor response to the therapy is observed by FDG-PET as early as 30 minutes after the treatment (64).

Clinically, FDG-PET has been increasingly used for evaluating the efficacy of therapies and predicting therapeutic outcomes (65–67). Therapeutic response is generally determined by visual analysis. Figure 5 shows the axial CT, [F-18]FDG PET, and merged CT-PET images of a patient with liver metastasis from GI stromal tumor before and one month after treatment with imatinib (68). The CT image does not show tumor volume reduction after the treatment, while FDG-PET image shows no appreciable glucose uptake, indicating response to the treatment. A standardized uptake value (SUV) has been recently proposed and is used as a semiquantitative biomarker assessing therapeutic response. SUV is calculated from the radioactivity in the tissue volume of interest and normalized to the injected activity and body weight or body surface area. It is expected that SUV can provide more reproducible assessment for the prognosis of anticancer therapies.

In addition to FDG, 3′-deoxy-3′-^{18}F-fluorothymidine (F-18 FLT) also shows promise to noninvasively visualize therapeutic response with PET based on DNA synthesis. FLT is taken up by cells through nucleoside transporters and phosphorylated by thymidine kinase-1 (TK1) to FLT monophosphate. The phosphorylated FLT is trapped in the cells, and only a small portion of FLT is incorporated into DNA. Nevertheless, TK1 activity directly correlates to the trapped FLT, which can be used as a biomarker for cellular proliferation. The direct correlation of FLT uptake to tumor cell proliferation has been shown in both preclinical and clinical studies (69–71). Several studies have shown that FLT-PET provides quantitative and reproducible measurement of the changes of tumor cell proliferation in response to therapies. It is believed that FLT-PET may be more sensitive than FDG-PET in assessing tumor response to therapies because FDG is not tumor specific, and high FDG uptake is also observed in inflammatory tissues and other noncancerous tissues and cells with increased glucose usage (72).

DYNAMIC CONTRAST-ENHANCED MRI

DCE-MRI measures the uptake kinetics of an MRI contrast agent in the tissue of interest. In oncology, tumor uptake kinetics can be correlated to tumor physiological properties, including microvessel blood flow, blood volume, and vascular permeability (73–75).

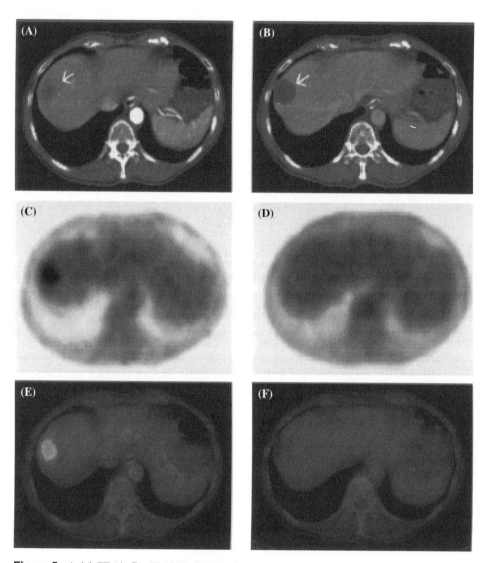

Figure 5 Axial CT (**A, B**), [F-18]FDG PET (**C, D**), and merged PET–CT images (**E** and **F**) of a patient with liver metastasis (*arrows* in **A** and **B**) from GI stromal tumor before (**A, C, E**) and one month after the treatment with imatinib therapy (**B, D, F**). High tumor metabolic activity is shown in the PET image and the merged image before the treatment. The metabolic activity reduces to normal after the treatment; even the tumor mass is still visible in the CT image. The reduced metabolic activity indicates response of the tumor to imatinib therapy (68). *Abbreviations*: GI, gastrointestinal; CT, computed tomography; FDG, 2-fluoro-2-deoxyglucose; PET, positron-emission tomography.

These physiological properties can be used to evaluate tumor response to therapies, including antiangiogenic therapy. DCE-MRI is feasible to evaluate therapeutic efficacy of drug dosage forms in both preclinical and clinical studies on the basis of changes in tumor vascular properties before and after the treatment. Generally, malignant tumors are highly vascularized and have high vascular permeability. Figure 6 shows the contrast enhancement time curves in tumor tissue of a low-molecular-weight contrast agent, Gd(DTPA-BMA), in a rat tumor model before and at various time points after the treatment with combretastatin, a vascular targeting agent (76). Tumor response to the

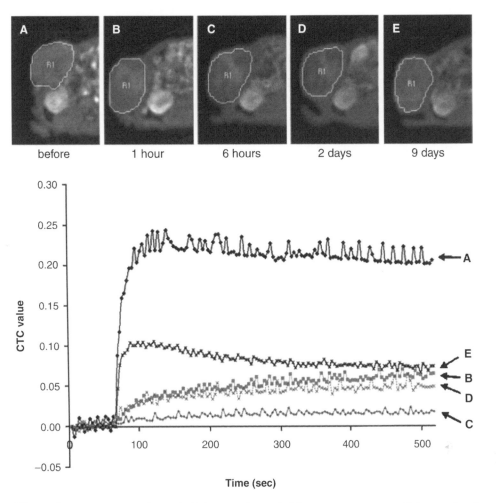

Figure 6 Axial contrast enhanced MR images of a rat rhabdomyosarcoma xenograft (*top row*) and contrast enhancement versus time curves (CTC, *bottom*) of the tumor tissue before (**A**) and 1 hour (**B**), 6 hours (**C**), 2 days (**D**), and 9 days (**E**) after the administration of combretastatin. The CTC curves correlate to the uptake kinetics of the contrast agent in the tumor. The treatment with combretastatin reduced tumor vascular permeability and resulted in low uptake kinetics (76). *Abbreviation*: MR, magnetic resonance.

treatment based on contrast agent uptake is shown as early as one hour after the treatment. Tumor uptake of the contrast agent is reduced to a minimal level six hours after the treatment and is then gradually recovered over time. The effectiveness of DCE-MRI with low molecular MRI contrast agents is shown in clinical studies for the noninvasive evaluation of therapeutic response.

DCE-MRI with macromolecular MRI contrast agents has also been developed for tumor characterization (77–80). Compared with low-molecular-weight contrast agents, macromolecular agents do not extravasate from vasculature and have prolonged blood circulation. Tumor accumulation of macromolecular contrast agents is mainly controlled by tumor vascular permeability. It is shown in animal models that DCE-MRI with macromolecular contrast agents provides more accurate measurement of tumor blood volume and vascular permeability. DCE-MRI with macromolecular agents is limited to preclinical studies in evaluating therapeutic response because no macromolecular MRI contrast agent is available for clinical applications. Several macromolecular MRI contrast agents are currently under development for clinical applications (81). It is possible in the future to use DCE-MRI with macromolecular MRI contrast agents for clinical studies when these agents are approved for human usage.

Data analysis of DCE-MRI results is a complicated process because it is difficult to accurately convert the MR signal to the concentration of the contrast agents. The MR signal or normalized signal versus time curves are commonly used for semiquantitative analysis of tumor vascular properties. The signal-tumor curves can be fitted in a commonly accepted two-compartmental model,

$$C_\mathrm{T}(t) = K^\mathrm{trans} \int_0^t C_\mathrm{p}(\theta) e^{-k_\mathrm{ep}(t-\theta)} d\theta + f_\mathrm{PV} C_\mathrm{p}(t),$$

where $C_\mathrm{T}(t)$ is the concentration or MR signal in tumor at any time point t, $C_\mathrm{p}(t)$ the blood concentration or signal, f_PV fractional tumor blood volume, k_ep back flow rate constant of contrast agent from tumor to blood, and K^trans the flow rate constant of contrast agent from blood to tumor (77). K^trans measures transport rate of a contrast agent from blood into tumor tissue, representing tumor vascular permeability. The transfer constant, K^trans, and fractional tumor volume, f_PV, obtained with the semiquantitative analysis correlates well with the tumor response to therapies, particularly for DCE-MRI with macromolecular contrast agents. MRI technologies are still under continuous improvement. More sensitive and quantitative MRI methods may be available in the future for accurate evaluation of pharmacodynamics of dosage forms. Nonetheless, DCE-MRI is considered as a valuable noninvasive tool in both preclinical and clinical study of the pharmacodynamics of dosage forms.

IN VIVO MAGNETIC RESONANCE SPECTROSCOPY

MRS quantitatively measures metabolites in the tissues of interest. It is capable of both characterizing the metabolites and quantitatively measuring the tissue concentration of each metabolite associated in the pathological–biochemical processes (82–85). The changes in metabolite concentration measured by MRS can be used as a pharmacodynamic biomarker for noninvasive evaluation of therapeutic response. The feasibility of MRS for evaluating therapeutic response has been shown in both preclinical and clinical studies. For example, choline and phosphocholine have an elevated concentration in tumor tissues as shown by ^{1}H and ^{31}P MRS. Quantitative measurement of choline and phosphocholine with MRS can be used as a biomarker for evaluation of the efficacy of choline kinase inhibitors in anticancer treatment. Figure 7 shows the in vivo ^{1}H and ^{31}P magnetic resonance spectra of HT29 human colon tumor xenografts in mice before and after the treatment with a choline kinase inhibitor, MN58b (85). The total choline concentration and phosphocholine concentration are significantly decreased in the tumor tissues after the treatment, showing the positive tumor response to the treatment. Clinical studies have shown that MRS is also effective to noninvasively evaluate biochemical-pathological changes of multiple sclerosis on the basis of NMR signal intensity of N-acetylaspartate (86). The change of metabolite concentration in the tissue of interest quantitatively determined by MRS is a valuable pharmacodynamic biomarker for noninvasive study of the efficacy of therapeutic dosage forms.

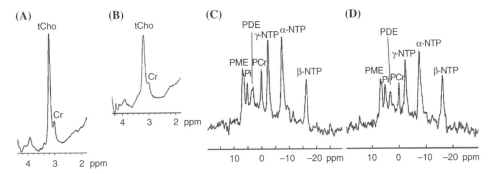

Figure 7 In vivo proton (**A** and **B**) and P-31 (**C** and **D**) magnetic resonance spectra of a HT29 xenograft in a mouse before (**A** and **C**) and after (**B** and **D**) the treatment with MN58b. The NMR peaks are assigned to tCho, Cr, PME, Pi, PDEs, PCr, and a-NTP, b-NTP, and c-NTP. *Abbreviations*: NMR, nuclear magnetic resonance; tCho, total choline; Cr, creatine; PME, phosphomonoesters; Pi, inorganic phosphate; PDE, phosphodiester; PCr, phosphocreatine; NTP, nucleoside triphosphate (85).

SUMMARY

Biomedical imaging provides noninvasive methods for in vivo study of kinetic, pharmacokinetic, and pharmacodynamic properties of therapeutic dosage forms in both preclinical and clinical drug development. The U.S. FDA is considering the use of imaging biomarkers and endpoints in drug discovery and development. Major pharmaceutical industries have established imaging branches alongside their discovery and development branches. The combination of diagnostic imaging and functional imaging will provide better patient care on the basis of timely and accurate determination of pharmacokinetics and pharmacodynamics of dosage forms. Personalized patient care or personalized medicine can be tailored by the physicians to achieve the maximum therapeutic outcome on the basis of early therapeutic response determined by noninvasive imaging. Up to now, biomedical imaging has not yet reached its full potential for noninvasive in vivo study of dosage forms. The continuous advancement of imaging technologies will have a revolutionary impact on more cost-effective drug development and better patient care.

REFERENCES

1. Kelloff GJ, Krohn KA, Larson SM, et al. The progress and promise of molecular imaging probes in oncologic drug development. Clin Cancer Res 2005; 11(22):7967–7985.
2. Workman P, Aboagye EO, Chung YL, et al. Minimally invasive pharmacokinetic and pharmacodynamic technologies in hypothesis-testing clinical trials of innovative therapies. J Natl Cancer Inst 2006; 98:580–598.
3. Gross S, Piwnica-Worms D. Molecular imaging strategies for drug discovery and development. Curr Opin Chem Biol 2006; 10(4):334–342.
4. Stephen RM, Gillies RJ. Promise and progress for functional and molecular imaging of response to targeted therapies. Pharm Res 2007; 24(6):1172–1185.
5. Hoskins P, Thrush A, Martin K, et al. Diagnostic Ultrasound: Physics and Equipment. London: Greenwich Medical Media Ltd., 2003.
6. Evans DH, McDicken WN. Doppler Ultrasound: Physics, Instrumental, and Clinical Applications. 2nd ed. New York: John Wiley & Sons, 2000.

7. Schutt EG, Klein DH, Mattrey RM, et al. Injectable microbubbles as contrast agents for diagnostic ultrasound imaging: the key role of perfluorochemicals. Angew Chem Int Ed Engl 2003; 42(28):3218–3235.

8. Klibanov AL. Ligand-carrying gas-filled microbubbles: ultrasound contrast agents for targeted molecular imaging. Bioconjug Chem 2005; 16(1):9–17.

9. Liang ZP, Lauterbur PC. Principles of Magnetic Resonance Imaging: A Signal Processing Perspective. New York: IEEE Inc., 2000.

10. Vlaardingerbroek MT, den Boer JA. Magnetic Resonance Imaging: Theory and Practice. 3rd ed. New York: Springer, 2002.

11. Merbach AE, Toth E. The Chemistry of Contrast Agents in Medical Magnetic Resonance Imaging. New York: John Wiley & Sons, 2001.

12. Caravan P, Ellison JJ, McMurry TJ, et al. Gadolinium(III) chelates as MRI contrast agents: structure, dynamics, and applications. Chem Rev 1999; 99(9):2293–2352.

13. Weissleder R, Ntziachristos V. Shedding light onto live molecular targets. Nat Med 2003; 9(1): 123–128.

14. Wang G, Cong W, Shen H, et al. Overview of bioluminescence tomography—a new molecular imaging modality. Front Biosci 2008; 13(1):1281–1293.

15. Chapman S, Oparka KJ, Roberts AG. New tools for in vivo fluorescence tagging. Curr Opin Plant Biol 2005; 8(6):565–573.

16. Seeram E. Computed Tomography: Physics Principles, Clinical Applications, and Quality Control. 2nd ed. Philadelphia: W.B. Saunders Company, 2008.

17. Kalender WA. Computed Tomography: Fundamentals, System Technology, Image Quality, Applications. Munich: Wiley-VCH, 2006.

18. Henwood S. Clinical CT: Techniques and Practice. London: Greenwich Medical Media Ltd., 1999.

19. Dawson P, Cosgrove DO, Grainger RG. Textbook of Contrast Media. Oxford: Isis Medical Media Ltd., 1999.

20. Saha GB. Physics and Radiobiology of Nuclear Medicine. 3rd ed. New York: Springer, 2006.

21. Wernick MN, Aarsvold JN. Emission Tomography: The Fundamentals of PET and SPECT. San Diego: Elsevier Academic Press, 2004.

22. Saha GB. Fundamentals of Nuclear Pharmacy. 5th ed. New York: Springer, 2004.

23. Phelps ME. PET: Molecular Imaging and its Biological Applications. New York: Springer, 2004.

24. Welch MJ, Redvanly CS. Handbook of Radiopharmaceuticals. New York: John Wiley & Sons, 2003.

25. von Schulthess GK. Molecular Anatomic Imaging? PET-CT and SPECT-CT Integrated Modality Imaging. Philadelphia: Lippincott Williams & Wilkins, 2006.

26. Oehr P, Biersack HJ, Coleman RE. PET and PET-CT in Oncology. New York: Springer, 2004.

27. Osman S, Rowlinson-Busza G, Luthra SK, et al. Comparative biodistribution and metabolism of carbon-11-labeled N-[2-(dimethylamino)ethyl]acridine-4-carboxamide and DNA-intercalating analogues. Cancer Res 2001; 61(7):2935–2944.

28. Spencer TJ, Biederman J, Ciccone PE, et al. PET study examining pharmacokinetics, detection and likeability, and dopamine transporter receptor occupancy of short- and long-acting oral methylphenidate. Am J Psychiatry 2006; 163(3):387–395.

29. Murthy R, Erlandsson K, Kumar D, et al. Biodistribution and radiation dosimetry of 11C-harmine in baboons. Nucl Med Commun 2007; 28(9):748–754.

30. Lu JQ, Ichise M, Liow JS, et al. Biodistribution and radiation dosimetry of the serotonin transporter ligand 11C-DASB determined from human whole-body PET. J Nucl Med 2004; 45(9): 1555–1559.

31. Scheinin NM, Tolvanen TK, Wilson IA, et al. Biodistribution and radiation dosimetry of the amyloid imaging agent 11C-PIB in humans. J Nucl Med 2007; 48(1):128–133.

32. Tipre DN, Fujita M, Chin FT, et al. Whole-body biodistribution and radiation dosimetry estimates for the PET dopamine transporter probe 18F-FECNT in non-human primates. Nucl Med Commun 2004; 25(7):737–742.

33. Saleem A, Aboagye EO, Matthews JC, et al. Plasma pharmacokinetic evaluation of cytotoxic agents radiolabelled with positron emitting radioisotopes. Cancer Chemother Pharmacol 2008; 61(5):865–873.

34. Sprague DR, Chin FT, Liow JS, et al. Human biodistribution and radiation dosimetry of the tachykinin NK1 antagonist radioligand [18F]SPA-RQ: comparison of thin-slice, bisected, and 2-dimensional planar image analysis. J Nucl Med 2007; 48(1):100–107.

35. Nye JA, Schuster DM, Yu W, et al. Biodistribution and radiation dosimetry of the synthetic nonmetabolized amino acid analogue anti-18F-FACBC in humans. J Nucl Med 2007; 48(6): 1017–1020.

36. Aboagye EO, Saleem A, Cunningham VJ, et al. Extraction of 5-fluorouracil by tumor and liver: a noninvasive positron emission tomography study of patients with gastrointestinal cancer. Cancer Res 2001; 61(13):4937–4941.

37. Ibekwe VC, Fadda HM, Parsons GE, et al. A comparative in vitro assessment of the drug release performance of pH-responsive polymers for ileo-colonic delivery. Int J Pharm 2006; 308 (1–2):52–60.

38. Newman SP, Pitcairn GR, Hirst PH, et al. Scintigraphic comparison of budesonide deposition from two dry powder inhalers. Eur Respir J 2000; 16(1):178–183.

39. Steingoetter A, Weishaupt D, Kunz P, et al. Magnetic resonance imaging for the in vivo evaluation of gastric-retentive tablets. Pharm Res 2003; 20(12):2001–2007.

40. Namur J, Chapot R, Pelage JP, et al. MR imaging detection of superparamagnetic iron oxide loaded tris-acryl embolization microspheres. J Vasc Interv Radiol 2007; 18(10):1287–1295.

41. Kopecek J, Kopecková P, Minko T, et al. HPMA copolymer-anticancer drug conjugates: design, activity, and mechanism of action. Eur J Pharm Biopharm 2000; 50(1):61–81.

42. Lammers T, Kühnlein R, Kissel M, et al. Effect of physicochemical modification on the biodistribution and tumor accumulation of HPMA copolymers. J Control Release 2005; 110(1): 103–118.

43. Mitra A, Nan A, Ghandehari H, et al. Technetium-99m-Labeled N-(2-hydroxypropyl) methacrylamide copolymers: synthesis, characterization, and in vivo biodistribution. Pharm Res 2004; 21(7):1153–1159.

44. Vasey PA, Kaye SB, Morrison R, et al. Phase I clinical and pharmacokinetic study of PK1 [N-(2-hydroxypropyl)methacrylamide copolymer doxorubicin]: first member of a new class of chemotherapeutic agents-drug-polymer conjugates. Clin Cancer Res 1999; 5(1):83–94.

45. Kobayashi H, Brechbiel MW. Dendrimer-based macromolecular MRI contrast agents: characteristics and application. Mol Imaging 2003; 2(1):1–10.

46. Ye F, Ke T, Lu ZR, et al. Noninvasive visualization of in vivo drug delivery of poly(L-glutamic acid) using contrast-enhanced MRI. Mol Pharm 2006; 3(5):507–515.

47. Wang Y, Ye F, Lu ZR, et al. Noninvasive visualization of pharmacokinetics, biodistribution and tumor targeting of poly[N-(2-hydroxypropyl)methacrylamide] in mice using contrast enhanced MRI. Pharm Res 2007; 24(6):1208–1216.

48. Lu ZR, Ye F, Vaidya A. Polymer platforms for drug delivery and biomedical imaging. J Control Release 2007; 122(3):269–277.

49. Zheng J, Liu J, Dunne M, et al. In vivo performance of a liposomal vascular contrast agent for CT and MR-based image guidance applications. Pharm Res 2007; 24(6):1193–1201.

50. Oku N, Tokudome Y, Asai T, et al. Evaluation of drug targeting strategies and liposomal trafficking. Curr Pharm Des 2000; 6(16):1669–1691.

51. Bao A, Goins B, Klipper R, et al. Direct 99mTc labeling of pegylated liposomal doxorubicin (Doxil) for pharmacokinetic and non-invasive imaging studies. J Pharmacol Exp Ther 2004; 308(2):419–425.

52. Harrington KJ, Mohammadtaghi S, Uster PS, et al. Effective targeting of solid tumors in patients with locally advanced cancers by radiolabeled pegylated liposomes. Clin Cancer Res 2001; 7(2):243–254.

53. Lanza GM, Wickline SA. Targeted ultrasonic contrast agents for molecular imaging and therapy. Prog Cardiovasc Dis 2001; 44(1):13–31.

54. Klibanov AL. Microbubble contrast agents: targeted ultrasound imaging and ultrasound-assisted drug-delivery applications. Invest Radiol 2006; 41(3):354–362.

55. Rapoport N, Gao Z, Kennedy A. Multifunctional nanoparticles for combining ultrasonic tumor imaging and targeted chemotherapy. J Natl Cancer Inst 2007; 99(14):1095–1106.

56. Leclercq F, Cohen-Ohana M, Mignet N, et al. Design, synthesis, and evaluation of gadolinium cationic lipids as tools for biodistribution studies of gene delivery complexes. Bioconjug Chem 2003; 14(1):112–119.

57. Medarova Z, Pham W, Farrar C, et al. In vivo imaging of siRNA delivery and silencing in tumors. Nat Med 2007; 13(3):372–377.

58. Iyer M, Berenji M, Templeton NS, et al. Noninvasive imaging of cationic lipid-mediated delivery of optical and PET reporter genes in living mice. Mol Ther 2002; 6(4):555–562.

59. Reske SN, Blumstein NM, Neumaier B, et al. Imaging prostate cancer with 11C-choline PET/CT. J Nucl Med 2006; 47(8):1249–1254.

60. Truong MT, Marom EM, Erasmus JJ. Preoperative evaluation of patients with malignant pleural mesothelioma: role of integrated CT-PET imaging. J Thorac Imaging 2006; 21(2):146–153.

61. Wachter S, Tomek S, Kurtaran A, et al. ^{11}C-acetate positron emission tomography imaging and image fusion with computed tomography and magnetic resonance imaging in patients with recurrent prostate cancer. J Clin Oncol 2006; 24(16):2513–2519.

62. Kelloff GJ, Hoffman JM, Johnson B, et al. Progress and promise of FDG-PET imaging for cancer patient management and oncologic drug development. Clin Cancer Res 2005; 11(8): 2785–2808.

63. Juweid ME, Cheson BD. Positron-emission tomography and assessment of cancer therapy. N Engl J Med 2006; 354(5):496–507.

64. Lapointe D, Brasseur N, Cadorette J, et al. High-resolution PET imaging for in vivo monitoring of tumor response after photodynamic therapy in mice. J Nucl Med 1999; 40(5):876–882.

65. Lin C, Itti E, Haioun C, et al. Early 18F-FDG PET for prediction of prognosis in patients with diffuse large B-cell lymphoma: SUV-based assessment versus visual analysis. J Nucl Med 2007; 48(10):1626–1632.

66. de Geus-Oei LF, van der Heijden HF, Visser EP, et al. Chemotherapy response evaluation with 18F-FDG PET in patients with non-small cell lung cancer. J Nucl Med 2007; 48(10):1592–1598.

67. Dose Schwarz J, Bader M, Jenicke L, et al. Early prediction of response to chemotherapy in metastatic breast cancer using sequential 18F-FDG PET. J Nucl Med 2005; 46(7):1144–1150.

68. Antoch G, Kanja J, Bauer S, et al. Comparison of PET, CT, and dual-modality PET/CT imaging for monitoring of imatinib (STI571) therapy in patients with gastrointestinal stromal tumors. J Nucl Med 2004; 45(3):357–365.

69. Sugiyama M, Sakahara H, Sato K, et al. Evaluation of 3'-deoxy-3'-18F-fluorothymidine for monitoring tumor response to radiotherapy and photodynamic therapy in mice. J Nucl Med 2004; 45(10):1754–1758.

70. Waldherr C, Mellinghoff IK, Tran C, et al. Monitoring antiproliferative responses to kinase inhibitor therapy in mice with 3'-deoxy-3'-18F-fluorothymidine PET. J Nucl Med 2005; 46(1): 114–120.

71. Chen W, Delaloye S, Silverman DH, et al. Predicting treatment response of malignant gliomas to bevacizumab and irinotecan by imaging proliferation with [18F] fluorothymidine positron emission tomography: a pilot study. J Clin Oncol 2007; 25(30):4714–4721.

72. Chen DL, Schuster DP. Imaging pulmonary inflammation with positron emission tomography: a biomarker for drug development. Mol Pharm 2006; 3(5):488–495.

73. Choyke PL, Dwyer AJ, Knopp MV. Functional tumor imaging with dynamic contrast-enhanced magnetic resonance imaging. J Magn Reson Imaging 2003; 17(5):509–520.

74. Leach MO, Brindle KM, Evelhoch JL, et al. The assessment of antiangiogenic and antivascular therapies in early-stage clinical trials using magnetic resonance imaging: issues and recommendations. Br J Cancer 2005; 92(9):1599–1610.

75. Jordan BF, Runquist M, Raghunand N, et al. The thioredoxin-1 inhibitor 1-methylpropyl 2-imidazolyl disulfide (PX-12) decreases vascular permeability in tumor xenografts monitored

by dynamic contrast enhanced magnetic resonance imaging. Clin Cancer Res 2005; 11(2 pt 1): 529–536.

76. Thoeny HC, De Keyzer F, Vandecaveye V, et al. Effect of vascular targeting agent in rat tumor model: dynamic contrast-enhanced versus diffusion-weighted MR imaging. Radiology 2005; 237(2):492–499.

77. Daldrup H, Shames DM, Wendland M, et al. Correlation of dynamic contrast-enhanced MR imaging with histologic tumor grade: comparison of macromolecular and small-molecular contrast media. AJR Am J Roentgenol 1998; 171(4):941–949.

78. Marzola P, Degrassi A, Calderan L, et al. In vivo assessment of antiangiogenic activity of SU6668 in an experimental colon carcinoma model. Clin Cancer Res 2004; 10(2):739–750.

79. Preda A, Novikov V, Möglich M, et al. MRI monitoring of Avastin antiangiogenesis therapy using B22956/1, a new blood pool contrast agent, in an experimental model of human cancer. J Magn Reson Imaging 2004; 20(5):865–873.

80. Cheng HL, Wallis C, Shou Z, et al. Quantifying angiogenesis in VEGF-enhanced tissue-engineered bladder constructs by dynamic contrast-enhanced MRI using contrast agents of different molecular weights. J Magn Reson Imaging 2007; 25(1):137–145.

81. Mohs AM, Lu ZR. Gadolinium(III)-based blood-pool contrast agents for magnetic resonance imaging: status and clinical potential. Expert Opin Drug Deliv 2007; 4(2):149–164.

82. Chung YL, Troy H, Banerji U, et al. Magnetic resonance spectroscopic pharmacodynamic markers of the heat shock protein 90 inhibitor 17-allylamino,17-demethoxygeldanamycin (17AAG) in human colon cancer models. J Natl Cancer Inst 2003; 95(21):1624–1633.

83. Glunde K, Ackerstaff E, Mori N, et al. Choline phospholipid metabolism in cancer: consequences for molecular pharmaceutical interventions. Mol Pharm 2006; 3(5):496–506.

84. Morse DL, Raghunand N, Sadarangani P, et al. Response of choline metabolites to docetaxel therapy is quantified in vivo by localized (31)P MRS of human breast cancer xenografts and in vitro by high-resolution (31)P NMR spectroscopy of cell extracts. Magn Reson Med 2007; 58(2): 270–280.

85. Al-Saffar NM, Troy H, Ramírez de Molina A, et al. Noninvasive magnetic resonance spectroscopic pharmacodynamic markers of the choline kinase inhibitor MN58b in human carcinoma models. Cancer Res 2006; 66:427–434.

86. De Stefano N, Filippi M, Miller D, et al. Guidelines for using proton MR spectroscopy in multicenter clinical MS studies. Neurology 2007; 69(20):1942–1952.

7

Chemical Kinetics and Drug Stability

David Attwood
School of Pharmacy and Pharmaceutical Sciences, University of Manchester, Manchester, U.K.

Rolland I. Poust
College of Pharmacy, University of Iowa, Iowa City, Iowa, U.S.A.

INTRODUCTION

In the rational design and evaluation of dosage forms for drugs, the stability of the active components must be a major criterion in determining their suitability. Several forms of instability can lead to the rejection of a drug product. First, there may be chemical degradation of the active drug, leading to a substantial lowering of the quantity of the therapeutic agent in the dosage form. Many drugs (e.g., digoxin and theophylline) have narrow therapeutic indices, and they need to be carefully titrated in individual patients so that serum levels are neither so high that they are potentially toxic nor so low that they are ineffective. For these drugs, it is of paramount importance that the dosage form reproducibly delivers the same amount of drug.

Second, although chemical degradation of the active drug may not be extensive, a toxic product may be formed in the decomposition process. There are several examples in which the products of degradation are significantly more toxic than the original therapeutic agent. For example, the conversions of tetracycline to epianhydrotetracycline, arsphenamine to oxophenarsine, and p-aminosalicylic acid to m-aminophenol in dosage forms give rise to potentially toxic agents that, when ingested, can cause undesirable effects. Nord et al. (1) reported that the antimalarial chloroquine can produce toxic reactions that are attributable to the photochemical degradation of the substance. Phototoxicity has also been reported to occur following administration of chlordiazepoxide and nitrazepam (2). Another example of an adverse reaction caused by a degradation product was provided by Neftel et al. (3), who showed that infusion of degraded penicillin G led to sensitization of lymphocytes and formation of antipenicilloyl antibodies.

Third, instability of a drug product can lead to a decrease in its bioavailability, rather than to loss of drug or to formation of toxic degradation products. This reduction in bioavailability can result in a substantial lowering in the therapeutic efficacy of the dosage form. This phenomenon can be caused by physical or chemical changes in the excipients in the dosage form, independent of whatever changes the active drug may have undergone.

Fourth, there may be substantial changes in the physical appearance of the dosage form. Examples of these physical changes include mottling of tablets, creaming of emulsions, and caking of suspensions. Although the therapeutic efficacy of the dosage form may be unaffected by these changes, the patient will most likely lose confidence in the drug product, which then has to be rejected.

In the present chapter, stability problems and chemical kinetics are introduced and surveyed. The sequence employed is as follows: first, an overview of the potential routes of degradation that drug molecules can undergo; then, a discussion of the mathematics used to quantify drug degradation; a delineation of the factors that can affect degradation rates, with an emphasis on stabilization techniques; a brief outline of the stability of solutions of proteins and peptides; and, finally, a description of the stability-testing protocols employed in the pharmaceutical industry. It is not the intent of this chapter to document stability data of various individual drugs. Readers are referred to the compilations of the stability data (4) and to literature on specific drugs (e.g., Ref. 5 and earlier volumes) for this kind of information.

CHEMICAL DECOMPOSITION OF DRUGS

Hydrolysis

In this type of reaction, the active drug undergoes decomposition following reaction with the solvent present. Usually, the solvent is water, but sometimes the reaction may involve pharmaceutical cosolvents, such as ethyl alcohol or polyethylene glycol. These solvents can act as nucleophiles, attacking the electropositive centers in drug molecules. The most common hydrolysis reactions encountered in pharmaceuticals are those involving "labile" carbonyl compounds, such as esters, lactones, and lactams (Table 1). Although all the functional groups cited are, in principle, subject to hydrolysis, the rates at which they undergo this reaction may be vastly different. For example, the rate of hydrolysis of a β-lactam ring (a cyclized amide) is much greater than that of its linear analog. The half-life (the time needed for half the drug to decompose) of the β-lactam in potassium phenethicillin at 35°C and pH 1.5 is about one hour. The corresponding half-life of penicillin G is about four minutes (6). In contrast, the half-life for hydrolysis of the simple amide propionamide in 0.18 molal H_2SO_4 at 25°C is about 58 hours (7). It has been suggested that the antibacterial activity of β-lactam antibiotics arises from a combination of their chemical reactivity and their molecular recognition by target enzymes. One aspect of their chemical reactivity is their acylating power and, although penicillins are not very good acylating agents, they are more reactive than simple, unsubstituted amides (8). Unactivated or "normal" amides undergo nonenzymatic hydrolysis slowly, except under the most extreme conditions of pH and temperature, because the N–C(O) linkage is inherently stable, yet when the amine function is a good leaving group (and particularly if it has a $pK_a > 4.5$), amides can be susceptible to hydrolysis at ordinary temperatures. A recent review by LePree and Connors gives a detailed account of the mechanisms involved in the hydrolytic degradation of drugs (9). Acyl transfer reactions in peptides, including the transfer to water (hydrolysis), are of fundamental importance in biological systems in which the reactions proceed at normal temperatures, and enzymes serve as

Table 1 Some Functional Groups Subject to Hydrolysis

Drug type		Examples
Esters	$RCOOR'$ $ROPO_3M_x$ $ROSO_3M_x$ $RONO_2$	Aspirin, alkaloids Dexamethasone sodium phosphate Estrone sulfate Nitroglycerin
Lactones		Pilocarpine Spironolactone
Amides	$RCON\,R'_2$	Thiacinamide Chloramphenicol
Lactams		Penicillins Cephalosporins
Oximes	$R_2C = NOR$	Steroid oximes
Imides		Glutethimide Ethosuximide
Malonic ureas		Barbiturates
Nitrogen mustards		Melphalan

catalysts; the chemical degradation of proteins and peptides is discussed in section "Protein Stability."

The most frequently encountered hydrolysis reaction in drug instability is that of the ester, but certain esters can be stable for many years when properly formulated. Substituents can have a dramatic effect on reaction rates. For example, the *tert*-butyl ester of acetic acid is about 120 times more stable than the methyl ester, which, in turn, is approximately 60 times more stable than the vinyl analog (10). Structure-reactivity relationships are dealt with in the discipline of physical organic chemistry. Substituent groups may exert electronic (inductive and resonance), steric, or hydrogen bonding effects that can drastically affect the stability of the compounds. Interested students are referred to a review by Hansch et al. (11), and to the classic reference text written by Hammett (12).

A dramatic decrease in ester stability can be brought about by intramolecular catalysis. This type of facilitation is affected mostly by neighboring groups capable of exhibiting acid-base properties (e.g., $-NH_2$, $-OH$, $-COOH$, and $COO-$). If neighboring group participation leads to an enhanced reaction rate, the group is said to provide anchimeric assistance (13). For example, the ethyl salicylate anion undergoes hydrolysis in alkaline solution at a rate that is 10^6 times greater than the experimental value for the uncatalyzed cleavage of ethyl *p*-hydroxybenzoate. The rate advantage is attributed to intramolecular general base catalysis by the phenolate anion (14).

Since hydrolysis is frequently catalyzed by hydrogen ions (specific acid catalysis) or hydroxyl ions (specific base catalysis), the most usual method of controlling drug decomposition is to determine the pH of maximum stability from kinetic experiments at a range of pH values and to formulate the product at this pH. Problems may, however, be encountered when adjusting pH because of catalysis by the acidic and basic species that are commonly encountered as components of buffers (general acid-base catalysis). Alteration of the dielectric constant by the addition of nonaqueous solvents such as alcohol, glycerin, or propylene glycol may in many cases reduce hydrolysis (see section "Liquid Dosage Forms"). Since only that portion of the drug which is in solution will be hydrolyzed, it is possible to suppress degradation by making the drug less soluble. Swintosky et al. (15), for example, reduced the solubility of penicillin in procaine penicillin suspensions by using additives such as citrates, dextrose, sorbitol, and gluconate and, in so doing, significantly increased the stability. Higuchi and Lachman (16) suggested adding a compound that forms a complex with the drug as a means of increasing stability. The addition of caffeine to aqueous solutions of benzocaine, procaine, and amethocaine was shown to decrease the base-catalyzed hydrolysis of these local anesthetics in this way. Solubilization of a drug by surfactants in many cases protects against hydrolysis, as discussed in section "Liquid Dosage Forms."

Modification of chemical structure using appropriate substituents is a possible method for reducing chemical degradation, provided of course that such modification does not reduce therapeutic efficiency. The Hammett linear free energy relationship for the effect of substituents on the rates of aromatic side-chain reactions, such as the hydrolysis of esters, is given by

$$\log k = \log k_0 + \sigma\rho \qquad (1)$$

where k and k_0 are the rate constants for the reaction of the substituted and unsubstituted compounds, respectively, σ is the Hammett substituent constant (which is determined by the nature of the substituents and is independent of the reaction), and ρ is the reaction constant which is dependent on the reaction, the conditions of the reaction, and the nature of the side chains undergoing the reaction. According to equation (1), a plot of $\log k$ against the Hammett constant [values are readily available in the literature (17)] will be linear with a slope of ρ. This concept has been used, for example, in the production of the best substituents for allylbarbituric acids to obtain optimum stability (18).

Oxidation

Although after hydrolysis, oxidation is the next most common pathway for drug breakdown, the oxidative degradation of drugs has received comparatively little attention. In most cases where simultaneous hydrolytic and oxidative degradation can occur, the oxidative process has usually been eliminated by storage under anaerobic conditions without an investigation of the oxidative mechanism. Recent reviews by Hovorka and Schöneich (19) and Pezzuto and Park (20) give details on the theory and mechanisms involved in the oxidative degradation of drugs.

Oxidation involves the removal of an electropositive atom, radical, or electron, or the addition of an electronegative atom or radical. Oxidative degradation can occur by *autoxidation*, in which reaction is uncatalyzed and proceeds quite slowly under the influence of molecular oxygen, or may involve *chain processes* consisting of three concurrent reactions—initiation, propagation, and termination. The mechanisms are, however, generally complex and involve multiple pathways for these three stages. Initiation can be via free radicals formed from organic compounds by the action of light, heat, or transition metals such as copper and iron, which are present in trace amounts in almost every buffer. Many autoxidation reactions are initiated by trace amounts of impurities, such as metal ions or hydroperoxides. Thus, ferric ion catalyzes the degradation reaction and decreases the induction period for the oxidation of the compound procaterol (21). As little as 0.0002 M copper ion will increase the rate of vitamin C oxidation by a factor of 10^5 (22). Hydroperoxides contained in polyethylene glycol suppository bases have been implicated in the oxidation of codeine to codeine-*N*-oxide (23). Peroxides apparently are responsible for the accelerated degradation of benzocaine hydrochloride in aqueous cetomacrogol solution (24) and of a corticosteroid in polyethylene glycol 300 (25,26). Many oxidation reactions are catalyzed by acids and bases (27).

The propagation stage of the reaction involves the combination of molecular oxygen with the free radical $R^{\bullet}$ to form a peroxy radical $ROO^{\bullet}$, which then removes H from a molecule of the organic compound to form a hydroperoxide, ROOH, and in so doing creates a new free radical. A simplified representation of the reaction process is

Initiation: $X^{\bullet} + RH \rightarrow R^{\bullet} + XH$

Propagation: $R^{\bullet} + O_2 \rightarrow ROO^{\bullet}$

$ROO^{\bullet} + RH \rightarrow ROOH + R^{\bullet}$

Termination: $ROO^{\bullet} + ROO^{\bullet} \rightarrow$ stable product

$ROO^{\bullet} + R^{\bullet} \rightarrow$ stable product

$R^{\bullet} + R^{\bullet} \rightarrow$ stable product

The reaction proceeds until the free radicals are destroyed by inhibitors or side reactions, which eventually break the chain. The rancid odor, a characteristic of oxidized fats and oils, is due to aldehydes, ketones, and short-chain fatty acids, which are the breakdown products of the hydroperoxides. Peroxides (ROOR′) and hydroperoxides (ROOH) are photolabile, breaking down to hydroxyl ($HO^{\bullet}$) and/or alkoxyl ($RO^{\bullet}$) radicals, which are themselves highly oxidizing species. The presence of residual peroxides in polyoxyethylene glycols is a cause for concern when these excipients are used in formulation, as for example in the case of fenprostalene (28).

A list of some functional groups that are particularly sensitive to oxidation is shown in Table 2. Some examples of drugs and excipients that are subject to oxidative degradation by the possession of these or other functional groups will be considered.

The possession of carbon-carbon double bonds can render a drug molecule susceptible to oxidation because of the addition of peroxyl radicals to these alkene moieties, as for example in the case of steroids and sterols. Addition of peroxyl radicals to the conjugated double bonds of the cholesterol-lowering agent simvastatin may lead to the formation of polymeric peroxides [simvastatin polymerizes up to a pentamer (29)], cleavage of which produces epoxides that may further degrade into aldehydes or ketones. Similarly, polyene antibiotics, such as amphotericin B, which contains seven conjugated double bonds (heptaene moiety), are subject to attack by peroxyl radicals leading to aggregation and loss of activity (30).

Table 2 Some Functional Groups Subject to Autoxidation

Funtional group		Examples
Phenols		Phenols in steroids
Catechols		Catecholamines (dopamine, isoproterenol)
Ethers	R–O–R′	Diethylether
Thiols	RCH$_2$SH	Dimercaprol (BAL)
Thioethers	R–S–R′	Phenothiazines (chlorpromazine)
Carboxylic acids	RCOOH	Fatty acids
Nitrites	RNO$_2$	Amyl nitrite
Aldehydes	RCHO	Paraldehyde

Polyunsaturated fatty acids, commonly used in drug formulations, are particularly susceptible to oxidation, and care must be exercised to minimize degradation in formulations containing high concentrations of, for example, vegetable oils (31).

The oxidation of phenothiazines to the sulfoxide involves two single-electron transfer reactions involving a radical cation intermediate; the sulfoxide is subsequently formed by reaction of the cation with water (32).

The ether group in drugs such as econazole nitrate and miconazole nitrate is susceptible to oxidation. The process involves removal of hydrogen from the C–H bonds in the α-position to the oxygen to produce a radical, which further degrades to α-hydroperoxides and eventually to aldehydes, ketones, alcohols, and carboxylic acids (33).

An obvious precaution to minimize oxidation is to avoid contact of the drug with ions such as iron, cobalt, or nickel that are initiators of the oxidation process. Similarly, the oxygen above the formulation should be replaced with nitrogen or carbon dioxide. Even traces of oxygen are, however, sufficient to initiate oxidation, and because it is difficult to remove all of the oxygen from a container, it is common practice to add low concentrations of antioxidants and chelating agents to protect drugs against autoxidation. Mechanistically, some antioxidants, such as ascorbic acid, ascorbyl palmitate, sodium bisulfite, sodium metabisulfite, sodium sulfite, acetone sodium bisulfite, sodium formaldehyde sulfoxylate, thioglycerol, and thioglycolic acid, act as reducing agents. They are easily oxidized, preferentially undergo autoxidation, thereby consuming oxygen and protecting the drug or excipient. They are often called oxygen scavengers because their autoxidation reaction consumes oxygen. They are particularly useful in closed systems in which the oxygen cannot be replaced once it is consumed. Primary or true antioxidants act by providing electrons or labile H, which will be accepted by any free radical to terminate the chain reaction. In pharmaceuticals, the most commonly used primary antioxidants are butylated hydroxytoluene (BHT), butylated hydroxyanisole (BHA), the tocopherols (vitamin E), and propyl gallate. Chelating agents act by forming complexes with the heavy metal ions that are often required to initiate oxidation reactions. The chelating agents used most often are ethylenediaminetetraacetic acid (EDTA) derivatives and salts, citric acid, and tartaric acid.

Photolysis

Normal sunlight or room light may cause substantial degradation of drug molecules. The energy from light radiation must be absorbed by the molecules to cause a photolytic reaction, and if that energy is sufficient to achieve activation, degradation of the molecule is possible. Saturated molecules do not interact with visible or near-ultraviolet light, but molecules that contain π-electrons usually do absorb light throughout this wavelength range.

Tønnesen (34) has reviewed the mechanisms of photodecomposition of drugs, and an extensive list of common photoreactions of drug substances has been compiled by Greenhill and McLelland (35). Certain chemical functions are known to introduce photoreactivity, including carbonyl, nitroaromatic and *N*-oxide functions, aryl halides, alkenes, polyenes, and sulfides. Nevertheless, it is difficult to predict which drugs are likely to be susceptible to photodegradation. Examples of drugs that are known to degrade when exposed to light include the phenothiazine tranquillizers, hydrocortisone, prednisolone, riboflavine, ascorbic acid, and folic acid. Not only is there a loss of potency of the drug when photodegradation occurs, but there is often discoloration of the product or onset of precipitation. Because sunlight is able to penetrate the skin to a sufficient depth to cause photodegradation of drugs circulating in the surface capillaries or in the eyes of patients receiving the photolabile drug, photodecomposition might occur not only during storage, but also during usage of the product. An additional problem is that excipients in the formulation (so-called photosensitizers) may absorb radiation and transfer this absorbed energy to the drug causing its degradation. Consequently, when assessing photosensitivity of a pharmaceutical product, it is necessary to consider the formulation as a whole and not just the drug itself (36).

Photolysis reactions are often associated with oxidation because the latter category of reactions can frequently be initiated by light. But photolysis reactions are not restricted to oxidation. The mechanisms of photodegradation are of such complexity as to have been fully elucidated in only a few cases. For example, the photodegradation of ketoprofen (36) (Scheme 1) can involve decarboxylation to form an intermediate (reaction 1), which then undergoes reduction (reaction 2), or dimerization of the ketoprofen itself (reaction 3).

The photodegradation of sodium nitroprusside, $Na_2Fe(CN)_5NO\cdot2H_2O$, in aqueous solution is believed to result from loss of the nitro-ligand from the molecule, followed by electronic rearrangement and hydration. Sodium nitroprusside is administered by IV infusion for the management of acute hypertension. On being exposed to normal room

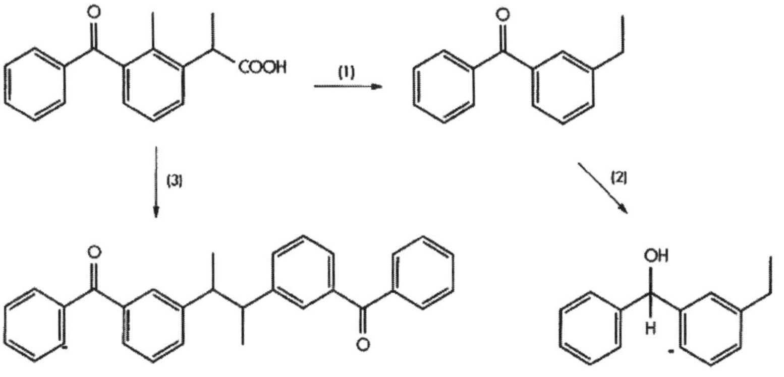

Scheme 1 Photodegradation of ketoprofen.

light, a sodium nitroprusside solution has a shelf life of only four hours (37), but when protected from light by wrapping in an aluminum foil, sodium nitroprusside 50 or 100 μg/mL was found to be stable in 5% glucose, lactated Ringer's, and normal saline solutions for 48 hours (38).

Pharmaceutical products can be adequately protected from photo-induced decomposition by the use of colored glass containers and storage in the dark. Amber glass excludes light of wavelength <470 nm and so affords considerable protection of compounds sensitive to ultraviolet light. In the clinical administration of solutions of sodium nitroprusside, for example, the infusion container should be opaque or protected with foil, but an amber-giving set may be used, to allow visual monitoring (39). Coating tablets with a polymer film containing ultraviolet absorbers has been suggested as an additional method for protection from light. In this respect, a film coating of vinyl acetate containing oxybenzone as an ultraviolet absorber has been shown (40) to be effective in minimizing the discoloration and photolytic degradation of sulfasomidine tablets.

Racemization

The racemization of pharmacologically active agents is of interest because enantiomers often have significantly different absorption, distribution, metabolism, and excretion, in addition to differing pharmacological actions (41). The best-known racemization reactions of drugs are those that involve epinephrine, pilocarpine, ergotamine, and tetracycline. In these drugs, the reaction mechanism appears to involve an intermediate carbonium ion or carbanion that is stabilized electronically by the neighboring substituent group. For example, in the racemization of pilocarpine (42), a carbanion is produced and stabilized by delocalization to the enolate. In addition to the racemization reaction, pilocarpine is also degraded through hydrolysis of the lactone ring.

Most racemization reactions are catalyzed by an acid or a base. For example, the isomerization of cephalosporin esters, which are widely used as intermediates in cephalosporin synthesis and as prodrugs for oral administration of parenteral cephalosporins, is base-catalyzed according to the following mechanism (43) (Scheme 2). A proton in the 2-position is abstracted by a base (B), and the resulting carbanion can be reprotonated in the 4-postion, giving a Δ2-ester. On hydrolysis, Δ2-cephalosporin esters yield Δ2-cephalosporins, which are biologically inactive.

A notable exception to the generality of acid-base–catalyzed reaction is the "spontaneous" racemization of the diuretic and antihypertensive agent, chlorthalidone, which undergoes facile S_N1 solvolysis of its tertiary hydroxyl group to form a planar carbonium ion. Chiral configuration is then restored by nucleophilic attack (S_N2) of a molecule of water on the carbonium ion, with subsequent elimination of a proton (44).

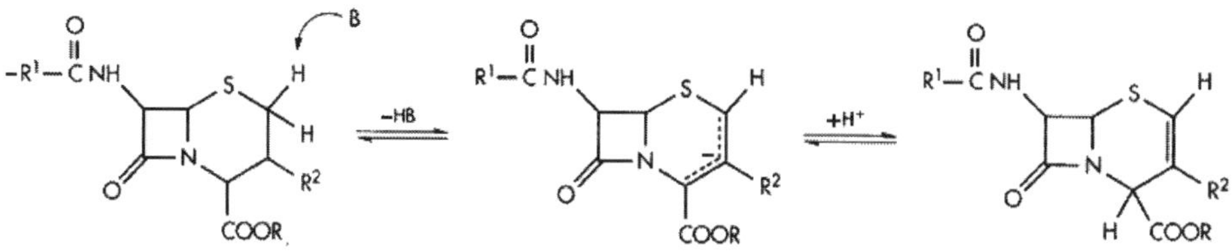

Scheme 2 Proposed mechanism for the base-catalyzed isomerization of cephalosporin esters.

Polymerization

A few examples have been cited of drugs that undergo polymerization during storage in solution. For example, Bundgaard (45) has shown that a polymerization process occurs during the storage of concentrated aqueous solutions of amino-penicillins, such as ampicillin sodium. The reactive β-lactam bond of the ampicillin molecule is opened by reaction with the side chain of a second ampicillin molecule, and a dimer is formed. The process can continue to form higher polymers. Such polymeric substances have been shown to be highly antigenic in animals, and they are considered to play a part in eliciting penicilloyl-specific allergic reactions to ampicillin in man. The dimerizing tendency of the amino-penicillins increases with the increase in the basicity of the side-chain group, the order, in terms of increasing rates, being cyclacillin $<<$ ampicillin $<$ epicillin $<$ amoxycillin.

Incompatibilities

Not only is it important to be aware of chemical instability of the drug itself, but it is also necessary to consider possible instability of the product caused by chemical interactions between two or more drug components in the same dosage form, or between an active ingredient and a pharmaceutical adjuvant. An example of drug-drug incompatibility is the inactivation of cationic aminoglycoside antibiotics, such as kanamycin and gentamicin, by anionic penicillins in IV admixtures. The formation of an inactive complex between these two classes of antibiotics occurs not only in vitro, but apparently also in vivo in patients with severe renal failure (46). Thus, when gentamicin sulfate (GS) was given alone to patients on long-term hemodialysis, the biological half-life of gentamicin was greater than 60 hours. But when carbenicillin disodium (CD) was given with GS in the dose ratio CD/GS 80:1, the gentamicin half-life was reduced to about 24 hours.

QUANTITATION OF THE RATE OF DEGRADATION

Before a discussion of the mathematics involved in the determination of reaction rates is undertaken, it is necessary to point out the importance of proper data acquisition in stability testing. Applications of rate equations and predictions are meaningful only if the data used in such processes are collected using valid statistical and analytical procedures. It is beyond the scope of this chapter to discuss the proper statistical treatments and analytical techniques that should be used in a stability study. But some perspectives in these areas can be obtained by reading the comprehensive review by Meites (47) and from the section on statistical considerations in the stability guidelines published by the FDA in 1987 (48).

Kinetics of Chemical Decomposition in Solution

Consider the reaction

$$a\mathrm{A} + b\mathrm{B} \rightarrow m\mathrm{M} + n\mathrm{N} \qquad (2)$$

where A and B are the reactants, M and N the products, and a, b, m, and n the stoichiometric coefficients describing the reaction. The rate of change of the concentration (denoted by square brackets) of any of the species can be expressed by the differential notations, $-d[\mathrm{A}]/dt$, $-d[\mathrm{B}]/dt$, $d[\mathrm{M}]/dt$, and $d[\mathrm{N}]/dt$. Note that the rates of change for the reactants are preceded by a negative sign, denoting a decrease in the concentration relative to time (rate of disappearance). In contrast, the differential terms for the products are positive in sign, indicating an increase in the concentration of these species as time increases (rate of appearance). The rates of disappearance of A and B and the rates of appearance of M and N are interrelated by equations that take into account the stoichiometry of the reaction:

$$-\frac{1}{a}\frac{d[A]}{dt} = -\frac{1}{b}\frac{d[B]}{dt} = \frac{1}{m}\frac{d[M]}{dt} = \frac{1}{n}\frac{d[N]}{dt} \tag{3}$$

The Rate Expression

The rate expression is a mathematical description of the rate of the reaction at any time t in terms of the concentration(s) of the molecular species present at that time. By using the hypothetical reaction $aA + bB \rightarrow$ products, the rate expression can be written as

$$-\frac{d[A]}{dt} = -\frac{d[B]}{dt} \, \alpha \, [A]_t^a [B]_t^b \tag{4}$$

Equation (4) in essence states that the rate of change of the concentration of A at time t is equal to that of B, and that each of these rate changes at time t is proportional to the product of the concentrations of the reactants raised to the respective powers. Note that $[A]_t$ and $[B]_t$ are time-dependent variables. As the reaction proceeds, both $[A]_t$ and $[B]_t$ will decrease in magnitude. For simplicity, these concentrations can be denoted simply by $[A]$ and $[B]$, respectively,

$$-\frac{d[A]}{dt} = -\frac{d[B]}{dt} = k[A]^a[B]^b \tag{5}$$

where k is a proportionality constant, commonly referred to as the reaction rate constant or the specific rate constant. The format for rate expressions generally involves concentration terms of only the reactants and very rarely those of the products. The latter occurs only when the products participate in the reaction once it has been initiated.

The order of the reaction, n, can be defined as $n = a + b$. Extended to the general case, the order of a reaction is the numerical sum of the exponents of the concentration terms in the rate expression. Thus, if $a = b = 1$, the reaction just described is said to be second order overall, first order relative to A, and first order relative to B. In principle, the numerical value of a or b can be integral or fractional.

Experimentally we can monitor the rate of breakdown of the drug either by its decrease in concentration with time or alternatively by the rate of appearance of one of the breakdown products. So if we represent the initial concentration of drug A as a mol/L and if we find experimentally that x mol/L of the drug has reacted in time t, then the amount of drug remaining at a time t is $(a - x)$ mol/L and the rate of reaction is

$$-\frac{d[A]}{dt} = -\frac{d(a - x)}{dt} = \frac{dx}{dt} \tag{6}$$

Notice that the term a is a constant and therefore disappears during differentiation. We will use dx/dt to describe the reaction rate in this section.

Simple Reactions

Reactions are classified according to the number of reacting species whose concentration determines the rate at which the reaction occurs, that is, the *order of the reaction*. This chapter concentrates mainly on *zero-order* reactions, in which the breakdown rate is independent of the concentration of any of the reactants; *first-order* reactions, in which the reaction rate is determined by one concentration term; and *second-order* reactions, in which the rate is determined by the concentrations of two reacting species.

It is obvious that to quantify the rate expression, the magnitude of the rate constant k needs to be determined. Proper assignment of the reaction order and accurate determination of the rate constant is important when reaction mechanisms are to be deduced from the kinetic data. The integrated form of the reaction equation is easier to use in handling kinetic data, and the integrated kinetic relationships commonly used for zero-, first-, and second-order reactions are summarized below.

Zero-order reactions In this type of reaction, the decomposition proceeds at a constant rate and is independent of the concentrations of any of the reactants. Zero-order reactions can often occur in suspensions of poorly soluble drugs. In these systems, the suspended drug slowly dissolves as the drug decomposes and so a constant drug concentration is maintained in the solution. Many decompositions in the solid state also apparently follow zero-order kinetics.

The rate equation is given by

$$\frac{dx}{dt} = k_0 \tag{7}$$

Integration of equation (7), noting that $x = 0$ at $t = 0$, gives

$$x = k_0 \times t \tag{8}$$

and hence the zero-order rate constant, k_0, may be determined from the gradient of a linear plot of the amount remaining as a function of time.

The time taken for half of the reactant to decompose is referred to as the *half-life* of the reaction, $t_{1/2}$. An expression for $t_{1/2}$ for a zero-order reaction may be derived from equation (8), noting that when $t = t_{1/2}$, $x = a/2$, hence

$$t_{1/2} = \frac{a}{2k_0} \tag{9}$$

First-order reactions The rate of first-order reactions is determined by one concentration term and may be written as

$$\frac{dx}{dt} = k_1(a - x) \tag{10}$$

Integration of equation (10) within the limits $x = 0$ when $t = 0$ gives

$$k_1 = \frac{2.303}{t} \log \frac{a}{a - x} \tag{11}$$

Rearranging into a linear form gives

$$t = \frac{2.303}{k_1} \log a - \frac{2.303}{k_1} \log(a - x) \tag{12}$$

The first-order rate constant k_1 may be obtained from the gradient, $-k_1/2.303$, of the linear plot of the logarithm of the amount of drug remaining (as ordinate) as a function of time (as abscissa). k_1 has units of time^{-1}.

An expression for the half-life of a first-order reaction may be derived from equation (11):

$$t_{1/2} = \frac{2.303}{k_1} \log \frac{a}{a/2} \tag{13}$$

Thus

$$t_{1/2} = \frac{2.303}{k_1} \log 2 = \frac{0.693}{k_1} \tag{14}$$

The half-life is therefore independent of the initial concentration of the reactants unlike the case of a zero-order reaction.

Even when a reaction involves more than one reacting species, the rate may still follow first-order kinetics. The most common example of this occurs in the reaction between an ester and water (hydrolysis) in a predominantly aqueous environment. If the initial concentration of the ester is 0.5 M or less, complete hydrolysis of the ester will bring about a corresponding decrease in the concentration of water of 0.5 M or less. Since the initial water concentration is 1000/18, which is about 55 M for an aqueous solution, the loss of water through reaction is insignificantly small and its concentration can be considered a constant throughout the entire course of the reaction. The reaction is thus apparently first order relative to ester and zero order relative to water; the overall reaction is known as a pseudo–first-order reaction. This type of kinetics is observed whenever the concentration of one of the reactants is maintained constant, either by a vast excess initial concentration, or by rapid replenishment of one of the reactants. Thus, if one of the reactants is the hydrogen ion or the hydroxide ion, its concentration, though probably small when compared to that of the drug, can be kept constant throughout the reaction by using buffers in the solution.

Second-order reactions The rate of a second-order reaction is determined by the concentrations of two reacting species. If the initial concentrations of reactants A and B are a and b, respectively (where $a \neq b$), the general rate equation may be written as

$$\frac{dx}{dt} = k_2(a-x)(b-x) \tag{15}$$

where x is the amount of A and B decomposed in time t. Integration of equation (15) by the method of partial fractions yields the following expression for the second-order rate constant k_2:

$$k_2 = \frac{2.303}{t(a-b)} \log \frac{b(a-x)}{a(b-x)} \tag{16}$$

Rearranging into a linear form suitable for plotting gives

$$t = \frac{2.303}{k_2(a-b)} = \log \frac{b}{a} + \frac{2.303}{k_2(a-b)} \log \frac{(a-x)}{(b-x)} \tag{17}$$

k_2 can then be obtained from the gradient, $2.303/k_2(a-b)$, of a plot of t (as ordinate) against $\log[(a-x)/(b-x)]$ (as abscissa). The units of k_2 are concentration^{-1} time^{-1}.

For reactions in which the initial concentrations of the two reactants are the same ($a = b$),

$$\frac{dx}{dt} = k_2(a-x)^2 \tag{18}$$

Integration of equation (18) between the limits of t from 0 to t and of x from 0 to x yields

$$t = \frac{1}{k_2}\left[\frac{1}{a-x} - \frac{1}{a}\right] = \frac{x}{k_2 a(a-x)} \tag{19}$$

from which it is seen that a plot of t (ordinate) against $x/a(a-x)$ (abscissa) yields a linear plot of slope $1/k_2$.

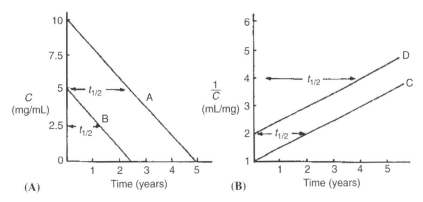

Figure 1 Effect of initial concentration on the half-life of (**A**) a zero-order and (**B**) a second-order reaction. (**A**) $k = 2$ mg/yr-mL; curve A, initial concentration $C_0 = 10$ mg/mL, $t_{1/2} = 2.5$ years; curve B, $C_0 = 5$ mg/mL, $t_{1/2} = 1.25$ years. (**B**) $k = 0.5$ mL/mg-yr; curve C, $C_0 = 1$ mg/mL, $t_{1/2} = 2$ years; curve D, $C_0 = 0.5$ mg/mL, $t_{1/2} = 4$ years.

The half-life of a reaction that follows equation (19) is given by

$$t_{1/2} = \frac{1}{k_2 a} \tag{20}$$

No simple expression can be derived for the half-life of a second-order reaction with unequal initial concentrations.

As with zero-order reactions, the half-life of a second-order reaction in which the initial concentrations of the reactants are equal is dependent on the initial concentration of the reactants. There is, however, an interesting difference in the concentration dependence in these two cases as shown in Figure 1 in which a zero-order reaction (Fig. 1A) and a second-order reaction (Fig. 1B) are plotted with two initial concentrations. It is readily seen that for a zero-order reaction, $t_{1/2}$ increases with a higher initial concentration. Conversely, for a second-order reaction, $t_{1/2}$ decreases with increasing initial concentration. For a reaction obeying first-order kinetics, $t_{1/2}$ is independent of the initial concentration of the reactant.

Determination of the order of reaction There are several ways by which the order of a reaction may be determined, the most obvious of which is to substitute the experimental data into the integrated equations for zero-, first-, and second-order reactions and observe which equation gives the most consistent value of k for a series of time intervals. Alternatively, the data may be displayed graphically according to the linear equations for the various orders of reactions until a linear plot is obtained. Thus, for example, if the data yield a linear graph when plotted as t against $\log (a - x)$, the reaction is then taken to be first order.

These methods, however, produce misleading results if a fractional order of reaction applies. In such cases, it may be necessary to determine the half-life for a series of initial drug concentrations, C_0, and substitute these values into equation (21).

$$\log t_{1/2} = \log \left[\frac{2^{n-1} - 1}{k(n-1)} \right] + (1 - n) \log C_0 \tag{21}$$

The order of the reaction, n, is then calculated from the gradient of plots of $\log t_{1/2}$ as a function of $\log C_0$.

Complex Reactions

In many instances, drug decomposition does not follow the simple reaction schemes outlined above because, for example, the reaction proceeds simultaneously by more than one pathway or involves several consecutive breakdown steps. In such cases, it is necessary to modify the rate equations as shown in the following examples of the most common types of complex reaction.

Parallel first-order reactions In many instances, the drug may degrade through more than one pathway, the preferred route being dependent on the reaction conditions.

$$A$$
$$k_A \nearrow$$
$$X$$
$$k_B \searrow$$
$$B$$

The composite rate equation for a parallel reaction is the sum of the rate constants for each pathway. Assuming that each of the decomposition processes follows first-order kinetics, the rate equation is

$$-\frac{d[X]}{dt} = (k_A + k_B)[X] = k \exp [X] \tag{22}$$

where k_A and k_B are the rate constants for the formation of A and B, respectively, and k_{exp} is the experimentally determined rate constant. Values of the rate constants k_A and k_B may be evaluated separately if it is possible to monitor the concentration of drug X and that of the breakdown products A and B as a function of time. The rate of formation of A can be expressed as

$$\frac{d[A]}{dt} = k_A[X] = k_A[X]_0 e^{-k_{exp}t} \tag{23}$$

where [A] is the concentration of the product A at time t, and $[X]_0$ is the initial concentration of the drug. It is reasonable to assume that the initial concentration of product A is zero and therefore integration of equation (23) gives

$$[A] = \frac{k_A}{k_{exp}}[X]_0(1 - e^{-k_{exp}t}) \tag{24}$$

Similarly, for product B,

$$[B] = \frac{k_B}{k_{exp}}[X]_0(1 - e^{-k_{exp}t}) \tag{25}$$

According to equations (24) and (25), plots of [A] or [B] against $(1 - e^{-k_{exp}t})$ should be linear with gradients $k_A[X]_0/k_{exp}$ and $k_B[X]_0/k_{exp}$, respectively, from which values of the rate constants k_A and k_B may be determined.

Reversible Reactions

Treatment of the kinetics of a reversible reaction involves two rate constants—one, k_f, to describe the rate of the forward reaction and the other, k_r, to describe the rate of the reverse reaction. The simplest example is one in which both of these reactions are first order, that is

$$A \underset{k_r}{\overset{k_f}{\rightleftharpoons}} B \tag{26}$$

It is important to note that equation (26) represents an approach to equilibrium in which the concentration of A decreases to form B and some of B reverts to A; a true equilibrium situation requires that the concentration of both A and B does not change with time.

According to equation (26), the net rate of decomposition of reactant A is given by the rate at which A decreases in the forward step minus the rate at which it increases in the reverse step, that is

$$\frac{-d[A]}{dt} = k_f[A] - k_r[B] \tag{27}$$

Equation (27) may be integrated noting that $[A]_0 - [A] = [B]$ and introducing the equilibrium condition $k_f[A]_{eq} = k_r[B]_{eq}$ to yield

$$t = \frac{2.303}{(k_f + k_r)} \log \frac{[A]_0 - [A]_{eq}}{[A] - [A]_{eq}} \tag{28}$$

where $[A]_0$, $[A]$, and $[A]_{eq}$ represent the initial concentration, the concentration at time t, and the equilibrium concentration of reactant A, respectively. Equation (28) indicates that a plot of t (as ordinate) against $\log\{([A]_0 - [A]_{eq})/([A] - [A]_{eq})\}$ should be linear with a slope of $2.303/(k_f + k_r)$. k_f and k_r may be calculated separately if the equilibrium constant K is also determined, since

$$K = \frac{[B]_{eq}}{[A]_{eq}} = \frac{(1 - [A]_{eq})}{[A]_{eq}} = \frac{k_f}{k_r} \tag{29}$$

where $[B]_{eq}$ is the equilibrium concentration of product B.

Consecutive Reactions

In its simplest form, a consecutive reaction may be described by a sequence

$$A \xrightarrow{k_A} B \xrightarrow{k_B} C$$

where each step is a nonreversible first-order reaction. The rate of decomposition of A is

$$\frac{-d[A]}{dt} = k_A[A] \tag{30}$$

The rate of change of the concentration of B is

$$\frac{d[B]}{dt} = k_A[A] - k_B[B] \tag{31}$$

and that of C is

$$\frac{d[C]}{dt} = k_B[B] \tag{32}$$

Integration of the rate of equation (30) yields

$$[A] = [A]_0 e^{-k_A/t} \tag{33}$$

Substitution of equation (33) into equation (31) gives

$$\frac{d[B]}{dt} = k_A[A]_0 e^{-k_A/t} - k_B[B] \tag{34}$$

which upon integration gives

$$[B] = \frac{k_A[A]_0}{(k_B - k_A)} [e^{-k_A t} - e^{-k_B t}] \tag{35}$$

Since at any time

$$[A]_0 = [A] + [B] + [C] \tag{36}$$

then

$$[C] = [A]_0 - [A] - [B] = [A]_0 \left[1 + \frac{1}{k_1 - k_2} \left(k_2 e^{-k_A t} - k_1 e^{-k_B t} \right) \right] \tag{37}$$

Equations (33), (35), and (37) may be used to estimate the rate constants k_A and k_B and also the concentration of the breakdown product C.

Kinetics of Chemical Decomposition in Solid Dosage Forms

It is only relatively recently that mechanisms that were developed to describe the kinetics of decomposition of pure solids have been applied to pharmaceutical systems and some rationalization of decomposition behavior of solid dosage forms has been possible (49,50). It is convenient to simplify this complex topic by dividing single-component systems into two categories—those solids that decompose to a solid product and a gas, and those that decompose to give a liquid and a gas.

Solids That Decompose to Give a Solid and a Gas

An example of this category is *p*-aminosalicylic acid, which decomposes to a solid (*p*-aminophenol) and a gas (carbon dioxide):

$$NH_2C_6H_3(OH)COOH \rightarrow NH_2C_6H_4OH + CO_2$$

The decomposition curves that result from such a reaction can be categorized into those in which there is (*i*) an initial rapid breakdown followed by a more gradual decomposition rate, which are accounted for by *topochemical* (or contracting geometry) models, or (*ii*) sigmoidal curves with an initial lag period, which are described by *nucleation* theories.

The model used in the treatment of topochemical decomposition is that of a cylinder or sphere in which it is assumed that the radius of the intact chemical substance decreases linearly with time. For the contracting cylinder model, the mole fraction x decomposed at time t is given by

$$(1 - x)^{1/2} = 1 - \left(\frac{k}{r_0} \right) t \tag{38}$$

For the contracting sphere model,

$$(1 - x)^{1/3} = 1 - \left(\frac{k}{r_0} \right) t \tag{39}$$

The decomposition of aspirin at elevated temperatures has, for example, been shown to decompose by topochemical reaction; linear plots were produced when data were plotted according to equation (38).

A similarity between equations (38) and (39) and the first-order rate equations was pointed out by Carstensen (49) who suggested that this similarity might account for the fact that many decompositions in solid dosage forms appear to follow first-order kinetics.

A model proposed by Prout and Tompkins may be used to interpret the sigmoidal decomposition curves. It is assumed in this model that the decomposition is governed by the formation and growth of active nuclei, which occur on the surface as well as inside the crystals. As decomposition product is formed, further strains develop in the crystal, since the surface array of product molecules has a different unit cell from the original substance, and these strains are relieved by the formation of cracks. Reaction takes place at the mouth of these cracks due to lattice imperfections and spreads down into the crevices. Decomposition on these surfaces produces further cracking and so the chain reaction spreads.

The equation proposed to describe decomposition by this process is of the form

$$\ln\left[\frac{x}{(1-x)}\right] = \left(\frac{k}{r_0}\right)t + C \tag{40}$$

where C is a lag-time term.

Sigmoidal curves were reported by Kornblum and Sciarrone (51) for the decomposition of powdered p-aminosalicylic acid, which produced linear plots when the data were plotted according to equation (40). Stability measurements made inadvertently in the lag periods of this type of decomposition would suggest zero-order kinetics.

Solids That Decompose to Give a Liquid and a Gas

The decomposition of p-aminobenzoic acid into aniline and carbon dioxide causes a layer of liquid to form around the solid, which dissolves the solid. The development of this liquid layer results in an initial lag period in the decomposition curves. Subsequently, the plot is linear, representing first-order decomposition of the solid in solution in its liquid decomposition products. There are thus two rate constants, that for the initial decomposition of the solid itself, and that for the decomposition of the solid in solution (52).

THE ARRHENIUS EQUATION AND ACCELERATED STABILITY TESTING

The equation that describes the effect of temperature on decomposition and which may be used to calculate the rate of breakdown at room temperature from measurements at much higher temperatures is the Arrhenius equation.

$$k = A\,e^{-E_a/RT} \tag{41}$$

or

$$\log k = \frac{E_a}{2.303RT} \tag{42}$$

where E_a is the activation energy, that is the energy barrier which has to be overcome if reaction is going to occur when two reactant molecules collide. A is the frequency factor and this is assumed to be independent of temperature for a given reaction, R is the gas constant (8.314 J/mol K), and T is the temperature in kelvins. A plot of $\log k$ as a function of $1/T$, referred to as the Arrhenius plot, is linear according to equation (42), if E_a is independent of temperature. Figure 2 shows a typical Arrhenius plot for the degradation of metronidazole under conditions of controlled pH and ionic strength (53). Thus, it is possible to conduct kinetic experiments at elevated temperatures and obtain estimates of rate constants at lower temperatures by extrapolation of the Arrhenius plot.

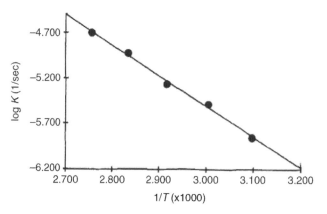

Figure 2 Arrhenius plot of the degradation of metronidazole (0.4 mg/mL) in pH 3.1 acetate buffer (0.1 M) solution and at an ionic strength of 0.5. *Source*: From Ref. 53.

This procedure, commonly referred to as accelerated stability testing, is most useful when the reaction at ambient temperatures is too slow to be monitored conveniently and when E_a is relatively high. For example, for a reaction with an E_a of 105 kJ/mol, an increase from 25°C to 45°C brings about a 14-fold increase in the reaction rate constant. In comparison, a rate increase of just threefold is obtained for the same elevation in temperature when E_a is 40 kJ/mol. The magnitude of E_a for a reaction can be obtained from the slope of its Arrhenius plot. Hydrolysis reactions typically have an E_a of 40 to 120 kJ/mol, whereas oxidation and photolysis reactions have smaller energies of activation.

An approximate method for estimation of decomposition rates at room temperature (T_1) when the rate constant at a single higher temperature (T_2) is known is to use equation (43), which assumes that the log A term is the same at each temperature,

$$\log\left[\frac{k_2}{k_1}\right] = -\frac{E_a}{2.303R}\left[\frac{1}{T_2} - \frac{1}{T_1}\right] \tag{43}$$

or

$$\log\left[\frac{k_2}{k_1}\right] = \frac{E_a(T_2 - T_1)}{2.303RT_2T_1} \tag{44}$$

Application of equations (43) and (44) requires a value of E_a; if only a rough estimation of k_1 is required, then a mid-range value of E_a, say 75 kJ/mol, may be assumed for these calculations.

An underlying assumption of the Arrhenius equation is that the reaction mechanism does not change as a function of temperature (i.e., E_a is independent of temperature). Since accelerated stability testing of pharmaceutical products normally employs a narrow range of temperature (typically, 35°C to at most 70°C), it is often difficult to detect nonlinearity in the Arrhenius plot from experimental data, even though such nonlinearity is expected from the reaction mechanism. Non-Arrhenius behavior has been observed in pharmaceutical systems (54). This may be attributed to the possible evaporation of solvent, multiple reaction pathways, change in physical form of the formulation, and so on, when the temperature of the reaction is changed (55). An interesting example of non-Arrhenius behavior is the increased rate of decomposition of ampicillin on freezing. Savello and Shangraw (56) showed that for a 1% sodium ampicillin solution in 5% dextrose, the percentage of degradation at four hours is approximately 14% at −20°C compared to 6% at 0°C and 10% at 5°C. This decrease in stability in frozen solutions is most frequently observed when the reaction obeys second- or higher-order kinetics. For example, the formation of nitrosomorpholine from morpholine and nitrite obeys third-order kinetics (57), and the rate of nitrosation is drastically enhanced in frozen solutions. A marked acceleration in the hydrolytic degradation of methyl, ethyl, and n-propyl-4-hydroxybenzoates in the frozen state has also been reported by Shija et al. (58). These authors found that although pseudo–first-order conditions found in the liquid state are also observed in the frozen state, the rate of reaction under frozen-state conditions showed very much less dependency on the initial hydroxide ion concentration.

The mechanism for rate enhancement in frozen solutions has been reviewed by Pincock (59). In reactions following second- or higher-order kinetics, an increase in rate may be brought about by concentration of the reactants in the liquid phase, the solute molecules being excluded from the ice lattice when the solution freezes. Occasionally, an increase in rate may be due to a change in pH on freezing. Fan and Tannenbaum (57) reported that citrate-sodium hydroxide and citrate-potassium phosphate buffers do not change pH on freezing, but citrate-sodium phosphate buffer at pH 8 decreases to pH 3.5 and sodium hydrogen phosphate at pH 9 decreases to pH 5.5 on freezing. A possible explanation for this phenomenon has been suggested by Murase et al. (60). Monosodium phosphate forms supersaturated solutions on cooling that become amorphous, with no precipitation of the salt. The disodium and monopotassium salts, on the other hand, readily precipitated when the initial solution concentration was > 0.2 M. The possibility of a pH change and rate acceleration should be considered when evaluating the stability of freeze-dried products. As discussed in section "Protein Stability," proteins are particularly sensitive to changes in pH, folding or unfolding to varying degrees in response to such changes. Proteins tend to be most stable at their isoelectric point owing to electrostatic interactions; however, when a solution is adjusted to the optimum pH for stability at room temperature with buffers, that pH may not be maintained throughout the lyophilization cycle, and the protein may aggregate or undergo denaturation.

Considerable interest has been generated in the use of accelerated stability testing that is based on a single condition of elevated temperature and humidity. For Abbreviated New Drug Applications (ANDAs), the FDA stability guidelines (48) suggest that a tentative expiration date of 24 months may be granted for a drug product if satisfactory stability results can be documented under a stressed condition of 40°C and 75% relative humidity. The simplicity of such a guideline is naturally attractive because a substantial saving in time can be obtained in advancing a drug product to the marketplace. However, the reliability of prediction can be subjected to question under certain circumstances. An analysis of the use and limitation of this approach has been presented elsewhere, and interested readers may refer to it for further information (61).

It is interesting to note that many authors have found that the effect of temperature on decomposition rate of solid dosage forms can be described by an Arrhenius-type equation, that is, plots of log k against $1/T$ are linear, so enabling the stability to be predicted at room temperature from measurements made at elevated temperatures. This is a surprising finding in view of the many possible complications that can arise on heating this type of formulation. The drug or one of the excipients may, for example, melt or change its polymorphic form as the temperature is increased, or it may contain loosely bound water, which is lost at higher temperatures. Although an apparent activation energy, E_a, can be calculated from the gradient of the plots, this does not, of course, have the same meaning as the activation energy for reactions in solution and will be affected, for example, by changes not only in the solubility of the drug in the moisture layer but also in the intrinsic rate of reaction.

ENVIRONMENTAL FACTORS THAT AFFECT REACTION RATE

A rational way to develop approaches that will increase the stability of fast-degrading drugs in pharmaceutical dosage forms is by a thorough study of the factors that can affect such stability. In this section, the factors that can affect decomposition rates are discussed; it will be seen that, under certain conditions of pH, solvent, presence of additives, and so on, the stability of a drug may be drastically affected. Equations that may allow prediction of these effects on reaction rates are discussed. Although most of the emphasis is placed on decomposition in the aqueous phase, reflecting the large body of literature in this area, some discussion is included of studies of environmental factors influencing the decomposition of semisolid and solid dosage forms.

Liquid Dosage Forms

pH

The pH of a drug solution may have a very dramatic effect on its stability. Depending on the reaction mechanism, a change of more than 10-fold in the rate constant may result from a shift of just 1 pH unit. When drugs are formulated in solution, it is essential to construct a pH versus rate profile, so that the optimum pH for stability can be located. Many pH versus rate profiles are documented in the literature, and they have a variety of shapes.

The study of the influence of pH on degradation rate is, however, complicated by the influence of the buffer components on the degradation rate. If the hydrolysis rate of the drug in a series of solutions buffered to the required pH is measured and the hydrolytic rate constant is then plotted as a function of pH, a pH-rate profile will be produced, but this will almost certainly be influenced by the buffers used to prepare the solutions, and it is probable that a different pH-rate profile would be obtained using a different buffer. Considering the simplest case of a nonionizable drug, it is necessary to consider not only the catalytic effect of hydrogen and hydroxyl ions, the so-called *specific acid-base catalysis*, but also the possible accelerating effect of the components of the buffer system, which is referred to as *general acid-base catalysis*. These two types of acid-base catalysis can be combined together in a general expression as follows.

$$k_{obs} = k_0 + k_{H^+} [H^+] + k_{OH} [OH^-] + k_{HX}[HX] + k_{X^-} [X^-] \qquad (45)$$

In this equation, k_{obs} is the experimentally determined hydrolytic rate constant, k_0 is the uncatalyzed or solvent catalyzed rate constant, k_{H^+} and k_{OH^-} are the specific acid- and base-catalysis rate constants, respectively, k_{HX} and k_{X^-} are the general acid- and base-catalysis rate constants, respectively, and [HX] and [X$^-$] denote the concentrations of protonated and unprotonated forms of the buffer. In a complete evaluation of the stability of the drug, the catalytic coefficients for specific acid and base catalysis and also the catalytic coefficients of possible buffers used in the formulation are determined.

By way of illustration we can consider a specific example of a stability study that has been reported for the antihypertensive vasodilating agent, ciclosidomine (62). Experiments carried out at constant temperature and constant ionic strength using a series of different buffers over the pH range 3 to 6 produced the graphs shown in Figure 3.

These plots show a marked effect of buffer concentration on the hydrolysis rate, particularly as the pH is increased from 3 to 4. The effect of the phosphate buffer on this system became less pronounced at higher pH and was found to have a negligible effect above pH 7.5. To remove the influence of the buffer, the reaction rate is measured at a

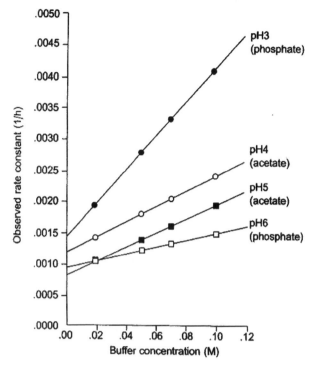

Figure 3 Effect of buffer concentration on the hydrolytic rate constant for ciclosidomine at $60°C$ as a function of pH. *Source*: From Ref. 62.

series of buffer concentrations at each pH and the data extrapolated back to zero concentration as shown in Figure 3. A buffer-independent pH-rate profile is then obtained by plotting these extrapolated rate constants as a function of pH.

A simple type of pH-rate profile reported for codeine sulfate (63) is illustrated in Figure 4. This drug is very stable in unbuffered solution over a wide pH range but degrades relatively rapidly in the presence of strong acids or bases. Since the influence of buffer components has been removed, the rate constants for specific acid and base catalysis can be calculated. Removing the terms for the effect of buffer from equation (45) gives

$$k_{obs} = k_1[H^+] + k_2 + k_3[OH^-] \qquad (46)$$

Consequently, a plot of measured rate constant k_{obs} against the hydrogen ion concentration $[H^+]$ at low pH has a gradient equal to the rate constant for acid catalysis. Similarly, a plot of k_{obs} against $[OH^-]$ at high pH gives the rate constant for base-catalyzed hydrolysis. For example, when $k_3[OH^-] > k_2 >> k_1[H^+]$, a log k_{obs} versus pH profile such as the one depicted in Figure 5A may result. On the other hand, if $k_1[H^+]$ and $k_3[OH^-]$ are both much greater than k_2, a log k_{obs} versus pH profile may resemble the curve shown in Figure 5B. When $k_1[H^+] > k_2 >> k_3[OH^-]$, the log k_{obs} versus pH profile will be a mirror image of Figure 5A, and when $k_2 >> k_1[H^+] + k_3[OH^-]$, the rate constant will be pH independent.

The degradation of codeine is particularly susceptible to the effect of buffers; for example, the hydrolysis rate in 0.05 M phosphate buffer at pH 7 is almost 20 times faster than in unbuffered solution at this pH. In phosphate buffers of neutral pH, the major buffer species are $H_2PO_4^-$ and HPO_4^{2-}, either of which may act as a catalyst for codeine

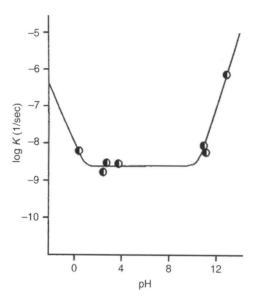

Figure 4 Log rate-pH profile for the degradation of codeine sulfate in buffer-free solutions at 60°C. *Source*: From Ref. 63.

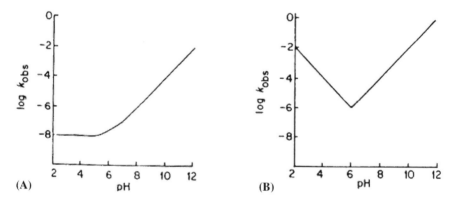

Figure 5 Log k_{obs} vs. pH profiles of nonionizable drugs.

degradation. Values of the catalytic coefficients of these two species may be determined from the experimental data in the following way. In neutral pH solutions, the observed rate constant, k_{obs}, is given by

$$k_{obs} = k_2 + k_{H_2PO_4^-}[H_2PO_4^-] + k_{HPO_4^{2-}}[HPO_4^{2-}] \qquad (47)$$

or

$$k_{obs} = k_2 + k'B_T \qquad (48)$$

where $k_{H_2PO_4^-}$ and $k_{HPO_4^{2-}}$ are the rate constants for catalysis by $H_2PO_4^-$ and HPO_4^{2-} ions, respectively, and B_T is the total concentration of phosphate buffer. The terms for specific acid and base catalysis have little effect at this pH and need not be considered in this treatment.

From equation (48), a plot of k_{obs} against B_T will have an intercept, k_2, and a gradient k'. To find values for the two catalytic coefficients, the equation is rearranged into the following linear form

$$k' = \frac{k_{obs} - k_2}{B_T} = \frac{k_{H_2PO_4}[H_2PO_4^-]}{B_T} + k_{HPO_4^2} \left\{ \frac{(B_T - [H_2PO_4^-])}{B_T} \right\} \qquad (49)$$

A second plot of the apparent rate constant k' against the fraction of the acid buffer component present, that is, $[H_2PO_4^-/B_T]$ will have an intercept at $[H_2PO_4^-/B_T] = 0$ equal to $k_{HPO_4^2}$. Furthermore, the k' value at $[H_2PO_4^-/B_T] = 1$ is the other catalytic coefficient $k_{H_2PO_4}$.

The relationship between the ability of a buffer component to catalyze hydrolysis, denoted by the catalytic coefficient, k, and its dissociation constant, K, may be expressed by the Brönsted catalysis law as

$$k_A = aK_A^\alpha \quad \text{for a weak acid} \qquad (50)$$

and

$$k_B = bK_B^\beta \quad \text{for a weak base} \qquad (51)$$

where a, b, α, and β are the constants characteristic of the reaction, the solvent, and the temperature (64,65). α and β are positive and vary between 0 and 1.

Because codeine has a pK_a of 8.2 at 25°C, its ionization state will change over the pH range 6 to 10, with potential implications for its stability. With this particular drug there are no appreciable stability problems associated with changes in its ionization, but this is not the case with many drugs, and complex pH-rate profiles are often produced because of the differing susceptibility of the unionized and ionized forms of the drug molecule to hydrolysis. In such cases, a detailed analysis of the reaction of each of the molecular species of the drug with hydrogen ion, water, and hydroxide ion as a function of pH allows the rationalization of the pH versus rate profile. When the drug is either monoacidic or monobasic, an equation similar to equation (46) can be written. Here, however, three kinetic terms are written for the acidic form of the drug, HA, and three terms for the basic form, A (electronic charges on HA and A are not designated here because either HA or A can be charged):

$$k_{obs} = k_1[H^+]f_{HA} + k_2f_{HA} + k_3[OH^-]f_{HA} + k_4[H^+]f_A + k_5f_A + k_6[OH^-]f_A \qquad (52)$$

where

$$f_{HA} = \frac{[HA]}{[HA] + [A]} = \frac{[H^+]}{[H^+] + K_a} \qquad (53)$$

and

$$f_A = \frac{[A]}{[HA] + [A]} = \frac{K_a}{[H^+] + K_a} \qquad (54)$$

Again, equation (52) can be analyzed by considering each individual term as a function of pH. Since the magnitudes of both f_{HA} and f_A are dependent on the relative magnitudes of K_a and H^+, the kinetic terms can be evaluated under three conditions: (i) when $[H^+] \gg K_a$, (ii) when $[H^+] = K_a$, and (iii) when $[H^+] \ll K_a$ (Table 3). The log k_{obs} versus pH profile for each kinetic term is shown in Figure 6, using a hypothetical pK_a of 6 and the condition that $k_{H^+} = 10^7$, $k_2 = k_3 = k_4 = 10^7$, $k_5 = k_6 = 1$. The profiles in Figure 6 show one break each in the lines, with a change of slope of 1 unit at the breaks. It is also seen that term (B) is equivalent to term (D) and that term (C) is equivalent to term (E), as far as

Table 3 Kinetic Expressions for Each Term in Equation (52)

Logarithm of kinetic term	When $[H^+] \gg K_a$	When $[H^+] = K_a$	When $K_a \gg [H^+]$
$\log k_1[H^+]f_{HA}$	$\log k_1 - pH$	$\log \frac{k_1 K_a}{2}$	$\log \frac{k_1}{K_a} - 2pH$
$\log k_2 f_{HA}$	$\log k_2$	$\log \frac{k_2}{2}$	$\log \frac{k_2}{K_a} - pH$
$\log k_3[OH^-]f_{HA}$	$\log k_3 K_w + pH$	$\log \frac{k_3 K_w}{2K_a}$	$\log \frac{k_3 K_w}{K_a}$
$\log k_4[H^+]f_A$	$\log k_4 K_a$	$\log \frac{k_4 K_a}{2}$	$\log k_4 - pH$
$\log k_5 f_A$	$\log k_5 K_a + pH$	$\log \frac{k_5}{2}$	$\log k_5$
$\log k_6[OH^-]f_A$	$\log k_6 K_w K_a + 2\,pH$	$\log \frac{k_6 K_w}{2K_a}$	$\log k_6 K_w + pH$

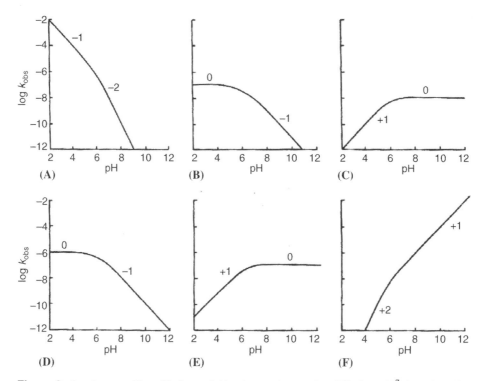

Figure 6 Log k_{obs} vs. pH profile for each kinetic term in equation (52): $k_1 = 10^7$, $k_2 = k_3 = k_4 = 10^7$, $k_5 = k_6 = 1$; $K_a = 10^{-6}$. Each number next to the curve indicates the slope of that portion of the curve.

their dependency on pH is concerned (Table 3 and Fig. 6). These terms, therefore, are kinetically equivalent and are indistinguishable from each other in a rate expression. Equation (52), then, can be reduced to a combination of only four terms. The shape of the overall log k_{obs}/pH profile of any drug is determined by the relative magnitudes of the four kinetic terms over the pH range considered. Each log k_{obs} versus pH profile of a monoacidic or monobasic drug can be adequately described by a combination of no more than four terms. Figure 7 illustrates this principle by showing the log k_{obs} versus pH profiles of idoxuridine (66) and acetylsalicylic acid (67). The hydrolysis of idoxuridine (Fig. 7A) as a function of pH can be rationalized by the equation $k_{obs} = k_2 f_{HA} + k_5 f_A^- + k_6[OH^-]f_A^-$ (three kinetic terms), whereas the hydrolysis of acetylsalicylic acid (Fig. 7B)

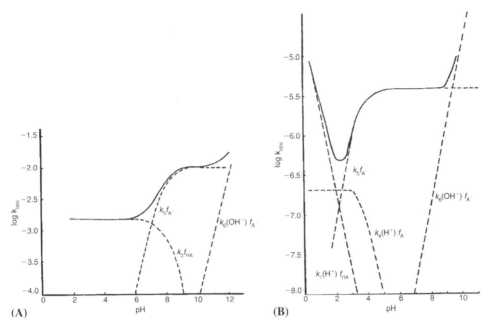

Figure 7 pH vs. log hydrolysis rate constant profile of (**A**) idoxuridine at 60°C (*solid line*) and (**B**) acetylsalicylic acid (*solid line*). The dashed lines indicate the individual contribution of each kinetic term.

can be decided only by using all four kinetic terms ($k_{obs} = k_1[H^+]f_{HA} + k_4[H^+]f_A^- + k_5f_A^- + k_6[OH^-]f_A^-$).

Some compounds exhibit pH behavior in which a bell-shaped curve is obtained with maximum instability at the peak (68). The peak corresponds to the intersection of two sigmoidal curves that are mirror images. The two inflection points imply two acid and base dissociations responsible for the reaction. For a dibasic acid (H_2A) for which the monobasic species (HA) is most reactive, the rate will rise with pH as [HA] increases. The maximum rate occurs at pH = (pK_1 + pK_2)/2 (the mean of the two acid dissociation constants). Where an acid and base react, the two inflections arise from the two different molecules. The hydrolysis of penicillin G catalyzed by 3,6-bis(dimethylaminomethyl) catechol (69) is a typical example.

Although the emphasis has been on the pH-dependent decomposition of drugs that undergo hydrolysis, it should also be noted that the oxidative degradation of some drugs in solution may be pH dependent; for example, the oxidation of prednisolone is base-catalyzed, and the oxidation of morphine occurs more rapidly in alkaline or neutral solution than in acid. The reason for this may be the effect of pH on the oxidation-reduction potential, E_0, of the drug. The photodegradation of several drugs is also pH dependent. For example, the photochemical decomposition of the benzodiazepine derivative midazolam increases with pH (70), and ciprofloxacin is most sensitive to photodegradation at slightly basic pH where the drug is in zwitterionic form, the stability increasing when the pH is lowered to 4 (71) (Fig. 8).

Solvent

In many pharmaceutical dosage forms, it may be necessary to incorporate water-miscible solvents to solubilize the drug. These solvents are generally low molecular weight alcohols, such as ethanol, propylene glycol, and glycerin, or polymeric alcohols, such as

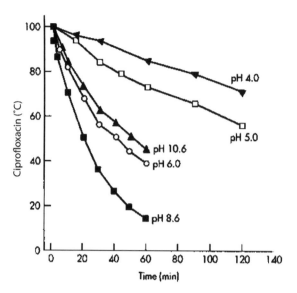

Figure 8 Effect of pH on the photodegradation of ciprofloxacin. Radiation source: Mercury lamp at a wavelength of 313 nm. *Source*: From Ref. 71.

the polyethylene glycols. Solvent effects can be quite complicated and difficult to predict. In addition to altering the activity coefficients of the reactant molecules and the transition state, changes in the solvent system may bring about concomitant changes in such physicochemical parameters as pK_a, surface tension, and viscosity, which indirectly affect the reaction rate. In some cases, an additional reaction pathway may be generated, or there may be a change in the product mix. The angiotensin-converting enzyme inhibitor, moexipril, undergoes hydrolysis as well as a cyclization reaction, leading to the formation of diketopiperazines. In mixed solvent (75–90% ethanol) systems, the hydrolysis reaction is suppressed, but the rate of the cyclization reaction increases by 5.5- to 29-fold (72). In the presence of increasing concentrations of ethanol in the solvent, aspirin degrades by an extra route, forming the ethyl ester of acetylsalicylic acid (73). On the other hand, a solvent change may bring about stabilization of a compound. The hydrolysis of barbiturates occurs 6.7-fold faster in water than in 50% ethanol, and 2.6-fold faster in water than in 50% glycerol (74).

Many approaches have been used to correlate solvent effects. The approach used most often is based on the electrostatic theory, the theoretical development of which has been described in detail by Amis (75). The reaction rate is correlated with some bulk parameter of the solvent, such as the dielectric constant or its various algebraic functions. A simple linear equation for prediction of the effect of the solvent on the hydrolysis rate is

$$\log k = \log k_{\varepsilon=\infty} - \frac{K z_A z_B}{\varepsilon} \tag{55}$$

In this equation, K is a constant for a given system at a given temperature. A plot of $\log k$ as a function of the reciprocal of the dielectric constant, ε, of the solvent should be linear with a gradient $K z_A z_B$ and an intercept equal to the logarithm of the rate constant in a theoretical solvent of infinite dielectric constant. When the drug ion and the interacting ion are of opposite signs, the slope will be positive and the choice of a nonpolar solvent will only result in an increase in decomposition. On the other hand, if the charges on the drug ion and the interacting species are the same, then the gradient of the line will be negative and replacement of water with a solvent of lower dielectric constant could theoretically have the desired effect of reducing the reaction rate. Although the solvent effect on the reaction rate could, in principle, be large, the limited availability of nontoxic solvents suitable for pharmaceutical products has rendered this stabilization approach somewhat impractical in most circumstances.

Solubility

As mentioned earlier in this chapter, penicillins are very unstable in aqueous solution by virtue of hydrolysis of the β-lactam ring. A successful method of stabilizing penicillins in liquid dosage forms is to prepare their insoluble salts and formulate them in suspensions. The reduced solubility of the drug in a suspension decreases the amount of drug available for hydrolysis. An example of improved stability of a suspension over that of a solution is illustrated in Figure 9, in which a hypothetical drug is formulated as a 10 mg/mL solution (curve A) and as a suspension containing the same total amount of drug, but with a saturated solubility of 1 mg/mL (curve B). It is seen that the drug in solution undergoes first-order degradation with a half-life of one year. In the suspension, the drug degrades through zero-order kinetics until there is no more excess solid present, after which point first-order kinetics is operative.

Additives

Buffer salts In most drug solutions, it is necessary to use buffer salts to maintain the formulation at the optimum pH. In addition to the promotion of drug degradation by buffer salts through general acid or general base catalysis, which was discussed above, buffer salts can affect the rate of drug degradation in other ways. First, a *primary salt effect* results because of the effect salts have on the activity coefficient of the reactants. At

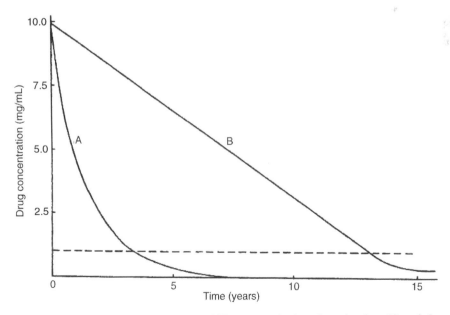

Figure 9 Solubility effects on drug stability: curve A, drug formulated as 10 mg/mL solution ($t_{1/2} = 1$ year); curve B, drug formulated as a suspension with a saturated solubility of 1 mg/mL ($t_{1/2} = 7.3$ years).

relatively low ionic strengths, the rate constant, k, is related to the ionic strength, μ, according to the Brønsted–Bjerrum equation,

$$\log k = \log k_0 + 2A z_A z_B \sqrt{\mu} \qquad (56)$$

In this equation, z_A and z_B are the ionic charges of the two interacting ions and A is a constant for a given solvent and temperature. According to equation (56), a plot of $\log k$ as a function of $\sqrt{\mu}$ should have an intercept of $\log k_0$ and a gradient of $2A z_A z_B$, which, in theory, should always be an integer for reactions in water at 25°C because both z_A and z_B are integral numbers and $A = 1.02$. In practice, however, the gradient is often fractional. The sign of the gradient is sometimes informative in identifying the reactants that participate in the rate-limiting step in the reaction mechanism, since reactions between ions of similar charge, for example, the acid-catalyzed hydrolysis of a cationic drug ion, will produce plots of positive slope (i.e., the reaction rate will be increased by electrolyte addition), whereas the base-catalyzed hydrolysis of positively charged drug species will produce negative gradients. But one must avoid drawing such conclusions in instances where a choice is to be made between kinetically equivalent rate terms (76).

Linear plots of $\log k$ against $\sqrt{\mu}$ are frequently found even in solutions of high ionic strength, although equation (56) is strictly valid only for ionic strengths of less than 0.01. At higher ionic strengths (up to about 0.1), it is preferable to use a modified form of the Brønsted–Bjerrum equation in which $\log k$ is plotted against $\sqrt{\mu}/(1 + \sqrt{\mu})$.

$$\log k = \log k_0 + 2A z_A z_B \left(\frac{\sqrt{\mu}}{(1 + \sqrt{\mu})} \right) \qquad (57)$$

Figure 10 shows linear plots when the data for the effect of added electrolyte on the decomposition of metronidazole at two pH values are plotted according to equation (57); the slope is positive as expected for the acid-catalyzed hydrolysis of this cationic drug and decreases as the pH increases from 3.1 to 7.4 because of the decrease in the hydrogen ion concentration and the reduced fraction of ionized metronidazole (53).

Buffer salts also can exert a *secondary salt effect* on drug stability. From Table 3 and Figure 7, it is clear that the rate constant for an ionizable drug is dependent on its pK_a. Increasing salt concentrations, particularly from polyelectrolytes such as citrate and phosphate, can substantially affect the magnitude of the pK_a, causing a change in the rate

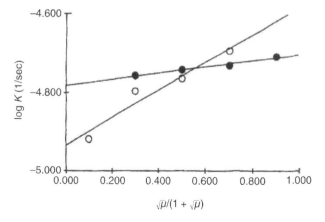

Figure 10 Effect of ionic strength on the degradation kinetics of metronidazole (0.04 mg/mL) in 0.1 M buffer solutions at 90°C plotted according to equation (57). (○) pH 3.1 acetate buffer; (●) pH 7.4 phosphate buffer.

constant. (For a review of salt effects containing many examples from the pharmaceutical literature, see Ref. 77.)

Surfactants The presence of surfactants in micellar form has a modifying effect on the rate of hydrolysis of drugs, the magnitude of which depends on the difference in the rate constant when the drug is in aqueous solution and when it is solubilized within the micelle, and also on the extent of solubilization. Thus

$$k_{obs} = k_m f_m + k_w f_w \tag{58}$$

where k_{obs}, k_m, and k_w are the observed, micellar, and aqueous rate constants, respectively, and f_m and f_w are the fractions of drug associated with the micelles and aqueous phase, respectively. The value of k_m is dependent on the location of the drug within the micelle; nonpolar compounds solubilized within the lipophilic core are likely to be more effectively removed from the attacking species than those compounds that are located close to the micellar surface. Where the drug is located near to the micellar surface, and therefore still susceptible to attack, the ionic nature of the surfactant is an important influence on decomposition rate. For base-catalyzed hydrolysis, solubilization into anionic micelles affords an effective stabilization due to repulsion of OH^- by the micelles. Conversely, solubilization into cationic micelles might be expected to cause an enhanced base-catalyzed hydrolysis. The hydrolysis of aspirin in the plateau region (pH 6–8) is inhibited by the presence of micelles of cetyltrimethylammonium bromide and cetylpyridinium chloride, whereas in the region where the normal base-catalyzed reaction occurs (pH > 9), the reaction is catalyzed by micelles of these same surfactants. The mechanism of hydrolysis in the plateau region involves intramolecular general base catalysis by the adjacent ionized carboxyl group, both in the presence and absence of micelles. This reaction is inhibited in the presence of micelles because the substrate molecules are solubilized into the micelle, and water is less available in this environment than in normal aqueous solutions (78).

Many drugs associate to form micelles in aqueous solution (79), and several studies have been reported of the effect of this self-association on stability. In micellar solutions of penicillin G (500,000 units/mL), the apparent rate of the hydrogen ion–catalyzed degradation was increased twofold, but that of water-catalyzed and hydroxide ion–catalyzed hydrolysis was decreased two- to threefold (80). Consequently, the pH profile was shifted to higher pH values, and the pH of minimum degradation was found to be 7.0 compared to 6.5 for monomeric solution (8000 units/mL). When compared at the respective pH-rate profile minima, micellar penicillin G was reported to be 2.5 times as stable as the monomeric solutions under conditions of constant pH and ionic strength.

Complexing agents Higuchi and Lachman (81) pioneered the work of improving drug stability by complexation. They showed that aromatic esters can be stabilized in aqueous solutions in the presence of xanthines such as caffeine. Thus, the half-lives of benzocaine, procaine hydrochloride, and tetracaine are increased by approximately two- to fivefold in the presence of 2.5% caffeine. This increase in stability is attributed to the formation of a less reactive complex between caffeine and the aromatic ester. Connors has written a comprehensive textbook that describes methods for the measurement of binding constants for complex formation in solution—along with discussions of pertinent thermodynamics, modeling statistics, and regression analysis (82). The various experimental methods useful for measuring equilibrium constants are also discussed. A good deal of attention has also been directed at the use of derivatives of cyclodextrin for the solubilization and stabilization of pharmaceuticals (83). One cautionary note: complexation may adversely affect the dissolution or permeability characteristics of the drug, thereby possibly decreasing drug bioavailability.

Light

The mathematical relationship between light intensity and drug degradation is much less developed than that describing pH and temperature effects. Part of the reason, perhaps, is that light effects on stability can be substantially avoided by using amber containers that shield off most of the ultraviolet light. Regulatory authorities usually require a statement on the photostability of products and the means of protection, if required. Often both daylight and artificial light sources are employed for tests on drug substances (84).

Semisolid Dosage Forms

The chemical stability of active ingredients incorporated into ointments or creams is frequently dependent on the nature of the ointment or cream base, and these should be chosen carefully during the formulation of the dosage form. For example, the reported shelf life of hydrocortisone in polyethylene glycol base (85,86) is only six months, which makes manufacture on a commercial basis an unreasonable proposition, considering the length of time involved in distribution of the drug from wholesaler to patient.

Similar care should be exercised if the ointment is diluted at a later stage as a means of reducing the potency of highly active topical preparations, particularly steroids. The pharmaceutical and biopharmaceutical dangers of this procedure, particularly its implications for drug stability arising from the inappropriate choice of diluents, have been stressed by Busse (87). For example, if betamethasone valerate cream is diluted with a cream base having a neutral to alkaline pH, the 17-ester may be converted to the less-active betamethasone 21-ester. Similarly, diluents containing oxidizing agents could cause chemical degradation of fluocinolone acetate to less-active compounds.

Changes in the stability of drugs following incorporation into gel formulations have been reported. For example, there was an increased degradation of penicillin G sodium in hydrogels of various natural and semisynthetic polymers (88).

Solid Dosage Forms

Moisture
Moisture is considered to be one of the most important factors that must be controlled to minimize decomposition in solid dosage forms, particularly when water-soluble drugs are present in the formulation. Such drugs will dissolve in the moisture layer on the surface and will then be influenced by many of the factors discussed above when dealing with liquid dosage forms. The problem is most pronounced with hygroscopic drugs or with drugs that decompose to give hygroscopic products, so much so that it may even be worth trying to prepare a less hygroscopic salt of the drug.

Care should be taken to minimize access of moisture during manufacture and also in the selection of packaging. The correct choice of packaging is not always straightforward. For example, tablets containing a water-labile drug were found to be more stable in a water-permeable blister package at 50°C than in a sealed glass bottle and yet the situation was reversed at room temperature and 70% relative humidity (89). The reason for this behavior was attributed to the loss of considerable amounts of water through the film at 50°C, so improving the stability, and the reverse diffusion at room temperature, so decreasing the stability.

Excipients

Excipients can affect the stability of solid dosage forms either by increasing the moisture content of the formulation or by interacting chemically with its components. Some excipients, particularly starch and povidone, have high water contents (povidone contains about 28% equilibrium moisture at 75% relative humidity), but whether this high moisture level has an effect on stability depends on how strongly it is bound and whether the moisture can come into contact with the drug. Magnesium trisilicate causes increased hydrolysis of aspirin in tablet form because, it is thought, of its high water content (90).

Several examples of the chemical interaction between components in solid dosage forms leading to increased decomposition effects have been reported in the pharmaceutical literature. A notable example was that observed when the phenacetin in compound codeine and APC tablets was replaced by paracetamol (acetaminophen) in NHS formulations in Australia in the 1960s (because of its undesirable side effects). An unexpected decrease in stability of the tablets occurred, which was later attributed to a transacetylation reaction between aspirin and paracetamol and also a possible direct hydrolysis of the paracetamol (91).

The increased generation of free salicylic acid at 37°C in the tablets containing paracetamol is seen in Figure 11. This figure also highlights the influence of tablet excipients on the stability; addition of 1% talc caused only a minimal increase in the decomposition, while 0.5% magnesium stearate increased the breakdown rate dramatically. Similar stability problems have been noted with stearate salts (92), and it has been suggested that these salts should be avoided as tablet lubricants if the active component is subject to hydroxide ion–catalyzed degradation. The degradative effect of the alkali stearates is inhibited in the presence of malic, hexamic, or maleic acid due, it is thought, to competition for the lubricant cation between the drug and the additive acid (93).

The stability of drugs when incorporated into suppositories can often be affected by the nature of the suppository base, particularly when polyoxyethylene glycols are used. For example, aspirin undergoes pseudo–first-order decomposition in several

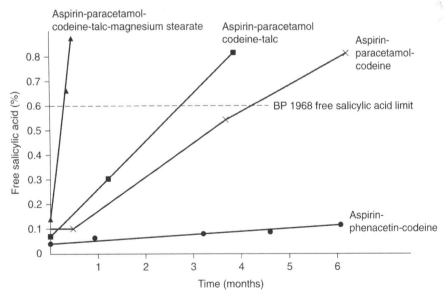

Figure 11 Development of free salicylic acid in aspirin-paracetamol-codeine and aspirin-phenacetin-codeine tablets at 37°C. *Source*: From Ref. 91.

polyoxyethylene glycols due in part to its transesterification to salicylic acid and acetylated polyethylene glycol (94). The rate of decomposition was considerably greater than when a fatty base such as cocoa butter was used (95). Analysis of commercial batches of 100 mg indometacin–polyethylene glycol suppositories (96) showed that approximately 2%, 3.5%, and 4.5% of the original amount of indometacin was esterified with polyoxyethylene glycol 300 after storage times of one, two, and three years, respectively.

The photostability of tablet formulations can be affected by excipients, in many cases because of the impurities present in the excipients (36). For example, phenolic impurities in tablet-binding agents such as povidone, disintegrants such as crospovidone, and viscosity-modifying agents such as alginates can lead to photodegradation through free radical reactions (97). Similarly, colored products may be formed by the reaction of aldehydes formed during spray-drying or autoclaving of lactose with primary amine groups in the product (98).

Humidity

Humidity is a major determinant of drug product stability in solid dosage forms. Elevation of relative humidity usually decreases the stability, particularly for those drugs highly sensitive to hydrolysis. For example, Genton and Kesselring have demonstrated a linear relationship between the logarithm of the rate constant for the decomposition of nitrazepam in the solid state and the relative humidity (99) (Fig. 12). In addition, increased humidity can also accelerate the aging process (100,101) through interaction(s) with excipients. Humidity does not always affect drug stability adversely. Cyclophosphamide, in lyophilized cakes containing mannitol or sodium bicarbonate, undergoes rapid ($t_{90} \approx 15$ days) degradation in the solid state. The cyclophosphamide was in the amorphous state in these formulations. However, on exposure to high humidity,

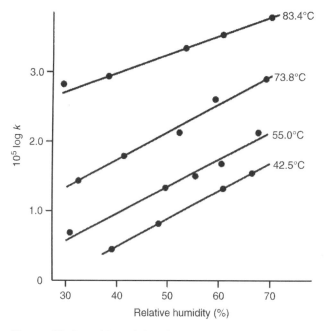

Figure 12 Logarithm of the nitrazepam decomposition constant, k, as a function of relative humidity at various temperatures. *Source*: From Ref. 99.

the cyclophosphamide was converted to the crystalline monohydrate form, which exhibited greatly improved stability (102). Reviews dealing with the effects of moisture on the physical and chemical stability of drugs are available (103,104). As peptides and proteins have become more important as therapeutic agents, the role residual moisture plays in their stabilization has attracted a good deal of attention (105,106).

The need for consideration of the effect of moisture on stability has been stressed by Carstensen (49), who stated that stability programs should always include samples that have been artificially stressed by addition of moisture.

PROTEIN STABILITY

Chemical Degradation

Chemical instability can involve one or more of a variety of chemical reactions including the following (107,108):

- *Deamidation*: the sole chain linkage in a glutamine (Gln) or asparagine (Asn) residue is hydrolyzed to form a carboxylic acid.
- *Oxidation*: the side chains of histidine (His), methionine (Met), cysteine (Cys), tryptophan (Trp), and tyrosine (Tyr) residues in proteins are potential oxidation sites.
- *Racemization*: all amino acid residues except glycine (Gly) are chiral at the carbon atom bearing the side chain and are subject to base-catalyzed racemization.
- *Proteolysis*: the cleavage of peptide (ZCO-NHY) bonds is involved.
- *β-Elimination*: high-temperature treatment of proteins leads to destruction of disulfide bonds as a result of β-elimination from the cystine residue.
- *Disulfide formation*: the interchange of disulfide bonds can result in an altered three-dimensional structure.

Protein Deamidation

In the deamidation reaction, the side-chain amide linkage in a Gln or Asn residue is hydrolyzed to form a free carboxylic acid, the Asn peptides being more susceptible to deamidation than the Gln peptides (109).

The rate of deamidation is strongly influenced by the sequence of residues in the peptide molecule, and the reader is referred to the comprehensive review by Cleland et al. (108) for a detailed account of this topic. The deamidation of Asn and Gln residues of proteins is an acid-and base-catalyzed hydrolysis reaction, which can occur rapidly under physiological conditions. The acid-catalyzed step involves protonation of the amide-leaving group, and the base-catalyzed step involves nucleophilic attack of the amide carbonyl carbon by hydroxide or conjugate base. The transition state is thought to be oxyanion tetrahedral intermediate as shown in Scheme 3. As with all acid-base–catalyzed reactions, there will be a particular pH for minimum reaction rate. In peptides where the Asn residue is next to a Gly, deamidation is believed to proceed through a cyclic imide intermediate by nucleophilic attack of the side-chain carbonyl group of Asn by the main-chain peptide nitrogen from the adjacent C-terminal residue. Deamidation of Gln residues does not readily occur by this route because the extra carbon in the Gln side chain hinders the formation of the cyclic structure. The breakdown of the imide itself is base-catalyzed producing either isoaspartate or aspartate (Asp) (depending on which of the nitrogen-carbonyl bonds is hydrolyzed) as outlined in Scheme 4.

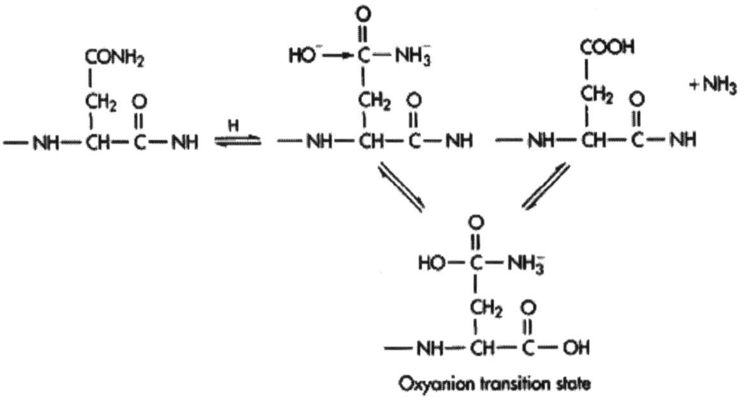

Scheme 3 General acid and base catalysis of deamidation.

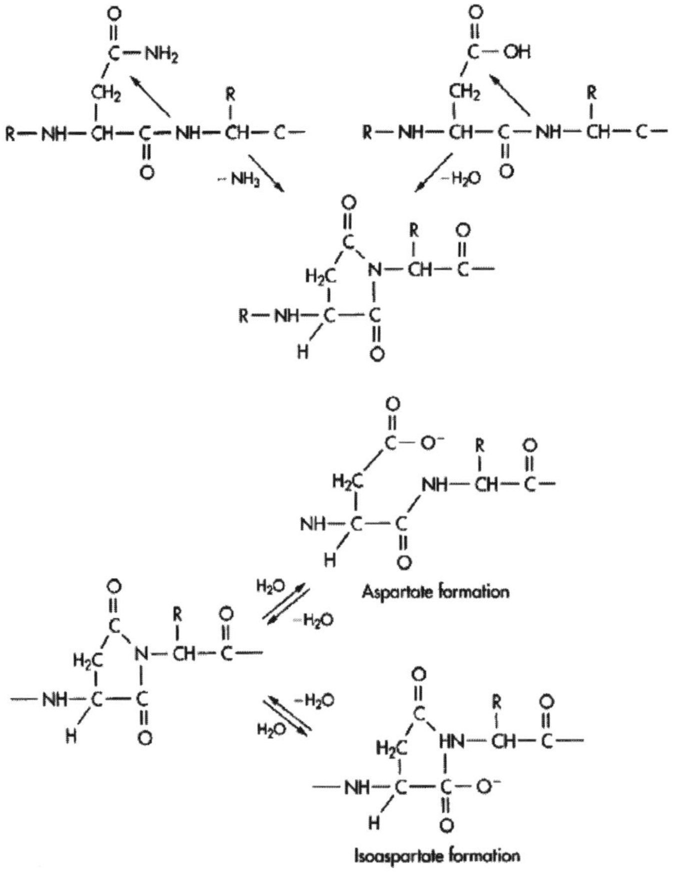

Scheme 4 Mechanisms for deamidation by cyclic imide formation and subsequent hydrolysis of the imide to form either aspartate or isoaspartate.

The hydrolysis reactions are completely reversible, that is, the final products of deamidation can interconvert through the cyclic imide intermediate. Since the succeeding amino acid is involved in the formation of the cyclic imide, the size and physicochemical properties of the neighboring amino acid side chain are expected to influence its rate of formation. Thus, the rate of cyclic imide formation of the Asn-Leu-hexapeptide at pH 7 was approximately 50 times slower than that of the Asn-Gly-hexapeptide because of steric hindrance by the leucine (Leu) side chain (110). Deamidation via the cyclic imide can occur when the adjacent residue is serine (Ser) or alanine (Ala) but to a lesser extent than when this residue is Gly.

For any particular protein it is necessary to determine experimentally the influence of deamidation on the therapeutic activity, since this is generally unpredictable. For many proteins, including insulin and interleukin-1α, deamidation has no measurable effect, whereas for proteins such as cytochrome c, interleukin-1β, lysozyme, and adrenocorticotropin, there is a decrease in activity on deamidation. Deamidation can have pronounced effects on conformation because of its effect on the surface charge at the site of modification. If deamidation results in irreversible unfolding of the protein molecule, there will be a greater susceptibility of that protein to irreversible aggregation, whereas the modification of the charge following deamidation may result in greater repulsion of adjacent protein molecules and a reduced tendency for aggregation.

Protein Oxidation

Oxidation is one of the major causes of protein degradation and has been widely studied. The side chains of histidine (His), methionine (Met), cysteine (Cys), tryptophan (Trp), and tyrosine (Tyr) residues in proteins are potential oxidation sites. The reactive oxygen species include singlet oxygen $^1O_2$, superoxide radical O_2^-, alkyl peroxide ROOH, hydrogen peroxide H_2O_2, hydroxy radicals (HO$^\bullet$ or HOO$^\bullet$), and halide complexes (CLO$^-$). The order of reactivity of these oxidants is

$$HO^\bullet, HOO^\bullet > O_2^- > ROOH, H_2O_2 > {}^1O_2, CLO^- > O_2$$

Although much is known about the reactive oxygen species, there are problems in predicting the probable extent of oxidation because it is often not known whether initiators are present or not. In most cases oxidation results in a complete or partial loss of activity, although antigenicity is not affected except in the relatively few instances in which the protein undergoes gross conformational changes. It is clear that minimizing protein oxidation is essential for maintaining the biological activity of most proteins and avoiding the immunogenic response caused by degraded proteins.

Methionine is very susceptible to oxidation and reacts with a variety of oxidants to give methionine sulfoxide (RS(OO)CH$_3$) or, in highly oxidative conditions, methionine sulfone (RS(O)CH$_3$) (Scheme 5). Whether or not methionine residues are susceptible to oxidation depends to a large extent on their exposure to the solvent. In proteins such as myoglobin and trypsin, these residues are buried within the hydrophobic regions of the protein and are relatively inert under conditions of mild oxidation. In contrast, in proteins such as ribonuclease A, chymotrypsin, pepsin, and lysozyme, the methionine residues are partially exposed to the solvent and the oxidation rate is very much faster.

The thiol group of cysteine readily reacts with oxygen to yield successively a sulfenic acid (RSOH), a disulfide (RSSH), a sulfinic acid (RSO$_2$H), and finally, a sulfonic (cystic) acid (RSO$_3$H) depending on reaction conditions. An important factor determining the extent of oxidation is the spatial positioning of the thiol groups in the proteins. Where contact between thiol groups within the protein molecule is hindered or when the protein contains only a single thiol group, intramolecular disulfide bonds are not formed. Factors that influence oxidation rate include the temperature, the pH, the buffer medium, the type of catalyst, and the oxygen tension.

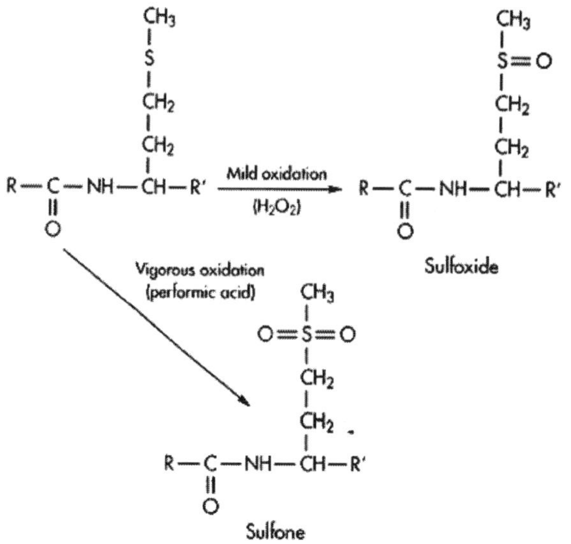

Scheme 5 Mechanism of oxidation of methionine-containing peptide under mild and strong conditions.

Histidine is susceptible to oxidation in the presence of metals, primarily by reaction with singlet oxygen, and this constitutes a major cause of enzyme degradation. Both histidine and tryptophan are highly susceptible to photooxidation.

Racemization

All amino acid residues except Gly are chiral at the carbon bearing the side chain and are subject to base-catalyzed racemization. Scheme 6 shows the mechanism involved. In alkaline solution the hydrogen of the α-methine is removed by the base to form a

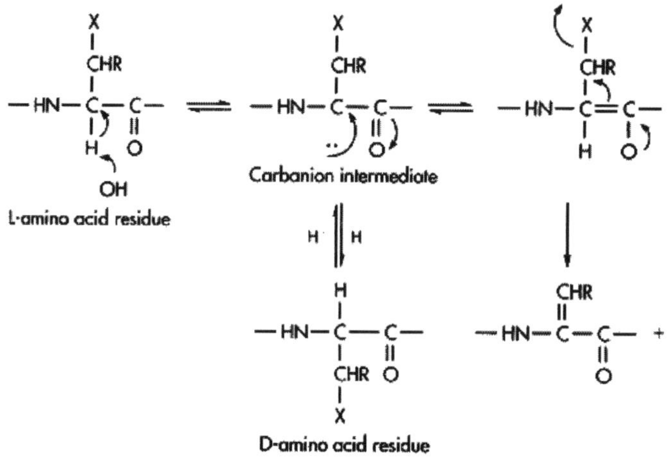

X = H, OH, O-glycosyl, O-phosphoryl, SH, SCH$_2$–R, aliphatic or aromatic residue. R = H or CH$_3$.

Scheme 6 Mechanism of β-elimination and racemization reactions in alkaline media.

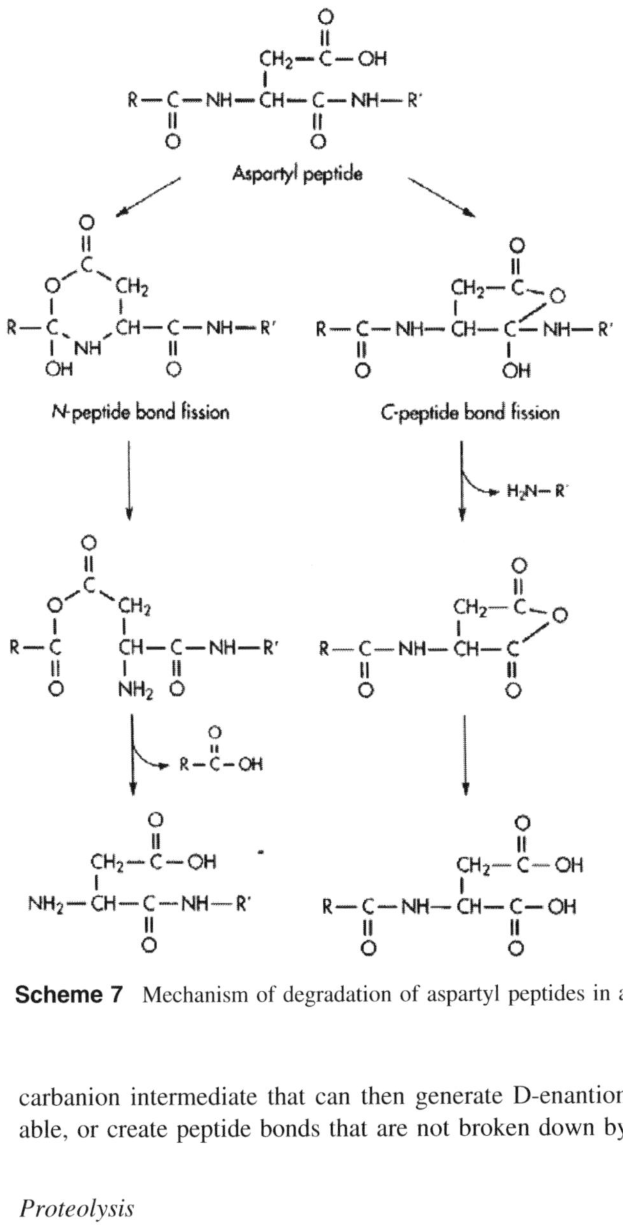

Scheme 7 Mechanism of degradation of aspartyl peptides in acidic media.

carbanion intermediate that can then generate D-enantiomers, which are nonmetaboliz-able, or create peptide bonds that are not broken down by proteolytic enzymes.

Proteolysis

The amino acid residue that is by far the most susceptible to proteolysis is Asp; the cleavage of the peptide bonds in dilute acid proceeds at a rate at least 100 times that of other peptide bonds. The hydrolysis can occur at the N-terminal and/or the C-terminal peptide bonds adjacent to the Asp residue (Scheme 7). Cleavage of the N-terminal peptide bond proceeds via an intermediate with a six-membered ring, while cleavage of the C-terminal peptide bond is thought to involve a five-membered ring. Such peptide bond cleavage can result in protein inactivation.

β-Elimination

The inactivation of proteins at high temperatures is often due to β-elimination of disulfides from the cystine residue, although other amino acids including Cys, Ser, Thr,

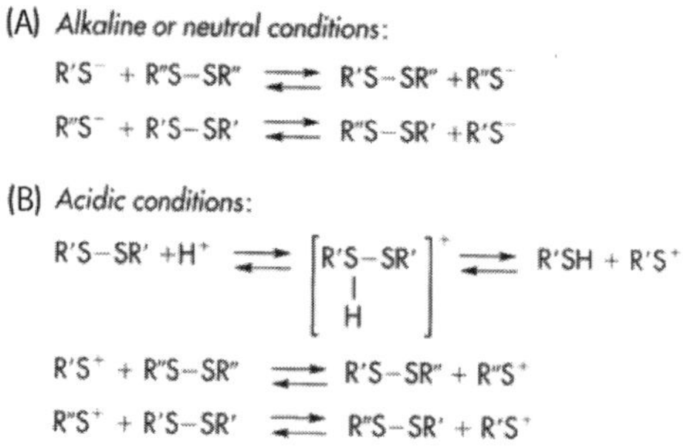

(A) *Alkaline or neutral conditions*:

$$R'S^- + R''S-SR''' \rightleftharpoons R'S-SR'' + R'''S^-$$

$$R''S^- + R'S-SR' \rightleftharpoons R''S-SR' + R'S^-$$

(B) *Acidic conditions*:

$$R'S-SR' + H^+ \rightleftharpoons \left[\begin{array}{c} R'S-SR' \\ | \\ H \end{array} \right]^+ \rightleftharpoons R'SH + R'S^+$$

$$R'S^+ + R''S-SR''' \rightleftharpoons R'S-SR'' + R'''S^+$$

$$R''S^+ + R'S-SR' \rightleftharpoons R''S-SR' + R'S^+$$

Scheme 8 Mechanism of disulfide exchange in (**A**) alkaline or neutral media and (**B**) acidic media.

Phe, and Lys can be degraded via β-elimination as seen from Scheme 6. The inactivation is particularly rapid under alkaline conditions and is also influenced by the presence of metal ions.

Disulfide Formation

The interchange of disulfide bonds can result in incorrect pairings with consequent changes in the three-dimensional structure and loss of catalytic activity. The mechanism is thought to be different in alkaline and acid conditions. In alkaline and neutral solutions, the reaction involves the nucleophilic attack on a sulfur atom of the disulfide (Scheme 8A). This reaction is catalyzed by thiols and can be prevented if thiol scavengers such as *p*-mercuribenzoate, *N*-ethylmaleimide, or copper ions are present. In acidic conditions the disulfide exchange takes place through a sulfenium cation, which is formed by attack of a proton on the disulfide bond (Scheme 8B). The sulfenium cation carries out an electrophilic displacement on a sulfur atom of the disulfide. Addition of thiols can inhibit this exchange by scavenging the sulfenium ions.

Formulation and Protein Stabilization

The physical stability of a protein may be improved through formulation by consideration of the many factors influencing chemical decomposition including pH, additives, and solvent; the particular effect that each of these has on stability is dependent on the nature of the decomposition. In addition, there are several general precautions common to most proteins, which should be considered during formulation and usage of the products.

Optimization of pH

For proteins undergoing deamidation, the choice of pH for optimum stability of the formulation is determined by the nature of the deamidation reaction. If this occurs by a general acid-base mechanism, then the optimum pH for a peptide formulation will usually be about 6, where both rates are at their minimum. If deamidation occurs through the cyclic imide intermediate, it is, in principle, preferable to formulate at a low pH since this type of deamidation is base-catalyzed. Other routes of degradation tend to predominate at lower pH, however, and a compromise pH must then be selected. Buffer components, particularly the phosphate anion (111), have a marked influence on deamidation rate, and these must be chosen with care.

The rate of oxidation may be pH dependent; for example, as the pH is decreased the rate of the hydrogen peroxide–catalyzed oxidation of cysteine decreases whereas that of methionine oxidation increases (112). Although the determination of the pH of maximum stability is of primary importance in the formulation of proteins susceptible to oxidation, it is also, of course, essential to exclude oxygen from the headspace of the container and where necessary to include antioxidants in the formulation where they may act by inhibition of oxidation, by removing trace metal ions or scavenging oxygen.

Choice of Solvent

Although studies on the influence of solvent on the rates of deamidation have generally involved solvents unsuitable for use in formulation, it is interesting to note a reported dependence of the rate on the dielectric constant of the solvent. The rate of deamidation of N-terminal-blocked Boc-Asn-Gly-Gly was decreased in ethanol (113). Similarly, the deamidation rate of the hexapeptide Val-Thr-Pro-Asn-Gly-Ala decreased with decrease in the dielectric constant of the solvent, an effect that was attributed to the destabilization of the deprotonated peptide bond nitrogen anion, which is involved in the formation of the cyclic imide intermediate (114).

Temperature

The decomposition of proteins susceptible to oxidative degradation can generally be minimized by temperature reduction either by refrigeration or by freezing, although the effect may be small because of the low activation energies involved. There are exceptions to this; for example, the oxidation of proteins with cysteine residues may increase as a consequence of increased intra- or intermolecular disulfide exchange because of the increase in the concentration of the protein by its exclusion from the ice matrix that forms during the freezing process.

Ionic Strength

An increase in the ionic strength of aqueous solutions of glutaminyl and asparaginyl pentapeptides has been reported to result in an increased rate of deamidation (113). Similar results have been noted in an earlier study on cytochrome c (115), although a lack of effect of ionic strength on stability was observed (116) in a series of pentapeptides Val-Ser-Asn-X-Val and Val-X-Asn-Ser-Val, where X is an amino acid. The ionic strengths of most parenteral formulations of proteins in which sodium chloride is used to adjust the tonicity are sufficiently low so that increased deamidation rates resulting from electrolyte addition will not be a major problem.

Prevention of Adsorption

The surface of glass is conducive to adsorption leading to protein denaturation, and it is preferable, if possible, to use more hydrophilic surfaces. In situations when the use of glass cannot be avoided, components may be added to the protein solution to prevent adsorption to the glass surface. These additives can act by coating the surface of the glass or by binding to the proteins. For example, serum albumin can be included in the formulation, since it will compete with the therapeutic protein for the binding sites on the glass surface and so reduce its adsorption. Similarly, surfactants such as poloxamers and polysorbates may be added to the protein solution, although consideration must be given to the effects of the surfactants on the pharmacology of the protein and to the toxicological effects of the surfactant itself.

Minimization of Exposure to Air

Significant denaturation of proteins can occur when the protein solutions are exposed at the air/solution interface, the extent of denaturation being dependent on the time of exposure of the protein at the interface. Denaturation may also occur as a result of agitation of protein solutions in the presence of air or application of other shear forces such as those that occur when the solutions are filtered or pumped. Again, the inclusion of surfactants can reduce denaturation arising from these processes. Stability testing of protein-containing formulations often involves subjecting the solutions to shaking for several hours and the subsequent assessment of the protein configuration. If the protein has retained its native state and has not aggregated, the formulation is considered to be stable against surface or shear-induced denaturation.

Addition of Cosolvents

Some excipients and buffer components added to the protein solution are able to minimize denaturation through their effects on solvation. These compounds, referred to as cosolvents, include polyethylene glycols and glycerol and may act either by causing the preferential hydration of the protein or alternatively by binding to the protein surface. Preferential hydration results from an exclusion of the cosolvent from the protein surface due to steric effects (as in the case of polyethylene glycols), surface tension effects (as with sugars, salts, and amino acids), or some form of chemical incompatibility such as charge effects. As a result more water molecules pack around the protein to exclude the additive, and the protein becomes fully hydrated and stabilized in a compact form (Fig. 13). Alternatively, the cosolvent may stabilize the protein molecule by binding to it either nonspecifically or to specific sites on its surface.

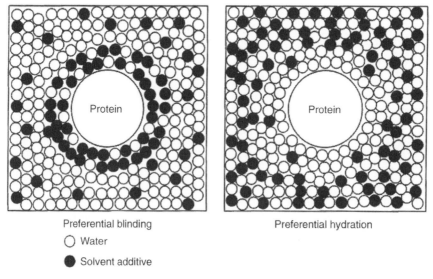

Preferential blinding   Preferential hydration

○ Water

● Solvent additive

Figure 13 Schematic illustration of preferential binding and preferential hydration by solvent additives; in preferential binding the additive occurs in the solvation shell of the protein at a greater local concentration than in the bulk solvent, while preferential hydration results from the exclusion of the additive from the surface of the protein. *Source*: From Ref. 117.

Accelerated Stability Testing of Protein Formulations

There have been relatively few reports of the influence of temperature on the rate of deamidation. Deamidation of peptides containing Gln and Asn (113) has been reported to proceed at a higher rate as the temperature was increased. From a study of the deamidation rates of an Asp residue in a model hexapeptide (118), it was concluded that the Arrhenius equation was obeyed over the temperature range 25°C to 70°C at pH 5.0 and 7.5.

In view of the complexity of the processes involved in the degradation of proteins, the mechanisms of degradation at higher temperatures may not be the same as at lower temperatures, and the application of the Arrhenius equation in the prediction of protein stability will be more uncertain than with formulations of small-molecule drugs. Nevertheless, many workers have attempted to use the Arrhenius approach with some degree of success. In general, this approach appears to be applicable when only the activity is monitored. In most of these studies degradation was due to thermal denaturation, and loss of activity was a consequence of conformational changes rather than covalent chemical reaction. Although the product of this reaction may involve many different unfolded forms of the protein, these forms will be inactive and indistinguishable from each other by activity assay (108). Deviation from the Arrhenius equation occurs, however, if the protein exists in multiple conformational forms that retain activity during unfolding. Where degradation occurs by deamidation or oxidation, it may still be possible to apply the Arrhenius equation if protein activity only is monitored since the final activity loss will be determined by the fastest reaction.

STABILITY TESTING IN THE PHARMACEUTICAL INDUSTRY

Stability testing of drug substances and drug products begins as part of the drug discovery/synthesis development/preformulation effort and ends only with the demise of the compound or commercial product. Activities include testing of drug substance; of compatibility with excipients; of preclinical formulations; of Phase I formulations and modifications; of the final, NDA (commercial) formulation; and of postapproval formulation changes. The regulatory basis for the various aspects of stability testing is established in 21 CFR 211.137, 211.160, 211.170, 211.190, 314.50, 314.70, and 314.81 (119–125).

While the Code of Federal Regulations establishes the statutory basis for carrying out stability testing, the U.S. Food and Drug Administration and the Expert Working Group of the International Conference on Harmonization (ICH) of Technical Requirements for the Registration of Pharmaceuticals for Human Use have published guidances for conducting the actual studies (126–131). These guidances provide definitions of key terms and principles used in the stability testing of drug substances and drug products as well as biotechnology products. Certain aspects of these guidances will be discussed later in this presentation.

Another valuable source of information on the establishment and maintenance of stability testing programs can be found in Carstensen's and Rhodes' book (132).

Resources

Personnel

The number and types of personnel are dictated by the size of the program, the functions contained within the program, and the nature of the program. Some companies maintain separate development and commercial product programs; others integrate the two. It is important, both for operating efficiency and regulatory compliance, that all personnel, regardless of their function, receive adequate and well-documented training both in Current Good Manufacturing Practices (cGMPs) and in the technical aspects of their jobs.

Education and experience The program is generally headed by a professional with several years of experience in the company. Experience in some aspect of formulation development or in the stability testing program itself may be of equal importance to the educational level of the person heading the program. People with a bachelor degree in pharmacy, chemistry, or related science as well as people with masters or doctoral level degrees have led successful programs. If the size of the program warrants, intermediate-level scientists, usually at the bachelor level, may assume responsibility for specific functions within the program, for example, chemical and physical testing, documentation, etc. Technicians generally have a high-school education or equivalent with clerical and/or scientific experience or interest. Clerical and data entry personnel have traditional training and experience in their respective areas.

Organization Functions are often divided into testing (chemical, physical, and biological), documentation, and clerical/computer operations, if the information system is computerized. Successful manual or paper systems are possible without the aid of computers. However, custom-designed software or commercially available database programs can also be programmed to automate the program. The documentation function usually consists of one or more persons who prepare the stability sections of regulatory documents. Persons specifically trained in technical writing or scientists with an interest and talent in document preparation generally perform well in this capacity.

Facilities

Storage chambers Several chambers capable of accurately maintaining different temperatures and combinations of temperature and humidity are needed. For most drug products, these include, as outlined in a recent ICH guidance (126), chambers ranging in temperature from $-20°C \pm 5°C$ to $40°C \pm 2°C/75\%$ RH $\pm 5\%$. For liquid products stored in semipermeable containers subject to water loss, exposure to lower humidities, for example, $25°C \pm 2°C/40\%$ RH $\pm 5\%$, $30°C \pm 2°C/65\%$ RH $\pm 5\%$, $40°C \pm 2°C$, is needed. Further details about the specific temperatures and humidities needed for specific dosage forms can be found in the ICH guidance (126). Also, a high-intensity light cabinet and a cycling chamber capable of cycling both temperature and humidity are needed. These chambers should be calibrated periodically according to a standard operating procedure, and records of these calibrations should be maintained in a logbook for each chamber.

For drug products normally stored at room temperature, long-term stability testing should be done at $25°C/60\%$ RH or $25°C/40\%$ RH. Stress testing should be done at $40°C/75\%$ RH or $40°C/(NMT)$ 25% RH for six months. If "significant change" occurs at these stress conditions, then the products should be tested at an intermediate condition, that is, $30°C/65\%RH$. Significant change is defined in the guidelines. If a lower temperature, for example, $-20°C$ or $5°C$, is needed for long-term storage, then the next highest temperature is used for stress testing.

Storage chambers should be validated with respect to their ability to maintain the desired conditions, and, if so equipped, the ability to sound an alarm if a mechanical or electrical failure causes the temperature to deviate from preestablished limits. They should also be equipped with recording devices, which will provide a continuous and permanent history of their operation. Logbooks should be maintained, and frequent readings of mercury-in-glass, National Institute of Science and Technology-traceable thermometers should be recorded.

Bench space Adequate laboratory bench, desk, and file space are needed for physical, chemical, and microbiological testing; for documentation; and for storing records, respectively.

Equipment

Chemical testing Adequate instrumentation for a variety of different test methods should be available. Most stability-indicating chemical assays are performed by high-pressure liquid chromatography. Occasionally, gas chromatography, infrared spectrophotometry, or spectrofluorimetry are used. Test methods should be validated (133–136) and stability indicating, that is, able to distinguish the active ingredient from its degradation products so that the active can be accurately measured. Also, methods are needed for identifying and quantitating degradation products that are present at levels of 0.1% or greater.

Biological testing A portion of the laboratory may be reserved for biological testing, or this work can be done by the company's microbiological laboratory. The ability to perform sterility, pyrogen, LAL, preservative challenge, and bioburden tests is needed to support the stability program. As is the case for chemical assays, test methods should be validated and operator familiarity should be documented.

Physical testing Equipment and trained personnel should be available for performing such tests as pH, tablet hardness, etc. One important and sometimes overlooked aspect of physical testing is the recording of product appearance. Carefully defined descriptions of appearance and standard descriptions of changes in appearance should be developed, especially when there is a high probability that the person who made the observation at the previous sampling time will not be the person making the observation at the next sampling time. Some companies maintain samples at a lower-than-label storage condition, for example, refrigeration, to use as standards, assuming that minimal or no appearance change will occur at this condition. The same argument for standard nomenclature applies to other test parameters that are subjective in nature.

Computers A certain number of personal computers are necessary for report generation and regulatory submission preparation. In addition, these may be useful for record keeping, depending on the type of stability information system that the company chooses to use. Alternatively, if the information system is intended to be accessible (read only) to many users, it may be more efficient to develop a local area network of minicomputers. The size of the database will help determine the nature of the software/hardware configuration used for this function.

Program

Scope and Goals

Activities encompassed by the stability program include sample storage of either development or production batches (or both), data collection and storage/retrieval, physical, chemical, and microbiological testing, document preparation of regulatory submissions, and package evaluation. In certain companies, personnel in separate departments may perform some of these functions, for example, regulatory document preparation. Nonetheless, the function is part of the company's overall stability program.

Protocols

FDA/ICH guidelines (126) are rather detailed regarding sampling times, storage conditions, and specific test parameters for each dosage form. Generally, samples stored at the product label storage condition, controlled room temperature for most products, are tested initially and after 3, 6, 9, 12, 18, and 24 months, and annually thereafter. Accelerated testing is generally done more frequently and for a shorter duration, for example, one, two, three, and six months. Three batches should be tested to demonstrate batch-to-batch uniformity. The number 3 represents a compromise between a large number desired for statistical precision and the economics of maintaining a manageable program. Generally, real-time data obtained at the label storage conditions on the final formulation in the final packaging configuration(s) are needed for an NDA. Supportive data obtained from drug substance stability studies, preformulation studies, and investigational formulations tested during clinical trials and formulation development may be used to supplement primary stability data. Requirements for the IND are less defined, the only requirement being that there should be adequate data to support the clinical batch(es) for the duration of the trials.

There are instances, especially in the case of solid, oral dosage forms, where several package types and configurations are desired by marketing and three or more strengths are needed for flexibility in dosing. In these situations, it may be feasible to apply the principles of bracketing and/or matrixing (129) to reduce the amount of testing. Bracketing refers to reduced testing of either an intermediate dosage strength or package size when the formulation characteristics of all strengths are virtually identical or when the same container/closure materials are used for all package sizes. Matrixing refers to reduced testing regardless of the strength or container in situations where there are similarities in formulation or container/closure. Bracketing and matrixing are acceptable only when the product is chemically and physically very stable and does not interact with the container/closure. Demonstration of this chemical and physical stability must be documented by preformulation, drug substance stability, and early formulation stability data. Although not as common, it may be possible to utilize bracketing and matrixing with other types of dosage forms. In all cases, discussions of such strategies with FDA prior to implementation are imperative.

Documentation

The need for adequate documentation of laboratory operations is established not only by good science but also by regulatory requirements (122).

Documentation of all facets of the operation is necessary. This includes validation and periodic calibration of storage chambers, instrumentation, and computer programs. Logbooks for the storage chambers and instruments are also necessary. Standard operating procedures are needed for, among other things, the stability program itself, use of instrumentation, documentation of experiments and their results, determination of expiration dates, investigation of specification failures, and operation of a computerized record-keeping system.

Many companies have developed or purchased computer software for the purpose of storing stability data for a large number of studies. Examples of commercially available systems are "SLIM" (137) and "Stability System" (138). These systems can perform other functions as well, including work scheduling, preparation of summaries of selected or all studies in the system, tabulation of data for individual studies, label printing, statistical analysis and plotting, and search capabilities. Such systems should be validated to keep pace with current regulatory activity (139).

Regulatory Concerns

cGMP Compliance

cGMPs (120) establish the requirements for maintaining a stability program and require that most pharmaceutical dosage forms have an established expiration date supported by test data (119). There are few allowable exceptions.

FDA Stability Guidelines

The guidelines under which stability programs operate and corresponding documentation is best described in ICH guidance (126). Although the agency emphasizes that these are guidelines and not regulations, it is generally prudent to follow specific recommendations as indicated in the guidelines. Deviations or omissions should be addressed, and the reasons should be supported with data where applicable.

Regulatory Submissions

An easy-to-read stability summary document will go a long way toward rapid approval of any regulatory submission. Such a document should include a number of items. A clear statement of the objective(s) of the studies included in the submission and the approach that was taken to achieve the objective(s) is critical. This statement of objective(s) should accompany basic information including product and drug substance names, dosage forms and strengths, and type(s) of container/closure systems. Although the objective is usually stated in the summary letter accompanying the submission, a brief reminder to the reviewing chemist is helpful.

A discussion of each of the parameters that were tested in the course of the evaluation, including test methods and specifications for each, should then follow. These parameters should follow those recommended in the stability guidelines (126) for the specific dosage form. It is especially important to provide a rationale for those parameters not studied. Next should come the study design itself, which should include a list of batch identification number, size, and date of manufacture as well as packaging configuration, storage conditions, and sampling times for each batch. The strategy and rationale for any bracketing or matrixing should also be presented.

The actual data, including replicates, mean, and range, in tabular form should follow accompanied by a brief discussion of the data. It is important to explain any out-of-specification data. Statistical analyses for all parameters, which lend themselves to such analyses along with conclusions, should be incorporated into the document at this point. These statistical analyses should be accompanied by the results of experiments conducted to determine the "poolability" of batches, or commonality of slopes and intercepts of individual batches. Graphs of these data should be included as part of the documentation.

Protocols for these batches and a commitment to continue them along with a "tentative" expiry date should also be included. Approval of these protocols will allow extension of the expiry date without a special supplement as long as the data remain within specifications. These data will ultimately be reported to FDA as part of periodic reports following NDA approval. Protocols intended for use on commercial batches should also be submitted.

Finally, the three-part commitment to mount studies for the first three production batches and a statistically determined number (at least one) each year, to update current studies in annual reports, and to withdraw any lots not meeting specifications should appear in the submission. Statistical sampling of production batches is usually based on $\log N$, $\sqrt{N}$, etc., where N is the number of batches produced per year. These batches are generally spread over various package types and manufacturing campaigns. There should be a standard operating procedure to handle specification deviations including confirmation of the result, cause and effect investigation, impact analysis, final report to management, and field alert or batch recall notice to FDA.

Annual Product Review

Once a product gains FDA approval for marketing, the sponsor should maintain a readily retrievable profile of commercial batches. This includes individual batch release data and stability data. These data should be compiled throughout the year and tabulated prior to the anniversary of NDA approval for submission in the annual product report to FDA. By maintaining an ongoing database, which is reviewed as new information is added, changing trends in the data can be observed and management notified if any of these trends are unfavorable.

REFERENCES

1. Nord K, Karisen J, Tønnesen HH. Int J Pharm 1991; 72:11–18.
2. Cornelissen PJG, Beijersbergen van Henegouwen GMJ, Gerritsma KW. Int J Pharm 1978; 1:173–181.
3. Neftel KA, Walti M, Spengler H, et al. Lancet 1982; 319:986–988.
4. Connors KA, Amidon GL, Stella VJ. Chemical Stability of Pharmaceuticals: A Handbook for Pharmacists. 2nd ed. New York: John Wiley & Sons, 1986.
5. Brittain HG, ed. Analytical Profiles of Drug Substances and Excipients. Vol 28. San Diego: Academic Press, 2001.
6. Schwartz MA, Granatek AP, Buekwalter FH. J Pharm Sci 1962; 51:523–526.
7. Krieble VK, Holst KA. J Am Chem Soc 1938; 60:2976–2980.
8. Casey LA, Gait R, Page MI. J Chem Soc Perkin Trans 2 1993; 23–28.
9. LePree JM, Connors KA. Hydrolysis of drugs. In: Swarbrick J, ed. Encyclopedia of Pharmaceutical Technology. 3rd ed. New York: Informa Healthcare, 2006:2040–2047.
10. Mark HB Jr., Rechnitz GA. In: Elving PJ, Kolthoff IM, eds. Chemical Analysis. Vol 24. New York: Wiley-Interscience, 1970.
11. Hansch C, Leo A, Taft RW. Chem Rev 1991; 91:165–195.
12. Hammett LP. Physical Organic Chemistry. 2nd ed. New York: McGraw-Hill, 1970.
13. Capon B, McManus SP. Neighboring Group Participation. New York: Plenum Press, 1976.
14. Khan MN, Gambo SK. Int J Chem Kinet 1985; 17:419–428.
15. Swintosky JV, Rosen E, Robinson MJ, et al. J Am Pharm Assoc 1956; 45:34–37.
16. Higuchi T, Lachman C. J Am Pharm Assoc 1955; 44:521–526.
17. Wells PR. Chem Rev 1963; 63:171–219.
18. Carstensen JT, Serenson EG, Vance JJ. J Pharm Sci 1964; 53:1547–1548.
19. Hovorka SW, Schőneich C. J Pharm Sci 2001; 90:253–269.
20. Pezzuto JM, Park EJ. Autoxidation and antioxidants. In: Swarbrick J, ed. Encyclopedia of Pharmaceutical Technology. 3rd ed. New York: Informa Healthcare, 2006:139–154.
21. Chen TM, Chafetz L. J Pharm Sci 1987; 76:703–706.
22. Pinholt P, Kristiansen H, Krowczynski L, et al. J Pharm Sci 1966; 55:1435–1438.

23. Schulz J, Bauer K-H. Acta Pharm Technol 1986; 32:78–81.
24. Hamburger R, Azaz E, Donbrow M. Pharm Acta Helv 1975; 50:10–17.
25. McGinity JW, Hill JA, La Via AL. J Pharm Sci 1975; 64:356–357.
26. McGinity JW, Patel TR, Naqvi AH, et al. Drug Dev Commun 1976; 2:505–519.
27. Gu L, Chiang H-S, Johnson DM. Int J Pharm 1988; 41:105–113.
28. Johnson DM, Taylor WF. J Pharm Sci 1984; 73:1414–1417.
29. Smith GB, DiMichele L, Colwell LF, et al. Tetrahedron 1993; 49:4447–4462.
30. Lamy-Freund MT, Ferreira VFN, Faljoni-Alário A, et al. J Pharm Sci 1993; 82:162–166.
31. Halbaut L, Barbé C, Aroztegui M, et al. Int J Pharm 1997; 147:31–40.
32. Underberg WJM. J Pharm Sci 1978; 67:1133–1138.
33. Oyler AR, Naldi RE, Facchine KL, et al. Tetrahedron 1991; 47:6549–6560.
34. Tønnesen HH. Photodecomposition of drugs. In: Swarbrick J, ed. Encyclopedia of Pharmaceutical Technology. 3rd ed. New York: Informa Healthcare, 2006:2859–2865.
35. Greenhill JV, McLelland MA. Prog Med Chem 1990; 27:51–121.
36. Tønnesen HH. Int J Pharm 2001; 225:1–14.
37. Frank MJ, Johnson JB, Rubin SH. J Pharm Sci 1976; 65:44–48.
38. Mahony C, et al. J Pharm Sci 1984; 73:838–839.
39. Lyall D. Pharm J 1988; 240:5.
40. Matsuda Y, Inouye H, Nakanishi R. J Pharm Sci 1978; 67:196–201.
41. Jamali F, Mehvar R, Pasutto FM. J Pharm Sci 1989; 78:695–715.
42. Nunes MA, Brochmann-Hanssen E. J Pharm Sci 1974; 63:716–721.
43. Richter WF, Chong YH, Stella VJ. J Pharm Sci 1990; 79:185–186.
44. Severin G. Chirality 1992; 4:222–226.
45. Bundgaard H. Acta Pharm Suec 1976; 13:9–26.
46. Riff LJ, Jackson GG. Arch Intern Med 1972; 130:887–891.
47. Meites L. CRC Crit Rev Anal Chem 1979; 8:1–53.
48. Guidelines for Submitting Documentation for the Stability of Human Drugs and Biologics. Rockville, MD: Center for Drugs and Biologics, Food and Drug Administration; February 1987.
49. Carstensen JT. J Pharm Sci 1974; 63:1–14.
50. Carstensen JT. Drug Stability. Principles and Practices. 2nd ed. New York: Marcel Dekker, Inc., 1995.
51. Kornblum SS, Sciarrone BJ. J Pharm Sci 1964; 53:935–941.
52. Carstensen JT, Musa MN. J Pharm Sci 1972; 61:1112–1118.
53. Wang D-P, Yeh M-K. J Pharm Sci 1993; 82:95–98.
54. Pikal MJ, Lukes AL, Lang JE. J Pharm Sci 1977; 66:1312–1316.
55. Woolfe AJ, Worthington HEC. Drug Dev Commun 1974; 1:185.
56. Savello DR, Shangraw RF. Am J Hosp Pharm 1971; 28:754–759.
57. Fan T-Y, Tannenbaum SR. J Agric Food Chem 1973; 21:967–969.
58. Shija R, Sunderland VB, McDonald C. Int J Pharm 1992; 80:203–211.
59. Pincock RE. Acc Chem Res 1969; 2:97–103.
60. Murase N, Echlin P, Franks F. Cryobiology 1991; 28:364–375.
61. Fung H-L, King S-YP. Pharm Tech Conference '83 Proceedings, Aster Publishing, Springfield, Oregon, 1983.
62. Carney CF. J Pharm Sci 1987; 76:393–397.
63. Powell MF. J Pharm Sci 1986; 75:901–903.
64. Cox BG, Kresge AJ, Sørensen PE. Acta Chem Scand 1988; A42:202–213.
65. Kresge AJ. Chem Soc Rev 1973; 2:475–503.
66. Ravin LJ, Simpson CA, Zappala AF, et al. J Pharm Sci 1964; 53:1064–1066.
67. Garrett ER. J Am Chem Soc 1957; 79:3401–3408.
68. Wells JI. Pharmaceutical Preformulation. West Sussex, UK: Ellis Horwood, 1988.
69. Schwartz MA. J Pharm Sci 1964; 53:1433.
70. Andersin R, Tammilehto S. Int J Pharm 1995; 123:229–235.
71. Torniainen K, Tammilehto S, Ulvi V. Int J Pharm 1996; 132:53–61.

72. Gu L, Strickley RG. Int J Pharm 1990; 60:99–107.

73. Garrett ER. J Org Chem 1961; 26:3660–3663.

74. Thoma K, Struve M. Pharm Ind 1985; 47:1078–1081.

75. Amis FS. Solvent Effects on Reaction Rates and Mechanisms. New York: Academic Press, 1966.

76. Connors KA. Chemical Kinetics: The Study of Reaction Rates in Solution. New York: VCH Publishers, 1990:411.

77. Carstensen JT. J Pharm Sci 1970; 59:1140–1143.

78. Broxton TJ. Aust J Chem 1982; 35:1357–1363.

79. Attwood D, Florence AT. Surfactant Systems, Their Chemistry, Pharmacy and Biology. London: Chapman and Hall, 1983.

80. Ong JTH, Kostenbauder HB. J Pharm Sci 1975; 64:1378–1380.

81. Higuchi T, Lachman L. J Am Pharm Assoc (Sci Ed) 1955; 44:521–526.

82. Connors KA. Binding Constants: The Measurement of Molecular Complex Stability. New York: John Wiley & Sons, 1987.

83. Bekers O, Uijtendaal EV, Beijnen JH, et al. Drug Dev Ind Pharm 1991; 17:1503–1549.

84. Anderson NH, Johnson D, McLelland MA, et al. J Pharm Biomed Anal 1991; 9:443–449.

85. Allen AE, Das Gupta V. J Pharm Sci 1974; 63:107–109.

86. Das Gupta V. J Pharm Sci 1978; 67:299–303.

87. Busse MJ. Pharm J 1978; 220:25.

88. Ullmann E, Thoma K, Zelfel G. Pharm Acta Helv 1963; 38:577–586.

89. Tingstad J, Dudzinski J. J Pharm Sci 1973; 62:1856–1860.

90. Maudling HV, Zoglio MA, Pigois FE, et al. J Pharm Sci 1969; 58:1359–1362.

91. Boggiano BG, Drew R, Hancock RD. Aust J Pharm 1970; 51:S14–S16.

92. Kornblum SS, Zoglio MA. J Pharm Sci 1967; 56:1569–1575.

93. Zoglio MA, Maudling HV, Haller RM, et al. J Pharm Sci 1968; 57:1877–1880.

94. Jun HW, Whitworth CW, Luzzi LA. J Pharm Sci 1972; 61:1160–1162.

95. Whitworth CW, Luzzi LA, Thompson BB, et al. J Pharm Sci 1973; 62:1372–1374.

96. Ekman R, Liponkoski L, Kahela P. Acta Pharm Suec 1982; 19:241–246.

97. Smidsroed O, Haug A, Larsen B. Acta Chem Scand 1963; 17:1473–1474.

98. Buxton PC, Jahnke R, Keady S. Eur J Pharm Biopharm 1994; 40:172–175.

99. Genton D, Kesselring UW. J Pharm Sci 1977; 66:676–680.

100. Horhota ST, Burgio J, Lonski L, et al. J Pharm Sci 1976; 65:1746–1749.

101. Chemburkar PB, Smyth RD, Buehler JD, et al. J Pharm Sci 1976; 65:529–533.

102. Kovalcik TR, Guillory JK. J Parenter Sci Technol 1988; 42:29–37.

103. Carstensen JT. Drug Dev Ind Pharm 1988; 14:1927–1969.

104. Ahlneck C, Zografi G. Int J Pharm 1990; 62:87–95.

105. Chen T. Drug Dev Ind Pharm 1992; 18:1311–1354.

106. Hageman MJ. Drug Dev Ind Pharm 1988; 14:2047–2070

107. Manning M, Patel K, Borchardt RT. Pharm Res 1989; 6:903–918.

108. Cleland JL, Powell MF, Shire SJ. Crit Rev Ther Drug Carrier Syst 1993; 10:307–377.

109. Robinson AB, Rudd CJ. Deamidation of glutaminyl and asparaginyl residues in peptides and proteins. In: Horecker BL, Stadtman ER, eds. Current Topics in Cellular Regulation. Vol 8. New York: Academic Press, 1974:247–295.

110. Geiger T, Clarke S. J Biol Chem 1987; 262:785–794.

111. Capasso S, Mazzarella L, Zagari A. Pept Res 1991; 4:234–238.

112. Mears GE, Feeney RE. Chemical Modification of Proteins. San Francisco: Holden-Day Inc., 1971:35.

113. McKerrow JH, Robinson AB. Anal Biochem 1971; 42:565–568.

114. Brennan TV, Clarke S. Protein Sci 1993; 2:331–338.

115. Flatmark T. Acta Chem Scand 1966; 20:1487–1496.

116. Tyler-Cross R, Schirch V. J Biol Chem 1991; 266:22549–22556.

117. Timasheff SN, Arakawa T. In: Creighton TE, ed. Protein Structure: A Practical Approach. Oxford: IRL Press, 1989:331–345.

118. Patel K, Borchardt RT. Pharm Res 1990; 7:703–711.
119. Code of Federal Regulations, Title 21, Food and Drugs, Part 211, Current good manufacturing practice for finished pharmaceuticals, Subpart G, §211.137 Expiration dating.
120. Code of Federal Regulations, Title 21, Food and Drugs, Part 211, Current good manufacturing practice for finished pharmaceuticals, Subpart I, §211.166 Stability testing.
121. Code of Federal Regulations, Title 21, Food and Drugs, Part 211, Current good manufacturing practice for finished pharmaceuticals, Subpart I, §211.170 Reserve samples.
122. Code of Federal Regulations, Title 21, Food and Drugs, Part 211, Current good manufacturing practice for finished pharmaceuticals, Subpart J, §211.194 Laboratory records.
123. Code of Federal Regulations, Title 21, Food and Drugs, Part 314, Applications for FDA approval to market a new drug or antibiotic drug, Subpart B, §314.50 Content and format of an application.
124. Code of Federal Regulations, Title 21, Food and Drugs, Part 314, Applications for FDA approval to market a new drug or antibiotic drug, Subpart B, §314.70 Supplements and other changes to an approved application.
125. Code of Federal Regulations, Title 21, Food and Drugs, Part 314, Applications for FDA approval to market a new drug or antibiotic drug, Subpart B, §314.81 Other postmarketing reports.
126. ICH Expert Working Group. Q1A (R2) Stability Testing of New Drug Substances and Products. International Conference on Harmonisation of Technical Requirements for the Registration of Pharmaceuticals for Human Use, 2003.
127. ICH Expert Working Group. Q1B Photostability Testing of New Drug Substances and Products. International Conference on Harmonisation of Technical Requirements for the Registration of Pharmaceuticals for Human Use, 1996.
128. ICH Expert Working Group. Q1C Stability Testing for New Dosage Forms. International Conference on Harmonisation of Technical Requirements for the Registration of Pharmaceuticals for Human Use, 1996.
129. ICH Expert Working Group. Q1D Bracketing and Matrixing Designs for Stability Testing of New Drug Substances and Products. International Conference on Harmonisation of Technical Requirements for the Registration of Pharmaceuticals for Human Use, 2003.
130. ICH Expert Working Group. Q1E Evaluation of Stability Data. International Conference on Harmonisation of Technical Requirements for the Registration of Pharmaceuticals for Human Use, 2004.
131. ICH Expert Working Group. Q5C Stability Testing of Biotechnological/Biological New Drug Substances and Products. International Conference on Harmonisation of Technical Requirements for the Registration of Pharmaceuticals for Human Use, 1995.
132. Carstensen JT, Rhodes CT. Drug Stability, Principles and Practices. 3rd ed. New York: Marcel Dekker, Inc., 2000.
133. Guideline for Submitting Samples and Analytical Data for Methods Validation. Rockville, MD: Center for Drugs and Biologics, Food and Drug Administration; February 1987.
134. ICH Expert Working Group. Q2B validation of analytical procedures: methodology. International Conference on Harmonisation of Technical Requirements for the Registration of Pharmaceuticals for Human Use, 1996.
135. Debesis E, Boehlert JP, Givand TE, et al., Submitting HPLC methods to the compendia and regulatory agencies. Pharm Tech 1982; 6(9):120–137.
136. United States Pharmacopeia 30, <1225> Validation of Compendial Methods, 2007:680–683.
137. Stability Lab Information Manager, Metrics, Inc., Greenville, NC.
138. Stability System, ScienTek Software, Inc., Tustin, CA.
139. Tetzlaff RF. GMP documentation requirements for automated systems: Part 3, FDA inspection of computerized laboratory systems. Pharm Tech 1992; 16(5):70–83.

8

The Solid State

Alastair J. Florence
*Strathclyde Institute of Pharmacy and Biomedical Sciences,
University of Strathclyde, Glasgow, U.K.*

INTRODUCTION

Many active pharmaceutical ingredients (APIs) can exist in more than one solid-state form, including crystalline polymorphs, solvates, salts, cocrystals, and noncrystalline or amorphous solids (Fig. 1; Table 1). Hence, assessment and control of the solid-state structure of APIs is necessary to ensure efficient and reproducible processing, manufacturing, and storage; to satisfy regulatory authorities; to protect intellectual property; and ultimately to deliver safe, effective, and high-quality medicinal products. This section introduces key practical aspects of solid-state pharmaceuticals, with a specific emphasis on crystalline solids and their preparation, handling, and analysis, particularly in the context of preclinical drug development and pharmaceutical manufacture.

Tablets and capsules are the most widely manufactured dosage forms, being relatively cheap to manufacture, effective at delivering many drugs via oral administration and are convenient for patients to take. The properties of these solid products are determined to a large extent by the solid-state form, or structure, of the component powders used in their manufacture. The physical form, or crystal structure, of an API determines many important pharmaceutical properties, including solubility, morphology, and hygroscopicity, which can in turn influence many processing and manufacturing properties such as filtration, compressibility, and long-term physical stability and can potentially impact the oral bioavailability of the product. Hence, in commercial solid-state development, it is important to identify all possible solid forms of the API, and the associated conditions that give rise to them, as early as possible in the development cycle and establish effective means of controlling physical form during production of raw material and subsequent processing.

Despite significant advances in the theoretical understanding of crystalline solids in recent years (3,4), it is not yet possible to predict crystal structure or physical properties reliably from a knowledge of molecular structure alone, particularly for molecules with the typical structural complexity of many APIs (that include significant conformational flexibility and/or counterions). Solid-state surveys therefore rely on experimental

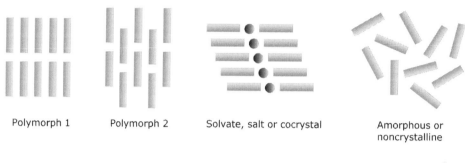

Polymorph 1   Polymorph 2   Solvate, salt or cocrystal   Amorphous or
                                                                              noncrystalline

API molecule

solvent molecule, counter-ion or cocrystal former

Figure 1 Schematic illustration of molecular arrangements in different types of organic solids showing ordered molecular arrangements in crystalline forms and molecular disorder in amorphous solids. The terminology used is outlined in Table 1.

Table 1 Outline of the Potential Range of Solid Forms of Relevance to Pharmaceuticals and Their Composition

Type	Description	Composition
Crystalline solid	Solid form displaying highly ordered molecular packing. This long-range three-dimensionally ordered structure will give rise to Bragg diffraction of X-rays.	API
Polymorph	Chemically identical crystalline forms in which the constituent molecules adopt different packing arrangements.	API
Crystalline solvate	Solid in which solvent, typically from the crystallization process, is incorporated within the crystal lattice with the solute. The term "pseudopolymorph" is also sometimes used. Lattice comprises API plus solvent.	API plus solvent
Crystalline salt	Ionic crystalline solid formed between an ionized API and counterion.	Charged API plus counterion
Cocrystal	Crystalline solid comprising nonionized API plus additional chemical entity. Also termed "multicomponent crystal" (1) or molecular complex. As for solvate, though cocrystallizing agent is a solid itself at room temperature (2).	API plus cocrystal former
Amorphous	A noncrystalline solid that possesses no long-range order (i.e., crystal lattice) and so does not give rise to Bragg diffraction of X rays.	API

crystallization approaches and physical form analysis techniques to identify all physical forms and their physical properties, structure, and relative stabilities (Fig. 2). This information is vital to inform selection of the optimal crystalline form (polymorph, solvate, or salt) of the API for use in the final product. With the considerable potential that exists for structural variation in the solid state, a knowledge of crystal structure can be of significant value in understanding the chemical and physical properties of the material.

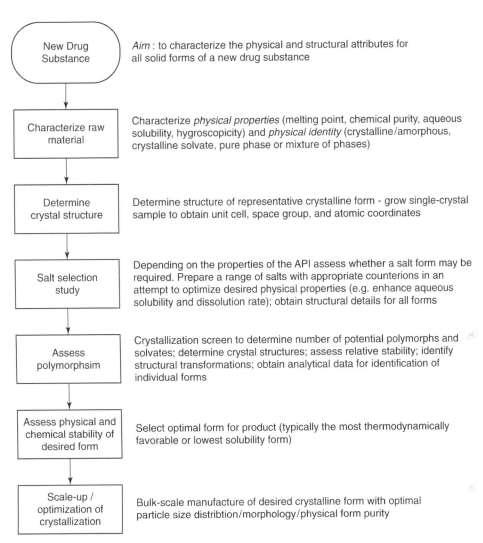

Figure 2 An overview of the main stages in the characterization and development of solid-state pharmaceutical materials.

Regulatory Considerations

As the solid-state form and physical stability of APIs may impact on product safety, efficacy, and quality, it is necessary for pharmaceutical companies to demonstrate to regulatory authorities that they have adequate control over solid form of new drug substances. The International Conference on Harmonisation of Technical Requirements for Registration of Pharmaceuticals for Human Use (ICH; www.ich.org) provides a range of guidance for registration processes in the EU, United States, and Japan that include specific recommendations for dealing with polymorphism. Guideline Specification Q6A (Specifications for New Drug Substances and Products: Chemical Substances; October 1999) (5) outlines various regulatory requirements on physical form and polymorphism for new chemical entities being submitted for approval and provides decision trees outlining logical steps to assist in satisfying these requirements. Salts are treated as separate chemical entities in this context.

Physical Form and Intellectual Property

The background and implications of physical form patenting of pharmaceuticals has been discussed in detail elsewhere (6,7). However, it is worth highlighting that in the context of the commercial exploitation of crystalline pharmaceuticals the value of identifying the complete range of solid-state structures and properties associated with an API extends beyond improved control of formulation and manufacturing processes. Innovator companies may use solid-state patents to defend, extend, and manage their intellectual property protection for a molecule discovered and developed by them, while generic manufacturers, having identified weaknesses in existing physical form patents, may attempt to use such issues to gain access to lucrative product markets. Polymorphic forms have been the basis of several high-profile litigation cases, with ranitidine hydrochloride being perhaps the most widely reported (8). In summary, a comprehensive knowledge of the extent of solid-state diversity can therefore add value to product development by protecting intellectual property and maximizing the revenue-earning life cycle of a new API.

CRYSTALLINE PHARMACEUTICALS

The majority of APIs will be encountered, at least in some stage in the production of medicinal products, in the solid state, and typically in the form of polycrystalline powders. As already stated, the size, shape, structure, and properties of the individual crystallites comprising the powder have significant influence over the properties of the final dosage form and therefore characterization, and control of solid-state forms is an important aspect of drug development (9–11). Solid-state form is not only of relevance to APIs; many excipients, including lactose (12), mannitol (13), and calcium hydrogen phosphate, for example, are also crystalline materials and can display a variety of crystalline forms, which if uncontrolled, may impact upon the performance of the final product. Excipients can also influence the physical stability of APIs during processing. For example, hydroxypropylmethylcellulose has been shown to inhibit the anhydrous-to-hydrate transformation of ciprofloxacin (14) and theophylline (15) during wet granulation steps, while PVPK12 enhanced the rate of formation of carbamazepine dihydrate from the anhydrous form of the drug in powder blends exposed to elevated humidity (16). Such physical interactions are not readily predictable and emphasize the need to monitor physical form, particularly during the development of new formulations and processes.

The range of solid-state forms of an API can be significant and both unpredicted, as with polymorphs or solvates, or deliberately encouraged, as in the intentional formation of crystalline salts. Regardless of the method of preparation of the form, the significance of such diversity arises from the change in molecular packing in each structure. As molecules adopt different packing arrangements and/or conformations in each form, the intermolecular interactions and Gibbs free energy of the materials will differ (17). As a consequence, each unique solid-state form can display a range of different physical properties. Comprehensive experimental approaches targeted at revealing the extent of physical form diversity for a given API therefore aim to identify both the structure and key properties of all forms to enable the optimal form to be selected.

Crystal structure details are largely determined using X-ray crystallographic methods; however, the detail of these techniques is beyond the scope of this text, and the interested reader is directed to the many specialist crystallography textbooks that provide an excellent introduction to the subject (see Refs. 18 and 19 for example). Here we will restrict ourselves to covering the basic terminology necessary to interpret crystal structure data in the context of solid-state pharmaceuticals.

The Crystalline State

The internal structure of a crystalline solid is highly ordered, with molecules packed in a periodic three-dimensional array known as the crystal lattice. The smallest assembly of molecules that can generate the full lattice by only translation of its contents is termed "the unit cell" (Fig. 3). This is of fundamental importance in experimental surveys of solid form as it can be determined routinely from diffraction data and used to identify each discrete crystalline phase unambiguously (Table 2).

The symmetry of the unit cell defines the crystal system (18), of which there are seven classes, ranging from cubic (high-symmetry structures, e.g., NaCl; lattice constants $a = b = c$; $\alpha = \beta = \gamma = 90°$) to the lowest symmetry triclinic system (lattice constants $a \neq b \neq c$; $\alpha \neq \beta \neq \gamma$). Pharmaceutical molecules, owing to their relatively complex molecular shapes, tend to crystallize in the lower symmetry orthorhombic, monoclinic, and triclinic systems. Indeed, the monoclinic space group $P2_1/c$ is the most frequently occurring space group in the Cambridge Structural Database (CSD) (20), a database of published organic and organometallic crystal structures, which at January 1, 2008, contained details of over 430,000 structures. The CSD represents a valuable information resource for molecular structure, conformation, and intermolecular packing for those concerned with the organic solid state.

The structure of a crystalline material can be described by reference to its crystal system, six unit cell parameters (Fig. 3), the symmetry operators, or space group (21), describing the symmetrical arrangement of molecules within the unit cell and the atomic positions (fractional coordinates) of each atom within the asymmetrical unit. These data therefore comprise a unique description, or fingerprint, of a crystal structure and can be used to identify specific crystalline forms. The entire three-dimensional crystal lattice is constructed by simple translation of the unit cell contents along each of the three lattice axes (Fig. 4).

The regularity of the molecular packing within a crystalline solid confers well-defined physical properties to the bulk material, such as sharp melting points, and is also reflected in the external morphology of individual crystals, with samples displaying flat faces, sharp edges, and well-defined interfacial angles (Fig. 5).

Polymorphism and Pharmaceuticals

Many organic materials can crystallize in more than one crystalline form, yielding chemically identical solids that differ only in their packing arrangements (8,10,28). The differences in lattice energies that arise from the altered intermolecular noncovalent

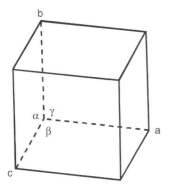

Figure 3 A schematic diagram showing a unit cell with lattice parameters describing its size and shape. The unit cell lengths are defined as a, b, and c and are in Ångstrom units (10^{-10} m) and the angles α, β, and γ intersecting the lattice axes are in degrees.

Table 2 Crystal Structure Data for Different Crystalline Forms of the Analgesic Paracetamol ($C_8H_9NO_2$; Mol. Wt. = 151.1)

	Paracetamol (form I) (22)	Paracetamol (form II) (22)	Paracetamol dioxane hemisolvate (23)	Paracetamol methanol solvate (24)	Paracetamol dihydrate (25)	Paracetamol trihydrate (26)
Formula	$C_8H_9NO_2$	$C_8H_9NO_2$	$C_8H_9NO_2, 0.5(C_4H_8O_2)$	$C_8H_9NO_2, CH_4O$	$C_8H_9NO_2, 2(H_2O)$	$C_8H_9NO_2, 3(H_2O)$
Crystal system	Monoclinic	Orthorhombic	Monoclinic	Monoclinic	Monoclinic	Orthorhombic
Space group	$P2_1/n$	$Pbca$	$P2_1/c$	$P2_1/c$	$P2_1/c$	$Pbca$
a (Å)	7.094	17.166	12.325	7.630	6.684	7.332
b (Å)	9.232	11.777	11.965	17.209	12.475	12.590
c (Å)	11.620	7.212	13.384	7.371	10.736	22.636
α (°)	90.0	90.0	90.0	90.0	90.0	90.0
β (°)	97.821	90.0	92.010	115.520	107.387	90.0
γ (°)	90.0	90.0	90.0	90.0	90.0	90.0
Cell volume (Å³)	753.937	1458.018	1972.506	873.419	854.296	2089.640

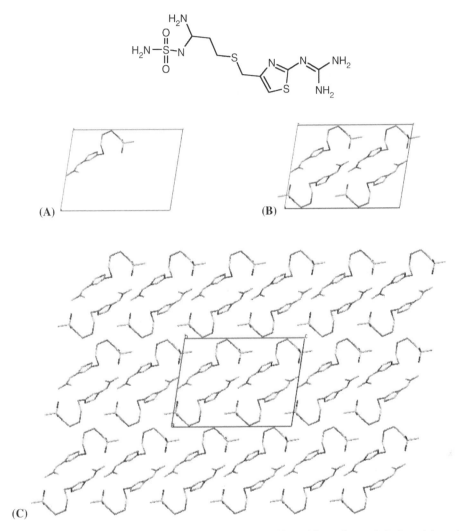

Figure 4 Packing diagram illustrating the crystal lattice of famotidine polymorph A viewed down the *b*-axis (*top*) [monoclinic, $P2_1/c$, $a = 17.762(1)$ Å, $b = 5.329(1)$ Å, $c = 18.307(1)$ Å, $\beta = 123.61(1)°$, volume $= 1443.14$ Å^3, $Z = 4$] (27). The structure is described by (**A**) one molecule of famotidine within the asymmetric unit of the unit cell ($Z' = 1$); (**B**) the space group symmetry operators generate a further three symmetry-related molecules within the unit cell to give a total of four ($Z = 4$); (**C**) the unit cell being repeated in three dimensions by translation along the cell axes *a*, *b*, *c* to produce the three-dimensional crystal lattice (as drawn, the *b*-direction lies above/below the plane of the page).

interactions within these different arrangements can have significant effects on important material properties, including aqueous solubility, morphology, melting point, hygroscopicity, density, and chemical stability (see Table 3).

For a compound that exhibits polymorphism, only one of the forms, having the lowest Gibbs free energy, will be the most thermodynamically favorable at room temperature. Thus, once samples of different polymorphs of a compound become available, the relative thermodynamic stability of each form should be determined to identify the most favourable polymorphic form. This form will display the lowest solubility among all the potential polymorphic forms (17), and solubility measurements are therefore a useful method of identifying the relative favorability of multiple forms at

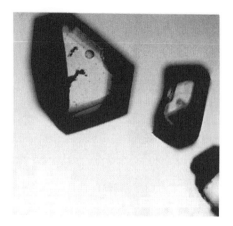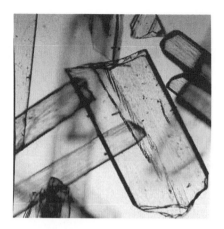

Figure 5 Photomicrographs showing well-defined crystals of famotidine with form A adopting an isometric prismatic morphology (*left*) and form B a platy morphology (*right*).

room temperature. An important proviso with such measurements is that the physical identity of the solid form present at equilibrium should be confirmed to rule out the possibility that a solution-mediated transformation has occurred (29). Solution-mediated transformations can occur because of solubility differences between polymorphs, where a solution in contact with a metastable polymorph (more soluble) is supersaturated with respect to a more stable (less soluble) form (30). Under these conditions, solute molecules can crystallize from solution and adopt the more favorable structure, although the kinetics of any transformation can be affected by the degree of agitation and temperature of solution, solubility, and properties of the solvent (31). The process will proceed until complete transformation of all of the original solid phase has occurred. The solubility profile shown in Figure 6 typifies solution-mediated transformations, although the timescales for the transformation to occur can vary from a few minutes to many hours, depending on the kinetics of transformation and nucleation and growth of the lower solubility form. This process can be exploited in slurrying experiments designed to obtain the most thermodynamically favorable form under a specific set of conditions (see section "Other Approaches to Physical Form Discovery").

A series of rules developed by Burger and Ramberger is widely used to characterize the relative stabilities and thermodynamic relationships between polymorphs employing thermal, spectroscopic, or density data (17,33). Let us consider a compound with two polymorphs, where at room temperature, form I is the most thermodynamically stable polymorph and form II is metastable. If form I is heated, it will ultimately melt to form a liquid at the melting point, T_m, unless it undergoes a phase transformation to form II, at $T_{trans} < T_m$. For this transformation to occur, the Gibbs free energy profiles for the two forms must intersect below T_m (Fig. 7A). In this case, forms I and II are enantiotropically related, and the relative stabilities below T_m are dependent on temperature. The two polymorphs are monotropically related if form I has the lowest Gibbs free energy at all temperatures below T_m and no form I → form II transition is observed prior to the melt. In a monotropic pair, form II is metastable to form I at all temperatures below T_m, and so the occurrence of a direct transformation of form II to form I will depend on the kinetics of the transformation. Form I cannot transform directly into form II on heating, but it can be obtained, for example, through recrystallization from solution.

The desired polymorph, from the point of view of product development, is usually the most stable form, conferring thermodynamic stability. However, which form will be

Table 3 Melting Point Data for Various Polymorphs of Organic Compounds

Compound	Polymorph	Value (°C)
Venlafaxine hydrochloride salt, $C_{17}H_{27}NO_2 2.HCl$	Form I (34); blocks orthorhombic, $Pca2_1$ $a = 26.230$ (5) Å; $b = 5.8810$ (12) Å; $c = 11.448$ (2) Å	209–213 (35) and references cited therein 208–210 (36)
	Form 2 (37); needles monoclinic, $P2_1/n$ $a = 5.797$ (6) Å; $b = 26.074$ (7) Å; $c = 11.722$ (3) Å $\beta = 100.72$ (5)°	210–221 (35) and references cited therein 208–210 (36)
	Form 6 (36); monoclinic, $P2_1/n$ $a = 5.887$ (10) Å; $b = 19.37$ (3) Å; $c = 31.41$ (5) Å $\beta = 92.16$ (3)°	219–220 (36)
4-bromobenzophenone, $C_{13}H_9BrO$	Form I (38); needles monoclinic, $P2_1/c$ $a = 12.092$ (2) Å; $b = 14.343$ (3) Å; $c = 7.293$ (2) Å $\beta = 97.26$ (3)°	82 (38)
	Form II (38); plates triclinic, $P\bar{1}$ $a = 6.106$ (1) Å; $b = 6.124$ (1) Å; $c = 12.100$ (2) Å $\alpha = 98.20$ (2)°; $\beta = 98.74$ (2)°; $y = 91.11$ (1)°	81 (38)
Indomethacin, $C_{19}H_{16}ClNO_4$	Form α (39); blocks monoclinic, $P2_1$ $a = 5.462$ (2) Å; $b = 25.310$ (9) Å; $c = 18.152$ (7) Å $\beta = 94.38$ (3)°	157 (40)
	Form γ (41); plates triclinic, $P\bar{1}$ $a = 9.236$ (5) Å; $b = 9.620$ (5) Å; $c = 10.887$ (5) Å $\alpha = 69.897$ (5)°; $\beta = 87.328$ (5)°; $\gamma = 69.501$ (5)°	163 (40)
Levofloxacin $C_{18}H_{20}FN_3O_4$	Form γ (42) No structure available	226 (42)
	Form α (42) No structure available	234 (42)

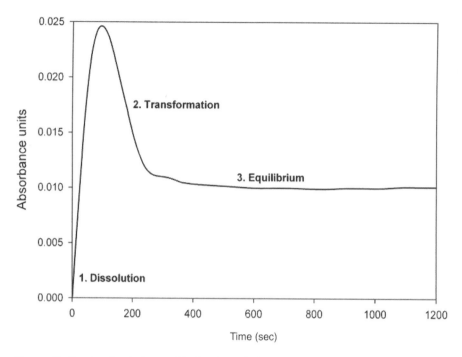

Figure 6 Powder dissolution profile showing solution UV absorbance at $\lambda = 275$ nm versus time for an excess of anhydrous theophylline in water at 22°C (data from Ref. 32). UV absorbance measurements were taken using an in situ sapphire ATR fiber-optic probe and Zeiss UV spectrometer. The characteristic profile shape can be broken into three main phases: (1) dissolution of anhydrous theophylline up to a maximum absorbance of ~ 0.024 A units; (2) a decreasing solubility phase corresponding with the solution-mediated phase transformation of excess solid theophylline from the anhydrous to the monohydrate form; the transformation is complete within approximately five minutes; and (3) the solution is now in equilibrium contact with solid theophylline monohydrate. The equilibrium absorbance value (~ 0.011) is less than 50% that of the maximum value observed for anhydrous theophylline. The physical identity of the starting and end solids was confirmed by X-ray powder diffraction.

obtained under a particular set of crystallization conditions depends on many factors, and crystallization screening therefore largely remains an empirical process. Hence, a significant amount of time and effort is often invested into solid-form selection to characterize the crystallization conditions that will yield the desired form plus characterize and identify all possible crystalline forms that may be relevant to the efficacy, processing, manufacture, and stability of the product.

Polymorphism can affect many aspects of product development from bulk powder flow properties, formulation, and tableting through to bioavailability. The orthorhombic form II of paracetamol, for example, offers potential advantages over the monoclinic form I used in commercial manufacture, being suitable for direct compression (22). Variability in the tableting properties of different batches of the hypnotic compound, zopiclone, was found to be due to the presence of mixtures of two polymorphs and a dihydrate in the raw material (43). Monoclinic zopiclone form I is hygroscopic and readily transforms to the dihydrate upon exposure to high humidity, while the orthorhombic form II, produced by heating form I, is non-hygroscopic. Hence, inadequate control of polymorphic form, that is, mixtures of forms I and II, combined with exposure to humidity can lead to variable mixtures of the three crystalline forms of the API and consequent variability in process performance.

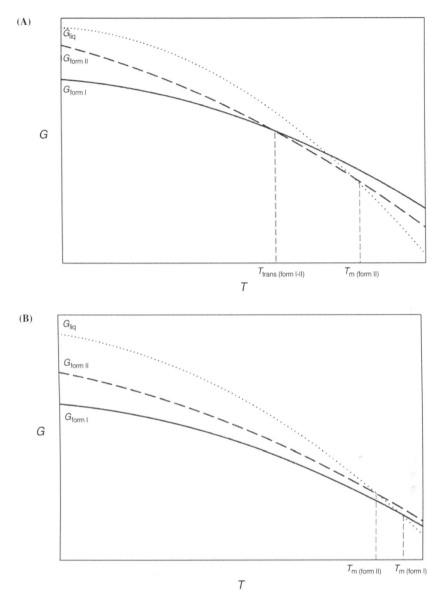

(A)

(B)

Figure 7 Schematic diagram showing the Gibbs free energy change as a function of T at constant pressure for two polymorphs, form I and form II, where (**A**) both forms are enantiotropically related and (**B**) forms I and II are monotropically related. (See Ref. 17 and references therein.)

A high-profile example of the potential impact of polymorphism on pharmaceutical products is that of Abbott Laboratories' HIV protease inhibitor, ritonavir, marketed as Norvir. The API was formulated as semisolid capsules containing a water/ethanol solution of ritonavir; however, the formulation had to be removed from the market and reformulated following the unexpected appearance of new, more thermodynamically stable form II (44). This form had a significantly lower solubility than the original form I (Table 4) and precipitated within the capsules, reducing the dissolution rate and oral

Table 4 Relative Solubilities of Two Polymorphs of the HIV Protease Inhibitor, Ritonavir ($C_{36}H_{46}N_6O_5S_2$) in Various Ethanol/Water Mixtures

Polymorph	Solubility (mg/mL) in ethanol/water ratio		
	99/1	90/10	75/25
Form I	90	234	170
Form II	19	60	30

Form I [monoclinic, $P2_1$, $a = 13.433$ (1) Å, $b = 5.293(2)$ Å, $c = 27.092$ (4) Å, $\beta = 103.102$ (9)°] and form II [orthorhombic, $P2_12_12_1$, $a = 10.0236$ (3) Å, $b = 18.6744$ (4) Å, $c = 20.4692$ (7) Å].
Source: From Ref. 44.

bioavailability of the product. Significantly, this new polymorph had not been observed during the initial development phase of the drug substance or formulated products (45).

Solvates, Cocrystals, and Salts

The nomenclature of crystal structures has, on occasion, stirred debate among those concerned with crystalline organic materials (46). Here, solvates, cocrystals, and salts are grouped into one section that could be described as multicomponent crystal system, that is, crystalline solids comprising API plus one or more chemical entities. In this sense, the only distinction is whether the additional chemical entity within the crystal lattice is solvent of crystallization, cosolute, or solution counterion. Their relevance comes from the potential to manipulate the physical properties of the solid form of the API, for example, to increase solubility or reduce hygroscopicity.

Solvates and Hydrates

If during crystal nucleation, the solvent of crystallization becomes incorporated alongside the drug molecule within the crystal lattice, a crystalline solvate is formed (Fig. 8). Where the solvent is water, the form is termed a "hydrate." The solvate stoichiometry (molar ratio, solvent:API) is also usually reflected in the name of the form such as dihydrate (2:1), monohydrate (1:1), or hemihydrate (1:2). The term "pseudo-polymorph" is also used in the literature to describe crystalline solvates, and while there has been some debate over this nomenclature, the term is still in widespread use (47–50).

The inclusion of solvent within the lattice (distinct from physical inclusions of microscopic droplets of liquid solvent within crystals) occurs to facilitate favorable hydrogen bonding interactions between the API and solvent molecules within the lattice, to stabilize packing arrangements by filling void space in an otherwise unstable arrangement, or to complete the coordination sphere around metal ions in salt structures (51,52). Solvents with strong hydrogen bond donor and/or acceptor groups have increased opportunity to form attractive, multipoint interactions (e.g., N−H···O, O−H···O and C−H···O) with the API molecule, and this tends to favor solvate formation (53). A survey of organic solvate crystals structures in the CSD identified *N,N*-dimethylformamide

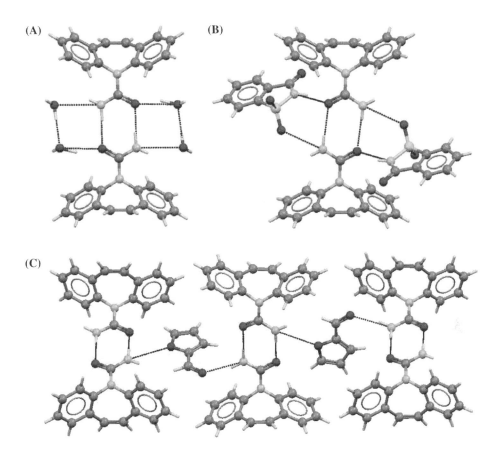

Figure 8 Packing diagrams illustrating the molecular packing arrangements within the crystal structures of three different multicomponent crystals of carbamazepine. The dashed lines indicate hydrogen bonds between carbamazepine and (**A**) water molecules in the dihydrate (63), (**B**) saccharin molecules in the 1:1 cocrystal (64), and (**C**) furfural molecules in the furfural hemi-solvate (65). In each of these multicomponent crystal structures the carbamazepine molecules hydrogen bond to one another to form a dimer motif, and solvent molecules in (**A**) and (**C**) form hydrogen bonds to the free N–H donor on the adjacent carbamazepine dimer. In the saccharin cocrystal (**B**), the saccharin molecules form double hydrogen bonds to both N–H donor and O acceptor atoms on the carbamazepine dimer.

(DMF), dimethylsulfoxide (DMSO), and 1,4-dioxane as solvents having a high propensity to yield crystalline solvates relative to other solvents such as ethylacetate and hexane, that have reduced hydrogen-bonding potential (53). The close-packing principle (54) states that void space in crystal structures is unfavorable, and so the inclusion of solvent molecules within a lattice even in the absence of strong intermolecular interactions can stabilize structures that would otherwise be unlikely to form. Solvent molecules may occupy the cavities or channels that the API molecules create when trying to adopt a close-packed arrangement and so stabilize a structure that would otherwise not form. Indeed, the increased number of solvate and hetero-solvate (i.e., more than one type of solvent included in the lattice) structures in the CSD since the 1960s has been attributed to the increasing size and complexity of new organic compounds that are being synthesized (52). Thus, the use of mixed solvent systems can potentially be exploited when attempting to obtain suitable single-crystal samples for the purposes of structure determination, where molecules resist forming nonsolvated structures.

Solvate formation can occur during crystallization of raw material, particularly during a solution crystallization screen or inadvertently during pharmaceutical processes that involve the introduction of liquids to the powder, such as wet granulation (13,14,16,55–57). Although there have been limited advances in the prediction of solvate formation for specific molecules and solvents based on computational methods (58) and from retrospective statistical modeling of crystallization searches (59), it is not currently possible to predict the likely number of crystalline solvates that a given molecule will form. Hence, as is the case with polymorphs, the total number of solvates that a molecule can form can only be reliably determined through experiment. Sulfathiazole, for example, has been reported to form over 100 solvates (60), illustrating the significant potential that exists for crystalline solvate formation.

Crystalline solvates differ in both their crystal structure and chemical identities from nonsolvated forms and display distinct physicochemical properties that may be potentially desirable in the context of product development. For example, crystalline solvates of the oral hypoglycemic agent glibenclamide have significantly higher solubility and dissolution rates compared with nonsolvated polymorphs of the drug (Table 5) (61). However, while solvates will often display increased aqueous solubility compared with a hydrate or nonsolvated form, their use in pharmaceutical products may be limited by poor physical stability to desolvation or potential toxicity of the solvent released upon dissolution of the solid. Only crystalline solvates involving class 2 or class 3 solvents (62) can be considered for administration to humans.

Hydrates are a particularly common form of solvate with organic compounds and of particular pharmaceutical relevance (52). Ampicillin, for example, is marketed as the crystalline trihydrate, despite being 50% less soluble in water (10.8 mg/mL) than the anhydrous form (5.4 mg/mL) (66). The water is well suited to solvate formation (67) as a result of having both hydrogen bond donor and acceptor capability and a relatively small size (~ 20–40 $\text{\AA}^3$ per molecule in the solid state). There is also a great deal of opportunity for hydrate formation with APIs due to the likelihood that they will come into contact with water, either in liquid or vapor form, at some stage during crystallization, processing, or storage. Some examples of compounds forming hydrates are shown in Table 6.

Hydrates and solvates may lose solvent from the lattice via desolvation, leading to a structural transformation (Fig. 9). Various factors including temperature, pressure, %RH, and changes in the identity and amount of solvent present can all influence desolvation processes (56,74). It is therefore essential that the physical stability of a crystalline solvate

Table 5   Relative Aqueous Solubilities at 37°C of Two Polymorphs and the Pentanol and Toluene Solvates of Glibenclamide ($C_{23}H_{28}ClN_3O_5S$)

Polymorph	Aqueous solubility (mg/100 mL) at 37°C
Form I	0.66
Form II	1.06
Toluene solvate	2.51
Pentanol solvate	33.70

Source: From Ref. 61.

Table 6   Crystal Structure Details for a Range of Pharmaceutical Hydrates

Compound	Polymorph
Ampicillin trihydrate, $C_{16}H_{19}N_3O_4S \cdot 3H_2O$	Powder study (68) Orthorhombic, $P2_12_12_1$ $a = 15.52275\ (16)$ Å; $b = 18.9256\ (3)$ Å; $c = 6.67375\ (8)$ Å
Ciprofloxacin hexahydrate, $C_{17}H_{20}FN_3O_3 \cdot 6H_2O$	Single-crystal study (69) Triclinic, $P\bar{1}$ $a = 9.5273\ (10)$ Å $b = 9.972\ (2)$ Å $c = 11.249\ (2)$ Å $\alpha = 94.794\ (13)°$ $\beta = 100.304\ (10)°$ $\gamma = 91.354\ (11)°$
Cephalexin hydrate, $C_{19}H_{16}ClNO_4$	Single-crystal study (70) Monoclinic, $C2$ $a = 31.548\ (2)$ Å $b = 11.8574\ (9)$ Å $c = 15.6654\ (22)$ Å $\beta = 112.364\ (7)°$
Morphine hydrochloride hydrate, $C_{17}H_{20}NO_3Cl \cdot 3H_2O$	Single-crystal study (71) Orthorhombic, $P2_12_12_1$ $a = 13.019\ (7)$ Å $b = 20.750\ (10)$ Å $c = 6.941\ (4)$ Å
Naloxone hydrochloride dihydrate $C_{19}H_{22}NO_4Cl \cdot 2H_2O$	Single-crystal study (72) Orthorhombic, $P2_12_12_1$ $a = 7.833\ (3)$ Å $b = 13.185\ (5)$ Å $c = 18.569\ (5)$ Å
Rosiglitazone maleate hydrate	Single-crystal study (73) Triclinic, $P\bar{1}$ $a = 9.3145\ (8)$ Å $b = 12.3555\ (10)$ Å $c = 20.8280\ (17)$ Å $\alpha = 105.475\ (2)°$ $\beta = 96.330\ (3)°$ $\gamma = 92.276\ (2)°$

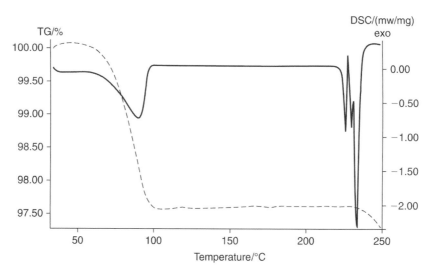

Figure 9   The effect of heating a polycrystalline sample of levofloxacin hemihydrate from 30°C to 250°C at 10°C/min using simultaneous DSC (*solid line*) and TGA (*dashed line*). The DSC curve shows a broad endotherm, with $T_{onset} = 70.0°C$ corresponding to dehydration of the hemihydrate form to the γ-polymorph. The γ-polymorph melts with $T_{onset} = 225.0°C$ and a small exothermic peak is observed, consistent with a melt-recrystallization of β-levofloxacin. A third endotherm ($T_{onset} = 229.6°C$) is associated with the $\beta \rightarrow \alpha$ transformation, with the α-polymorph melting at $T_{onset} = 232.2°C$. The TGA curve shows a weight loss of 2.47% associated with the desolvation endotherm and is in good agreement with the calculated weight loss for hemihydrate stoichiometry. Data (A Johnston and AJ Florence, unpublished results) interpreted in accord with reference (42). *Abbreviations*: DSC, differential scanning calorimetry; TGA, thermal gravimetric analysis.

be monitored during all stages of processing and production to identify any occurrence of desolvation and retain control of the desired form and its associated properties. Desolvation of solvates can, however, also be used to advantage in terms of physical form discovery as a potential route to obtaining new polymorphic forms. For example, by varying the rate of desolvation of an ethanol solvate of spironolactone, two nonsolvated polymorphs, I (75) and II (76), can be obtained selectively (77).

Pharmaceutical Cocrystals

Recent years have seen a considerable amount of interest in API cocrystals as potential pharmaceutical solids (78,79). The distinction between cocrystals and crystalline solvates is that a cocrystal comprises an API plus a pharmaceutically acceptable cocrystal former that is a solid at room temperature, rather than a liquid (as in a solvate) (2). The aim of cocrystal formation is to obtain a crystalline solid that comprises more than one component and by manipulation of both chemical and crystal structure as with salt formation, alter the physical properties of the API. Outcomes from cocrystallization attempts can vary from a physical mixture of the starting materials, a salt involving proton exchange between molecules introducing ionic interactions into the structure or, a cocrystal in which the molecules are un-ionized and the strongest directional noncovalent interactions involve hydrogen bonds. As with other crystalline pharmaceuticals, cocrystals are also prone to exhibit polymorphism (80).

Cocrystal screening approaches have sought to develop a rational design approach to the selection of potential cocrystal formers through the application of crystal

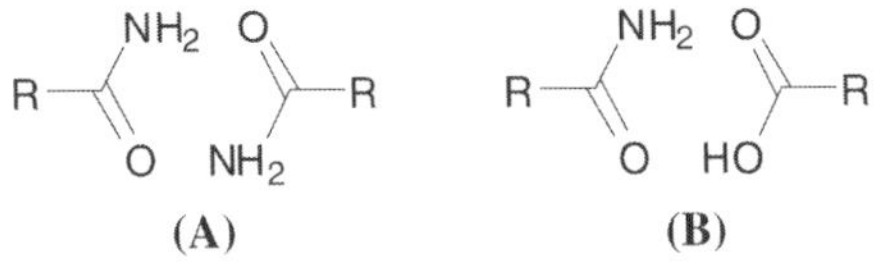

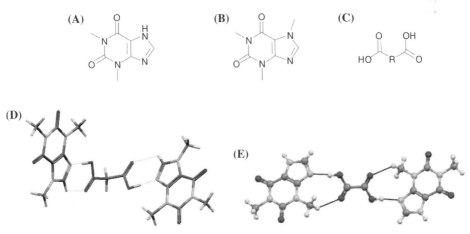

(A)   **(B)**

Figure 10 Potential bimolecular hydrogen bonded motifs or synthons formed between **(A)** carboxamide ... carboxamide groups and motif **(B)** carboxamide ... carboxylic acid interaction—this motif could involve a pair of carbamazepine molecules or carbamazepine plus a primary amide. Motif **(B)** carboxamide ... carboxylic acid interactions. In both motifs, the NH_2 group has a donor hydrogen atom that remains available for further hydrogen bonding interactions.

engineering methodology (81,82). This involves targeting potential cocrystal formers possessing complementary hydrogen bond donor and acceptor arrangements to the available hydrogen bonding groups on the API molecule. The aim is to exploit robust intermolecular motifs, or synthons, that will direct the formation of stable crystal packing arrangements. Additional considerations include the pharmaceutical acceptability and physical properties of the cosolute. For example, novel cocrystals and solvates of carbamazepine were obtained by cocrystallization with a range of compounds, including saccharin (Fig. 8B), nicotinamide, acetic acid, formic acid, butyric acid, trimesic acid, 5-nitrosophthalic acid, and adamantane-1,3,5,7-tetracarboxylic acid (64). The structural rationale in this study targeted the formation of complementary hydrogen-bonded motifs between molecules of carbamazepine and carboxylic acids (Fig. 10).

Cocrystallization of caffeine (83) and theophylline (84) with a range of dicarboxylic acids, including oxalic acid, malonic acid, maleic acid, and glutaric acid, respectively yielded six and four novel cocrystal structures, which demonstrated superior stability upon exposure to high humidity relative to the parent compounds. The dicarboxylic acids targeted in these studies sought to exploit the intermolecular interactions shown in Figure 11.

Figure 11 (*Top*) Molecular structures of **(A)** theophylline ($C_7H_8N_4O_2$), **(B)** caffeine ($C_8H_{10}N_4O_2$), and **(C)** dicarboxylic acids. (*Bottom*) Intermolecular packing interactions (O–H ... N and C–H ... O contacts shown as *dashed lines*) in the crystal structures of **(D)** caffeine-malonic acid cocrystal [(2:1); orthorhombic, *Fdd2*, $a = 30.399(1)$ Å, $b = 31.285(1)$ Å, $c = 4.674(1)$ Å] and **(E)** theophylline-oxalic acid cocrystal [(2:1); monoclinic, $P2_1/c$, $a = 5.821$ (1) Å, $b = 16.609$ (3) Å, $c = 9.806$ (2) Å, $\beta = 99.83$ (3)°].

Pharmaceutical Salts

Approximately two-thirds of APIs are weakly acidic or basic entities, and salt formation therefore provides a significant opportunity to alter the physicochemical properties of the API in the solid state (85). The decision whether to pursue a salt form is usually taken early in the development process on the basis of the known properties of the uncharged molecule. Salt formation will often be considered where the API has one or more unfavorable properties, including low aqueous solubility (<10 μg/mL), poor chemical stability, hygroscopicity, low melting point ($<80°C$), poor crystallization (e.g., forms oils or amorphous solids on crystallization attempts) or displays multiple polymorphs (85,86). A significant number of counterions are suitable for pharmaceutical salt selection studies of weakly acidic or basic APIs, and there is therefore a broad range of opportunity to obtain different salts with improved properties (Tables 7 and 8). Saccharin, for example, has been proposed as a suitable counterion for salts of bitter basic drugs, such as quinine and vincamine, to mask the unpleasant taste and improve patient compliance (87).

Table 7 Summary of Anionic Pharmaceutical Salts in Use at 1993 with Frequency of Occurrence as a Percentage of All Anionic Salt Forms

Anion	Percent	Anion	Percent
Aceglumate	0.07	Edisylate	0.20
Acephyllinate	0.26	Estolate	0.13
Acetamidobenzoate	0.07	Esylate	0.13
Acetate	2.09	Ethylbromide	0.07
Acetylasparaginate	0.07	Ethysulfate	0.07
Acetylaspartate	0.07	Fendizoate	0.07
Adipate	0.13	Formate	0.07
Aminosalicylate	0.13	Fosfatex	0.07
Anhydromethylenecitrate	0.07	Fumarate	0.92
Ascorbate	0.13	Gluceptate	0.13
Aspartate	0.33	Gluconate	0.52
Benzoate	0.20	Glucoronate	0.13
Besylate	0.26	Glutamate	0.07
Bicarbonate	0.07	Glycerophosphate	0.52
Bisulphate	0.13	Glycinate	0.13
Bitartrate	0.52	Glycollylarsinilate	0.07
Borate	0.26	Glycyrrhizate	0.07
Bromide	3.79	Hippurate	0.07
Butylbromide	0.07	Hemisulphate	0.13
Camphorate	0.01	Hexylresorcinate	0.07
Camsylate	0.59	Hybenzate	0.20
Carbonate	0.46	Hydrobromide	1.37
Chloride	3.53	Hydrochloride	43.99
Chlorophemoxyacetate	0.07	Hydroiodide	0.07
Citrate	2.81	Hydroxybenzenesulfonate	0.07
Closylate	0.07	Hydroxybenzoate	0.07
Cromesilate	0.07	Hydroxynapthoate	0.07
Cyclamate	0.13	Iodide	1.11
Dehydrocholate	0.07	Isethionate	0.52
Dihydrochloride	1.37	Lactate	0.98
Dimalonate	0.07	Lactobionate	0.07
Edetate	0.07	Lysine	0.65

Table 7 Summary of Anionic Pharmaceutical Salts in Use at 1993 with Frequency of Occurrence as a Percentage of All Anionic Salt Forms (*Continued*)

Anion	Percent	Anion	Percent
Malate	0.26	Polistirex	0.85
Maleate	3.14	Pyridoxylphosphate	0.07
Mandalate	0.13	Polygalacturonate	0.20
Mesylate	3.20	Propionate	0.13
Methylbromide	0.39	Saccharinate	0.20
Methyliodide	0.20	Salicylate	0.78
Methylnitrate	0.13	Stearate	0.20
Methylsulphate	0.98	Stearylsulphate	0.07
Monophosadenine	0.07	Subacetate	0.07
Mucate	0.07	Succinate	0.52
Napadisylate	0.13	Sulfate	5.82
Napsylate	0.20	Sulfosalicylate	0.07
Nicotinate	0.13	Tannate	0.85
Nitrate	1.18	Tartate	2.68
Oleate	0.13	Teprosilate	0.07
Orotate	0.26	Terephthalate	0.07
Oxalate	0.26	Teoclate	0.33
Oxoglurate	0.13	Thiocyanate	0.20
Pamoate	1.37	Tidiacicate	0.07
Pantothenate	0.07	Timonaciate	0.07
Pectinate	0.07	Tosylate	0.39
Phenylethylbarbiturate	0.13	Triethiodide	0.07
Phosphate	2.48	Undecanoate	0.13
Picrate	0.07	Xinafoate	0.07
Policrilix	0.07		

Source: From Ref. 94.

Table 8 Summary of Cationic Pharmaceutical Salts in Use at 1993 with Frequency of Occurrence as a Percentage of All Cationic Salt Forms

Cation	Percent	Organic cation	Percent	Metallic cation	Percent
Ammonium	1.95	Hydroxyethylpyrrolidone	0.15	Aluminium	1.35
Benethamine	0.15	Imidazole	0.30	Bismuth	0.30
Benzathine	0.45	Meglumine	2.41	Calcium	12.18
Betaine	0.15	Olamine	0.45	Lithium	0.90
Carnitine	0.15	Piperazine	0.90	Magnesium	4.51
Clemizole	0.15	4-Phenylcyclohexylamine	0.51	Neodymium	0.15
Chlorcylizine	0.15	Procaine	0.15	Potassium	9.77
Choline	0.60	Pyridoxine	0.15	Rubidium	0.15
Dibenzylamine	0.15	Triethyanolamine	0.15	Sodium	57.74
Diethanolamine	0.45	Tromethamine	0.90	Strontium	0.30
Diethylamine	0.60			Zinc	1.05
Diethylammonium	0.15				
Eglumine	0.15				
Erbumine	0.15				
Ethylenediamine	0.15				
Heptaminol	0.15				
Hydrabamine	0.15				

Source: From Ref. 94.

The selection of suitable counterions for inclusion in a salt selection search is dependent on safety considerations, for example, chloride and sodium ions are regarded as safe to administer and well tolerated (88), and the physical properties of the species involved. Counterions' selection often uses the pK_a values for the acid and base involved to estimate the likelihood of successful salt formation. Generally, a pK_a difference of at least 3 between the acid and base is required for salt formation to occur, although even when this criterion is met the formation of a crystalline product is not guaranteed and is also dependent upon successful nucleation and crystal growth. Where pK_a differences are less than 3, cocrystal formation (i.e., a structure comprising non-ionised molecules) may result. Given the empirical nature of the selection process, automated parallel crystallization approaches are often adopted in commercial screening operations, with the aim of identifying at least one crystalline salt that demonstrates superior properties to that of the parent compound (89). In commercial pharmaceutical solids development, only small amounts of drug material will usually be available at this stage for salt screening (~ 0.1–1 g) (86,90), hence the drive toward the adoption of high-throughput crystallization screening methodologies. These techniques enable many small-scale experiments to be carried out in parallel yielding rapid results from small sample amounts (91).

Regardless of the scale of the method, API and counterions are mixed in a suitable solvent and crystallization induced by cooling, solvent evaporation, or the addition of antisolvent. It is advisable to avoid aqueous solutions because of the potentially high aqueous solubility of the salt form. If salt formation takes place in an organic solvent, the product is more likely to precipitate within a reasonable time frame. The products from each test crystallization are then identified and characterized using suitable analytical methods, including optical microscopy to identify birefringence from crystalline products, Raman spectroscopy, DSC, and X-ray powder diffraction (XRPD) to distinguish novel crystalline product from raw materials (92). In a salt formation study on the selective estrogen receptor modulator drug, tamoxifen ($C_{26}H_{29}NO$) (Fig. 12A), salt formation with 6 acid counterions in 12 solvents was assessed using a 96-well plate system (93). Polarizing light microscopy identified 114 crystalline products from 132 crystallizations, and Raman spectroscopy confirmed salt formation by comparison of the crystalline product spectra with those for the free base and acid compounds. Several of the salts were found to crystallize in multiple polymorphs and solvates from the different solvents included in the search.

A salt selection study for the investigational drug RPR 127963 ($C_{16}H_{21}N_3O_2$) aimed to identify crystalline salt forms suitable for use in high-dose tablet and injection formulations (90). The free base form ($pK_a = 4.10$) of the molecule (Fig. 12B) formed multiple hydrate forms and displayed a relatively low melting point (119–123°C). Five crystalline salts were identified from the salt formation screen, including the hydrochloride, mesylate, citrate, tartrate, and sulfate. The relevant properties of each of these

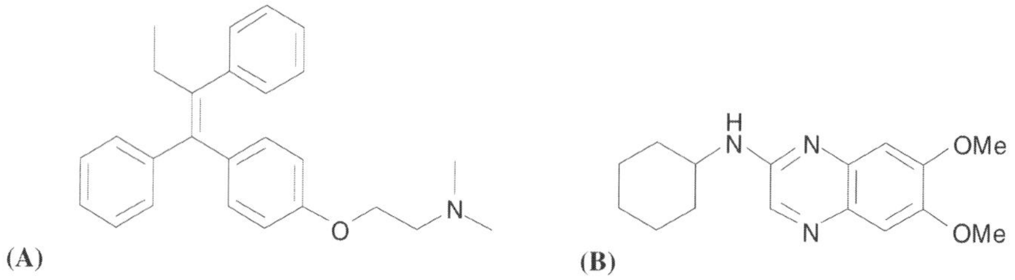

(A)   (B)

Figure 12 Molecular structures of the free base forms of (**A**) tamoxifen and (**B**) RPR 127963.

Table 9 Physical Properties for a Series of Salt Forms Assessed During Salt Selection Study on RPR 127963 (Fig. 12)

	HCl	Mesylate	Citrate	Tartrate	Sulfate
Melting point ($^\circ$C)	166, 191, 275	280.9–282/2	130.2–134.4	198.5–201.6	305.7–308.9
Crystalline forms	3	1	2	2	1
Solubility[a] (mg/mL)	3.92	108	0.83	0.89	∼50
Hygroscopicity	–	–	–	+++	–

[a]Measured in demineralized water at 25°C.
Source: From Ref. 90.

salt forms are summarized in Table 9, and on the basis of these results, the sulfate salt was selected for further development.

Crystal Structure Prediction

It has long been recognized that there is a need for reliable methods of predicting organic crystal structures (95). However, the complexity of accurately identifying all naturally occurring crystalline forms from a knowledge of molecular structure alone still poses a significant scientific and technical challenge (96). This is particularly true for molecules with significant conformational flexibility, as is the case for many APIs, and those with multiple chemical fragments in the asymmetric unit such as salts or solvates. For such molecules, the scale of the computational search of low-energy conformers and favorable packing arrangements, drawing on accurate models for intermolecular interactions, becomes impractical with current technology. However, the challenge of developing methods for crystal structure prediction (CSP) is being actively pursued by many researchers through a series of Blind Test challenges to the structure prediction community, demonstrating a significant progress in this field (3,97,98). While there have been considerable developments in this area in recent years (3,58,99–101), the capability to predict all observable crystal structures for organic molecules of the complexity of 'typical' pharmaceutical APIs remains elusive. Although CSP does not currently offer a complete view of the range of actual crystal structures that a particular molecule will adopt, it does produce a range of thermodynamically feasible structures containing favorable intermolecular packing arrangements. Knowledge of the range of hypothetical structures can also provide opportunities to manipulate crystallization conditions that may favor structures with particular hydrogen-bonding motifs (102,103) or be of value in interpreting the crystal energy landscape of small organic molecules revealed by experimental crystallization (104).

PRACTICAL APPROACHES TO CRYSTALLIZATION OF SOLID FORMS

General Principles of Crystallization

Crystallization of pharmaceuticals may be carried out for a variety of reasons that include (*i*) growing single-crystal samples for crystal structure determination, for example, to confirm chemical identity or to determine absolute configuration; (*ii*) crystallization screening aimed at identifying all potential crystalline forms, including salts; and (*iii*) the production of large quantities of the polycrystalline raw material with well-defined morphology and particle size distributions for use in production-scale manufacture. The process of crystallization involves the nucleation and growth of a solid crystalline phase, which can occur from gases (crystallization from the vapor phase), liquids (crystallization from solution or the melt), or solids (solid-solid transformations in amorphous or crystalline solids). The following sections will introduce some of the practical aspects of crystallization by various routes, with an emphasis on their application in physical form discovery.

Nucleation and Crystal Growth

Crystallization proceeds in two phases. The first phase, termed "nucleation," involves the formation of stable aggregates of molecules, termed "nuclei" or "crystal embryos" (17,105). These are the first, ordered molecular arrangements to appear out of a supersaturated solution and only become stable once they have reached a critical size, r_{crit}. As further molecular collisions occur and aggregation proceeds, clusters with a size less than r_{crit} will dissolve as they do not possess significant cohesive energy to overcome the surface free energy increase required to expand against the surrounding solution (105). As clusters with $r > r_{crit}$ emerge from the addition of molecules and further collision and aggregation of clusters, crystal growth ensues with molecules orienting and attaching at the surface of nuclei until visible crystals are formed. Key parameters that can influence nucleation and crystal growth processes, and hence the polymorphic form obtained, include the degree of supersaturation, the interfacial energy between the expanding nucleus and surrounding medium, temperature, solution viscosity, and the extent of agitation (105). The use of different solvents and antisolvents and the addition of additives such as surfactants can therefore impact on crystal formation and are frequently exploited during crystallization screens for physical form discovery in an attempt to vary the outcome (106). The addition of polymers during high-throughput crystallization studies on paracetamol, sulfamethoxazole, and carbamazepine has been demonstrated to yield different polymorphs due to heteronucleation (107,108). Ultimately, the specific crystalline form [polymorph(s) or solvates] obtained from a particular set of crystallization conditions is dependent on the relative thermodynamic favorability of each of the possible forms and their relative rates of nucleation and/or growth (109). Thus, the product can be under either thermodynamic or kinetic control, and changes in one or more parameters may influence the crystalline form produced.

Ostwald's rule of stages states that the first form observed from solution will be the one whose free energy is closest to the starting free energy state of the system (110). Hence when crystallizing from solution, the first product observed may be expected to be a metastable form. This can then transform to a more stable form until ultimately the most thermodynamically stable polymorph is produced. This is, however, a heuristic rule and many systems do not comply, inferring that such crystallizations are under kinetic control. For example, the most stable polymorph may nucleate very quickly, but if crystal growth of that form is relatively slow, other faster-growing forms may dominate the final product. It can therefore be difficult to apply generalisations to crystallisation processes as they may be under either thermodynamic or kinetic control.

Crystallization in Processes and Products

The majority of crystallizations of organic molecules are carried out from solution, for example, as a precipitation at the end of a synthetic route or as a fractional crystallization to separate a compound from other impurities (105,111). The crystallization of bulk API is clearly an important step in controlling the physical form ultimately introduced into the product. In industrial-scale processes, there is therefore a need to control nucleation and crystal growth in order to obtain the desired product. Changes in the regulatory environment, with a movement toward adoption of quality-by-design approaches in pharmaceutical manufacture coupled with advances in process analytical technologies (PATs) relevant to the control of crystallization, provide new opportunities for improved control and understanding of crystallization processes (112). These improvements promise to contribute to better control of raw material manufacture and improved methods for controlling API solid form.

Crystallization of API from solution can also occur unintentionally in liquid formulations. The antiepileptic compound phenytoin can precipitate during the preparation of infusion fluids because of changes in pH of the vehicle (113). Changes in pH resulting from mixing trimethoprim solutions with phosphate buffer can also lead to crystallization (114). Crystallization of drug substances in vivo can also be problematic, and compounds including acylcovir, indinavir, triamterene, and ciprofloxacin have been reported to cause drug-induced crystal nephropathy as a result of precipitation within the renal tubules (115).

Solution Crystallization Studies

A typical solution crystallization experiment will involve some or all of the basic steps outlined in Figure 13. A solute (or solutes for salt or cocrystal formation) will be dissolved in a suitable solvent and the resultant solution filtered to remove any seed crystals of the starting form. Supersaturation is then induced in the particle-free solution to induce nucleation or to support the growth of seed crystals that have been deliberately introduced into the solution to control the identity of the form produced.

Given the importance of solution crystallization, it is worthwhile to briefly review the typical parameters used to control this process (Fig. 14). Line 1 (Fig. 14) shows an idealized solubility curve, rising with increasing temperature. Below this line, point A in Fig. 14, the solution is undersaturated ($C < C_s$) and so no crystallization can occur (dissolution will occur if additional solid is added). Line AB shows the effect of cooling solution A. As the temperature falls, the solution concentration remains constant, becoming saturated at line 1 (i.e., $C = C_s$). As cooling progresses, the solution becomes supersaturated, and the concentration exceeds the solute solubility ($C > C_s$). This is a prerequisite for nucleation and crystal growth to occur.

While the concentration of the solution lies within the metastable zone between lines 1 and 2 (Fig. 14), nucleation of new crystallites does not occur, despite the solution being supersaturated. However, growth of seed crystals added to a metastable solution will occur and, indeed, this can exploited to obtain good quality single-crystal samples for

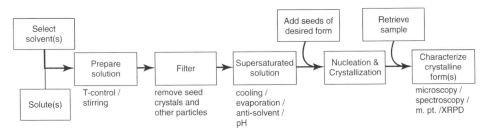

Figure 13 Basic steps in solution crystallization experiments aimed at obtaining crystalline samples (either single crystals or polycrystalline powder).

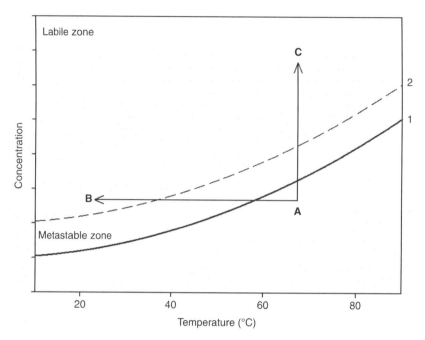

Figure 14 A schematic plot showing a rise in equilibrium saturation solubility, line 1 (—) with increasing temperature. The dashed line, line 2 (- - -), corresponds to the upper concentration limit of the metastable zone. The lines AB and AC show the change in state of the solution as a result of cooling and isothermal evaporation, respectively.

a diffraction study via solution seeding. As the degree of supersaturation increases on continued cooling, the solution enters the labile zone (above line 2), and nucleation and crystal growth can occur. Similarly, if a solution at point A is subjected to controlled solvent evaporation at constant temperature, the concentration will rise and the solution will become sequentially saturated, metastable, and labile as evaporation continues.

The metastable zone width is an important parameter for defining crystallization processes and can vary widely depending on the particular solute, solvent, and experimental conditions (105). It can provide valuable information on the ease of nucleation of crystalline forms under specific conditions and inform subsequent crystallization experiments. It is usually impractical to enumerate individual metastable zone widths for large numbers of different crystallization conditions before embarking on solution crystallization experiments as part of a physical form screen. However, a knowledge of the metastable zone width and the factors that influence it can be of significant value when attempting to secure accurate control over crystallization as in, for example, batch crystallization operations and polymorph control (116–119). Some readily implemented strategies to influence crystallization outcomes based on the concepts outlined in this section are outlined in Table 10.

Single-Crystal Growth for X-Ray Structural Analysis

When single-crystal samples are required for X-ray diffraction analysis, it is often necessary to carry out specific crystallizations aimed at achieving crystals of the required quality and size, typically not less than approximately 100 µm on edge. Generally the aim in such experiments is to reduce the rate of nucleation so as to minimize the number of nuclei formed and maximize the growth of individual crystallites. It can be helpful to

Table 10 Some General Relationships Between Crystallization Conditions and Crystallization Outcome

Crystallization condition	Crystallization outcome
Low degree of supersaturation	Reduced extent of nucleation and crystal growth
Slow cooling/evaporation	Obtain large single crystals
High degree of supersaturation	Increased extent of nucleation
Rapid cooling/evaporation	Obtain larger number of smaller crystallites
	Possibility of metastable polymorphs
Increased agitation	Increase/decrease rate of nucleation
	Smaller particles
Reduce agitation of the crystallization solution	Quiescent solutions best for larger crystal growth, e.g., for single-crystal structure determination
Introduce seed crystals	Increase size of existing crystals
	Increase amounts of the seed crystal form due to secondary seeding and growth

filter solutions to remove dust and other particles that may be acting as heterogeneous nucleation sites. If nucleation is not occurring, scratching the surface of the crystallization vessel may be all that is required to induce crystallization. If the material forms oil, crystallization at a higher temperature may encourage nucleation. Controlled cooling or slow evaporation of solutions is often ideal, with best results for single-crystal growth obtained from unstirred solutions with conditions designed to yield slower growth. If sufficient material is available, then it may be worth recrystallizing the compound from a range of solvents to assess whether more desirable morphologies (e.g., isometric, prismatic crystals) can be obtained (120). Note, however, such approaches may also give rise to alternative crystalline forms, that is, polymorphs or solvates. There are numerous alternative approaches that alter the environment in which nucleation and crystal growth occur and may favor improved quality single-crystal samples. These include trying different solvents, solvent mixtures, and temperatures, or other methods such as vapor diffusion (121,122), liquid-liquid diffusion or layering (123), thermal gradients (124), sublimation (125,126), growth from the melt (126,127), and crystallization from gels (128,129). If initial attempts are unsuccessful, it is worth persevering—patience can be the key. If these attempts fail, at least within the timescales imposed by the experiment, then structure determination from polycrystalline powder samples may be an attractive alternative to securing crystal structure data (see section "Structure Determination from Powder Data").

Seeding

Seeding can be used for the growth of large high-quality single-crystal samples, for diffraction analysis, or for the control of batch crystallization processes. Suspending a small seed crystal of the desired form in a metastable supersaturated solution will often promote growth of the seed, yielding a larger individual crystal. Pure phase samples of form IV carbamazepine can be obtained by seeding methanol solutions with seed crystals obtained from mixed phase samples originally crystallized from methanol solutions containing hydroxypropylcellulose (130). The polymer is necessary for the initial formation of this polymorphic form of carbamazepine, however, in the presence of seeds, pure phase samples can be obtained from methanol solution. Also, accurate control of the polymorphic form of L-glutamic acid batch crystallizations can be achieved by seeding solutions with seed crystals of the desired form (131).

Parallel Crystallization Approaches to Physical Form Discovery

The application of automation technology to crystallization processes facilitates a systematic approach to be applied to experimental searches for crystalline forms, enabling many crystallizations to be implemented in parallel with accurate, reproducible control over all steps. Ideally, all the steps from the traditional, manual crystallization process (Fig. 13) are automated to minimize any manual intervention during the workflow from raw API to analytical data and maximize efficiency. System hardware requirements are summarized in Table 11, with an illustration of the implementation of these elements on a commercial platform in Figure 15. Automated crystallization methods also draw on a range of software tools for the design and implementation of workflows (system control and design of experiments), multivariate analysis tools for the collation, and classification of analytical data associated with unique forms and mixtures produced plus information management tools for archival and retrieval of data and to provide access to the large volumes of data accumulated during the search for subsequent analysis and data mining. The main goals of automated crystallization methods are to (*i*) maximize the coverage of crystallization chemical space in the minimum amount of time, (*ii*) secure a comprehensive knowledge of the physical form diversity of a compound, and (*iii*) identify all forms and the conditions under which they are produced. Once all samples have been identified, further physical and structural analysis can be applied to characterize the forms, their structure, properties and thermodynamic relationships.

Several commercial systems are available from companies including Anachem, Avantium, Bruker, Chemspeed, and Zinsser that can implement automated crystallization workflows across a range of solution volumes (microliter to milliliter scale) in large numbers for application in polymorph, solvate, salt and cocrystal searches. High-throughput crystallization systems often utilize 96-well plate designs to support large

Table 11 System Requirements for Automated Crystallization

Component	Objective
Solid dispensing	Accurate dispensing of raw compound for dissolution
	Addition of multiple solid components for salt and cocrystal screening
Liquid dispensing	Prepare solutions for accurate dispensing of single or mixed solvent systems
	Addition of buffer solutions to control/vary pH
	Addition of antisolvent
Temperature control	Control of solution temperature at dissolution and crystallization
Agitation	Facilitate dissolution using magnetic stirring, orbital shaking or sonication under temperature control
Filtration	Remove undissolved solid to prevent seeding by starting form
	Retrieve recrystallized solid
Sample retrieval and transfer	Identify presence of solid (e.g., turbidity/optical inspection)
	Transfer samples for analysis/identification
Sample analysis	Collect characteristic data to distinguish between solid forms
	Methods used include microscopy, spectroscopy, and XRPD

Abbreviation: XRPD, X-ray powder diffraction.

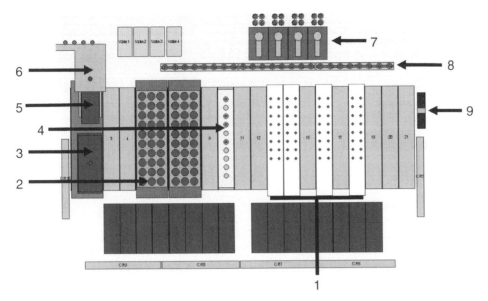

Figure 15 Schematic of the main elements of a parallel crystallization platform taken from the system control software. (1) Crystallization vessels arranged in four blocks of eight pairs of pre- and postfiltration 13-mL vessels. The crystallization blocks are located on an orbital shaker, allowing the programmed vortexing of all crystallization vessels in the range 0 to 1400 rpm. (2) Solvent library held in individual rubber septum glass vials across two racks. (3) SDU home station. The SDU comprises an overhead balance that dispenses solid (weighing by difference) into crystallization vessels to a precision of 0.1 mg. (4) Solution rack for larger solvent volumes (50–100 mL). (5) Home station for four-channel needle head. (6) Four-channel needle head; the exchange and movement of solid and liquid handling tools is controlled by a robotic arm. (7) Four 10-mL glass syringes for liquid aspiration and dispensing via the four-channel needle head. The syringes provide dosing precision of 0.04%. (8) Solid dosing extruder rack. The robotic arm selects powders from the rack. Each extruder comprises a plastic vial and extruder mechanism, enabling the precise flow of powders. (9) Rinse station for four-channel needle head, to eliminate cross-contamination between vessels. *Abbreviation*: SDU, Solid-dispensing unit. *Source*: From Ref. 138.

numbers of small-volume solutions and are based on hardware platforms (e.g., multichannel liquid dispensers) that have been available for many years for use in high-throughput biological screening and protein crystallization applications. Such systems enable extensive screens to be implemented, applying combinatorial approaches to examine the influence of solvent, supersaturation, additives, temperature, heating/cooling rates, antisolvent, evaporation, and mixing on crystallization outcome (91,105). On the basis of such small-volume approaches, parallel crystallization searches can easily be tailored to accommodate availability of API material down to milligram quantities.

Inclusion of a diverse range of polar and nonpolar solvents (and mixtures thereof) in the experimental library can introduce significant diversity into the crystallizations search and a significant increase in the number of crystallizations and concurrent analyses required (106). Ideally, design of experiments (DOE) approaches can be applied to assist in the selection of process variables for the search, taking into consideration the equipment capabilities (e.g., liquid handling volume constraints) and any relevant prior knowledge (e.g., chemical properties of solutes and solvents) (91). Clustering of solvents based on their physicochemical descriptors can be used to reduce the number of crystallizations required while in principle retaining the same breadth of chemical diversity in the search

(132–135). Quantum mechanics calculations of the hydrogen bonding properties of class 2 and class 3 solvents have also been applied to attempt to rationalize the impact of solvent on crystallization outcomes for ranitidine hydrochloride and stearic acid (136). It is desirable to maximize diversity yet exclude redundant crystallization conditions (e.g., solvents that are essentially identical in terms of their properties relevant to crystallization), but given the difficulties in modeling ab initio what the outcome of any crystallization may be (137), retrospective analysis of the results from crystallization screens can also be used to estimate the completeness of the experimental search (59).

For smaller-scale studies, there are also various benchtop systems, often based on parallel reactors for chemical synthesis, capable of implementing crystallization under computer control. Typically, these offer control over temperature, evaporation, and stirring without the sophistication of liquid or solid dispensing, in-line filtration, or retrieval of sample (Fig. 16). However, these systems can provide a useful complement to both small-scale manual crystallization and high-throughput methods.

(A)

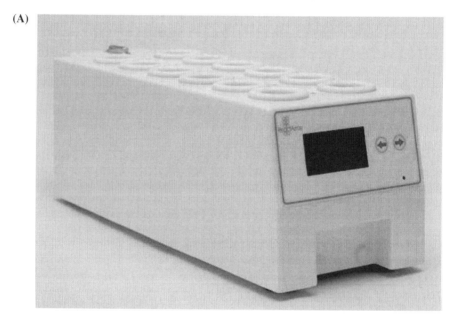

(B)

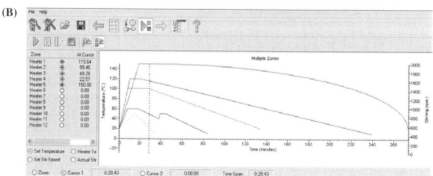

Figure 16 Pictures showing: (**A**) a typical small-scale, benchtop parallel reactor device. The unit comprises 12 independent wells that can hold solutions volumes varying from <1 to 30 mL with T-control in the range −30°C to 150°C and stirring; (**B**) a computer control interface allows control and data logging of each crystallization vessel. Plot shown illustrates five different heating and cooling profiles applied simultaneously to different crystallizations.

The method of analysis used to assess the crystallization product is an important practical consideration when implementing a crystallization search strategy (Table 12). The potentially large numbers and small amounts of solid recovered from high-throughput methods require sensitive and rapid analytical tools, such that the acquisition of data is on a timescale commensurate with the study. It is also important that characterization data are collected soon after the initial appearance of solid to avoid missing metastable forms that may transform over time.

Table 12 Information and Details on Various Techniques of Value in the Physical and Structural Analysis of Pharmaceutical Solids Highlighting Typical Applications of Each Technique

	Method	Information provided
X-ray diffraction	Single crystal	Unit cell, space group atomic coordinates, atomic displacement parameters (ADPs)
		3-D molecular conformation and intermolecular packing
		Absolute configuration
		Variable temperature and high-pressure studies
	XRPD	Pattern fingerprint from polycrystalline sample
		Quantitative phase analysis of mixtures
		Unit cell, space group atomic coordinates, and atomic displacement parameters
		3D molecular conformation and intermolecular packing
		%crystallinity in amorphous/crystalline mixed phase samples
		Monitor in situ solid-solid transformations as a function of %RH and T
Spectroscopy	Mid FT-IR	Characteristic absorption spectrum for polymorphs
		Avoid residual solvent/damp samples
		Distinguish nonsolvated and solvate structures
		Distinguish amorphous and crystalline forms
		Avoid KBr disks—risk of transformation
		Quantification of mixtures
	Raman	Characteristic Raman spectrum for crystalline and amorphous forms
		Can be used with wet (aqueous) samples
		Noncontact and immersion probes available for in situ measurements
		Rapid measurements from small samples—ideal for high-throughput screening applications
		Track lattice changes as a function of T and pressure
	Solid-state NMR	Determine Z′ (number of unique formula units in unit cell)
		Fingerprint forms from chemical shifts
		3D arrangements of atoms in solid
		Solid-state tautomerism
		Dynamic disorder
	Terahertz spectroscopy	3D molecular conformation and intermolecular packing

Table 12 Information and Details on Various Techniques of Value in the Physical and Structural Analysis of Pharmaceutical Solids Highlighting Typical Applications of Each Technique (*Continued*)

	Method	Information provided
Thermal analysis	DSC	Temperatures of transformations (desolvation, crystallization, Tg, melt)
		Heat capacity
		Relative stabilities of polymorphs
		Heats of transition, ΔH
	TGA	Quantify weight loss associated with desolvation
		Enable calculation of solvate stoichiometry
	Melting point	Measure characteristic melting points for all crystalline forms
		Influence of impurities
	Hot-stage microscopy	Changes in particles as a function of T
		Structural transformations
		Melting point
		Crystallization from melt
		Desolvation (evolution of gas bubbles from samples held under oil)
Physical	Microscopy	Morphology
		Identify crystalline forms from characteristic indices of refraction, birefringence
		ID polymorphs from mixed morphologies
		Particle size distributions
		Visualize crystallization or solution-mediated phase transformations in droplets of solution
	DVS	Assess hygroscopicity; stability
		Moisture uptake at constant T as a function of %RH
		Identify structural transformations (anhydrous → $n$hydrate; $n$hydrate → anhydrous)
		Organic vapor DVS also to study solvate formation
		Weight loss on drying
	Inverse-phase gas chromatography	Measurement of surface energy
		Quantification of amorphous content
		Humidity induced crystallization
	TSC	Measurement of Tg in amorphous solids
		Identify transitions between crystalline forms
	Solubility/dissolution	Equilibrium saturation solubility
		Influence of pH on solubility
		Influence of T on solubility—identify phase transformations
		Solution-mediated phase transformations
		Dissolution rate (intrinsic dissolution rate)
		Influence of crystal structure on solubility and dissolution
	SEM	Morphology and surface structure of particles and different crystalline and amorphous forms
		Influence of processing on particles
		Agglomeration of particles
		Influence of T and %RH on particle morphology

Abbreviations: XRPD, X-ray powder diffraction; DSC, differential scanning calorimetry; FT-IR, Fourier Transform Infrared; TGA, thermal gravimetric analysis; DVS, dynamic vapor sorption; NMR, nuclear magnetic resonance; TSC, thermally stimulated currents; SEM, scanning electron microscopy.

Though some pharmaceutical companies have invested in developing automated crystallization systems in-house (92), the cost of development and maintenance of the necessary specialized equipment and software can be significant. There are, however, several contract research organizations that have been established to serve the needs of pharmaceutical industry in this field.

Other Approaches to Physical Form Discovery

A range of alternative crystallization approaches potentially suitable for crystallizing APIs is listed in section "Single-Crystal Growth for X-Ray Structural Analysis," however these are not only of interest for single-crystal growth. By varying the nucleation and crystallization conditions as widely as possible, the chances that an alternative crystalline form is obtained is increased. Solvent drop grinding has also been used to obtain polymorphs of anthranilic acid and succinic acid (139), which had previously only been obtained via crystallization from the melt and via high-temperature transformation, respectively. Mechanical grinding has also been used to obtain a new solid form of barbituric acid (140). Various techniques, in addition to cocrystallization from solution (141), have been applied to cocrystal formation, including liquid-assisted grinding (142–145) and melt growth techniques (146). These techniques potentially offer a rapid and efficient means of screening for novel forms that require only small amounts of material and yield sufficient sample for analysis by XRPD, for example. Slurrying is also a common method applied to assessing physical form diversity. It involves agitating a suspension of solid in a saturated solution in an attempt to obtain more thermodynamically stable polymorphs or solvates. If a metastable form is placed in a suspension, over time it can transform to a more stable form via a solution-mediated transformation.

High-pressure studies where solutions of drug are recrystallized under high pressures (GPa) in a diamond anvil cell have also been demonstrated as being successful in finding new polymorphs and hydrates of pharmaceuticals (25,147,148). Once a crystal has formed, the anvil cell can be mounted on diffractometer and the crystal structure obtained. High-pressure crystallization, in addition to providing further structural information on the diversity of experimental forms a particular molecule can adopt, can also be used to obtain bulk quantities of the new form, in the event that suitable seed crystals can be recovered at ambient pressure.

Influence of Impurities

The presence of small concentrations of related chemical impurities in the crystallization solution can be of particular relevance when working with material from early discovery chemistry. The impurities may inhibit the nucleation of a particular form, possibly even the most stable form, such that it is only observed later in the development process once chemical purity has improved (149). Impurities can also adsorb at the growing faces of crystals altering their morphology by effectively poisoning further growth of the affected face (150).

STRUCTURAL ANALYSIS OF SOLID-STATE PHARMACEUTICALS

A wide variety of analytical methods may be used to determine the physical properties and structure of pharmaceutical solids (151,152). It is often necessary to use data from several complementary techniques to fully characterize a material, including defining structural parameters for polymorphs and defining each individual form's physical properties. Techniques can be classified as crystallographic, spectroscopic, thermal analysis, microscopy, and physical measurements and an overview of various methods is summarized in Table 12.

X-Ray Diffraction

Since the first crystal structures of simple inorganic salts were determined in the early 20th century (153), X-ray diffraction has become an invaluable tool for the structural analysis of organic molecules. A number of excellent textbooks are available for interested readers to obtain more detail on X-ray crystallography and diffraction data analysis (18,19,154–159). In the context of routine analysis of crystalline pharmaceuticals, we shall focus on single-crystal and XRPD methods using laboratory instruments and introduce the basic concepts of diffraction required to apply X-ray diffraction to the identification and structural characterization of pharmaceutical solids.

The diffraction of X-rays by a crystal lattice arises from constructive interference of X-rays, usually described as having been reflected from repeating planes of electron density within the lattice. Bragg's law (equation 1) describes the geometric conditions under which reflected X-rays experience constructive interference and give rise to diffraction, where λ (Ångstroms) is the radiation wavelength, and θ (degrees) is the scattering angle of the diffracted beam. The interplanar spacing, d (Ångstroms) is thus calculated from the Bragg equation (equation 1) (Fig. 17).

$$n\lambda = 2d \sin \theta \tag{1}$$

In most laboratory diffraction experiments, a known fixed wavelength of X-ray radiation is used. The X-ray wavelength is determined by the anode's composition in the X-ray tube, typically Cu (CuKα1 radiation, $\lambda = 1.54056$ Å) or Mo (MoKα1 radiation, $\lambda = 0.71073$ Å). The intensity of the incident beam is partly dependent on the voltage and current applied across the anode (typical values = 30–50 kV; 30–40 mA). The sample is bathed in the incident beam of X-rays, and a detector scans around the sample identifying the position and intensity of the diffracted radiation.

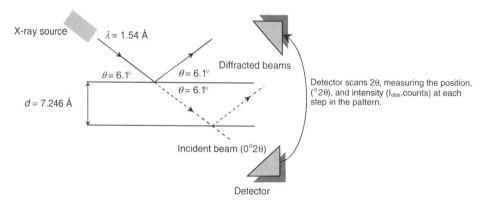

Figure 17 Schematic illustration showing the geometric conditions for Bragg diffraction. The parallel lines illustrate repeating planes in the lattice of a crystalline solid that has a d-spacing of 7.246 Å. X rays ($\lambda = 1.54$ Å) pass through the sample, and a proportion of the incident radiation is reflected from each plane. When $\lambda = 2d \sin \theta$, the reflected beams will be in phase and give rise to constructive interference, resulting in an observed Bragg reflection at 12.2° 2θ.

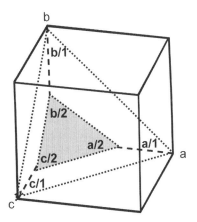

Figure 18 Plot illustrating the planes defined by Miller indices (222) (*gray*) and (111) (*dotted lines*) relative to the unit cell axes. The labels, *a*/1, *b*/1, *c*/1, etc., indicate the intercepts of the two planes on each of the cell axes.

The crystal planes within a lattice are defined by their Miller indices (*hkl*), where *h*, *k*, and *l* are integers that are defined such that a plane with Miller indices (*hkl*) intercepts the unit cell axes *a*, *b*, and *c* at *a*/*h*, *b*/*k*, and *c*/*l*. For example, a lattice plane with Miller indices (241) intercepts the *a*, *b*, and *c* axes at *a*/2, *b*/4, and *c*/1, respectively (Fig. 18).

The position of each diffracted beam relates to the dimensions of the unit cell, while the intensity of the diffracted beams is determined by the position and identity of atoms within the unit cell. In a crystal structure determination, the aim is to regain this information from the diffraction data by calculating the electron density at all points within the unit cell, with the regions of highest electron density corresponding to the atomic positions. The electron density throughout the cell can be calculated by a Fourier synthesis (equation 2) summed over all Bragg's reflections, *hkl*, using the experimental structure amplitudes, $|F_{hkl}^{obs}|$ (obtained from the square of the observed intensities, I_{obs}), and the reflection phases, α_{hkl}. *V* is the unit cell volume.

$$\rho(xyz) = \frac{1}{V} \sum_{hkl} |F_{hkl}^{obs}| \cos[2\pi(hx + ky + lz) - \alpha_{hkl}] \tag{2}$$

The phases of the reflected waves cannot be recovered during a diffraction measurement and so must be estimated to calculate the electron density and obtain the three-dimensional coordinates of all atoms, *x*, *y*, *z*, within the crystal structure. Several methods can be used to estimate the phases of the observed reflections, and *direct method* is typically the first approach to be tested (160,161). Once the initial electron density has been successfully determined by solving the phase problem, a preliminary model with atoms assigned to various positions within the unit cell is obtained. The best fit to all the observed data is obtained by subsequent least-squares refinement of the initial structure against the data in which the atomic coordinates (*x*, *y*, *z*) and atomic displacement parameters (ADPs) (1 isotropic parameter, U_{iso}, or 6 parameters for anisotropic displacements, U_{aniso}) are optimised. The ADPs describe the displacement of atoms arising from thermal motion around their mean position. A measure of the quality of the final refinement is obtained by calculating a residual or *R*-factor. While these are not an infallible indicator, good quality, accurate structure refinements will typically yield values up to 5% (0.05). *R*-factor values of greater than 10% often indicate a problem with the single-crystal structure.

Single-Crystal X-Ray Diffraction: Practical Considerations

Single-crystal X-ray diffraction is the routine method for crystal structure determination and is responsible for over 430,000 experimental crystal structure determinations available as of January 2008 in the CSD (20). Modern laboratory instruments are widely available and offer automated collection of good quality data to atomic resolution (<1 Å), as required by the direct methods approach commonly applied to structure determination of organic materials. Ideally, the ratio of observed intensities to the number of parameters to be determined should be at least 10:1 for an accurate structure refinement, typically requiring measurement of several thousand reflections (Fig. 19). Crystal structure data are now routinely presented in a crystallographic information file (.cif) format, and several freely available applications are available for visualizing crystal structures (162,163).

Single-crystal samples of at least 100 µm are usually required for modern laboratory instruments, though smaller crystals may be used in some cases. For smaller, weakly scattering crystals, high-powered rotating anode laboratory sources or synchrotron instruments may be able to collect sufficiently good data to allow structure determination (164). In addition to small size, other sample problems that may impede successful structure determination include disorder and twinning. Where such problems are encountered, it is worth attempting to recrystallize the sample in an attempt at improving sample diffraction quality (see section "Single-Crystal Growth for X-Ray Structural Analysis"). Samples are usually cooled during data collection using a temperature-controlled nitrogen gas stream to between 100 and 150 K. The low temperature reduces the thermal motion of the atoms in the crystal, improving the accuracy of the measured intensities. However, if the material undergoes a structural transformation during cooling, then the crystal may crack or disintegrate, rendering it useless for further measurement. Single crystals of pyrene form I, for example, shatter on cooling because of a solid-solid transformation to the low temperature form II at approximately 100 K (165).

X-Ray Powder Diffraction

Single-crystal diffraction is the routine method for crystal structure determination. However, for the successful application of the technique, suitable diffraction quality single-crystal samples must be available. If crystals of a particular API form (polymorph,

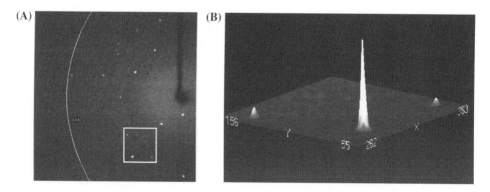

Figure 19 A single frame from a two-dimensional area detector on a laboratory single-crystal diffractometer (Mo radiation) showing: (**A**) diffraction spots corresponding to individual Bragg reflections from a single crystal sample that extend out to a resolution of 0.84 Å (*white line*) and (**B**) a three-dimensional view of the reflections in the region highlighted in (**A**), showing the relative intensities of the three peaks.

solvate, salt, or cocrystal) are too small or otherwise yield poor single-crystal diffraction data, structure determination from powder data (SDPD) is a valuable alternative approach that can be applied (166). XRPD is widely applied to the characterization and identification of the components in a polycrystalline powder produced during a crystallization search or in a batch of raw material received from a supplier or process. Single-crystal diffraction provides structural information collected from an individual particle selected from a sample, and XRPD data, collected from a sample of powder, is also of use where the interest is to confirm the structural form of particles comprising the bulk sample. XRPD therefore has wide application to the structural characterization of polycrystalline pharmaceutical samples and can be used to address a range of questions that commonly arise during studies of solid-state pharmaceuticals:

Q1. Is the sample crystalline or amorphous?

Q2. Are multiple samples the same or different crystalline forms?

Q3. Does the sample contain a single phase, or is it a mixture of crystalline phases?

Q4. Is the single-crystal structure representative of the bulk material?

Q5. What is the crystal structure of the material, considering no single crystals are available?

An XRPD experiment involves placing a sample of powder (i.e., many small crystallites) into an X-ray beam and measuring the position and intensity of the Bragg's reflections arising from the simultaneous diffraction from all crystalline particles present. An XRPD pattern (Fig. 20) is therefore a convenient means of visualizing a "fingerprint"

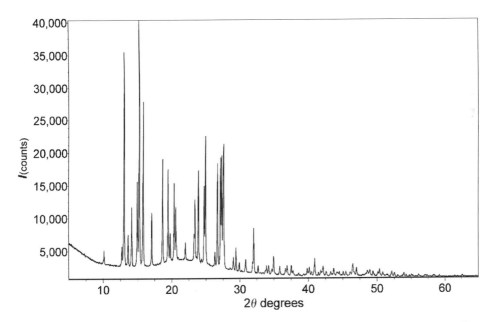

Figure 20 An XRPD pattern collected from a sample of carbamazepine form III in the range $5°$ to $70°\ 2\theta$ on a Bruker-AXS Advance D8 powder diffractometer with primary monochromator (CuKα1 radiation, $\lambda = 1.54056$ Å) and PSD. The sample was held in a rotating 0.7-mm borosilicate glass capillary during data collection. The pattern displays the sharp diffraction peaks characteristic of a polycrystalline sample. The high background at low 2θ values is due to air scatter and the rise in background between ~ 18 and $30\ °2\theta$ arises from the scattering produced by the glass capillary. A significant fall-off in reflection intensities is observed above $\sim 30\ °\ 2\theta$. *Abbreviations*: XRPD, X-ray powder diffraction; PSD, position-sensitive detector.

of the crystalline components of the sample, as all crystallites in the sample contribute to the observed diffraction profile. A significant consequence of simultaneous diffraction from many randomly oriented crystallites is that the individual diffraction spots (Fig. 19), corresponding to each of the lattice planes that satisfy Bragg's law during the experiment, become overlapped. This is particularly significant for APIs that crystallize in large unit cells and in low-symmetry space groups and has important consequences for the analysis of XRPD data. In the context of crystal structure determination from powder data reflection overlap results in a reduction in intensity information that can be extracted from the pattern in comparison to a single-crystal experiment. There are, however, various means of overcoming this limitation, and it is therefore increasingly common to apply XPRD, not just for pattern comparison or fingerprinting but also to extract valuable structural information, including crystal symmetry, unit cell parameters, atomic positions, lattice strain crystallite size.

Powder diffractometers have benefited from continued development over recent years, particularly with high-quality optics, monochromators, and high-sensitivity solid-state position-sensitive detectors. It is therefore relatively straightforward to collect high-quality laboratory data from a modern, well-specified, and accurately aligned instrument using a correctly prepared sample.

XRPD: practical considerations The objectives of a powder diffraction experiment are essentially to measure accurate peak positions ($°2\theta$) and/or to record accurate peak intensities for many Bragg's reflections. Commercial laboratory powder diffractometers are widely available in a range of configurations to meet the varied demands of different applications, though careful sample preparation can also be decisive in securing high-quality data. In simple terms, powder diffractometers comprise an X-ray source, sample holder, and X-ray detector combined with a varied range of optics to achieve a monochromatic beam, minimize axial divergence of the beam, optimize angular resolution (measured by peak full width half maximum, full-width half-maximum (FWHM) in $°2\theta$), and minimize background scattering in the pattern. Means of controlling sample environment including temperature and %RH are also available. The appropriate choice of each of these elements allows instruments to be tailored to a particular experimental requirement.

Where XRPD is used to analyze samples output from experimental crystallization searches, the objective is to identify all possible physical forms (polymorphs, solvates, salts, or cocrystals) as quickly and efficiently as possible. Hence, in the context of physical form screening, XRPD instruments must be able to handle small sample quantities with very little sample preparation, collect data rapidly, and provide good angular resolution and accurate peak positions (167). Multisample instruments provide an efficient means of collecting analytical data on large numbers of samples in varying quantities ($<$1–10s of milligrams).

Two common instruments configurations for the characterization of pharmaceuticals are based on reflection and transmission diffraction geometry. In reflection instruments, the sample is usually prepared as a thin layer in a metal sample holder and filled into the holder such as to present a flat surface to the incident beam. Care must be taken not to introduce preferred orientation into the sample at this stage by applying pressure while packing the sample. Use of an oriented Si crystal or "zero-background plate" sample holder reduces background and can overcome sample transparency effects that are often observed with organic compounds because of low absorbance of X-rays by the sample. Reflection geometry instruments are particularly useful when samples or their holders are opaque to X-rays (i.e., absorb the X-ray beam) and can provide accurate peak positions from small amounts of sample. Also, as both source and detector lie on the same side of the sample position, it is relatively straightforward to introduce a multisample device or sample environment chamber into the instrument. GADDS XRPD in reflection geometry allows standard 96-well plates from high-throughput automated crystallization screens, which are opaque to X-rays, to be used (168). The instrument can make measurements in a few minutes from only micrograms of material. Crystallites are automatically located within each well, and the sample height is adjusted and collects an XRPD pattern using a two-dimensional area detector to enable rapid acquisition and minimize sample preferred orientation effects. Simultaneous DSC-XRPD has also been developed using a reflection configuration to accommodate the fact that the sample is held in an Al pan (169,170).

Transmission geometry presents some advantages for structural analysis where, as with many organic pharmaceuticals, the materials are not strongly absorbing (171). Transmission instruments used in pharmaceutical applications generally fall into two categories: foil or flat plate transmission and capillary transmission geometries. The former have particular value in the context of physical form screening as they require only small sample amounts (~ 10 mg is sufficient); minimal sample preparation is required, and they provide good quality data with good signal-to-noise, low FWHM, and excellent positional accuracy of peaks. Positional accuracy is particularly important where there is an interest in powder pattern indexing of low-symmetry structures that require accurate measurement of the first 20 reflections in the pattern. Although the use of a primary monochromator will reduce the intensity of the primary beam affecting data collection times and signal-to-noise ratio, monochromatic radiation ensures that only a single wavelength of radiation contributes to the observed pattern and can simplify data analysis. However, with a position-sensitive detector (PSD) and monochromatic radiation, 40 to 45 minutes per sample typically yields good signal-to-noise across the range $3°$ to $35°$ 2θ, which would allow a single instrument to collect XRPD data from ~ 30 samples per day.

Samples can either be sandwiched between two X-ray transparent foils (such as Kapton® or Mylar®) or placed on top of a horizontal foil base (Fig. 21A). The former offers better reproducibility over sample thickness and therefore the positional accuracy of peaks, while the latter requires minimal preparation and also offers the opportunity to mount suspensions or solutions in situ and monitor the emergence of crystalline solid over

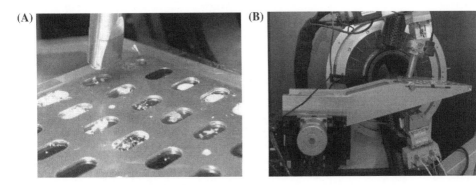

Figure 21 (A) Close-up view of a multiwell foil-transmission plate configured for 28 samples. Each well contains a sample of polycrystalline held on a Kapton film. (B) The plate is mounted on an automated *x-y* stage that moves each well into the beam for data collection and oscillates the samples in the *x-y* plane. The X-ray tube stand is seen at the top RHS of the picture and the PSD detector at the bottom RHS. *Abbreviations*: PSD, position-sensitive detector; RHS, right-hand side.

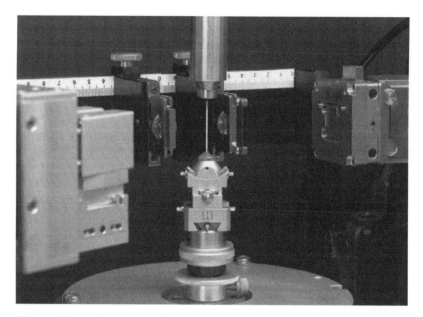

Figure 22 A 0.7-mm borosilicate glass capillary containing a polycrystalline sample on a laboratory XRPD instrument. The sample is rotated continuously during data collection and is aligned so that it lies at the center of the diffractometer and remains in the beam throughout the measurement. X-rays emerge from the monochromator housing (*RHS of the image*) and strike the sample. Diffracted beams are collected by the PSD (*front of PSD visible on LHS of image*) as it scans round 2θ. The silver tube located at the top of the capillary is a cryostream device for accurate sample temperature control. *Abbreviations*: XRPD, X-ray powder diffraction; PSD, position-sensitive detector; RHS, right-hand side; LHS, left-hand side.

time. Foil transmission is also readily amenable to multisample applications by using an automated sample base to enable many samples to be collected sequentially (Fig. 21B). A comparison of two multisample foil-transmission laboratory powder instruments confirmed that the data were of a high quality (FWHM down to 0.06° 2θ) and enabled successful pattern indexing of a range of pharmaceutical compounds (167).

Capillary transmission geometry is used for applications where (*i*) there is a need to obtain accurate reflection intensities, such as for SDPD; or (*ii*) where there is a need to protect a sensitive sample from air or humidity (Fig. 22). For SDPD applications, an effective instrumental configuration includes primary monochromated radiation, capillary sample holder, and PSD. The sample is filled into a glass capillary (typically 0.5–1.0 mm diameter, borosilicate or quartz glass) and rotated continuously during data collection. This effectively reduces preferred orientation effects and maximizes the number of crystallites contributing to the diffraction pattern during the data collection (Fig. 22).

Preferred orientation A potential drawback of reflection and foil-transmission configurations is that the data are particularly prone to preferred orientation effects (Table 13). Preferred orientation can arise where particles within a sample stack preferentially along certain directions and can be particularly problematic with needle or plate morphologies. It impacts on the observed peak intensities as particles in the sample are not randomly oriented, and so the relative intensities that are measured will be related not only to crystal structure but also to sample presentation. Careful sample preparation and the appropriate

Table 13 March–Dollase Correction of Intensities for Preferred Orientation in Data Collected from Samples of Six Pharmaceutical Compounds Using Both Foil-Transmission (Foil) and Capillary Transmission Geometry (Capillary)

Compound	Dir	r (foil)	r (capillary)
Sotalol.HCl	[010]	0.91	0.98
Hydroflumethiazide	[010]	0.90	0.97
Verapamil.HCl	[100]	0.78	0.92
Captopril	[001]	0.94	0.96
Clomipramine.HCl	[100]	1.39	1.09
Famotidine	[100]	1.66	1.04

"Dir" is the crystallographic direction and "r" is the magnitude of the correction. An r value of 1.0 indicates no preferred orientation. Note that while the extent of preferred orientation is significantly lower for the capillary data sets, it is still present.
Source: From Ref. 167.

selection of instrument geometry is key to minimizing preferred orientation, but may not always eliminate it. While accurate intensities may not be important for pattern comparison or pattern-indexing approaches based only on peak positions, if an analysis requires accurate intensity information, then any preferred orientation effects on the intensities must be taken into consideration. Several mathematical models have been developed that can accurately correct the effects of preferred orientation during, for example, structure determination and refinement. The most widely used method is the March–Dollase correction (172), though other correction methods based on spherical harmonics are also available (173).

However, prevention is better than cure, and so it is desirable to minimize preferred orientation effects in the sample where possible, for example, by sprinkling or lightly packing the sample into the sample holder (flat plate, well, or capillary) rather than firmly pressing it in. Light grinding of samples in a mortar and pestle can also be effective in improving highly anisotropic particle morphologies, though care must be taken when grinding potentially sensitive samples, such as metastable polymorphs or crystalline solvates, that grinding does not induce a structural transformation in the sample. Also, excessive grinding or particle size reduction may lead to peak broadening due to size and/or lattice strain effects (159) and even to the formation of amorphous material. As shown in Table 13, preferred orientation effects may also be observed in capillary data, albeit at a reduced level.

Applications of XRPD to Pharmaceutical Solids

Sample Characterization by XRPD
Often the first structural property to be established for a solid sample is to determine whether it is crystalline (Fig. 1). While several analytical techniques can be used to distinguish crystalline and amorphous forms, X-ray diffraction can be particularly useful, as crystalline solids give rise to Bragg diffraction of X-rays while amorphous solids, lacking any long-range internal order, produce only a diffuse scattering halo and no Bragg diffraction peaks (Fig. 23). The term "diffraction amorphous" is often used to describe a sample that has not shown any X-ray diffraction peaks. This term emphasizes that the sample contains no crystalline material within the limits of detection of the method. Where there is a requirement to quantify particularly small amounts of amorphous material within a sample, other more sensitive analytical methods should be used (Table 12).

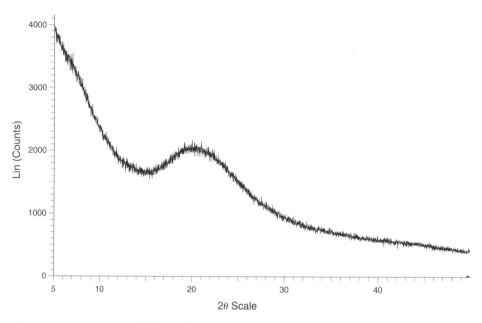

Figure 23 Characteristic XRPD profile collected from an amorphous sample. There is a complete absence of Bragg peaks and a broad "hump" in the background between ∼15° and 30° 2θ. *Abbreviation*: XRPD, X-ray powder diffraction.

Knowing whether a solid material is amorphous or crystalline is important, as the amorphous form is thermodynamically metastable relative to the crystalline form. While this may confer some advantages, such as increased aqueous solubility, unless the amorphous form has sufficient kinetic stability it may be of limited use, as it will transform to a more favorable, and less soluble, crystalline phase. Many pharmaceutical processes such as milling or spray drying may destroy crystalline structure and produce an amorphous component within the product (174–176), and significant effort has gone in to establishing means of accurately quantifying amorphous content of pharmaceutical powders (177–183). In some processes, such as lyophilization, amorphous material is desirable as it produces enhanced dissolution rates during reconstitution of the freeze-dried powder; however, in the context of solid-dosage forms the uncontrolled presence of amorphous content may be problematic.

Sample Identification

Fingerprinting—XRPD pattern comparison Sample "fingerprinting" is readily achieved by simply comparing the XRPD patterns from one or more samples to identify similar forms. The accuracy of the measured peak positions is therefore important. The position of each peak corresponds with the *d*-spacing from a set of planes within the lattice, and so a given crystalline form will always yield the same representative peaks at the same 2θ values when collected using the same wavelength radiation and sample temperature. Data collected using different wavelengths can be similarly compared by applying equation (1) to convert 2θ values into *d*-spacings for each pattern. A match between diffraction peak positions across multiple patterns confirms that each sample comprises the same polycrystalline phase or mixture of phases. Typically, when the diffraction patterns arise from samples comprising different polycrystalline polymorphs or solvates, or mixtures thereof, then the patterns will be easily distinguishable based on differences in the peak positions. With small numbers of patterns, fingerprinting can be easily done from direct visual comparison of the data; however, automated means of assessing the similarity between patterns are highly desirable where larger numbers of patterns are likely as in polymorph screening.

Fingerprinting is often done on a search/match basis by comparison of all the individual powder patterns collected from samples generated during a crystallization screen, and there are a range of software applications available to assist with this task. One widely used search/match tool is the Powder Diffraction File from the International Centre for Diffraction Data that uses *d*-spacing (*d*) and intensity (*I*) data derived from peak positions and intensities extracted from reference powder patterns (184). Other approaches do not require a data preparation step to extract *d*-spacings and/or intensity information and use full pattern comparisons on the raw data to identify and cluster similar sample patterns together (185). One commercial program, Poly-Snap, can compare hundreds of powder patterns simultaneously and enable clustering of the patterns based on dendrograms, metric multidimensional scaling, three-dimensional principal-component analysis, and scree plots (168). This method also has applications in distinguishing noncrystalline samples from crystalline forms from the relatively high background intensity and lack of diffraction peaks. Although these can be applied to any *x-y* data set, such as FT-IR, Raman, or DSC, XRPD data has the advantage of providing access to the crystal lattice dimensions as well. Hence, with suitably accurate data, it is possible to add value to the physical form screening process by determining lattice parameters and space group symmetry for any novel crystalline forms identified.

Comparison of XRPD data with a known crystal structure Where the crystal structure of a reference form is known, from single-crystal diffraction for example, this information can be used to identify a sample on the basis of its observed powder diffraction pattern. A Pawley-type fit (186) is a least-squares fit in which parameters describing the background, instrumental zero-point error, lattice parameters, peak shapes, and peak areas are refined to obtain a fit to the observed data (Fig. 24). A Pawley refinement can readily be applied to confirm whether a particular single-crystal structure is representative of a bulk sample. The experimental unit cell parameters and space group from a single-crystal structure are used as the starting point for a refinement against XRPD data collected from a polycrystalline sample. Where the calculated profile accounts for all the observed diffraction peaks and a good fit is achieved, it can be concluded that the polycrystalline sample comprises individual particles with the same structure (i.e., the single-crystal structure is representative of the bulk). Careful inspection of the final fit can also identify the presence of any contaminant crystalline phases in the sample. For example, in Figure 24, the Pawley refinement confirms that the sample largely comprises a polycrystalline sample of hydrochlorothiazide:DMSO 1:1 solvate (187), with a small amount of form I hydrochlorothiazide also present (188). The presence of the anhydrous form may have resulted from partial desolvation of the solvate prior to XRPD data collection.

Note the published unit cell parameters for the hydrochlorothiazide:DMSO solvate [triclinic; $P\bar{1}$, $a = 7.5068$ (4) Å, $b = 9.8272$ (5) Å, $c = 10.7311$ (6) Å, $\alpha = 85.639$ (3)°, $\beta = 73.896$ (3)°, $\gamma = 80.246$ (3)°] were determined at 123 K, whereas the XRPD data were collected at room temperature and yielded refined cell parameters $a = 7.5111(4)$ Å, $b = 9.8352(5)$ Å, $c = 10.7036(8)$ Å, $\alpha = 85.795(4)$°, $\beta = 73.920(4)$°, $\gamma = 79.982(4)$°. The increase in unit cell volume at room temperature is due to thermal expansion of the sample relative to 123 K.

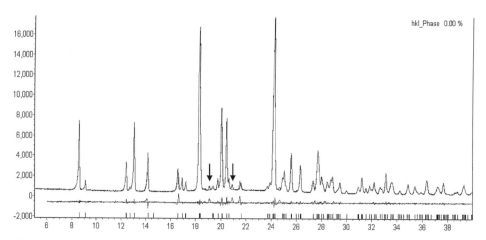

Figure 24 A Pawley fit to capillary XRPD data in the range 6° to 40° 2θ collected from a polycrystalline sample of hydrochlorothiazide recrystallized from DMSO carried out in TOPAS. The plot shows the observed, calculated, and difference (*bottom*) profiles for the final fit. The vertical tick marks along the bottom of the plot show the calculated reflection positions. The fit to the data are good as indicated by a low R_{wp} value (5.15) and the relatively flat difference profile. The published unit cell parameters at 123 K were used as the starting point for the refinement. The peaks at ∼ 19° and 21° 2θ (*arrows*) are not fitted by the calculated profile and do not correspond to the calculated peak positions. These peaks correspond to form I hydrochlorothiazide (data not shown). *Abbreviations*: XRPD, X-ray powder diffraction; DMSO, dimethylsulfoxide.

Freely available software, such as Mercury (189), is available for simulating powder patterns from single-crystal data using the unit cell dimensions, space group, and atomic coordinates from the known structure. Direct comparison of calculated powder patterns can be a useful way to compare crystal structures to confirm that they are different polymorphs (190,191). However, the change in reflection positions across the entire pattern due to thermal expansion of the structure can make it difficult to compare directly simulated patterns, calculated from a crystal structure determined at low temperature with powder patterns obtained at room temperature (192). Varying the low-temperature cell parameters to achieve a fit to the room temperature XRPD data using a Pawley refinement improves the chances of reliably confirming the sample identity and also yields the refined unit cell dimensions at room temperature. A further level of analysis would be to use a Rietveld refinement (193), which differs from a Pawley refinement in that the peak intensities, rather than being fitted by refining peak areas are calculated from the atomic coordinates of atoms within the crystal structure. However, where the aim is to identify whether observed diffraction peaks arise due to a particular crystalline phase with a known unit cell and space group, Pawley refinement is ideally suited. The applications of Pawley and Rietveld methods in structure determination and refinement are also discussed later in this chapter.

Structure Determination from Powder Data

While single-crystal methods remain the method of choice for crystal structure determination, in the absence of a suitable single-crystal sample of a particular crystalline form, SDPD using global optimization methods can prove to be invaluable. These methods have been successfully applied to solving the structures of a wide range of organic (194–197), inorganic (198–200), and organometallic (201–203) materials. With

Table 14 Various Factors for the Successful Application of SDPD Using Laboratory XRPD Data to Polycrystalline Pharmaceuticals

Requirements

Sample
Min. 10-mg sample of known composition (e.g., solvate or salt)
Minimal preferred orientation
Unit cell and space group should be known
Accurate 3D models of the molecular geometry

Instrument
Accurately aligned instrument to minimize zero-point error (e.g., using NIST SRM 640c (221))
Capillary geometry (e.g., sample in rotating 0.7 mm diameter borosilicate capillary)
Primary monochromated radiation (e.g., CuKα1, λ = 1.54056 Å)
Position-sensitive detector (e.g., Vantec, X'celerator, Lynxeye)
Sample temperature control for low T data collection and phase surveys

Data
Good signal-to-noise and good angular resolution (ca. 0.08° 2θ FWHM is typical for organics)
Step size between 0.01 and 0.015° 2θ ideal to allow accurate fitting of peak shapes
Capillary data set to at least 2Å resolution (data to 45° 2θ with CuKα1 radiation) for indexing and global optimization. Relatively long step times (5–10s) desirable to identify weak reflections at low angles for indexing stage
Capillary data to at least 1.3 Å resolution (variable count time data to 70° 2θ with CuKα1 radiation) for Rietveld refinement

Software
Indexing (e.g., DICVOL (222, 223), ITO (224), TREOR (225, 226), TOPAS (227), McMaille (228), and X-Cell (229))
Structure determination (e.g., DASH (230), Endeavour (231), ESPOIR (232), FOX (233), PowderSolve (234), PSSP (235), and TOPAS (236))
Structure refinement (e.g., GSAS (237), TOPAS)
Crystal structure analysis (e.g., Platon (162), Mercury (189), d-SNAP (238), Xpac (239), CrystalExplorer (240))

Abbreviations: XRPD, X-ray powder diffraction; FWHM, full-width half-maximum; SDPD, structure determination from powder data.

pharmaceuticals, SDPD has also been widely applied to solving the structures of polymorphs (43,204,205), solvates (68,206,207), salts (208–211), and cocrystals (212) of APIs as well as natural products (213) and crystalline excipients (214–216). The increased use of SDPD has been facilitated by the wide range of software implementing global optimization approaches that are now available (Table 14). For a detailed review of SDPD using global optimization methods see reference (217). In this section, we shall introduce the basic principles of SDPD and focus on practical approaches aimed at maximizing the chances of successfully solving an unknown crystal structure when only a polycrystalline sample is available. A schematic overview of the key stages in the application of SDPD is provided in Figure 25, and some of the requirements pertinent to these stages are listed in Table 14.

Traditional direct method approaches used in single-crystal diffraction are typically able to draw on thousands of individually measured reflection intensities to locate the position of individual atoms within the unit cell. However, a high-resolution laboratory powder diffraction pattern may only yield a few hundred reflection intensities as a result

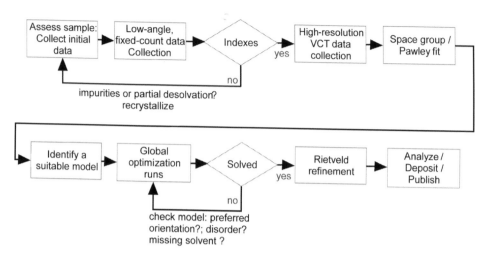

Figure 25 An overview of the key stages, and potential bottlenecks, in attempting crystal structure determination from powder diffraction data.

of peak overlap. Global optimization methods accommodate for this relative paucity of intensity information by enabling additional, nondiffraction data to be introduced into the structure determination process. This supplementary information is typically in the form of chemical structure details, such as molecular geometry (bond lengths, angles) describing the atomic connectivity within the molecular fragments or conformational constraints that have been derived from a structural database such as Mogul (218) or from solid-state NMR measurements (219).

XRPD Data collection To maximize the chances of successfully and accurately solving crystal structures from laboratory XRPD data, the following data requirements should be addressed: accurate measurement of reflection positions and intensities; high angular resolution (i.e., small FWHM) and spatial resolution (~ 2 Å or better); and good signal-to-background ratios across the full pattern and minimal preferred orientation effects. These requirements are best achieved in the laboratory with the sample mounted in a rotating capillary and the data collected in transmission geometry using monochromatic CuKα1 radiation. Linear one-dimensional PSDs combine excellent angular resolution with favorable count rates, and the development of modern solid-state PSDs offers the prospect of even greater improvements in performance with respect to low background, high sensitivity, and rapid data acquisition. It is desirable to utilize variable count time (220) (VCT) schemes for data collections for application in SDPD. These vary the step time with 2θ such that short counting times are used at low 2θ, where the average peak intensity is large, and progressively longer times are used at high 2θ values, where measured intensities are lower. VCT schemes improve the counting statistics [doubling the count time reduces the estimated standard deviation (ESD) on the observed counts by a factor of $\sqrt{2}$] and single-to-noise ratio and provides more accurate estimates of the reflection intensities.

Powder pattern indexing. With accurate data collected, the next step (Fig. 25) is to attempt to index the diffraction pattern. Indexing methods typically use the first 20 peak positions to determine the crystal system and unit cell dimensions of the sample. Indexing methods use different algorithms to search for combinations of lattice parameters that give the best match to the observed peak positions. Where accurate peak positions are

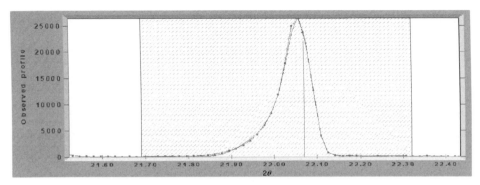

Figure 26 A diffraction peak fitted in DASH (230). The hatched area shows the data range used by DASH to obtain an accurate fit to the data. The vertical line indicates the calculated reflection position (22.069° 2θ) fitted using a combination of Lorentzian, Gaussian, and asymmetry functions to describe the observed peak shape. The peak maximum is at 22.057° 2θ; thus measuring the peak position from its maximum would introduce a potential error of approximately 0.01° 2θ, which is potentially significant for indexing procedures.

available, indexing programs (Table 14) tend to work extremely well, and so the chances of successful indexing are increased if the data are recorded from a well-prepared sample on a well-aligned instrument with a low zero-point displacement error. Peak positions must also be measured accurately from the data; ideally the line positions taken from the observed peaks should be based on accurate modeling of the peak shapes rather than by simply measuring the peak maximum (Fig. 26).

Indexing procedures tend to be intolerant of the presence of impurity peaks in the input peak listing. This is unsurprising, given that a set of peak positions that arise from two crystal lattices cannot be described by a single set of unit cell parameters. Some programs allow for this and enable the user to assign potential impurity peaks a lower weighting (e.g., based on weak intensities) or omit them completely from the search (223,227). The M_n (241) and F_n (242) figures of merit (Table 15) are commonly used to describe the quality of fit between the observed and calculated reflection positions for any cells returned by the indexing attempt, and some typical values returned from successful indexing attempts using laboratory XRPD data are shown in Table 15.

At this stage, it is also useful to estimate the validity of the cell using approximate molecular volumes of the constituent fragments to confirm that the proposed cell makes

Table 15 Some Typical Values of M_n and F_n Figures of Merit for The Correct Unit Cells Obtained from the First 20 Reflection Positions Measured in DASH from Laboratory Capillary XRPD Data Collected from Each Sample

Compound	$M(20)$	$F(20)$
Chlorpropamide	53.2	117.4
Creatine monohydrate	41.9	83.4
Diltiazem.HCl	37.6	103.1
Dopamine.HBr	92.8	188.0
Famotidine (form B)	32.3	88.6
Hydrochlorothiazide	87.1	160.8

Abbreviation: XRPD, X-ray powder diffraction.

good chemical sense. Also, visual comparison of the calculated reflection positions against the observed peaks confirms that all the observed diffraction peaks are accounted for by the cell. If indexing is unsuccessful, the process cannot proceed to structure determination (Fig. 25), and so if no suitable cells are returned from an indexing attempt, then it is worth exploring other options. One relatively straightforward approach might be to recrystallize the sample to sharpen the diffraction profile and better resolve overlapped reflections and/or to remove impurities.

Space group determination. The space group describing the crystallographic symmetry of molecules within the unit cell must also be known before attempting structure determination. This can be identified by visual comparison of the observed peak positions with those of reflection positions calculated using the unit cell for each appropriate space group within the relevant crystal system. The aim is to identify the space group whose systematic absences match the actual combination of observed reflections for the unit cell. It is useful to know at this stage if the sample is enantiomerically pure or a racemic mixture, as this may help to reduce the potential space group options to be checked. However, this can be a time-consuming process, particularly if many space groups have to be tested, as is the case for orthorhombic lattices. However, algorithms for space group selection based on probabilistic methods are also available to assist with this process (243). A Pawley fit (outlined in section "Comparison of XRPD Data with a Known Crystal Structure") (Fig. 24) can be used to provide final confirmation that the unit cell and space group assignment are accurate.

Intensity extraction. With unit cell and space group determined, the next step is to extract the individual intensities associated with each reflection from the observed diffraction peaks. The Le Bail (244) and Pawley (186) methods are most widely applied to dealing with intensity extraction from overlapped peaks (Fig. 27), although the Pawley method is mathematically more robust (245). The aim is to determine the reliable Bragg peak intensity estimates on the basis of the peak areas in the powder pattern by least-squares refinement of parameters that describe the background, zero-point error, peak shape, unit cell parameters, and peak area. The importance of good quality data cannot be overstated,

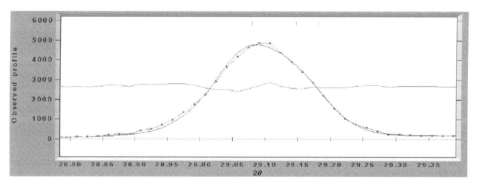

Figure 27 A challenge in exploiting XRPD data for SDPD is dealing with the loss of intensity information arising from reflection overlap. In the example shown, three reflections (*tick marks, top of plot*) overlap to give a single diffraction peak. Typically, during intensity extraction the intensities of each reflection are estimated by simply partitioning the total intensity across each contributing reflection. *Abbreviations*: XRPD, X-ray powder diffraction; SDPD, structure determination from powder data.

as the measured peak intensities dictate the accuracy of the extracted intensities available to the subsequent structure determination attempt. If these are inaccurate or contain systematic errors, this may inhibit the ability to solve the structure.

Global optimization methods for SDPD. In SDPD, global optimization strategies are frequently used to find the trial crystal structure (position, orientation, and conformation of molecular components in the unit cell) that gives the lowest-possible R-factor (i.e., best fit or global minimum) to the observed reflection intensities. Various search methods have been applied in this context, though genetic algorithms and simulated annealing are perhaps the most widely implemented in software packages for SDPD (Table 14). Of the available global optimization methods, simulated annealing has been widely adopted because of the relative ease of its implementation within software and its requirements for relatively straightforward control parameters. Global optimization methods are also amenable to parallelization and so can be readily be modified to take advantage of modern multicore processors or distributed computing grids. This can significantly reduce the time required to solve complex structures or assess multiple models, for example, when dealing with potentially disordered structures. With simulated annealing, many runs (typically hundreds) are implemented to assess the reproducibility with which the lowest R-factor structure is obtained and confirm that the global minimum has been correctly identified in the search.

In single-crystal methods, each atomic position is determined independently, whereas in global optimization approaches, the number of parameters to be determined is significantly reduced by applying prior knowledge of the atomic connectivity of the molecular fragments. A three-dimensional model, in the form of a z-matrix, is constructed for each structural fragment in which the bond lengths and angles defining the connectivity of atoms are constrained to standard values. A simple way to construct an accurate z-matrix is from a related crystal structure, such as a polymorph, salt, or solvate of the molecule of interest. In the absence of such a structure, mean values for bond lengths, covalent bond angles, and nonoptimizable torsion angles can be obtained from the CSD (20). Flexible torsions that define the conformation of the molecule are allowed to vary during the search. In this way, the crystal structure can be described by six variables describing the position (x, y, z) and orientation (θ, ϕ, ψ) of each molecular fragment in the structure plus an additional variable for each flexible torsion angle to describe molecular conformation. The crystal structure of chlorothiazide ($C_7H_6ClN_3O_4S_2$) (Fig. 28), for example, would require 69 parameters just to describe the coordinates of all 23 atoms in a direct methods analysis using single-crystal diffraction data. In contrast, for global optimization methods, only seven parameters (degrees of freedom) are necessary to describe the position, orientation, and conformation of the molecule (assuming 1 torsion angle varies). In this way, the number of parameters that are required to solve the crystal structure is greatly reduced. If the structure is a metal salt, the metal counterion is treated as single point requiring only three positional variables to describe its position. Similarly, as hydrogen atoms scatter X rays very weakly, it is common practice to describe water molecules in a hydrate structure as a single oxygen atom, thereby removing three orientational degrees of freedom from the search. Additional strategies can be applied to increase the chances of successfully solving a crystal structure using global optimization strategies, and some of these are highlighted in Table 16.

A survey of simulated annealing SDPD success rates with laboratory data across a series of 35 organic and organometallic crystal structures spanning a range of complexity (6–22 degrees of freedom) confirmed that structures with less than 10 degrees of freedom were essentially trivial problems and solved reliably and accurately (100% of individual

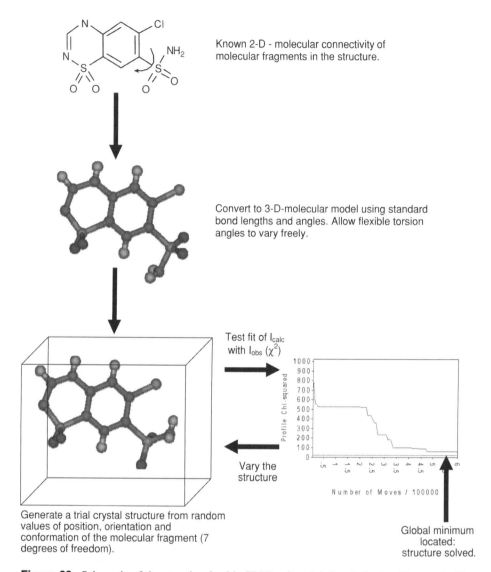

Known 2-D - molecular connectivity of molecular fragments in the structure.

Convert to 3-D-molecular model using standard bond lengths and angles. Allow flexible torsion angles to vary freely.

Test fit of I_{calc} with I_{obs} (χ^2)

Vary the structure

Generate a trial crystal structure from random values of position, orientation and conformation of the molecular fragment (7 degrees of freedom).

Global minimum located: structure solved.

Figure 28 Schematic of the steps involved in SDPD using global optimization illustrated with a molecule of chlorothiazide. A three-dimensional model is constructed, and random trial crystal structures varying each of the parameters describing the position, orientation, and conformation of the molecule are generated. The calculated intensities of each trial structure are compared with the observed intensities and the model further varied until the best fit to the data is identified. Once the global minimum has been located, the structure is solved. *Abbreviation*: SDPD, structure determination from powder data.

simulated annealing runs locate the global minimum). As structural complexity increased to over 15 degrees of freedom, the success rate with which the global minimum was located reduced significantly. Simulated annealing runs for an SDPD attempt on verapamil hydrochloride required 22 degrees of freedom to describe the structure and successfully returned the global minimum on only 5% of runs, reflecting the significant complexity of the search space (246). This said, SDPD has been used to solve the crystal structure of a variety of complex molecular structures using laboratory XRDP data. For

Table 16 Approaches for Optimizing Data Quality and Maximising the Chance of Successfully Solving Crystal Structures from Laboratory XRPD Data Using Simulated Annealing Global Optimization

Approach	Aim/advantage	Comment/reference
Recrystallization	Minimize intrinsic sample line width; improve angular resolution	Risk of phase transformation or texture effects
Low-temperature data collection	Improve signal-to-noise, particularly at high 2θ angles; improve accuracy of reflection intensities	Differential thermal expansion (247, 248) Risk of phase transformation
Variable count time data collection	As "low T data collection."	Improve accuracy of extracted intensities at high angles (249)
Optimize SA control parameters	Increase probability of locating global minimum	For example, reducing the cooling rate to avoid quenching (217)
Crystallographic constraints	Reduce number of degrees of freedom to be optimized during search; increase probability of locating global minimum	For example, in space groups such as $P1$, with floating origins, fixing the x, y, and z coordinates of an atom in the formula unit removes three degrees of freedom
Chemical constraints	As "crystallographic constraints"	For example, fixing amide torsion angle (H−N−C=O) to an exact value of $180°$, removing it from the optimization

Source: From Ref. 246.

example, a chlorothiazide:*N,N*-dimethylformamide solvate (1:2) with six independent molecules in the unit cell (42 degrees of freedom) was successfully solved by simulated annealing and a Rietveld refinement, using data collected to 1.4 Å resolution, yielded a final $R_{wp} = 2.0$ (Fig. 29). However, this method by no means represents the limit of structural complexity that can be tackled using this approach. For example, the crystal structure of the β_2-polymorph of monounsaturated triacylglycerol 1,3-distearoyl-2-oleoylglycerol [$C_{57}H_{108}O_6$; monoclinic, Cc, $a = 5.440$ (1), $b = 130.30$ (1), $c = 8.221$ (1), $\beta = 88.75$ (1), volume $= 5825.8$ (4), $Z = 4$] (250) was solved using laboratory XRPD data and a parallel tempering global optimization method. However, the significant conformational flexibility of the molecule arising from the long aliphatic chains required a stepped approach to be taken to structure determination. The location and orientation of the molecule were optimized on the basis of an assumed molecular conformation before gradually allowing torsion angles to vary and locate their actual values.

Rietveld refinement. The final stage of the structure determination process is normally a refinement of the crystal structure, obtained from the global optimization step, against high-resolution XRPD data, typically collected to a minimum of 1.3Å resolution ($\equiv 70°$ 2θ with CuKα1 radiation, minimum required for submission of a powder structure to *Acta Crystallographica*). This is known as Rietveld refinement (157,193) and involves least-squares refinement of the structure (atomic coordinates plus ADPs) and background,

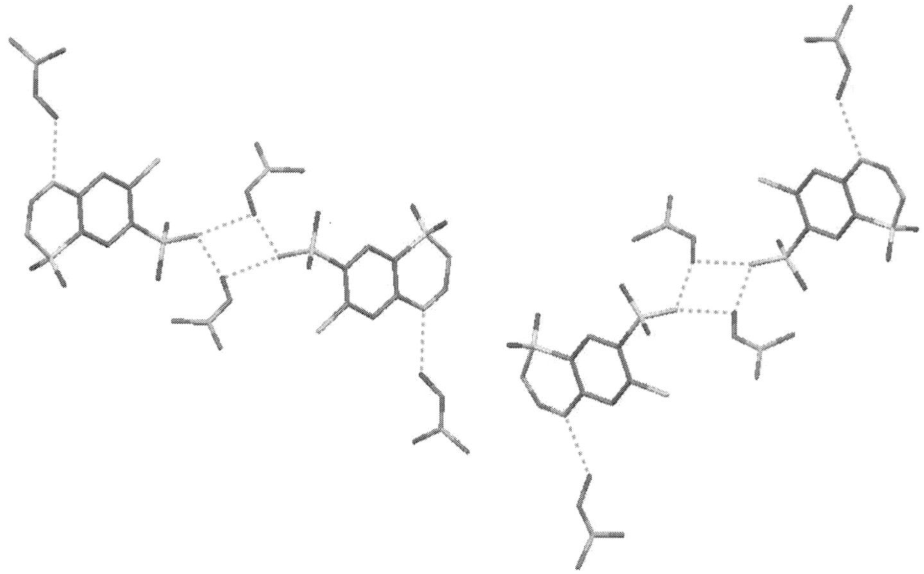

Figure 29 A packing diagram showing hydrogen-bonding interactions (*dashed lines*) between molecules of chlorothiazide and solvent within the crystal structure of the chlorothiazide: *N, N*-dimethylformamide (1:2) solvate. H-atoms omitted for clarity. [monoclinic, $P2_1/c$, $Z' = 4$, $a = 12.3586(2)$ Å, $b = 8.5619(2)$ Å, $c = 37.3043(7)$ Å, $\beta = 92.8786(13)°$, $V = 3942.29(13)$ Å^3]. *Source*: From Ref. 204.

zero-point error, unit cell, and peak-shape parameters to achieve the best possible fit to the entire diffraction pattern. Several software packages that implement Rietveld refinement algorithms are available (see Table 14 for examples). The aim is to obtain the most accurate representation of both molecular and crystal structure that is consistent with the observed diffraction pattern. The lack of intensity data due to peak overlap also impacts on refinement approaches such that it is common practice to apply slack constraints to the atomic positions during refinement. These restrict variation in bond lengths and angles during the refinement to within ranges close to the original, standard values derived from the z-matrix input at the global optimization stage. An alternative method is to treat the molecule as either a single rigid body or series of rigid bodies and vary only the position and orientation of the fragments plus any appropriate torsion angles. The accuracy of the final refined structure can be scrutinized by removing all constraints and allowing atoms to move freely, their position guided only by the fit to the data. Generally, it is expected that for an accurate structural model and high-resolution data, the positions of non-hydrogen atoms should not move significantly.

Variable temperature XRPD and SDPD. Capillary XRPD with temperature control is a particularly effective technique for tracking structural transformations in polycrystalline samples. The temperature range 80 to 500 K is routinely accessible using standard cryostream systems. The sample is heated in situ to monitor the transformation, such as a desolvation or solid-solid transition, and high-resolution capillary XRPD data can then be collected from the product, enabling the crystal structure to be solved and refined (Fig. 30). These types of transformations cannot usually be monitored using single-crystal diffraction as the structural rearrangement associated with the transition frequently results in a polycrystalline sample.

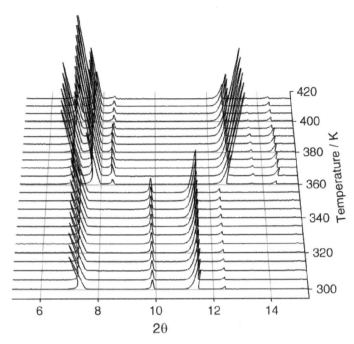

Figure 30 Plot showing the change in peak positions as a function of temperature during an in situ variable temperature XRPD study of the temperature-dependent transition between form I and form III of the diastereomeric (R)-1-phenylethylammonium (R)-2-phenylbutyrate salt (251). Note the abrupt change in peak positions above 360 K. *Abbreviation*: XRPD, X-ray powder diffraction.

The structure determination of form II cyheptamide (252) ($C_{16}H_{15}NO$) (Fig. 31) is an example of the application of SDPD, Rietveld refinement, and variable-temperature XRPD to good effect. A polycrystalline sample of the monoclinic form of cyheptamide, an analog of carbamazepine, was held in a rotating capillary and heated in situ, whereupon a transformation was observed at approximately 174°C. The sample of form II was subsequently cooled to −173°C, where it remained stable, and high-resolution data were collected, enabling the crystal structure of form II cyheptamide to be determined using simulated annealing and a z-matrix constructed from the form I crystal structure. The triclinic structure required 28 degrees of freedom to describe four independent molecules in the unit cell and one torsion angle per molecule. A rigid-body Rietveld refinement using 76 parameters [27 profile (including background, zero-point, peak shape), 6 unit cell parameters, 1 scale, 14 preferred orientation, 4 torsion angles, 12 position plus 12 rotation] returned a final $R_{wp} = 4.6$ (Fig. 31). The accuracy of the refined structure was inspected by allowing all atomic coordinates to refine without constraints. This increased the number of refined parameters to 444 and yielded an improved fit to the data with $R_{wp} = 1.5$. However, while the C, N and O atoms in the structure remained very close to their original positions, confirming the accuracy of the starting structure, the improved fit to the data was obtained at the expense of the weakly scattering hydrogen atoms moving to chemically nonsensical positions within the cell. It is critically important when evaluating the success of a Rietveld refinement that any improvement in fit achieved by the inclusion of additional parameters is not at the expense of the accuracy of the structure.

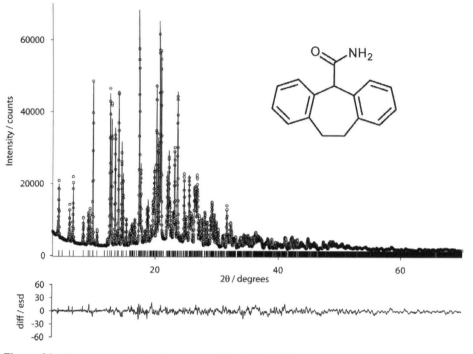

Figure 31 Final observed (*points*), calculated (*line*), and difference $[(y_{obs} - y_{calc})/\sigma(y_{obs})]$ profiles for the Rietveld refinement of cyheptamide (*inset*) form II [$a = 5.6491(1)$ Å, $b = 19.5639(4)$ Å, $c = 22.0741(5)$ Å, $\alpha = 84.2178(13)°$, $\beta = 88.4073(14)°$, $\gamma = 83.6001(13)°$, $V = 2411.72(9)$ Å^3, triclinic, $P\bar{1}$, $Z' = 4$], using laboratory XRPD data collected at 100 K to a resolution of 1.3 Å. The final fit to the data is excellent yielding an $R_{wp} = 4.6$. *Abbreviation*: XRPD, X-ray powder diffraction.

CONCLUDING REMARKS

Control and prediction of the structure and properties of solid-state pharmaceuticals remain significant challenges for those involved in the commercial development and manufacture of APIs and pharmaceutical products. An understanding of the basic science underpinning phenomena such as polymorphism and solvate formation is continually developing. However, in the absence of tools to predict reliably which crystalline forms will be observed, rigorous experimental investigation remains the only means of determining the individual forms, the conditions under which they may be produced and their physicochemical properties. Ultimately, the goal of those concerned with solid-state pharmaceuticals is to translate a comprehensive knowledge of the formation and stability of different solid-state forms into better control of pharmaceutical materials, processes and products.

REFERENCES

1. Stahly GP. Cryst Growth Des 2007; 7:1007–1026.
2. Aakeroy CB, Salmon DJ. Cryst Eng Comm 2005; 7:439–448.
3. Day GM, Motherwell WDS, Ammon HL, et al. Acta Crystallogr Sect B Struct Sci 2005; 61:511–527.

4. Price SL, Adv Drug Deliv Rev 2004; 56:301–319.
5. Giron D, Mutz M, Garnier S. J Therm Anal Calorim 2004; 77:709–747.
6. Miller SPF, Raw AS, Yu LX. In: Hilfiker R, ed. Polymorphism in the Parmaceutical Industry. Weinheim, Germany: Wiley-VCH, 2006:385–402; [Chichester, U.K.: John Wiley (distributor)].
7. Bernstein J. In: Hilfiker R, ed. Polymorphism in the Pharmaceutical industry. Weinheim, Germany: Wiley-VCH, 2006:365–382; [Chichester, U.K.: John Wiley (distributor)].
8. Bernstein J. Polymorphism in Molecular Crystals. New York, Oxford: Oxford University Press, 2002:297–307.
9. Bernstein J. Polymorphism in Molecular Crystals. New York: Oxford University Press, 2002:240–256.
10. Brittain HG, ed. Polymorphism in Pharmaceutical Solids. New York: M. Dekker, 1999.
11. Hilfiker R, Blatter F, von Raumer M. In: Hilfiker R, ed. Polymorphism in the Pharmaceutical Industry. Weinheim, Germany: Wiley-VCH, 2006:1–20.
12. Kirk JH, Dann SE, Blatchford CG. Int J Pharm 2007; 334:103–114.
13. Burger A, Henck JO, Hetz S, et al. J Pharm Sci 2000; 89:457–468.
14. Li XW, Zhi F, Hu YQ. Int J Pharm 2007; 328:177–182.
15. Wikstrom H, Carroll WJ, Taylor LS. Pharm Res 2008; 25:923–935.
16. Salameh AK, Taylor LS. J Pharm Sci 2006; 95:446–461.
17. David Grant JW. In: Brittain HG, ed. Polymorphism in Pharmaceutical Solids. New York: M. Dekker, 1999:1–33.
18. Glusker JP, Trueblood KN. Crystal Structure Analysis: A Primer. New York, Oxford: Oxford University Press, 1985.
19. Hammond C. The Basics of Crystallography and Diffraction. Oxford: Oxford University Press, 2001.
20. Allen FH. Acta Crystallogr Sect B Struct Sci 2002; 58:380–388.
21. Henry NFM, Kasper JS, Lonsdale KD, et al. In: Henry NFM, Lonsdale K, eds. International Tables for X-Ray Crystallography. Vol 1. Symmetry Groups. 1952: xi. 558.
22. Nichols G, Frampton CS. J Pharm Sci 1998; 87:684–693.
23. Vrcelj RM, Clark NIB, Kennedy AR, et al. J Pharm Sci 2003; 92:2069–2073.
24. Fabbiani FPA, Allan DR, Dawson A, et al. Chem Commun 2003; 3004–3005.
25. Fabbiani FPA, Allan DR, David WIF, et al. Cryst Eng Comm 2004; 6:504–511.
26. McGregor PA, Allan DR, Parsons S, et al. J Pharm Sci 2002; 91:1308–1311.
27. Ferenczy GG, Parkanyi L, Angyan JG, et al. J Mol Struct (Theochem) 2000; 503:73–79.
28. Hilfiker R, ed. Polymorphism in the Pharmaceutical Industry. Weinheim, Germany: Wiley-VCH, 2006; [Chichester U.K.: John Wiley (distributor)].
29. Shefter E, Higuchi T. J Pharm Sci 1963; 52:781–791.
30. Rodriguez-Hornedo N, Murphy D. J Pharm Sci 1999; 88:651–660.
31. Gu CH, Young V, Grant DJW. J Pharm Sci 2001; 90:1878–1890.
32. Florence AJ, Johnston A. Spectrosc Eur 2005; 16:24–27.
33. Burger A, Ramberger R. Mikrochim Acta 1979; 2:259–271.
34. Vega D, Fernandez D, Echeverria G. Acta Crystallogr Sect C Cryst Struct Commun 2000; 56:1009–1010.
35. Roy S, Aitipamula S, Nangia A. Cryst Growth Des 2005; 5:2268–2276.
36. Roy S, Bhatt PM, Nangia A, et al. Cryst Growth Des 2007; 7:476–480.
37. Sivalakshmidevi A, Vyas K, Rao SM, et al. Acta Crystallogr Sect E Struct Reports Online 2002; 58:O1072–O1074.
38. Strzhemechny MA, Baumer VN, Avdeenko AA, et al. Acta Crystallogr Sect B Struct Sci 2007; 63:296–302.
39. Chen XM, Morris KR, Griesser UJ, et al. J Am Chem Soc 2002; 124:15012–15019.
40. Urakami K, Shono Y, Higashi A, et al. Chem Pharm Bull 2002; 50:263–267.
41. Cox PJ, Manson PL. Acta Crystallogr Sect E Struct Reports Online 2003; 59:O986–O988.
42. Kitaoka H, Wada C, Moroi R, et al. Chem Pharm Bull 1995; 43:649–653.
43. Shankland N, David WIF, Shankland K, et al. Chem Commun 2001; 2204–2205.
44. Bauer J, Spanton S, Henry R, et al. Pharm Res 2001; 18:859–866.

45. Chemburkar SR, Bauer J, Deming K, et al. Org Process Res Dev 2000; 4:413–417.
46. Thayer AM. Chem Eng News 2007; 85:28–29.
47. Bernstein J. Cryst Growth Des 2005; 5:1661–1662.
48. Desiraju GR. Cryst Eng Comm 2003; 5:466–467.
49. Nangia A. Cryst Growth Des 2006; 6:2–4.
50. Seddon KR. Cryst Growth Des 2004; 4:1087–1087.
51. Vandersluis P, Kroon J. J Cryst Growth 1989; 97:645–656.
52. Gorbitz CH, Hersleth HP. Acta Crystallogr Sect B Struct Sci 2000; 56:526–534.
53. Nangia A, Desiraju GR. Chem Commun 1999; 605–606.
54. Kitaigorodskii AI. Organic Chemical Crystallography, New York: Consultants Bureau, 1961.
55. Khankari RK, Grant DJW. Thermochim Acta 1995; 248:61–79.
56. Morris KR, Griesser UJ, Eckhardt CJ, et al. Adv Drug Deliv Rev 2001; 48:91–114.
57. Tian F, Sandler N, Aaltonen J, et al. J Pharm Sci 2007; 96:584–594.
58. Cabeza AJC, Day GM, Motherwell WDS, et al. J Am Chem Soc 2006; 128:14466–14467.
59. Johnston A, Johnston BF, Kennedy AR, et al. Cryst Eng Comm 2008; 10:23–25.
60. Bingham AL, Hughes DS, Hursthouse MB, et al. Chem Commun 2001; 603–604.
61. Suleiman MS, Najib NM. Int J Pharm 1989; 50:103–109.
62. International Conference on Harmonisation of Technical Requirements for Registration of Pharmaceuticals for Human Use (ICH) ICH Harmonized Tripartite Guideline Q3C Impurities: Residual Solvents, 1997.
63. Harris RK, Ghi PY, Puschmann H, et al. Org Process Res Dev 2005; 9:902–910.
64. Fleischman SG, Kuduva SS, McMahon JA, et al. Cryst Growth Des 2003; 3:909–919.
65. Johnston A, Florence AJ, Kennedy AR. Acta Crystallogr Sect E Struct Rep Online 2005; 61: O1777–O1779.
66. Liu CL, Chang TC, Wu SM, et al. J Chin Chem Soc 2006; 53:851–856.
67. Infantes L, Fabian L, Motherwell WDS. Cryst Eng Comm 2007; 9:65–71.
68. Burley JC, van de Streek J, Stephens PW. Acta Crystallogr Sect E Struct Rep Online 2006; 62: O797–O799.
69. Turel I, Bukovec P, Quiros M. Int J Pharm 1997; 152:59–65.
70. Kennedy AR, Okoth MO, Sheen DB, et al. Acta Crystallogr Sect C Cryst Struct Commun 2003; 59:O650–O652.
71. Gylbert L. Acta Crystallogr Sect B Struct Sci 1973; B 29:1630–1635.
72. Sime RL, Forehand R, Sime RJ. Acta Crystallogr Sect B Struct Sci 1975; 31:2326–2330.
73. Cuffini SL, Faudone S, Ferro M, et al. Acta Crystallogr Sect C Cryst Struct Commun 2008; 64:O119–O122.
74. Bechtloff B, Nordhoff S, Ulrich J. Cryst Res Technol 2001; 36:1315–1328.
75. Dideberg O, Dupont L. Acta Crystallogr Sect B Struct Crystallogr Cryst Chem 1972; B 28:3014–3022.
76. Agafonov V, Legendre B, Rodier N. Acta Crystallogr Sect C Cryst Struct Commun 1989; 45:1661–1663.
77. Nicolai B, Espeau P, Ceolin R, et al. J Therm Anal Calorim 2007; 90:337–339.
78. Almarsson O, Zaworotko MJ. Chem Commun 2004; 1889–1896.
79. Zaworotko M. J Pharm Pharmacol 2006; 58:A91–A91.
80. Zaworotko M, Peddy V. Acta Crystallogr Sect A 2005; 61:c12–c13.
81. Braga D, Grepioni F. Making Crystals by Design: Methods, Techniques and Applications. Weinheim, Germany: Wiley-VCH, 2007.
82. Desiraju GR. Crystal Design: Structure and Function. Chichester, U.K.: Wiley, 2003.
83. Trask AV, Motherwell WDS, Jones W. Cryst Growth Des 2005; 5:1013–1021.
84. Trask AV, Motherwell WDS, Jones W. Int J Pharm 2006; 320:114–123.
85. Wermuth CG, Stahl PH. Handbook of Pharmaceutical Salts: Properties, Selection, and Use. In: Stahl PH, Wermuth CG, eds. Weinheim, Germany; Chichester, U.K.: Wiley-VCH, 2002:1–8.
86. Balbach S, Korn C. Int J Pharm 2004; 275:1–12.
87. Banerjee R, Bhatt PM, Ravindra NV, et al. Cryst Growth Des 2005; 5:2299–2309.

88. Pfannkuch F, Rettig H, Stahl PH. In: Stahl PH, Wermuth CG, eds. Handbook of Pharmaceutical Salts: Properties, Selection, and Use. Weinheim, Germany; Chichester, U.K.: Wiley-VCH, 2002:117–134.

89. Kumar L, Amin A, Bansal AK. Drug Discov Today 2007; 12:1046–1053.

90. Bastin RJ, Bowker MJ, Slater BJ. Org Process Res Dev 2000; 4:427–435.

91. Morissette SL, Almarsson O, Peterson ML, et al. Adv Drug Deliv Rev 2004; 56:275–300.

92. Storey R, Docherty R, Higginson PD, et al. Crystallogr Rev 2004; 37:243–252.

93. Kojima T, Onoue S, Murase N, et al. Pharm Res 2006; 23:806–812.

94. Berge SM, Bighley LD, Monkhouse DC. In: Swarbrick J, Boylan JC, eds. Encyclopedia of Pharmaceutical Technology. New York: Marcel Dekker, 1996:453–499.

95. Maddox J. Nature 1988; 335:201–201.

96. Price SL. Phys Chem Chem Phys 2008; 10:1996–2009.

97. Lommerse JPM, Motherwell WDS, Ammon HL, et al. Acta Crystallogr Sect B Struct Sci 2000; 56:697–714.

98. Motherwell WDS, Ammon HL, Dunitz JD, et al. Acta Crystallogr Sect B Struct Sci 2002; 58:647–661.

99. Cabeza AJC, Pidcock E, Day GM, et al. Cryst Eng Comm 2007; 9:556–560.

100. Hulme AT, Price SL. J Chem Theory and Comput 2007; 3:1597–1608.

101. Lancaster RW, Karamertzanis PG, Hulme AT, et al. Chem Commun 2006; 4921–4923.

102. Cross WI, Blagden N, Davey RJ, et al. Cryst Growth Des 2003; 3:151–158.

103. Florence AJ, Leech CK, Shankland N, et al. Cryst Eng Comm 2006; 8:746–747.

104. Johnston A, Florence AJ, Shankland N, et al. Cryst Growth Des 2007; 7:705–712.

105. Mullin JW. Crystallization. Oxford, Boston: Butterworth-Heinemann, 2001.

106. Florence AJ, Johnston A, Price SL, et al. J Pharm Sci 2006; 95:1918–1930.

107. Lang MD, Grzesiak AL, Matzger AJ. J Am Chem Soc 2002; 124:14834–14835.

108. Price CP, Grzesiak AL, Matzger AJ. J Am Chem Soc 2005; 127:5512–5517.

109. Yu L. Cryst Eng Comm 2007; 9:847–851.

110. Ostwald WZ. Z Phys Chem 1897; 22:289–330.

111. Florence AJ, Shankland N, Johnston A. In: Sarker SD, Latif Z, Gray AI, eds. Natural Products Isolation. Totowa, NJ: Humana Press, 2006:275–296.

112. Yu ZQ, Chew JW, Chow PS, et al. Chem Eng Res Des 2007; 85:893–905.

113. McDonald C, Muzumdar PP. J Clin Pharm Ther 1998; 23:235–239.

114. McDonald C, Faridah. J Parenter Sci Technol 1991; 45:147–151.

115. Yarlagadda SG, Perazella MA. Expert Opin Drug Saf 2008; 7:147–158.

116. Groen H, Roberts KJ. J Phys Chem B 2001; 105:10723–10730.

117. Liang KP, White G, Wilkinson D, et al. Ind Eng Chem Res 2004; 43:1227–1234.

118. Lu J, Wang XJ, Yang X, et al. J Pharm Sci 2007; 96:2457–2468.

119. Nagy ZK, Chew JW, Fujiwara M, et al. J Process Control 2008; 18:399–407.

120. Parmar MM, Khan O, Seton L, et al. Cryst Growth Des 2007; 7:1635–1642.

121. Field JS, Ledwaba LP, Munro OQ, et al. Cryst Eng Comm 2008; 10:740–747.

122. Toro R, de Delgado GD, Bahsas A, et al. Z Kristallogr 2007; 563–568.

123. Weatherhead-Kloster RA, Selby HD, Miller WB, et al. J Org Chem 2005; 70:8693–8702.

124. Watkin DJ. J Appl Crystallogr 1972; 5:250.

125. Ceolin R, Toscani S, Gardette MF, et al. J Pharm Sci 1997; 86:1062–1065.

126. Sarma B, Roy S, Nangia A. Chem Commun 2006; 4918–4920.

127. Bleay J, Hooper RM, Narang RS, et al. J Cryst Growth 1978; 43:589–596.

128. Henisch HK. Crystal Growth in Gels. London: Dover Publications; New York: Constable and Co., 1996.

129. Ramachandran E, Natarajan S. Cryst Res Technol 2006; 41:411–415.

130. Lang MD, Kampf JW, Matzger AJ. J Pharm Sci 2002; 91:1186–1190.

131. Yokota M, Mochizuki M, Saito K, et al. Chem Eng Commun 1999; 174:243–256.

132. Alleso M, Van Den Berg F, Cornett C, et al. J Pharm Sci 2008; 97:2145–2159.

133. Hosokawa K, Goto J, Hirayama N. Chem Pharm Bull 2005; 53:1296–1299.

134. Reichardt C. Org Process Res Dev 2007; 11:105–113.

135. Xu D, Redman-Furey N. Int J Pharm 2007; 339:175–188.
136. Mirmehrabi M, Rohani S. J Pharm Sci 2005; 94:1560–1576.
137. Gavezzotti A. Chem Eur J 1999; 5:567–576.
138. Florence AJ, Johnston A, Fernandes P, et al. J Appl Crystallogr 2006; 39:922–924.
139. Trask AV, Shan N, Motherwell WDS, et al. Chem Commun 2005; 880–882.
140. Chierotti MR, Gobetto R, Pellegrino L, et al. Cryst Growth Des 2008; 8:1454–1457.
141. Zhang GGZ, Henry RF, Borchardt TB, et al. J Pharm Sci 2007; 96:990–995.
142. Friscic T, Fabian L, Burley JC, et al. Chem Commun 2006; 5009–5011.
143. Trask AV, Jones W. Org Solid State React 2005; 254:41–70.
144. Wenger M, Bernstein J. Cryst Growth Des 2008; 8:1595–1598.
145. Basavoju S, Bostrom D, Velaga SP. Pharm Res 2008; 25:530–541.
146. Berry DJ, Seaton CC, Clegg W, et al. Cryst Growth Des 2008; 8:1697–1712.
147. Fabbiani FPA, Pulham CR. Chem Soc Rev 2006; 35:932–942.
148. Fabbiani FPA, Allan DR, Parsons S, et al. Cryst Eng Comm 2005; 7:179–186.
149. Gong YC, Collman BM, Mehrens SM, et al. J Pharm Sci 2008; 97:2130–2144.
150. Winn D, Doherty MF. AIChE J 2000; 46:1348–1367.
151. Threlfall TL. Analyst 1995; 120:2435–2460.
152. Yu L, Reutzel SM, Stephenson GA. Pharm Sci Technol Today 1998; 1:118–127.
153. Bragg WH, Bragg WL. X Rays and Crystal Structure. London: Bell & Sons Ltd, 1915.
154. Glusker JP, Lewis M, Rossi M. Crystal Structure Analysis for Chemists and Biologists. New York, Cambridge: VCH, 1994.
155. Ladd MFC, Palmer RA. Structure Determination By X-Ray Crystallography, New York, London: Kluwer Academic/Plenum Publishers, 2003.
156. George H. Stout and Lyle H. Jensen, X-Ray Structure Determination: A Practical Guide. New York: Wiley, 1989.
157. Young RA. The Rietveld Method. Oxford: Oxford University Press, 1993.
158. David WIF. Structure Determination from Powder Diffraction Data. Oxford: Oxford University Press, 2002.
159. Klug HP, Alexander LE. X-Ray Diffraction Procedures for Polycrystalline and Amorphous Materials. 2nd ed. New York, London: Wiley-Interscience [S.l.], 1974.
160. Sheldrick GM. Acta Crystallogr 1984; A 40(suppl S):C440.
161. Sheldrick GM. Acta Crystallogr Sect A 2008; 64:112–122.
162. Spek AL. J Appl Crystallogr 2003; 36:7–13.
163. Macrae CF, Edgington PR, McCabe P, et al. J Appl Crystallogr 2006; 39:453–457.
164. Clegg W, Teat SJ. Acta Crystallogr Sect C Cryst Struct Commun 2000; 56:1343–1345.
165. Frampton CS, Knight KS, Shankland N, et al. J Mol Struct 2000; 520:29–32.
166. David WIF, Shankland K, McCusker LB, et al. eds. Structure Determination from Powder Diffraction Data. Oxford: Oxford University Press, 2002.
167. Florence AJ, Baumgartner B, Weston C, et al. J Pharm Sci 2003; 92:1930–1938.
168. Barr G, Dong W, Gilmore CJ. J Appl Crystallogr 2004; 37:658–664.
169. Albers D, Galgoci M, King D, et al. Org Process Res Dev 2007; 11:846–860.
170. Nishimoto Y, Kaneki Y, Kishi A. Anal Sci 2004; 20:1079–1082.
171. Louër D. In: David WIF, ed. Structure Determination from Powder Diffraction Data. Oxford, New York: Oxford University Press, 2002:xvii, 337.
172. Dollase WA. J Appl Crystallogr 1986; 19:267–272.
173. Jarvinen M. J Appl Crystallogr 1993; 26:525–531.
174. Chikhalia V, Forbes RT, Storey RA, et al. Eur J Pharm Sci 2006; 27:19–26.
175. Heng JYY, Thielmann F, Williams DR. Pharm Res 2006; 23:1918–1927.
176. Lee AY, Myerson AS. MRS Bull 2006; 31:881–886.
177. Dilworth SE, Buckton G, Gaisford S, et al. Int J Pharm 2004; 284:83–94.
178. Lappalainen M, Pitkanen I, Harjunen P. Int J Pharm 2006; 307:150–155.
179. Lehto VP, Tenho M, Vaha-Heikkila K, et al. Powder Technol 2006; 167:85–93.
180. Strachan CJ, Rades T, Gordon KC, et al. J Pharm Pharmacol 2007; 59:179–192.
181. Vemuri NM, Chrzan Z, Cavatur R. J Therm Anal Calorim 2004; 78:55–62.

182. Young PM, Chiou H, Tee T, et al. Drug Dev Ind Pharm 2007; 33:91–97.

183. Zeitler JA, Taday PF, Newnham DA, et al. J Pharm Pharmacol 2007; 59:209–223.

184. Faber J, Fawcett T. Acta Crystallogr Sect B Struct Sci 2002; 58:325–332.

185. Barr G, Gilmore CJ, Paisley J. J Appl Crystallogr 2004; 37:665–668.

186. Pawley GS. J Appl Crystallogr 1981; 14:357–361.

187. Johnston A, Florence AJ, Kennedy AR. Acta Crystallogr Sect E Struct Rep Online 2006; 62:O2288–O2290.

188. Dupont L, Dideberg O. Acta Crystallogr Sect B Struct Crystallogr Cryst Chem 1972; B 28:2340–2347.

189. Bruno IJ, Cole JC, Edgington PR, et al. Acta Crystallogr Sect B Struct Sci 2002; 58:389–397.

190. Leech CK, Florence AJ, Shankland K, et al. Acta Crystallogr Sect E Struct Rep Online 2007; 63:O675–O677.

191. Karami S, Li Y, Hughes DS, et al. Acta Crystallogr Sect B Struct Sci 2006; 62:689–691.

192. Stephenson GA. J Pharm Sci 2006; 95:821–827.

193. Rietveld HM. J Appl Crystallogr 1969; 2:65–71.

194. Harris KDM, Cheung EY. Org Process Res Dev 2003; 7:970–976.

195. Fernandes P, Florence AJ, Shankland K, et al. Acta Crystallogr Sect E Struct Rep Online 2007; 63:O202–O204.

196. Hulme AT, Fernandes P, Florence A, et al. Acta Crystallogr Sect E Struct Rep Online 2006; 62:O3752–O3754.

197. Pagola S, Stephens PW, Bohle DS, et al. Nature 2000; 404:307–310.

198. Deem MW, Newsam JM. Nature 1989; 342:260–262.

199. Reinaudi L, Leiva EPM, Carbonio RE. J Chem Soc Dalton Trans 2000; 4258–4262.

200. Edgar M, Carter VJ, Grewal P, et al. Chem Mater 2002; 14:3432–3439.

201. Ivashevskaja SN, Aleshina LA, Andreev VP, et al. Acta Crystallogr Sect C Cryst Struct Commun 2002; 58:m300–m301.

202. Dinnebier RE, Wagner M, Peters F, et al. Z Anorg Allg Chem 2000; 626:1400–1405.

203. Espallargas GM, Hippler M, Florence AJ, et al. J Am Chem Soc 2007; 129:15606–15614.

204. Fernandes P, Shankland K, Florence AJ, et al. J Pharm Sci 2007; 96:1192–1202.

205. Florence A, Johnston A, Fernandes P, et al. Acta Crystallogr Sect E Struct Rep Online 2005; 61:O2798–O2800.

206. Fernandes P, Florence AJ, Shankland K, et al. Acta Crystallogr Sect E Struct Rep Online 2006; 62:O2216–O2218.

207. Florence AJ, Johnston A, Shankland K. Acta Crystallogr Sect E Struct Rep Online 2005; 61:O2974–O2977.

208. Chernyshev VV, Stephens PW, Yatsenko AV, et al. J Pharm Sci 2004; 93:3090–3095.

209. Stephenson GA. J Pharm Sci 2000; 89:958–966.

210. Lewis GR, Steele G, McBride L, et al. Cryst Growth Des 2005; 5:427–438.

211. Nishibori E, Ogura T, Aoyagi S, et al. J Appl Crystallogr 2008; 41:292–301.

212. Remenar JF, Peterson ML, Stephens PW, et al. Mol Pharm 2007; 4:386–400.

213. Pagola S, Tracanna MI, Amani SM, et al. Nat Prod Commun 2008; 3:759–764.

214. Nunes C, Suryanarayanan R, Botez CE, et al. J Pharm Sci 2004; 93:2800–2809.

215. Platteau C, Lefebvre J, Affouard F, et al. Acta Crystallogr Sect B Struct Sci 2004; 60:453–460.

216. van Mechelen JB, Peschar R, Schenk H. Acta Crystallogr Sect B Struct Sci 2008; 64:240–248.

217. Shankland K, David WIF. In: David WIF, Shankland K, McCusker LB, et al. eds. Structure Determination from Powder Diffraction Data. Oxford: Oxford University Press, 2002:252–285.

218. Bruno IJ, Cole JC, Kessler M, et al. J Chem Inf Comput Sci 2004; 44:2133–2144.

219. Middleton DA, Peng X, Saunders D, et al. Chem Commun 2002; 1976–1977.

220. Shankland K, David WIF, Sivia DS. J Materials Chem 1997; 7:569–572.

221. National Institute of Standards & Technology, Standard Reference Material® 640c: Silicon Powder Line Position and Line Shape Standard for Powder Diffraction, The certified lattice parameter for a temperature of 22.5°C is 0.54311946 nm ± 0.00000092 nm.

222. Boultif A, Louer D. J Appl Crystallogr 1991; 24:987–993.

223. Boultif A, Louer D. J Appl Crystallogr 2004; 37:724–731.

224. Visser J. J Appl Crystallogr 1969; 2:89–95.

225. Werner PE, Eriksson L, Westdahl M. J Appl Crystallogr 1985; 18:367–370.

226. Altomare A, Giacovazzo C, Guagliardi A, et al. J Appl Crystallogr 2000; 33:1180–1186.

227. Coelho AA. J Appl Crystallogr 2003; 36:86–95.

228. Le Bail A. Powder Diffr 2004; 19:249–254.

229. Neumann MA. J Appl Crystallogr 2003; 36:356–365.

230. David WIF, Shankland K, van de Streek J, et al. J Appl Crystallogr 2006; 39:910–915.

231. Putz H, Schon JC, Jansen M. J Appl Crystallogr 1999; 32:864–870.

232. Le Bail A. In Epdic 7. Eur Powder Diff 2001; (pts 1 and 2):65–70.

233. Favre-Nicolin V, Cerny R. J Appl Crystallogr 2002; 35:734–743.

234. Engel GE, Wilke S, Konig O, et al. J Appl Crystallogr 1999; 32:1169–1179.

235. Stephens PW, Huq A. Trans Am Crystallogr Assoc 2002; 27:127–144.

236. Coelho AA. J Appl Crystallogr 2000; 33:899–908.

237. Larson AC, Von Dreele RB. General Structure Analysis System (GSAS). Report LAUR 86-748. New Mexico, USA, Los Alamos National Laboratory, 2004.

238. Barr G, Dong W, Gilmore CJ, et al. J Appl Crystallogr 2005; 38:833–841.

239. Gelbrich T, Hursthouse MB. Cryst Eng Comm 2005; 7:324–336.

240. McKinnon JJ, Mitchell AS, Spackman MA. Chem Eur J 1998; 4:2136–2141.

241. de Wolff PM. J Appl Crystallogr 1968; 1:108–113.

242. Smith GS, Snyder RL. J Appl Crystallogr 1979; 12:60–65.

243. Markvardsen AJ, David WIF, Johnson JC, et al. Acta Crystallogr Sect A 2001; 57:47–54.

244. Le Bail A, Duroy H, Fourquet JL. Mater Res Bull 1988; 23:447–452.

245. David WIF, Sivia DS. In: David WIF, Shankland K, McCusker LB, et al. eds. Structure Determination from Powder Diffraction Data. Oxford: Oxford University Press, 2002:136–161.

246. Florence AJ, Shankland N, Shankland K, et al. J Appl Crystallogr 2005; 38:249–259.

247. Zachariasen WH, Ellinger FH. Acta Crystallogr 1963; 16:777–783.

248. Shankland K, David WIF, Csoka T. Z Kristallogr 1997; 212:550–552.

249. Madsen IC, Hill RJ. J Appl Crystallogr 1994; 27:385–392.

250. van Mechelen JB, Peschar R, Schenk H. Acta Crystallogr Sect B Struct Sci 2006; 62:1131–1138.

251. Karamertzanis PG, Anandamanoharan PR, Fernandes P, et al. J Phys Chem B 2007; 111:5326–5336.

252. Florence AJ, Shankland K, Gelbrich T, et al. Cryst Eng Comm 2008; 10:26–28.

9

Excipient Design and Characterization

Graham Buckton
School of Pharmacy, University of London, London, and Pharmaterials Ltd., Reading, U.K.

INTRODUCTION

With only a few exceptions, for example, some inhalation products, active pharmaceutical ingredients are converted to medicines through the thoughtful incorporation of excipients. A potentially valuable drug substance, which could bring life-changing benefits to millions of patients, can be rendered worthless by poor formulation, and equally, actives of moderate properties can become valuable medicines by optimized delivery methods. For the majority of medicines it can be expected that the combined excipient content in the formulation will greatly exceed the mass of active. The selection of suitable excipients and the proportions used will be determined on the basis of the desired route of administration, the dose, the physicochemical properties of the active (preformulation is covered elsewhere and will be the starting point for the process of excipient selection), and the proposed method of manufacture for the product.

Excipients are added for many reasons, which can broadly be divided into two, the first being to aid in the process of making a medicine and the second to ensure reproducible release of the active from the medicine at a desired rate. The ability to manufacture a product with suitable and reproducible properties (including uniformity of content of the active in the unit dose, suitable physical and chemical stability, etc.) and a controlled and reproducible dissolution rate combine to define the quality of the medicine, which is an essential part of determining the safety and efficacy of that medicine. Taking the example of an uncoated tablet formulation to be prepared by wet granulation, a reasonable list of excipients could be

In the granule:

1. Diluent (possible too with different compaction properties)
2. Binder
3. Disintegrant

In the tablet mixed after granulation:

4. Disintegrant
5. Antiadherent

6. Die wall lubricant
7. Surfactant

Of this list, excipients 1, 2, 5, and 6 are added to assist in the manufacturing process, and (possibly) 1, 3, and 7 can assist in the process of dissolution. What is certain is that the functionality of these excipients, the quantity used, and the way in which they are added will be central to the properties of the tablet produced. It is no exaggeration to say that the quality, safety, and efficacy of the medicine will be related to the way these excipients perform.

The chapters "The Solid State" and "Preformulation" in this volume reveal that a great deal of effort is taken to control the physicochemical nature of the active in any medicine, and that failure to do so will cause a great risk to the patient. It would be logical therefore for us to believe that excipients are chemically pure, well-controlled materials with well-known physicochemical properties; however, that is often not the case. Many excipients are manufactured in bulk to serve many industries, the pharmaceutical industry often being a very small part of the market. The specification of the excipient may therefore be very wide, allowing considerable variation. In this chapter, a few examples of variability in excipients will be described to demonstrate some of the problems that can be encountered.

The basis of this chapter will be to review examples of variability in excipients and to show that variability is often linked to changes in functionality and that therefore we need to better characterize and understand excipients with respect to the key properties that link to functionality.

EXCIPIENTS WITH VARIABILITY OR A HISTORY OF VARIABILITY

Simply by way of example, a small number of excipients are described below to demonstrate the enormous scope for variability in the properties of commonly used excipients. The examples are not the only ones that show variability; indeed, variability is the norm rather than the exception. The polydispersity of polymeric excipients, the changes in surface activity of surfactants due to impurities and degradation products, and many more issues are not described here. For detailed reviews of individual excipients, the reader should consult the *Handbook of Pharmaceutical Excipients* (1). Often a tablet formulation will contain the active, plus two diluents (often lactose and microcrystalline cellulose) and magnesium stearate as a lubricant, along with other excipients. As examples, these commonly used excipients will be discussed below.

Magnesium Stearte

Magnesium stearate is the die wall lubricant of choice and as such is present in the vast majority of tablet formulations to aid the removal of the compressed tablet from the die of the machine. Lubricants, by their nature, tend to be hydrophobic materials, and magnesium stearate is no exception. It is well known, for example, that addition of magnesium stearate will have a tendency to slow the dissolution rate of the active from the tablet. It has been found that a small amount of the lubricant should be added, which should be of controlled small particle size and mixed just before tabletting, with the time of mixing being critical, as too much mixing can coat the particles to such an extent that they become excessively hydrophobic. In short, this is a vital excipient, without which the tablet would break on ejection from the tabletting machine, but it carries with it a disadvantage that its use can and will be detrimental to drug release. For such a critical excipient, one may expect that the purity and physical form would be meticulously controlled and defined to ensure that tablets can be made with reproducible properties. The reality, however, is that magnesium stearate has a notorious history of batch-to-batch and supplier-to-supplier variability.

The *British Pharmacopoeia* (2) defines magnesium stearate as

> "a mixture of magnesium salts of different fatty acids consisting mainly of stearic acid and palmitic acid and minor proportions of other fatty acids. It contains not less than 4.0% and not more than 5.0% of Mg.... The fatty acid fraction contains not les than 40.0% stearic acid and the sum of stearic and palmitic acid is not less than 90.0%"

On the basis of this pharmacopoeial monograph, it is clear that magnesium stearate is not chemically pure.

A good review of research undertaken on magnesium stearate is available in the *Handbook of Pharmaceutical Excipients* (1) where it is reported that

> ≈ It has not been conclusively established which form of pure magnesium stearate possesses the best lubricating properties. Commercial lots of magnesium stearate consist of mixtures of crystalline forms....

Here, crystalline forms refer to the presence of different polymorphic forms and different hydrate forms of magnesium stearate. As mentioned previously (and as reported in chap. 8, "The Solid State," this volume), it would be quite unacceptable for the crystalline form of a hydrophobic active ingredient to be uncontrolled in a medicine; and given that magnesium stearate has a major role in defining the quality and dissolution of tablets, it is important that its variability does not go unchecked.

Further, it is reported in the *Handbook of Pharmaceutical Excipients* (1) that

> ≈ Physical properties of magnesium stearate can vary among batches from different manufacturers because the solid-state characteristics are influenced by manufacturing variables. Variations in the physical properties of different lots of magnesium stearate from the same vendor have also been observed. Presumably because of these variations it has not been possible to conclusively correlate the dissolution rate retardation with observed lubricity...physical properties of different batches of magnesium stearate such as specific surface area, particle size, crystalline structure, moisture content, and fatty acid composition have been correlated with lubricant efficiency.... The hydrophobic nature of magnesium stearate can vary from batch to batch owing to the presence of water soluble, surface active impurities such as sodium stearate....

Here we see that three general things can vary, the chemical composition, the solid-state form (polymorphs/hydrates), and the bulk forms (size/surface area). Each of these things has an impact; for example, the surface-active impurity that is often present can mitigate the dissolution retardation. Presence or absence of this impurity can therefore potentially alter bioavailability. The different materials present, and their different physical forms, give rise to variations in lubricant efficiency (and hence product quality) as well as alter the strength of the tablets that are produced.

Relatively recently, when it is considered that this excipient has been used for a generation, the interconversion between magnesium stearate in the amorphous, anhydrate, dihydrate, and trihydrate forms was reported (3). It has been shown that the existence of these different hydrate levels will result in a significant change in the functionality of the excipient. One way by which the hydrate level on new batches of magnesium stearate can be studied is to use near-infrared (IR) spectroscopy, which is a rapid analytical method that shows very clear peaks in the second derivative spectra for water, and which is able to differentiate hydrate water from that which is more loosely associated with the solid.

There are serious questions that must be asked about magnesium stearate and whether it is fit for the purpose. Is it right to allow an excipient whose chemical composition can vary so much? Should there be only one allowable physical form? Should there be tight specification for bulk properties such as size? Should pharmacopoeias be setting specifications for functionality? The answers to these questions are, however, not easy. For example, it has been shown that chemically pure magnesium stearate is not as good a lubricant as the commercially available material(s). It is known that some existing products will work well when anhydrous magnesium stearate is used, and other products require hydrate forms of magnesium stearate to function properly. From this we can learn that it is not possible to limit the specification of this excipient to one form, but rather to have awareness of what is needed to make a specific product function and to have suitable testing in place to define the specification of the excipients that are used in that product. Extending from this, it is clear that pharmacopoeias can provide advice on functionality, this being an area of much current debate, but fundamentally it is a requirement of the pharmaceutical product manufacturer, rather than necessarily the excipient manufacturer, to define the specification that will be suitable, and most importantly that which will be unsuitable to allow the manufacture of high-quality, safe, and effective medicines.

While magnesium stearate will be present as (often less than) 1% of the mass of a tablet, it has a profound impact on the product that is produced, altering the tablet tensile strength and dissolution rate and being a cause of batch-to-batch variability. This example shows that the understanding of such a complex excipient will present difficulties, and that it is not possible to use any batch of the excipient from any supplier and expect to be able to make a good product.

Lactose

Lactose is added as an excipient into many solid oral dosage forms as well as inhalation products. It is one of the most commonly used pharmaceutical excipients. It is a sugar that can exist as α and β forms through rotation of the ring structure. The α form can exist as an anhydrate and a monohydrate, and this monohydrate form is what is known as lactose in the *British Pharmacopoeia*. It is known that these different forms of lactose have different compression properties, and this can give rise to tablets with quite different properties. It follows that a measurement of whether the supplied material is crystalline β-lactose, α-lactose or α-lactose monohydrate (or indeed a mixture of these) is an important thing to measure.

A further complexity with respect to lactose is that the crystalline form readily converts to the amorphous form during energetic processing, such as milling (4). Partially amorphous lactose is also commercially available (sold as spray-dried lactose, which usually contains 15% to 20% amorphous lactose with the remainder being crystalline) and is purchased because the amorphous material has better compression properties than the crystalline lactose alone. The amorphous material is plastic in nature and the crystalline material brittle, giving a good combination when compressed together, resulting in a strong tablet. Even for tabletting use, and much more significantly for inhalation use, there must be a concern if there is an uncontrolled change from material that is intended to be crystalline such that it becomes amorphous, and vice versa. As mentioned, it is easy to

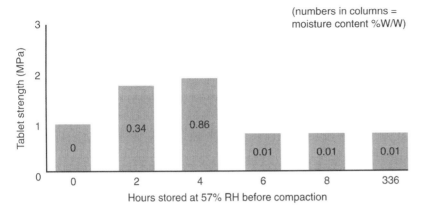

Figure 1 Schematic representation of the effect of water content on the compression properties of partially amorphous lactose. *Source*: From Ref. 5.

make crystalline lactose partially amorphous through processing, the recovery back to the crystalline state will be very rapid at humidity of 50% and above, but will be very slow at low humidity. This presence/absence of amorphous form (for lactose and indeed for many materials) can be a major cause of batch-to-batch variability.

Acknowledging that the purchase of spray-dried lactose (partially amorphous) is undertaken deliberately, and on the clear understanding that the partially amorphous excipient will compact in a preferred manner to crystalline lactose, it is important to consider how this thermodynamically unstable form will perform when exposed to humid conditions. Sebhatu et al. (5) showed that there was an immediate advantage of using partially amorphous lactose with respect to the strength of the tablet that was formed. In Figure 1, it can be seen that the strength of the tablets increased if the amorphous material was exposed to 57% relative humidity (RH) for up to four hours before the tabletting process. This was due to the increased water content (rising to 0.86%) causing the amorphous region to be plasticized (have increased mobility), which in turn has clearly facilitated the compaction process. However, if the material was stored at 57% RH for six hours or more, the tablets had lower strength, due to the fact that the amorphous lactose had crystallized prior to compaction, and thus the tablets were simply made from crystalline material. This raises an issue about how much of the material is amorphous and whether that material has crystallized during storage or during the processing (e.g., mixing, standing, transfer, and tabletting). If there is a goal to have uniform quality of product, then there is a need to study the physical form of the excipients and to know what is received into the production plant, and under what conditions that will change. The temperature and RH to which the sample is exposed, as well as the mass of material that has been stored, are significant to the tendency to crystallize. A small mass of sample (in milligram) will equilibrate rapidly with the environment and crystallize, whereas a 20-kg bag will have much slower equilibration. Buckton and Darcy (6) demonstrated this effect by investigating the rate of crystallization of amorphous lactose when stored in a 200 mL measuring cylinder. Rather than all spontaneously crystallizing when exposed to a humid environment, the sample crystallized gradually, taking 70 days for the material at the very bottom of the cylinder to crystallize (Fig. 2). This can be expected to happen in large containers of excipient, which are left open ready to use in manufacture; however, if agitated in a humid environment (during processing), it would be expected that

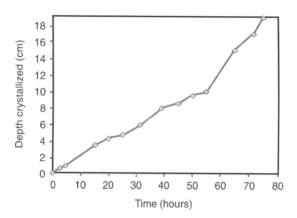

Figure 2 The depth of amorphous lactose that crystallizes in a 100 mL measuring cylinder when exposed to elevated humidity over 70 days. *Source*: From Ref. 6.

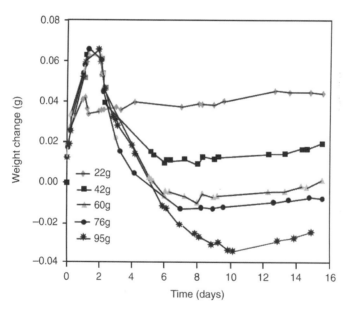

Figure 3 The mass change in a 100 mL measuring cylinder containing different masses of amorphous lactose, as a consequence of crystallization occurring gradually in the sample. *Source*: From Ref. 6.

crystallization would be much faster. Also of importance is the fact that a small amount of water is all that is needed to cause a large mass to crystallize. Darcy and Buckton (6) (Fig. 3) showed that the mass increase during bulk crystallization was not related to sample mass, with sample of 22 to 95 g all showing similar mass changes, which were much smaller than would be expected and which indicate that the surface saturates, crystallizes, and then passes the expelled water through the sample mass to be essentially reused, rather than a substantial water sorption throughout the sample mass prior to any crystallization onset, hence the properties of bulk samples are different from those of small ones, but only a small amount of water ingress can spoil a large sample of partially amorphous lactose eventually, causing the entire amorphous content to crystallize.

From this section, it should be clear that input materials of complex physical nature should be tested on receipt, prior to use, and the transitions that may occur during processing must be fully investigated and understood.

THE EVOLUTION OF EXCIPIENTS AND NEW HIGH-FUNCTIONALITY EXCIPIENTS

The regulatory consideration of excipients is such that approval will be given for the use of an excipient that has been used previously and demonstrated to be safe at the proposed level of exposure for the same duration (chronic vs. acute treatment) and by the same route of administration. An exception to this would be materials that have been used in foods for a long time and which are designated as "generally recognized as safe" (GRAS). It follows that an existing excipient used in a different way (e.g., different route of administration) or an entirely new excipient will be subject to requirements for extensive safety/toxicity testing. The International Conference on Harmonisation (ICH), in ICH S7A provides the required testing for a new excipient, which includes toxicity testing in rodents and nonrodent mammals, including adsorption, metabolism, and excretion studies; genetic toxicity studies; and reproductive toxicology testing, for periods that reflect the duration of intended use.

Regulatory authorities do not approve excipients, rather they consider applications for medicines that contain an active and an excipient. Thus the only way to get regulatory approval for a new excipient is to test it with an active and present that data to the authorities. Relatively few companies are willing to risk a new excipient with a new chemical entity, as it could conceivably slow the process of licensing (or at least be perceived to risk slowing the licensing process). It is not surprising then that the vast majority of products that come to market use well-established excipients. In rare cases, a company will take on the challenge of developing a new excipient and bringing it to market, with all the associated costs of safety testing. One such example in recent years is Captisol (sulfobutylether-β-cyclodextrin). Cyclodextrins are toroidal-shaped molecules formed by sugars that exhibit a hydrophilic outside and a hydrophobic internal face of the ring structure. As such these molecules are ideal to host a hydrophobic drug molecule into the ring and allow it to be dissolved in water. The increase in solubility in water can be by orders of magnitude, and this can make drugs of very low solubility become viable to deliver by parenteral and oral routes. Despite a number of cyclodextrins being in existence, the most regularly used is the β-form, which has been shown to be safe and used in licensed products. The development of Captisol came about as it was well suited to host the Pfizer compound. Cydex Inc. developed Captisol with significant assistance from Pfizer, who carried out the safety package with respect to the very insoluble antifungal drug voriconazole, which was required to be solubilized for intravenous (IV) formulation. An extensive review of the development of this excipient has been presented by Thompson (7), where it has been reported that the cost of undertaking the safety assessment for this new excipient was in excess of US$30 million. This level of investment can only be justified on rare occasions, in reality, when a major active pharmaceutical could not successfully come to market using any other available technology. Potentially an excipient manufacturer could consider the development of a new excipient of this sort alone, but there would need to be great confidence that the commercial value as a drug delivery tool was sufficiently exclusive (strong patent position) and valuable for the large costs to be recovered. Even then it is not obvious that many excipient companies would have the resources to invest this sort of money in a potential new excipient.

Given the major hurdle in bringing new excipients to market, excipient manufacturers have worked on combinations and adaptations of existing materials to enhance functionality. Adaptation of existing excipients includes not only the adaptation of solid-state properties, for example, the sale of spray dried, partially amorphous, lactose to enhance the compressibility but also changes in size, shape, surface area, porosity, etc. These different particle properties will alter flow (uniformity of content of solid dosage forms), compressibility, and also dissolution rates.

The advantage of coprocessed materials is that functionality can be changed, but as there is no covalent bonding between the materials, there is no new chemical entity formed, and thus no need for new toxicology. The development and use of coprocessed, high-functionality excipients raise interesting questions about control of functionality.

As mentioned above, excipients are generally poorly controlled (at least in comparison to the active), so if functionality can be enhanced by processing and adding small amounts of another material to an existing excipient [the example used below is silicified microcrystalline cellulose (SMCC)], then to what extent may the functionality of many other excipients change because of variation in chemical composition and modest control over the manufacturing processes? To be clear, there is no suggestion that well-manufactured and coprocessed materials are flawed or suffer from quality defects (indeed they are often controlled to very high standards in comparison to other excipients), but rather the argument being made is that coprocessing gives rise to major changes in properties (deliberately), which could easily be exhibited by batch variability in content or manufacture of other excipients (accidentally).

Silicified Microcrystalline Cellulose (Prosolv SMCC)

Microcrystalline cellulose has been used for many years as a tabletting excipient. It has a history of supplier-to-supplier variability and batch-to-batch variability, relating to the method of manufacture, but such concerns are no longer reported with excellent product being available from a number of well-established excipient suppliers. One reported change in microcrystalline cellulose is the reduction in compressibility following wet granulation (8). A proposed solution to this problem was the coprocessed excipient SMCC. Coprocessed excipients are attractive as the actives are chemically the same as materials that are used to date, but the functionality is claimed to be superior to simple physical mixtures, by way of some physicochemical interaction during the coprocessing stage.

Microcrystalline cellulose is prepared by spray drying, and when colloidal silica is introduced to this process (rather than physically mixing after preparation of the microcrystalline cellulose), it is claimed that there are benefits (9). Edge et al. (9) reported that unlubricated compacts of SMCC produced "enhanced strength . . . greater stiffness and required considerably more energy for tensile failure to occur. Comparison of the data with that obtained for a dry blend of silicon dioxide/microcrystalline cellulose suggested that the functionality benefits of silicification were not due to a simple composite material model."

JRS Pharma has a number of case studies of how SMCC results in changes in properties of products. One is a report of a tablet formulation for a high-dose active, which yielded weak tablets resulting in breakage in the coating pan. The tablets were oval shaped

9×20 mm^2, with height of 5.9 mm, and the mass was 1070 mg. The failing friable tablet was formulated with 8% microcrystalline cellulose, and the challenge was to optimize the formulation to reduce friability while maintaining tablet size (which was deemed to be as large as could be tolerated). The original formulation broke under a force of 30 N; addition of 25% microcrystalline cellulose resulted in a formulation that had sufficient strength (130 N breaking strength), but a formulation containing 12% SMCC had a breaking strength of 230 N. The 25% microcrystalline cellulose formulation had to be a larger tablet, whereas the 12% SMCC was the same size as the original failing formulation. These data indicate that the intentional addition of a small amount of colloidal silica resulted in a benefit for this formulation—improved strength, removed issued of failure during coating, and no increase in tablet size. This shows two things: the first is that coprocessing is an interesting way of enhancing excipient properties. The second is more of a concern and suggests that if intentional minor changes in excipients can have substantial effects on the product, then accidental (or uncontrolled) variability could likewise have major significance. Given what has been said earlier in this chapter about the poor control of many pharmaceutical excipients, it can be expected that variability will be common for many formulations and that the excipient variability may often cause batch-to-batch variability in the pharmaceutical product.

The development of coprocessed excipients has mostly been to address issues in tabletting, and especially to facilitate the economically favored approach of direct compression. The needs for direct compression are good flow properties, excellent compression, and then rapid disintegration and dissolution. Flow is largely optimized by control of particle size distribution and is thus enhanced by granulation. For direct compression, a goal would be to have excipients, which aid flow to such an extent that glidants are not required (colloidal silica is the most common glidant and comes with handling difficulties due to it slow bulk density and inhalation risk). A number of coprocessed excipients have shown improved flow in certain circumstances [e.g., Cellactose (10), a lactose and microcrystalline cellulose combination, and SMCC (11)]. The second important feature for direct compression is the improvements in compressibility feature. Here Cellactose, SMCC, and Ludipress (a lactose/polyvinylpyrrolidone product) have all been shown to have better properties than the respective physical mixtures of their components (12–14).

FUNCTIONALITY TESTING/QUALITY BY DESIGN

As described above, excipients are often not pure chemical entities and have complexity because of impurities, changes in polymorph, hydrate, solvate, amorphous form and variability in particle size and shape. Given that the pharmaceutical industry is highly regulated, it is not a surprise that there is a serious effort to improve the understanding of the key properties that link to functionality, indeed this has become an area that the pharmacopoeias have started to consider. There are, however, major challenges in this respect; for example, it is clear that the suitability of magnesium stearate to function as a lubricant will be affected greatly by the nature of the material. So the anhydrous and hydrate forms will have different functionality, but that does not mean that all formulations will be best served by using the hydrate or vice versa, rather the manufacturer will need to understand for their product(s), which will be the key parameters that must be controlled. This will to a greater or lesser extent be the same for all excipients. While there may be general characteristics that can be defined as critical (e.g., the surface area of magnesium stearate), the definition of good and bad material will be harder as that is formulation specific. While it is good that the key parameters will be defined by pharmacopoeias, it is right that these will not be mandatory. Further complications arise as a number of excipients are used for different functions and in different types of dosage forms. Lactose, for example, is often seen in tablets, hard-gelatin capsules, and dry powder inhaler formulations. Clearly the compaction properties that are essential for tablets do not form part of the requirement when the other two formulations are considered. Thus, different physicochemical properties are needed for each route and formulation. The very significant challenge ahead is that pharmaceutical manufacturers must define suitable functionality attributes for excipients and be able to guarantee these are sufficiently well controlled and measured to be certain that the product will be of the desired quality. This is an essential part of the quality by design concept and puts a great demand on pharmaceutical materials science as a discipline.

Excipient Characterization

Given that the quality of many excipients will not improve, the concept of quality by design demands that the characterization of excipients will become ever more important. At this time, the users of excipients may well only test incoming materials for identity and chemical purity, which is in keeping with traditional pharmacopoeial requirements. Obvious extensions to this would include the particle size distribution; for example, many excipients are sold by grades that relate to particle size (e.g., microcrystalline cellulose) and changes in size alter flow, compression properties, and tablet characteristics (such as breaking strength, friability, disintegration). Most probably the future will require in-house functionality tests for supplies of excipients; these will include size distribution, surface area, density measurements, and indications of compaction. The choice of method to assess compaction is wide, ranging from microindentation of crystals or compacts through to force compaction profiles using instrumented tablet presses or compaction simulators. From these data, a knowledge of the brittle/plastic and elastic nature of the materials will be obtained, and this will be used to make sure that the tablet is suitably balanced in properties to be a reliable product. None of these methods are without issues; for example, the notionally simple thing of measuring particle size is complicated where different methods give different challenges, all relating to the ability to disperse the particles and prevent aggregation without causing size reduction, followed by the arithmetic treatment of the measurement (where most methods assume spherical particles).

For dry powder inhalers, lactose is the most often used carrier, here the active is present in very small amounts due to the low-dose needs for the inhaled route. The carrier is there to allow uniform dose delivery and work by a weak adhesion of the active to the carrier (often long-range forces with strengths of 20–40 kJ/mol may be involved). It follows that the key properties that are required of lactose for inhalation will be those that cause good mixing and uniform adhesion of the active to the carrier and allow for reproducible drug release from the carrier when the patient inhales. This balance of adhesive and cohesive forces is influenced by the size, shape, and roughness of the surface of the carrier. Further factors such as changes in form (polymorphs, isomers, anomers, amorphous forms, hydrates) alter these interactions, at least in part due to changes in the surface energy.

The goal is to understand the material properties that will be critical and the interplay between the processing and the formulation components. By high-quality materials science and analysis and suitable data handling, it will become possible to improve our understanding of the key factors that influence product quality to such an extent that the requirements for the active and excipients will be defined, and the

Table 1 The Dispersive Surface Energy of Lactose Determined Using IGC

Sample	Dispersive surface energy (mJ/m^2)
Crystalline	31.2 ± 1.1
Spray dried (completely amorphous)	37.1 ± 2.3
Milled (0.7% amorphous)	41.6 ± 1.4
Physical mixture 99% crystalline and 1% amorphous	31.5 ± 0.4

Abbreviation: IGC, inverse phase gas chromatography.
Source: Ref. 15.

specifications set such that as long as they meet those requirements, the processing will result in product of suitable characteristics.

The complexity of testing needed for excipients will be product and process dependent. Newell et al. (15) have shown that the surface energy of a material changes when it is milled; these data are shown in Table 1, where it can be seen that the dispersive surface energy for crystalline lactose is substantially different from that for amorphous lactose and that milled lactose has a dispersive energy that is different again. The milled lactose has an amorphous content of about 1% and a surface energy very different from that of a mixture of 99% crystalline lactose and 1% amorphous lactose. This demonstrates that milling can make the surface of materials amorphous, and this will result in a change in surface energy, which in turn will alter functionality, such as mixing, granulation, inhalation performance, and potentially many others. Although this is a reasonable general statement, the practical reality is that some formulations will be more sensitive to the effects of changes in surface energy than others. A further complication will be the tendency of amorphous materials to change with time. This relaxation in the amorphous state (including the amorphous material on the surface of milled material) can result in morphological (16) and surface energy changes (17).

Formulation development, when undertaken using the principles of quality by design, will need to include an understanding of how materials and processes interact to provide potential effects on the product and to make the necessary measurements and studies to give understanding and control.

EXCIPIENT COMPATIBILITY TESTING

A key aspect of developing a formulation is to understand the balance between the functionality and stability. For example, often those formulation efforts that enhance solubility of an active can give stability problems. The final formulation may therefore be a trade off between those aspects that are needed to give adequate bioavailability and those which will give a suitably long shelf life without the need for unusual storage conditions. While the stability of the product will be dominated by the inherent stability of the active, it is also possible that an otherwise stable active can be destabilized by an interaction with one or more excipients.

Excipient compatibility studies are carried out during preformulation essentially to rule out excipients (or combinations) that are predicted to be too detrimental to the stability of the final product. The ultimate test of a product is what happens in real-time room temperature storage, and all other tests are accelerated to estimate with a greater or lesser degree of accuracy and predictive ability. There are a few well-known excipient interactions, and then there are many that are not reported and for which the mechanism is never studied. The Maillard reaction is the best known and occurs between lactose

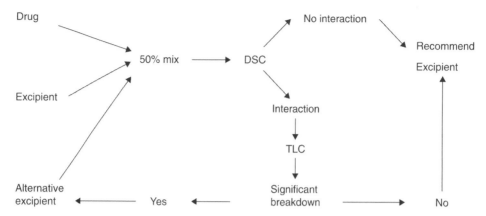

Figure 4 Schematic plan for excipient compatibility testing by DSC. This flow chart scheme is reported in many texts. *Abbreviation*: DSC, differential scanning calorimetry.

(more accurately reducing sugars) and primary amines, which should be avoided in combination in any product.

Conventional excipient compatibility testing is based on the fact that a reaction will more or less double in rate with each 10°C increase in temperature. The choice of conditions for a compatibility study is not defined by regulators (as they are concerned with the final product), which will vary between companies. Broadly, the higher the temperature of storage is, the more rapidly it will be possible to determine if an interaction has taken place. Assuming a good HPLC method is available, storage at 60°C for one to two months may be sufficient. This does obviously assume that the same reactions happen at room temperature as at the elevated temperature, which is an assumption that gets less reliable as the temperature of storage is raised. The alternative of storing samples at 50°C or 40°C will result in longer storage times before knowing if there are any issues. It follows that the data for excipient compatibility testing may well be rate limiting in formulation development, and as such there is a need for a rapid method. Differential scanning calorimetry (DSC) has long been proposed as a rapid method. The much-used schematic of this is shown in Figure 4.

DSC is a technique in which a sample and reference pan are heated, and any events that take place in one pan give rise to a heat change, which either alters the power needed to heat that pan (power compensation) or the heat flow from or to that pan (heat flux). Consequently any reactions that take place in the calorimeter pan may be detectable if the heat generation is adequate. As the heat flow in any calorimetric experiment (this being true for scanning calorimetry and isothermal calorimetry, although with the former method the scan rate will also have an effect) will relate to the enthalpy of the reaction, the rate of the reaction, and the concentration of the reactants, it will be complicated to interpret the data for unknown reactions. A real complexity for the design of the experiment is the concentration term. For liquid-state reactions we understand concentration well; however, for solid-state reactions the concentration relates to the area of point contacts between particles and will be altered by particle size, the degree of packing of the particles, and possibly the presence of moisture that may condense at these contact points (Fig. 5). It follows that the rate of reaction between an active and an excipient could change if the particle size and degree of consolidation (powder mix to granule to tablet) are altered. This alone makes it impossible to judge the consequence of a potential interaction in relation to the shelf life of a final product, from simple powder mixtures. A further complexity in calorimetric data interpretation is that the signal is a function of

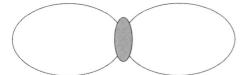

Figure 5 Schematic indication of the "concentration" term of a solid-state reaction. The actual mass of the sample is not all available, being limited to the areas of contact between particles. The contact area can be mediated by condensed water (*shown in shaded area*).

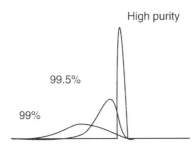

Figure 6 Schematic (and exaggerated to demonstrate the point) indication of how a melting point peak would tend to alter as purity is reduced.

reaction rate and enthalpy. As the enthalpy is unknown, there will be no observable difference between a fast reaction of low enthalpy and a slow reaction of high enthalpy, and clearly these have very different consequences for a product as a fast reaction has a greater impact on shelf life.

It is worthwhile to consider the value of DSC for excipient compatibility studies. The major advantage of DSC studies is that the results are available rapidly. An interaction would be shown by a comparison of data for the active and the excipient alone with the response that is measured when their mixture is run in the DSC. If a new peak is seen or any expected peak is lost or altered in shape, then a reaction is believed to be present. The basis for the measurement is in part linked to the fact that the purity of a material can be seen as a change in the measured melting response. In Figure 6, the effect of purity of a substance on the peak shape of the melt seen by DSC is shown (much exaggerated to demonstrate the concept). For most actives, the melting point will be higher than the melting point (if any) of the excipient, and if there is any degradation during the heating, then the melt of the active may be seen to change. This requires the acceleration of the reaction to have been very substantial, such that it is a measurable difference after a short (at most an hour or so) DSC experiment. The basis for this is the approximate doubling of reaction rate for a 10°C increase in temperature, so by the time the temperature has reached a melt at, for example, 250°C, the degradation will have been sufficiently fast to be measurable. The major disadvantage is that the data are not necessarily reliable. From the discussion above, it can be seen that the use of DSC provides, at best, an indication of the presence or absence of an interaction between a drug and an excipient and does not allow the investigator to judge the consequence of the interaction on the shelf life of the product with any great consequence; however, this is the least of the worries when using this method. Other concerns include the fact that the reaction may not be measurable due to limited particle contact, for example, this would give a false negative, that is, apparent stability when there may be a significant reaction. False positives are also possible; indeed these are common when using certain excipients. If we consider the test for an interaction between magnesium stearate and a crystalline hydrophobic drug with a melting point of 250°C, then the mixture (usually 50:50) of the two would be heated and the magnesium stearate would be seen to melt at around 88°C. The drug would then be expected to melt at 250°C, and any loss of this melt would be interpreted as an interaction. What will usually happen is that the drug will dissolve in the molten magnesium stearate (given that the drug is hydrophobic and will have some reasonable level of solubility in this molten wax), resulting in either the complete or partial loss of the melt response for the drug. This does not in fact tell us whether there was a chemical reaction between the two materials, but by applying the logic that the loss of the melting peak of the drug is an indication of interaction, this would result in the exclusion of what may be a perfectly good lubricant from the formulation. As a result of these false negatives, there is no real value in the study of hydrophobic drugs with waxy excipients, and certainly no justification for the exclusion of magnesium stearate on the basis of a DSC test. A further issue with magnesium stearate testing is that as a lubricant it will be used in very small mass in the final formulation (maybe 0.5%), but in an excipient compatibility test it will need to be studied in much high proportions to allow detection of any possible issue. This elevated concentration again gives a risk of detecting interactions that are false positives. In summary therefore, while DSC seems like an attractive option for excipient compatibility testing due to the speed with which data are generated, the occurrence of false positives and negatives makes the use of this method too unreliable for routine use. As such there remains a need for a more reliable rapid method to aid the formulation development process.

Isothermal microcalorimetry is a technique by which heat flow to or from a sample is studied as a function of time at a set temperature. Modern isothermal calorimeters are very sensitive and can achieve orders of magnitude of greater sensitivity than DSC experiments. It is appealing to consider use of such experiments to study compatibility whereby a powder mix can be stored in a sealed ampoule and studied as a function of time. The major issues here are whether a large-enough signal will be measured, and that will depend upon the $\approx$ concentration... (related to powder/powder contact area as discussed above), the enthalpy, and the rate of the reaction(s) taking place. While one might expect an oxidation reaction (usually high enthalpy) to be detected reasonably well, hydrolysis reactions often have much lower enthalpy change and may well be missed. A second issue with these experiments is that all processes that happen can be measured; so physical processes (e.g., redistribution of water) would also be detected and could be misinterpreted as a damaging reaction between active and excipient. A way to get around these issues is to consider isothermal measurements at a series of temperatures, with rapid changes between temperatures. The best way to do this is to use a high-sensitivity DSC with a large sample pan (e.g., 1–2 mL) so that interactions can be monitored at near room temperature and then the temperature increased sequentially to 40°C, 50°C, and 60°C with a suitably long holding time at each temperature to monitor the heat flow. If there is displacement from baseline and if that displacement is seen to accelerate, then an interaction can be predicted. In Figure 7, data are shown for an aspirin-containing tablet (to generate these unpublished data, a commercial aspirin tablet was ground up and mixed with extra excipient) and magnesium stearate, here we see that as the temperature of the experiment is increased, there is deviation of the heat flow from baseline. The complexity of the data is not something that is interpreted; rather it is the existence of a heat flow that shows an interaction. By contrast, when the same ground tablet is mixed with starch, for which no interaction is expected, there is no deviation from baseline (Fig. 8, unpublished

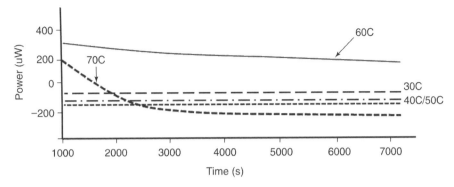

Figure 7 Interaction between magnesium stearate and an aspirin-containing formulation.

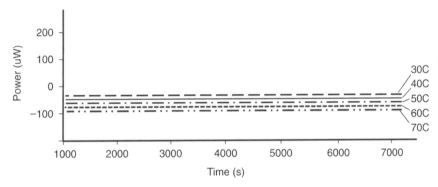

Figure 8 Excipient compatibility test of starch and an aspirin-containing formulation showing no interaction.

data). This approach is a more reliable method by which rapid assessment of compatibility can be determined. For the reasons discussed, all rapid methods have to be confirmed with analysis to assess the extent of reaction and to see if it is critical for the formulation, but this approach will allow development to progress with excipients that can reasonably be expected to yield stable product.

CONCLUSIONS

Increasingly over the year active pharmaceutical are getting harder to deliver by reasons of poor solubility and excipients are playing a more important role with respect to delivery of compounds. It will always be the case that the majority of excipients have greater tendency to be variable than the actives, and as such there needs to be an awareness of the critical parameters that influence functionality. Excipient manufacturers will utilize processing and coprocessing to produce high-value excipients that aid formulation.

Pharmaceutical manufacturers will have to understand the properties of excipients that influence product as part of the quality by design concept, and this will result in more extensive testing. The testing will initially be to show critical parameters that influence the processing and functionality and then will form part of the routine testing of input materials for processes.

Finally, there are advances in excipient-compatibility testing that can speed the progress to market.

The application of materials science to excipient development, the improvement of excipients, and their use in formulations will enhance the quality of the products that are made and reduce the tendency for batch failure, thus providing major economic benefits to the industry.

REFERENCES

1. Rowe RC, Sheskey P, Owen SC, eds. Handbook of Pharmaceutical Excipients. 5th ed. London: Pharmaceutical Press, 2006.
2. The British Pharmacopoeia, The Stationery Office, UK, 2008.
3. Bracconi P, Andres C, Ndiaye A. Structural properties of magnesium stearate pseudopolymorphs: effect of temperature. Int J Pharm 2003; 262:109–124.
4. Briggner L-E, Buckton G, Bystrom K, et al. The use of isothermal microcalorimetry in the study of changes in crystallinity induced during the processing of powders. Int J Pharm 1994; 105:125–135.
5. Sebhatu T, Elamin AA, Ahlneck C. Effect of moisture sorption on tabletting characteristics of spray dried (15% amorphous) lactose. Pharm Res 1994; 9:1233–1238.
6. Darcy P, Buckton G. Crystallization of bulk samples of partially amorphous spray-dried lactose. Pharm Dev Technol 1998; 3:503–507.
7. Thompson DO. Cyclodextrin—enabling excipients: a case study on the development of a new excipient—sulfobutylether-beta-cyclodextrin. In: Katdare A, Chaubal MV, eds. Excipient Development for Pharmaceutical, Biotechnology and Drug Delivery Systems. New York: Informa Healthcare, 2006:51–68.
8. Staniforth JN, Chatrath M. Towards a new class of high functionality tablet binders. I. Quasi-hornification of microcrystalline cellulose and loss of functionality. Pharm Res 1996; 12:S208.
9. Edge S, Steele DF, Chen A, et al. The mechanical properties of compacts of microcrystalline cellulose and silicified microcrystalline cellulose. Int J Pharm 2000; 200:67–72.
10. York P. Crystal engineering and particle design for the powder compaction process. Drug Dev Ind Pharm 1992; 18:677–721.
11. Allen JD. Improving DC with SMCC. Manuf Chemist 1996; 67:19–23.
12. Belda PM, Mielck JB. The tabletting behaviour of cellactose compared with mixtures of celluloses and lactose. Eur J Pharm Biopharm 1996; 42:325–330.
13. Sherwood B, Becker JW. A new class of high functionality excipients: silicified microcrystalline cellulose. Pharm Technol 1998; 22:78–88.
14. Schmidt PC, Rubensdorfer CJW. Evaluation of Ludipress as a "multipurpose excipient" for direct compression. Part 1. Powder characteristics and tabletting properties. Drug Dev Ind Pharm 1994; 29:2899–2925.
15. Newell HE, Buckton G, Butler DA, et al. The use of inverse phase gas chromatography to measure the surface energy of crystalline, amorphous, and recently milled lactose. Pharm Res 2001; 18:662–666.
16. Hogan SE, Buckton G. Water sorption/desorption—near IR and calorimetric study of crystalline and amorphous raffinose. Int J Pharm 2001; 227:57–69.
17. Newell HE, Buckton G, Butler DA, et al. The use of inverse phase gas chromatography to study the change of surface energy of amorphous lactose as a function of relative humidity and the processes of collapse and crystallisation. Int J Pharm 2001; 217:45–56.

10
Preformulation

Gavin W. Halbert
Cancer Research UK Formulation Unit, Strathclyde Institute of Pharmacy and Biomedical Sciences, University of Strathclyde, Glasgow, U.K.

INTRODUCTION

Drug discovery occurs in silico, in chemistry laboratories, in cell-free assays or tissue culture systems, or in vivo in animal models on a molecule synthesized by the chemist. Final drug usage however occurs in patients using tablets, creams, injections, or other products that are a combination of the drug and various excipients, which together constitute the final medicinal product intended to produce the desired therapeutic effect. Preformulation is the initial stage of the conversion of molecule to drug where various important pharmaceutical (physical, chemical, and biological) properties of the putative drug molecule are assessed. It is difficult to define fully what constitutes preformulation (Fig. 1) or where it starts and ends within a drug discovery/development program. In an innovator setting, studies will be conducted in an expedient fashion on the small experimental amounts of material available in competition with other equally or more important studies related to preclinical pharmacology. Assuming acceptable results and continuation of drug development the drug quantities available will increase and the range of preformulation studies (including pharmacology) expanded to encompass all aspects of preclinical and preformulation development of drugs. In a generic development setting, these restrictions in general will not apply since preexisting information may be available and compound supplies are already established. Excessive early studies in an innovator program on candidate drugs that may never progress beyond preclinical development is a resource drain. This development dilemma is an important consideration that controls the application of preformulation studies and is difficult to reconcile to minimize development time and resource waste, while maximizing success potential. In general the various studies will be conducted where possible in parallel with the most immediate required information generated as early as possible.

The aim of preformulation is to provide key pharmaceutical information during development permitting progress decisions and ultimately leading into formulation studies for the final marketed product. The requirement for rapid development and reduced times to market is blurring the boundary between drug discovery and development as more stages are performed in parallel and new techniques introduced to accelerate studies. The information required on preformulation will to a certain extent

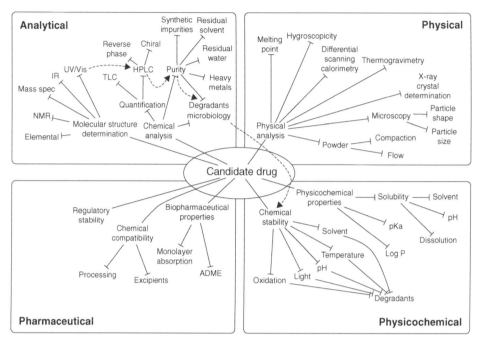

Figure 1 Preformulation Studies. Map of preformulation studies revolving around the candidate drug. Studies would commence in the Analytical segment and swing around to the Pharmaceutical segment as the compound's development progressed. Since early studies influence later studies the dotted arrow indicates one linkage, the determination of the UV/VIS spectrum feeding into HPLC method development, which is influenced by synthetic impurities and degradants, which then permits degradation studies to be conducted. Multiple relationships could be drawn indicating the linked nature of preformulation with drug discovery and later pharmaceutical development. *Abbreviations*: UV/VIS, ultraviolet/visible; HPLC, high-performance liquid chromatography.

be dictated by the final product, the proposed route of administration, and the company's development plan. A generic manufacturer will only require to cover aspects important to the particular product type under consideration, while an innovator will by necessity have to cover a range of product types. For an intravenous injection, aqueous solubility and stability will be important, while for a tablet, properties such as powder flow and compressibility are critical. If the marketed formulation for an innovator is a tablet, then in vivo studies (in humans) determining bioavailability will be required, which necessitates an intravenous formulation as a reference and therefore greater resource input. Since around 50% of marketed products are oral tablet formulations, the optimal goal of drug discovery and development is an oral product.

As preformulation forms the foundation for subsequent pharmaceutics and may influence preclinical pharmacology, it is crucial that it be comprehensive and no important features are overlooked. The recent example of the antiretroviral compound Ritonavir[TM] serves as a reminder of the importance of this stage. Ritonavir was marketed in 1996 as a solution capsule formulation (1) since the only known polymorph was not conducive to tableting. However, in 1998, a more stable and slower-dissolving polymorph appeared in the formulation, which required product removal from the market, loss of a quarter of a billion dollars in sales, and the expenditure of millions to resolve the problem. It is a moot point whether more extensive preformulation studies would have picked up this issue.

Small and Large Molecules

The vast majority of published preformulation information relates to small-molecule drugs with a molecular weight below approximately 1000 Da (2,3). Recent developments in recombinant DNA technology have permitted the production of macromolecular drugs such as peptides and proteins with higher molecular weights (4). These molecules are chemically and structurally more complex and presented in different formulations (5). However, the principles that follow are still applicable with suitable modification.

Regulatory Influences

If the drug does progress through development, it is important that the information gathered at all stages is comparable and will satisfy global regulatory authorities (6). The concept applied is that quality should be built into the product rather than tested after manufacture using quality control methods, which are based on an assumption of uniformity and would only sample and analyze 20 tablets of a batch of 500,000. The application of Quality Assurance under the heading of current Good Manufacturing Practice (cGMP) was originally applied to the manufacture of the marketed product but has now been extended to include the drug or active pharmaceutical ingredient (API). API has particular regulatory connotations and its development, scale-up, production, and control is a complex process (7). A globally marketed product could be manufactured at a level of 5 billion tablets annually, and if the dose is 100 mg, then 500,000 kg of API will be required. This quantity is multiple orders of magnitude greater than the initial synthesis levels, which may be measured in grams or even milligrams. To satisfy cGMP it is crucial to ensure that the API's properties are identical to the initial samples. This requires that the synthetic route is quickly defined and that analytical methods are available early in development, a process that is necessary since late changes could result in a repetition of early studies and costly delays to market.

IN SILICO PREFORMULATION

The majority of this text will focus on the individual molecular properties that require to be determined during preformulation. The traditional methods to measure these parameters involve wet chemistry experiments using milliliters of solvents and milligrams or grams of drugs. These are labor intensive and material intensive and only capable of processing low sample numbers. As detailed below the modern drug development paradigm requires the processing of high numbers of samples quickly to gain early access to key information involved in the decision-making process.

Computational Studies

Traditionally preformulation studies have required actual drug samples on which to perform the studies (8), even though theoretical models to predict, for example, solubility have existed for some time. The massive increase in computing power coupled with increased understanding of computational chemistry (9) is leading to a situation where a drug's molecular properties can be calculated even before synthesis.[a] Although some programs do require high-level computing facilities, Web-based systems are available (10) that will calculate a structure's physicochemical properties such as log P, solubility,

---

[a]There has always been a general feeling for molecular properties based on structure review coupled with suitable experience.

and pK_a. VCCLAB and Osiris calculate that the nonsteroidal anti-inflammatory fenoprofen has a log P value of 3.13, which agrees well with an experimentally derived value of 3.45 (11). However, the Osiris-calculated pK_a value of 4.30 is substantially different from the experimental value of 5.70. For preformulation requirements, computational calculations are still limited and have not yet attained the sophistication that would enable excipient compatibility, for example, to be assessed. It is unlikely that they will replace experimentally obtained results (12), but they do provide a rapid assessment of a drug's properties. Increasingly as computational techniques further improve, in silico preformulation will become a standard feature.

High-Throughput Preformulation

Drug discovery currently applies combinatorial and/or parallel chemistry synthesis techniques to generate large numbers of putative drug molecules that may be further tested for biological activity in high-throughput screening systems. These techniques have revolutionized the initial drug discovery stages producing large drug "sets" early in development. In response to this high throughput of samples, preformulation strategies have been developed using microtiter plates to determine solubility (13) and chromatography-based systems (14) to measure lipophilicity (log P) and also to examine crystal properties (15). While these techniques now have an established role in early drug discovery/development especially during candidate selection, they have yet to gain a wider regulatory acceptance. However, as computational techniques improve their application will certainly increase and further blur the boundary between drug discovery and development.

ANALYTICAL STUDIES

The foundation on which the majority of drug development stages are based is the ability to characterize and analyze the drug during testing. This ranges from the basic determination of molecular structure through separative methods capable of detecting subtle changes during synthesis, stability studies, or the minute quantities present in biological samples. The development and application of these analytical methods with increasing sensitivity and sophistication will be staged and synchronized during the development program in parallel to their application.

Molecular Identity and Characterization

A basic requirement is to ensure that the drug's molecular structure is identical to that proposed by the synthetic chemist; arguably, this should be performed before any form of testing. The armamentarium available will not be discussed in detail here, but it ranges from the determination of the ultraviolet/visible (UV/VIS), infrared (IR), and near-IR spectral properties to nuclear magnetic resonance spectra for hydrogen and carbon atoms to mass spectrometry data indicating molecular weight and fragmentation pattern and elemental analysis determining the percentage of the molecule attributable to a particular atom. Individually these tests will not absolutely confirm molecular structure but collectively they do. Although not essentially preformulation, these studies will form the basis for other analytical techniques. Simple UV/VIS analysis might be all that is required for early solubility and dissolution studies and will form the basis for detection in separative quantification methods such as high-performance liquid chromatography (HPLC). Mass spectrometry information may also be employed as a more sensitive and specific HPLC detection technique, while near-IR information might find a role in sample identification testing at the manufacturing stage.

Quantification

The complexity applied to drug quantification will vary depending on circumstances. If concentration determination is required in a simple system, for example, drug and buffer employed in solubility studies, then UV/VIS analysis will usually suffice or even turbidity measurements (16). If a more complex matrix is present, for example, microsomal enzymes, or the requirement is to differentiate between similar molecules present in the sample, then a more sophisticated separative technique such as HPLC (17) will be required. The key criterion for any separative method is specificity providing quantification without interference from impurities arising from the synthetic route or degradation products arising from chemical instability (18). Development of the analytical method is beyond this chapter (19), but the final assay performance should match regulatory expectations (20)[b] and validated for specificity, linearity, accuracy, and precision. The main peak representing the drug is not always the focus for these methods since drug is present. Of greater importance are the related substances, impurities, and degradation products, which should not be present or present in minimal amounts. This is analytically challenging, and in certain cases impurities require to be detected at very low levels, such as 0.03% by weight of the drug substance. These methods if so can be developed in combination with initial forced degradation stability studies, which deliberately stress the drug to induce degradation.

Purity

A key component of analytical development is purity determination, which is the actual percentage of the sample, usually by weight, that can be attributed to the drug. This is a simple calculation of weight of drug divided by total weight of drug plus other impurities ($\times 100$). Impurities however can range through organic impurities (synthetic intermediates, by-products, related impurities, and degradation products detected by separative quantification techniques), inorganic impurities (heavy metals, salts, and catalysts detected by pharmacopoeial or other methods), and residual solvents (quantified through gas chromatographic methods). The difficulty is that each necessitates the development of specific validated analytical techniques. Also of importance is enantiomeric purity, if the drug is chiral, and polymorphic purity, as discussed below.

Additional Analytical Requirements

Further testing will be required to determine microbiological contamination (21) by either viable organisms or nonviable entities in the form of pyrogen if the drug is required for parenteral administration. Other tests might include organoleptic properties such as taste and texture determination.

SOLID-STATE PROPERTIES

The solid state is the subject of chapter 8, but a summary of its importance in preformulation studies is given here. Chemical synthesis is conducted in a liquid medium, but the final drug product is usually a solid simply because solids generally have better

---

[b]International Conference on Harmonisation Web site contains regulatory accepted guidelines in the areas of quality, safety, and efficacy on subjects such as analytical method validation and impurities in new drug substances.

chemical stability, are more resistant to microbiological colonization, and solid dosage forms constitute the greatest proportion of marketed products. The first two criteria however also mean that even liquid products will at some stage pass through a solid phase. One of the first reports concerning the biopharmaceutical effects of variations in a drug's solid properties was by Aguiar in 1967 on the dissolution and oral absorption of chloramphenicol palmitate (22). It was discovered that this drug existed in two polymorphic forms A and B, with form B exhibiting the best oral absorption, and in mixtures absorption was controlled by the percentage of form B present. A study of commercial products indicated that they contained varying and uncontrolled mixtures of the forms, resulting in the introduction of a specification for this quality parameter. Ritonavir illustrates a more recent incident, and both highlight the importance and impact solid-state properties may have on pharmaceutical and subsequent biological performance. Therefore a drug's solid-state properties are paramount (23,24) and must be investigated in a systematic manner that will satisfy regulatory authorities (25) and ensure that sufficient data are obtained.

Salt Form

Generally small molecular drugs are either weak acids or bases and normally presented as a salt as a means of assisting crystallization and subsequent solubility (26). High solubility is desirable, since for oral administration a salt providing a higher solubility will generally have a higher bioavailability. However, excessive solubility can lead to hygroscopicity problems when the salt attracts moisture and influences stability and thus affects the ability to process on a commercial scale. Any biocompatible acid or base counterion maybe employed for salt formation; sodium (Na^+) and potassium (K^+) are common for carboxylic acids and hydrochloride and sulfate for bases (27). Fenoprofen-free acid, for example, is a low melting point solid ($40°C$), which cannot form tablets, butit can be converted into salts (8) with the Ca^{2+} salt employed pharmaceutically (Table 1). Amphoteric compounds can be processed by either route. Salt form choice lies at the interface between early discovery/development and preformulation, and it is important to optimize the selection. While counterion changes will not affect pharmacology (assuming molar equivalents are used), it will influence pharmaceutics and therefore should be determined early to avoid time-consuming changes and study repetition later in development.

Crystal Form and Polymorphism

Crystallization is a classical technique for compound purification from solution and generally the final step in the synthetic process leading to the drug (24). Crystallization conditions are crucial to a drug's pharmaceutical properties since they control the crystal form, habit, and size. The basic structure of a crystal is the unit cell, which contains a fixed number of drug molecules, and/or ions, which is then replicated in three dimensions to produce the crystal. Most pharmaceutical compounds can crystallize in one or more crystalline forms or polymorphs, which have the same chemical composition but different molecular arrangements, conformations, or packing in the unit cell. Pseudopolymorphs or solvates are also possible where the molecule cocrystallizes with solvent molecules (hydrates if the solvent is water). Note that in these instances chemical composition may vary. If the crystal is capable of losing the solvent to the atmosphere, a desolvated form may arise where the crystal has simply lost the solvent molecules. Since polymorphism is

Table 1 Physicochemical Data on Fenoprofen

Salt	Hydration	Form	Melting point (°C)	Aqueous solubility (mg/mL)	Weight change (%) Relative humidity (%)					
					10	20	40	60	70	93
Free acid	–	Oil	40	0.05	–	–	–	–	–	–
K$^+$	Unknown	Crystal	–	>200	Extremely hygroscopic					
Mg^{2+}	Dihydrate	–	–	>200	–	–	–	–	–	–
Al(OH)$^{2+}$	Dihydrate	Amorphous	–	0.1	0	–	0	–	–	0
Na$^+$	Anhydrous	Amorphous	–	>200	−0.5	+10.7	+12.5	–	+15.8	+36.5
Na$^+$	Dihydrate	Crystalline	80	>200	−11.4	+0.3	+0.4	–	+2.5	+9.3
Ca^{2+}	Anhydrous	Amorphous	–	2.5	+0.5	+1.7	+2.9	+3.7	–	+6.3
Ca^{2+}	Dihydrate	Crystalline	110	2.5	0	0	0	–	0	0

Source: From Ref. 8.

a structural rather than chemical difference, it influences the drug's pharmaceutical properties and is optimally detected and examined by physicochemical testing (28).

Pharmaceutical Effects of Polymorphism

Dissolution and solubility If a solid (solute) is to dissolve in a liquid (solvent), the attractive forces holding the solute together must be overcome by the attractive forces between the molecules of the solid and solvent. It follows therefore that if the arrangement of drug molecules in the solid varies (i.e., polymorphism), the attractive forces holding the solid together will also vary and consequently dissolution and solubility will vary (see section "Solubility"). There are multiple pharmaceutical examples (29), which illustrate the importance of this phenomenon, for example, oxytetracycline, carbamazepine, and glibenclamide.

Processing properties Polymorphism can affect the crystal's mechanical properties and therefore affect processing behavior such as mixing and compressibility during tableting. The ease of tablet formation by compressing crystals together is subject to a general (although not absolute) rule that the more physically stable of two polymorphs may provide weaker tablets. A simple rationale is that the more stable the polymorph, the more energy will be required to deform the crystal (during compression) and produce new surfaces that can form interparticle bonds that maintain the tablet.

Stability Polymorphism can influence stability either by a direct effect on chemical reactivity and therefore the drug's basic chemical stability or via instability of the polymorphic form itself. For example, furosemide (30) degradation by light stability is linked to polymorphic form. Stability issues may also arise from polymorphic changes occurring during processing of the API, for example wet granulation or drying stages, into the final product (31). Generally, the more stable the polymorph, the greater the chemical stability, attributable to higher crystal packing or density and maintenance of the molecule in an optimized stable orientation.

Amorphous Solids

Amorphous solids can be defined as materials that are not crystalline in nature and therefore have no defined long-range molecular structure. Because of this they are generally "energetic" solids with higher dissolution rates and solubilities along with better compression properties than their crystalline counterparts. However, they tend to be less stable both chemically and physically. The amorphous state is common with large flexible molecules such as proteins, sugars, and polymers; a protein can of course be an API, and sugars and polymers can be employed as excipients. In addition various standard pharmaceutical processes such as lyophilization, spray drying, and dehydration of hydrates can produce amorphous forms of normally crystalline materials (32).

Examination of Solid-State Properties

Since the differences between solid states are physical rather than chemical (with the exception of solvates), the examination of these properties relies on physical testing methods.

Melting Point

A basic property of solids is the temperature at which the solid melts to become a liquid. During this process thermal energy is initially required to heat the solid to the melting point, at which temperature the thermal energy overcomes the forces holding the crystals together and induces a phase change from a solid to a liquid. During melting the material must still absorb heat—the heat of fusion—to fully overcome the forces in the crystal. For crystals, melting point is defined, and although this implies precision, the melting process normally occurs over a range of a few degrees. For amorphous materials where there is no structure, there is no abrupt phase change at any specific temperature, rather a gradual change in properties. The determination of melting point by visually (either microscopically or by the naked eye) examining the material while it is being heated is a classical method of chemistry. However, other than for a basic characterization, this technique will not generally permit the discrimination between polymorphic forms.

Vibrational Spectroscopy

Infrared IR spectroscopy is applied by chemists as a structure determination technique for a molecule. IR absorption results in changes in a molecule's vibrational and rotational energy levels, which permits examination of the molecular bonds. If these are constrained because of differences in crystal structure and hence orientation, then the effects on the vibrational and rotational energy levels can be determined. The common method of analyzing a sample is to use Fourier transform IR coupled with a reflectance (either diffuse or total attenuated) technique so that the solid sample is not subjected to any processing that may alter polymorphic properties. Since this is a light-based technique, it can also be applied through a microscope.

Raman If a monochromatic source of light impinges on a sample, it interacts with the molecules to produce excited vibrational energy states, and the scattered light can be modified by this effect. If the interaction is such that the molecule returns to its original energy state, then Rayleigh scattering occurs, and the scattered light has the same wavelength as the incident light. If, however, the molecule does not return to its original energy state but a higher one, then the wavelength of the scattered light will also change producing Raman scattering. Only a very small percentage ($\approx 0.001\%$) of the incident light is Raman scattered, and since a small amount of energy has been absorbed by the sample, the scattered wavelength is at a lower wave number.

Comparison Both IR and Raman rely on the vibrational properties of bonds in the drug and therefore might seem to be similar techniques. However, vibrational changes during IR absorption are related to the molecular dipole, while during Raman, molecular polarizability is important. Thus the two techniques are complementary (28), with vibrations due to polar groups strongly IR absorbing and those due to symmetric and homopolar bonds strongly Raman. Both can therefore be used for the characterization of polymorphic behavior by comparing spectra to different polymorphic forms.

Differential Scanning Calorimetry

Differential scanning calorimetry (DSC) is a thermoanalytical technique that measures the difference in the amount of heat required to increase the temperature of a sample and reference as a function of a change in temperature, generally linearly increasing. Both the reference and the sample are maintained at the same temperature over the desired temperature range, and the reference must have a characterized heat capacity in the range. If the sample undergoes a physical change or a chemical change, for example, melting or degradation, then more (if the transition is endothermic) or less (if the transition is exothermic) heat will be required to maintain the sample temperature in comparison to the reference. By measuring heat flow against temperature it is possible to calculate the enthalpy of the phase transition and the temperature at which it occurs. This provides a very sensitive method of examining the physical properties of solid samples, which can be further improved by modulating the heat flow to discriminate between reversible and irreversible thermal effects (33). DSC is therefore a powerful research and analytical tool that is employed to characterize pharmaceutical solids and determine polymorphic behavior. DSC is one of a family of thermally based techniques such as differential thermal analysis (heat flow, rather than temperature, is maintained at a constant rate) or thermogravimetric analysis (sample weight is measured as a function of temperature) that can be employed to study solid pharmaceutical materials (34).

X-Ray Scattering Techniques

X rays are part of the electromagnetic radiation spectrum with wavelengths around 10^{-10} m or 1 Angstrom (Å). X-ray scattering techniques are a family of analytical methods that provide information about a solid's structure and chemical composition. X rays on passing through the solid are diffracted according to Bragg's law:

$$n\lambda = 2d \sin \theta$$

where λ is the wavelength of the incident X ray at an angle of θ, d is the distance between the planes in the crystal, and n is an integer representing the order of reflection. The interaction of waves with a crystal is described by the dynamical theory of diffraction, and the diffraction pattern obtained is a means of measuring distances between atoms or planes in the crystal. This means that the diffraction pattern obtained for every crystalline form of a compound is unique and can be employed to identify the compound and polymorphic forms and calculate the dimensions on the unit cell. The sample, which can either be a powder or a single crystal, is exposed to the X-ray source normally at ambient temperatures, and the method of sample preparation and presentation is important to ensure that no artifacts are introduced.

Scanning Probe Microscopy

A recent microscopic technique is the scanning probe or atomic force microscope, which scans a sample's surface at an atomic level (35). These have an obvious application in the characterization of solids and pharmaceutical polymorphs although limited only by the ability to examine the surface of the material under test.

Polymorph Discovery

The pharmaceutical importance of polymorphism during the drug development process and the requirement to detect, characterize, and control the phenomenon has led to a variety of techniques for the discovery of polymorphs.

High-Throughput Screening

Since polymorphism arises during crystallization, forced crystallization of drugs using ranges and mixtures of solvents, counterions, and experimental conditions should provide an avenue to polymorphs. This roulette of variables for a single compound lends itself to high-throughput techniques (36) on relatively small single-figure gram samples of the drug. These studies will, if polymorphism is possible, provide hits, which can be further examined by the techniques above.

Computational Screening

The intrinsic prediction of crystal structure and polymorphic potential from molecular structure would be a useful tool during the early stages of drug development. However, the complexity of drugs and the associated numbers of potential molecular orientations make this a nascent and very challenging field (37). The analysis of paracetamol calculated 14 potential polymorphs where only 2 are known (38). Undoubtedly future accuracy will improve through improved techniques and computing power.

Latent Polymorphism

Since there is no absolute method available to calculate the number of polymorphs for any compound and screening methods by their very nature are statistical, there is always the probability that an unknown polymorph will arise. The Ritonavir example illustrates the problems that this can cause and indicates that this aspect of preformulation possibly continues through the entire use of the drug!

Hygroscopicity

If a solid drug absorbs water from air, it is termed "hygroscopic," and conversely, if it loses water, it is termed "efflorescent." Both situations represent a type of physicochemical instability since variation in water content inevitably leads to variations in potency (i.e., the percentage of drug present for any given weight), which if uncontrolled makes drug handling difficult. In addition, variations in water content can lead to further physical and chemical instability. Since this is a dynamic phenomenon, it will be influenced by the relative humidity of the ambient air, which can vary from 0% (deserts and very cold environments) to 50% in temperate and 80% to 90% in tropical environments. These values are not fixed and will vary with weather conditions. If a drug is not affected by variations in relative humidity, it is termed "nonhygroscopic," which is the optimal property for new drugs (Table 1). There is an interesting paradox to this since nonhygroscopicity imparts stability, while hygroscopicity (or hydrophilic) properties are required for dissolution and solubility. To assess hygroscopicity, the drug is exposed to a range of relative humidities, with or without temperature variation, permitting both sorption and desorption of water to be measured. The effect is monitored by simple gravimetric measurement and termed "dynamic vapor sorption." It is difficult to change this particular property since it is a function of the drug, salt and crystal form. The results of the studies, however, should provide information on the optimal storage and handling conditions for the drug and indicate the type of packaging required, glass versus polyethylene.

Particle Size and Shape

A basic physical feature of a solid is that for any given weight of material as the diameter of the particles that constitute the material decreases, the surface area present increases. Since a solid's interaction with its external environment occurs at surfaces, particle size is an important characteristic controlling a variety of properties, for example, dissolution and adhesion. For very potent drugs formed into solid dosage forms, dose uniformity is inversely related to particle size, since the larger the numbers of drug particles, which constitute a dose, the greater the uniformity. If the compound is for pulmonary delivery via inhalation, only a particular size fraction, generally <10-μm diameter, will reach the lungs. Particle size is therefore an important parameter.

If powders consisted of spherical particles, a simple statement of radius would describe the particles. However, pharmaceutical powders consist of particles with varying nonspherical shapes and sizes, and any size measurement has to account for this. This is an interesting mathematical and statistical problem, which leads to the utilization of a variety of descriptors based on geometrical relationships, for example, using surface area or volume, of the particle under measurement and a nominally equivalent ideal sphere (39). Mathematically, a general shape factor (Γ) can be calculated as follows (3):

$$\text{Particle surface area} = \Gamma \times \text{particle volume}^{2/3}$$

For a sphere this value is 4.8, and the greater the value for a particle, the greater the deviation of its shape from spherical. Shape is an important factor along with size, since it has been demonstrated that the more spherical the particle, the easier its processing. Particle shape also influences the measurement of particle size through orientation effects of the particle during measurement. If the sample consists of disc-like particles (plates), which were viewed after placing in a suitable sample holder, they are gravitationally likely to adopt a flat orientation rather than standing on their sides, thus presenting their largest diameter for the measurement process.

Measurement of Particle Size

During preformulation the techniques available to measure particle size are restricted, and traditionally this has relied on optical microscopy, a field that has been revolutionized by the introduction of image analysis and laser light scattering–based methods. A key feature of any particle size measurement is the method adopted to present the particle in a stable non-agglomerated (i.e., as individual particles) format for measurement. If this is not attained, measurement by any method is suspect.

Optical Microscopy

This is the simplest technique and will visually provide an indication of crystallinity, shape, and other features such as surface smoothness. The classical optical determination of size relies on a comparison of the particles, under microscopic examination, with discs (usually a graticule within the eyepiece) of a known size and the counting or comparison of a statistically significant number ($n > 625$). This is a tedious process, and if the particles deviate from disc-like shapes, it also becomes difficult. The traditional manual method has however been replaced by the advent of computer-based image analysis systems (for example Morphologi G3 from Malvern Instruments), which remove human-based size comparison errors, greatly speed up the analysis, and permit rapid statistical data processing.

Laser Light Scattering

If a particle is suspended (in a liquid or gas) in a laser beam, it scatters the light, an effect dependent on the difference between the laser's wavelength and the size of the particle. If the particle is larger (generally 0.5–1000 μm diameter) than the wavelength, the light is forward scattered with only a small change in angle to produce a Fraunhofer diffraction pattern. This pattern is a summation of all the different particles within the incident beam and can be quantified using a photodetector. If the particle is smaller (0.001–5 μm diameter) than the wavelength, it will, due to its size, undergo Brownian motion. The scattered light fluctuates at a rate dependent on the particle size since smaller particles move faster. This is termed "dynamic light scattering" based on the Lorenz–Mie–Debye theory, and detection and quantification of the light fluctuation pattern yields the particles velocity of movement or diffusion coefficient. In both cases computer-based mathematical processing of the detected signal can then extract the particle size distributions.

Bulk Powder Properties

The manufacture of commercial product batches necessitates the handling of large quantities (kilograms) of drug, and therefore bulk powder properties are important for processing, for example, flow into dies during tablet production. These properties are primarily controlled by particle size and shape, a feature that can change during scale-up and should be measured as early as possible to ensure consistency.

Compression

The formulation of a tablet (see chap. 13) will depend on the proposed oral dose—a value that will only become apparent during preclinical pharmacology testing. However, early studies can be performed to determine the compressibility properties and potential routes to tablet formulations. Materials can be categorized as elastic, plastic, or brittle on the basis of behavior in simple tableting experiments utilizing a basic formulation (compound, lubricant, and diluent) and single-die hydraulic press similar to those employed to produce IR discs. Elastic materials (e.g., paracetamol) spring back after compression, and the compressed tablet will delaminate on storage, an effect that can be modified by excipients. Plastic materials deform on compression rather than create new surfaces, with the deformation related to the time under compression, tablet strength in these instances is increased by increasing compression time. Brittle materials create new surfaces on compression, and therefore "new" bonds between the particles producing tablets that do not delaminate are not improved by increased compression time or influenced by excipients. Brittle materials are therefore favored as the simplest route to tablet formation; however, in reality, application of suitable processing and formulation techniques will overcome most deficiencies.

Powder Flow

The simplest technique is to determine the "angle of repose" where the powder is allowed to flow/fall under gravity from a nozzle onto a flat surface, and the angle of incline of the resultant powder cone is measured. The lower the angle, the better the flow properties, with angles less than 30° constituting good flow. A related test is to compare a powder's poured density with the tapped density (details of such tests can be found in national pharmacopoeias) to calculate Carr's index:

$$\text{Carr's index} = \left(\frac{(\text{tapped density} - \text{poured density})}{\text{tapped density}} \right) \times 100$$

Values less than 15 indicate good flow properties. Both tests can be extended by determining either the rate of flow onto the surface using a balance or by serial determination of Carr's index during tapping. The latter provides information on consolidation, which is an essential feature during tablet die filling. If the properties are not adequate, the effect of glidants to improve flow can be determined via these techniques.

PHYSICOCHEMICAL PROPERTIES

The properties above are all related to the new drug presented in a solid form. To exert any biological activity a basic pharmaceutical requirement is that the compound must be able to dissolve in aqueous biological media. Once dissolved, the "solution" properties of the drug such as the ability to cross biological membranes and interact with proteins become critical. Preformulation aims to examine these properties to determine if the drug has an appropriate pharmaceutical balance.

Solubility

A key physicochemical property is solubility, particularly in aqueous media. Failures during drug development are often related to poor or insufficient solubility (40). In addition, particular products, for example, intravenous injections, require a solution. Therefore, solubility is a crucial parameter to determine since it influences multiple development studies.

Solution formation from separate solute and solvent phases must be thermodynamically favorable to occur spontaneously. A primary driving force for solution formation is entropy, which is a measure of the disorder brought about by mixing solute and solvent molecules. This can be expressed mathematically as ΔS_{mix}, the ideal entropy of mixing in an ideal binary system:

$$\Delta S_{mix} = -R(n_1 \ln X_1) + n_2 \ln X_2$$

where R is the ideal gas constant, n_1 is the number of moles of solvent, X_1 the mole fraction of solvent present, and n_2 and X_2 the same parameters for the solute. Since the mole fraction will always be less than 1, ΔS_{mix} is always positive and contributes to the spontaneity of solution formation. Although mixing is entropically favorable, the overall change in free energy (ΔG) must also be negative for a solution to arise spontaneously. This can be expressed in terms of changes in entropy ΔS and enthalpy ΔH on the formation of a solution through the equation:

$$\Delta G = \Delta H - T\Delta S$$

where T is the temperature in °K. In an ideal system of noninteracting molecules, there is no change in ΔH or enthalpy and therefore changes in ΔS drive solution formation. Drugs are not ideal and do interact, which means that $\Delta H \neq 0$ and enthalpy changes must be considered. Enthalpy changes arise since energy-dependent stages are involved in solution formation, mainly breaking the "bonds" holding both the solute and solvent molecules together in their respective solid and liquid phases, formation of the spaces required between the solvent molecules to accommodate the solute molecules, and the formation of new bonds between the solute and solvent molecules. These changes can be expressed as:

$$\Delta H = \Delta H_{crystal\ breakdown} + \Delta H_{solvation}$$

where $\Delta H_{crystal\ breakdown}$ is the enthalpy change involved in breaking the solute's crystal structure, which will always be positive since bonds are being broken, and $\Delta H_{solvation}$ the enthalpy change arising from the formation of new bonds between the solvent and solute molecules and therefore usually negative. If $\Delta H_{crystal\ breakdown} > \Delta H_{solvation}$, then the solution reaction will be endothermic, and conversely if $\Delta H_{crystal\ breakdown} < \Delta H_{solvation}$, solution formation will be exothermic.

The changes in enthalpy ΔH relative to changes in entropy $T\Delta S$ will have to be negative, zero, or less than $T\Delta S$ for solutions to form. This has led to the development of theories, based on calculations of ΔH and $T\Delta S$, to predict solubility from chemical structure–derived properties (41). The mobile order theory, for example, calculates solubility (determined as volume fraction ϕ) as the sum of six parameters, that is to say:

$$\ln \phi = -A_m + B - D - F + O - OH$$

where A_m relates to the melting of the crystal during dissolution, B the entropy of mixing, D the solution enthalpy when the solute solvent interaction energy is different from the solvent-solvent and solute-solute interactions, F hydrophobic effects of the solute on the solvent, which causes ordering of the solvent molecules through repulsion, and O and OH related to the formation of hydrogen bonds between the solute and solvent. The "O" and "OH" terms are complicated by the solute's ability to act either as a proton donor or acceptor or both during hydrogen bond formation. Alternative theories exist, but this illustrates the common approach of summing the various interactions. Practically the theories can be approximated by the statement that "like will dissolve like," and therefore polar solutes will dissolve in polar solvents and nonpolar solutes in nonpolar solvents.

Solution formation occurs at the solute-solvent interface and consists of two consecutive stages. The first is the interaction between the solute and solvent molecules that results in the "transfer" of a solute molecule from the solid phase into the solvent to form the solution. Since this occurs at the interface, it produces a layer of a saturated solute solution or *boundary layer*. Therefore, once in solution, the solute molecules must diffuse away through the boundary layer to the bulk solution (Fig. 2).

The overall rate of dissolution will be controlled by the slowest or rate-limiting step that generally is solute diffusion across the boundary layer. The Noyes–Whitney equation defines this process as:

$$\frac{dm}{dt} = \frac{DA[C_s - C]}{h}$$

where dm/dt is the rate of solute mass transfer from the solid surface (i.e., dissolution) into the bulk solution, D is the diffusion coefficient of the solute molecule, A is the surface area available for dissolution, $[C_s - C]$ is the concentration difference between the saturated concentration at the surface $[C_s]$ and the bulk of the solution concentration $[C]$, and h the thickness of the boundary layer. If $[C]$ is maintained at less than 10% of $[C_s]$, sink conditions are said to apply, and the equation simplifies to:

$$\frac{dm}{dt} = \frac{DA[C_s]}{h}$$

There are multiple methods available to determine dissolution rate either of the drug or its products under development. Only the former constitutes preformulation. The usual method is to compress the drug under investigation into a disc, around 1 cm in diameter, and measure dissolution from the surface into a suitable solute over time as either the disk is rotated or the solute stirred.

Solubility is expressed as a concentration term (i.e., mg/mL or mol/L) usually as a saturated value at a constant temperature in a specified solvent. Determination of saturated solubility is relatively easy and should be one of the first preformulation studies

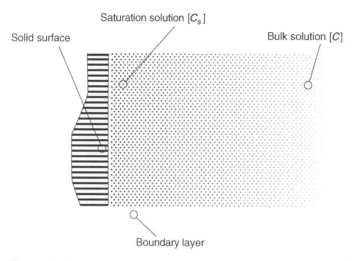

Figure 2 Schematic diagram of drug dissolution from a solid surface.

conducted. Solvent and solute (in excess) are placed in contact usually in a sealed container and mixed or agitated at a constant temperature until equilibrium is achieved. A sample of the solution is then extracted, ensuring that no solid is carried over, and this supernatant analyzed for the concentration of solute present. The analytical method must be capable of accurately measuring the concentration, and time allowed for equilibrium will depend on the dissolution behavior. Another method is to dissolve the solute in a water-miscible solvent such as dimethyl sulfoxide (DMSO) and add this solution to an aqueous system until precipitation occurs, a method suitable for high throughput but influenced to varying extents by the presence of DMSO.

Factors Affecting Solubility

Basic Factors
The temperature of solution formation is important, and the key temperature is 37°C; however, for processing, higher temperatures could be employed especially if they aid dissolution. Effects of temperature on solubility can be determined calorimetrically by measuring temperature changes (heat of solution, ΔH) on dissolution and applying the Van't Hoff equation.

As stated, *like will dissolve like*, and the solvent's physicochemical properties such as dielectric constant (ε), which is a measure of polarity, and its solubility parameter (δ), which is a numerical value that measures a solvent's "solvency" based on the strength of intermolecular attractive forces between the solvent molecules, are important. If the compound is nonionizable, these two parameters will be of overriding importance. For pharmaceutical processing, any suitable biocompatible solvent may be appropriate; however, the major biocompatible solvent is water, and hence aqueous solubility is a key parameter to determine.

The crystal properties are also important since this will control the value of the A_m term. In early preformulation when initial solubility experiments are conducted, polymorphic or solid-state properties maybe unknown or only poorly controlled. In these situations results should be treated with caution. However, since both solubility and polymorphism lend themselves to high-throughput approaches, these studies can now be conducted in parallel.

The Noyes–Whitney equation predicts that surface area influences dissolution, and therefore the particle size employed in solubility experiments is important. The basic relationship is that for any weight of compound the smaller the particle size, the greater the available surface area and therefore the greater the dissolution rate. In early preformulation solubility experiments particle size may not be well controlled, and results should be treated with caution. However, if required, particle size reduction, by milling, micronization, or even the formation of nanocrystals, can be utilized as a formulation technique to improve poor dissolution properties.

Effect of pH

If the drug has either weakly acidic or basic (or both) groups in its structure such as a carboxylic acid or primary amine, respectively, then these will be affected by pH in aqueous media. For a weak acid, alkaline pH values will promote dissociation or ionization of the acid group creating a charged molecule, which will increase solubility, through improved hydrogen bond formation, with the converse applicable to weak bases. This can be represented by the following equations for a monofunctional acid or base.

$$HA \Leftrightarrow H^+ + A^- \quad \text{or} \quad B + H^+ \Leftrightarrow BH^+$$

where HA represents a weakly acidic drug and B a weakly basic drug. Applying the law of mass action the ionization constant (K_a) maybe calculated (for an acid) as follows:

$$K_a = \frac{[H^+][A^-]}{[HA]}$$

where $[H^+]$, $[A^-]$, and $[HA]$ represent the concentrations of the hydrogen ion, acid anion, and free acid in solution. This can be further simplified by taking the logarithm of the equation to

$$pK_a = pH + \log\frac{[HA]}{[A^-]}$$

which can be expressed in the following format for weak acids:

$$pK_a = pH + \log\frac{[C_u]}{[C_i]}$$

also known as the Henderson–Hasselbalch equation, where pK_a is the ionization constant for the drug and $[C_u]$ and $[C_i]$ the concentration of unionized and ionized species, respectively. A similar equation can be developed for weak bases.

$$pK_a = pH + \log\frac{[C_i]}{[C_u]}$$

The equation predicts that solubility will be maximal for acidic compounds at higher pH values and for basic compounds at lower pH values. Note that it also predicts that when pH $= pK_a$, the compound will be present in a 50:50 mixture of ionized and unionized species and with 2 pH units on either side of the pK_a, the compound will either be 99% ionized or 1% ionized. Over a range of 4 pH units, which easily occurs in the gastrointestinal tract, there will therefore be a vast change in solubility and also dissolution (Fig. 3). The determination of the pK_a of a drug therefore is a key stage in preformulation.

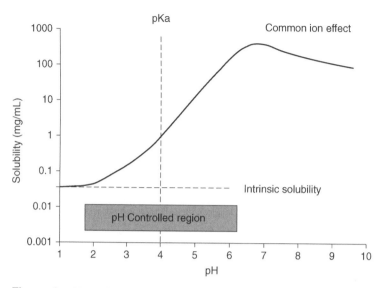

Figure 3 pH solubility for an acidic drug. Typical pH solubility profile for an acid drug (fenoprofen) pK_a 4.3 and intrinsic solubility 0.08 mg/mL. Note increasing solubility as pH increases due to increasing ionization.

Determination of pK_a

One simple method for determining pK_a is to titrate the compound with either an acid or a base and simply plot the quantity of titrant added against solution pH. When the pH $= pK_a$, the concentration of unionized and ionized species is equal, and this occurs at half neutralization, which can be determined graphically. Although simple, this does require the availability of reasonable quantities of drug but does not require an analytical method. The value can also be obtained spectrophotometrically if the UV/VIS absorption spectrum of the drug changes during ionization. The approach is similar to titration but can be conducted with smaller quantities of drugs, amenable to high-throughput techniques, and useful if the solubility is low and the pK_a values are low (<3) or high (>11). The drug, however, must exhibit changes in its absorption spectrum linked to ionization. Finally, pK_a can be determined using solubility measurements. If the compound is a weak acid, measurement of the saturation solubility $[C_u]$ in 0.1 M HCl should provide a value for [HA], sometimes termed "the intrinsic solubility," since ionization will be suppressed.

$$[C_u] = [HA]$$

Measurement of the saturation solubility $[C_s]$ at a higher pH, for example, between 6 and 8 will provide solubility information with contributions from both [HA] and $[A^-]$:

$$[C_s] = [HA] + [A^-]$$

therefore

$$[A^-] = [C_s - C_u]$$

which can then be substituted into the equation above to determine pK_a:

$$pK_a = pH_{(C_s measurement)} + \log \frac{[C_u]}{[C_s - C_u]}$$

Salt form

Drugs are normally processed as salts since this presents the compound in the ionized form, which has greater solubility and hence dissolution rate, thereby increasing solubility without the requirement to change pH. For a number of reasons, selection, however, should not simply be guided by the salt providing maximal solubility. Formulation issues may arise if the pH of the salt is at an extreme, which renders the solution unfit for ocular or parenteral administration.

The solubility of a salt in a saturated solution maybe represented by the equation where AB is the solid and A^- and B^+ the anion (acid-based drug) and cation (or salt, e.g., sodium), respectively.

$$[AB]_{solid} \Leftrightarrow [A^-]_{ion} + [B^+]_{ion}$$

and applying the law of mass action the equilibrium constant (K) for the reaction is given by:

$$K = \frac{[A^-][B^+]}{[AB]}$$

Since the concentration of solid can be considered constant then

$$K_{sp} = [A^-][B^+]$$

where K_{sp} is a constant termed "the solubility product." If the solubility product is exceeded, the concentrations in solution will shift to restore the equilibrium by the formation of fresh solid [AB]. In these situations an excess of a common ion (sodium in the above example, but could equally be chloride) will induce precipitation.

Partition Coefficient

If a drug is added to a system consisting of two immiscible solvents and is soluble in either of the solvents, it will naturally distribute itself or partition between the solvents and concentrate in the solvent that is most thermodynamically favorable. The drug's distribution ratio between the solvents can be used to determine the partition coefficient usually presented as a log value and defined as follows:

$$\log P_{o/w} = \log \left[\frac{C_o}{C_w} \right]$$

where P is the partition coefficient, $[C_o]$ is the drug's concentration in the nonaqueous phase, and $[C_w]$ the concentration in the aqueous phase. This ratio is not concentration or temperature dependent, although it will be influenced by the physicochemistry of the two solvents and drug. Normally the nonaqueous phase employed is *n*-octanol, and log P can also be referred to as log K_w^o. *n*-Octanol is employed since it is immiscible with water, has properties that mimic biological membranes, and through general use has a large information database available (42). If the drug is capable of ionization in the aqueous phase, then pH must be controlled since only the unionized form will partition into the nonaqueous phase. In these cases, $[C_w]$ must be the total concentration of both ionized and nonionized species. In these cases, log P will be pH dependent and is determined with a known aqueous phase pH. Log P provides a measure of the drug's lipophilicity or ability to dissolve in nonaqueous phases; the higher the log P, the more the compound will reside in lipid phases. For preformulation the utility of log P is that it provides a useful parameter, which can be used to determine solubility in both aqueous and mixed solvent systems. In development log P is an important preclinical measure of the drug's biopharmaceutical and pharmacodynamic properties. For example, during oral administration the compound must be absorbed from the aqueous intestinal contents through the epithelial lipid bilayers but it is not so lipophilic that it does not redissolve in the bloodstream to permit distribution around the body (43). Compounds with high log P values also tend to have higher volumes of distribution post administration, which affects pharmacokinetic properties. Finally, lipophilicity is a major driving force for the interaction of a drug with its receptor; log P is therefore useful during the drug design phase.

The simplest method "shake-flask method" to measure log P is to add the drug under test to a mixture of aqueous and n-octanol phases (n-octanol needs to be equilibrated with the aqueous phase for 24 hours prior to the experiment), permit the drug to equilibrate, at least 30 minutes, and then determine the concentration in each phase. This method is time consuming but can be automated and adapted for high throughput. The value can also be determined using HPLC if compounds with known log P values and similar chemical structures are available. The test compound's retention time is simply compared with a calibration graph constructed from known values. This does not require large quantities of material to perform and can be automated. Finally, since there is a large database of available information, it is possible to determine log P computationally on the basis of approaches such as functional group contributions or data mining using similar structures. Note that calculated values will not always equal experimental values but are useful initial estimates.

BIOPHARMACEUTICAL PREFORMULATION

Historically, preformulation consists of a barrage of chemical and physicochemical tests on a drug. It has now recognized that the drug's biopharmaceutical properties such as absorption, distribution, metabolism, and excretion (ADME) are of crucial importance in the development and decision-making process. Previously ADME could only be studied in whole-animal models and was therefore expensive and time consuming since only a single compound could be processed. However, tissue culture techniques are now available that allow in vitro assessments of ADME and therefore permit this type of information to be considered and factored into drug development programs earlier. Only absorption will be considered in this chapter.

Absorption Studies

The gastrointestinal tract is a complex organ with a mouth at one end, the rectum at the other, and several anatomical structures in between. A drug is therefore exposed to a range of conditions after oral administration that can affect its absorption into the bloodstream. For the majority of drugs, it is now recognized that the main site of absorption is the small intestine (44), and its physiology and anatomy has been well characterized. It is possible to grow intestinal epithelial cells, such as Caco-2, on membrane filter supports immersed in suitable tissue culture media. The cells divide and grow over time, normally around 21 days, assuming an identical structure and function to "normal" intestinal epithelial cells with microvilli on the apical (facing into the intestine) surface and tight junctions linking the cells (Fig. 4) (45). Once the cells have formed a functioning intestinal epithelial membrane, it is possible to add drugs to the media bathing

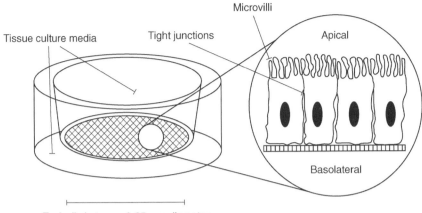

Typically between 6-25 mm diameter

Figure 4 Schematic diagram of Caco-2 intestinal cell monolayer. Cells grown on monolayer support bathed in tissue culture medium; once monolayer is functional, drugs can be added to either compartment and appearance in the opposing compartment measured.

the apical surface and measure the appearance in the basolateral compartment after transfer through the cell membrane. This permits a permeability value for the drug through the cell membrane to be calculated. A result in isolation using this system is not informative unless the system is "calibrated" using drugs with known oral bioavailability values. This permits a prediction of the drug's oral bioavailability, which does not require large amounts of compound or animals and maybe automated to permit high-throughput screening (46).

Biopharmaceutics Classification System

In the mid-1990s it was realised that a drug's oral absorption was primarily controlled by two features, basic solubility in aqueous media coupled with permeability through the gastrointestinal membrane. It is easy to visualize that if a drug is neither soluble nor permeable, then no oral absorption will occur after administration of a solid dosage form. For solubility, the aqueous media simulates conditions that the drug would meet on passage through the gastrointestinal tract. Drugs, where the highest administered dose strength dissolves in ≤250 mL of water between pH 1 and 7.5, are considered to have "high solubility" and those not meeting this specification considered to have "low solubility." Dissolution performance is also considered, and "rapidly dissolving" drugs are defined as those where ≥85% of the drug dissolves within 30 minutes during a pharmacopoeial dissolution test. This requirement involves the final formulation and therefore will not be applicable during preformulation testing. Permeability is measured using bioavailability with a "high-permeability" drug defined as a ≥90% absorption of the administered dose; those compounds not meeting this specification have a "low permeability." During preformulation permeability information can be obtained from in vitro permeation experiments across epithelial cell monolayers.

Drugs are then grouped into classes based on the definitions as in Table 2. Although the biopharmaceutics classification system (BCS) is generally for application to finished products, knowledge of a compound's likely classification as early as possible in the development process is useful. Since this can be obtained through solubility and in vitro

Table 2 Biopharmaceutics Classification System

	Solubility	
Permeability	High	Low
High	Class I Compounds well absorbed, good absorption rate, excellent candidates for oral administration, for example, metoprolol	Class II Compound absorption limited by solubility, formulations to increase solubility maybe required, for example, glibenclamide
Low	Class III Compound absorption limited by permeability that can be maximized by maximizing solubility, for example, cimetidine	Class IV Compounds with poor and variable oral absorption, for example, hydrochlorothiazide

measurements, it is easy to perform during preformulation. The ideal compounds fall into class I with increasing development issues related to the other classes.

STABILITY

A basic premise of development studies is that they are conducted on the "same" material, which requires a degree of drug stability post synthesis during testing. Chapter 7 in this volume addresses chemical kinetics and stability in some detail. Commercial pharmaceutical products require a shelf life measured in years (ideally up to 5 years) to ensure that the product's potency is identical throughout and provide a sensible time frame for manufacture, distribution, sale, and administration. A major element of preformulation is therefore aimed at investigating and understanding the drug's stability. This information is critical since it influences handling during preformulation studies, storage (including choice of container), formulation approaches (including excipient choices), and the processes that maybe employed during product manufacture, storage, and distribution. Throughout development stability studies will be applied to the solid drug and to solutions or other preparations, which maybe employed. The effort is aimed at determining known conditions under which the drug maybe stored and handled without any degradation arising.

What Constitutes Degradation?

During early preformulation a relatively loose specification will be applied, possibly limited by availability of analytical methods, for example, drug content $\geq 95\%$. As preformulation information develops, the specification will be refined to include a limit for individual degradants (e.g., $\leq 1\%$) and incorporating a limit for total detectable degradant levels (e.g., $\leq 3\%$). The development and setting of these specifications should be in combination with the identified degradants structures and their likely toxicity.

Physical Stability

Several aspects of physical instability such as hygroscopicity have been dealt with previously and will not be considered further.

Chemical Stability

The discovery of chemical instability relies on the availability of an analytical method capable of detecting small quantities of degradation products over time in the sample under test against the background of impurities already present. This requires a specific separative analytical method with a key focus on the degradation products and not on the parent drug. Degradant quantification rather than the parent compound is optimal since 1% degradation will only change the parent from 100% to 99%, a change that analytically will be difficult to quantify, while the degradant will change from 0% to 1%, which is easily detected and quantified. In addition, chemical identification of the degradants is beneficial since it permits discovery of the degradation pathway(s) and potential routes for avoidance. Chemical degradation occurs by three main chemical processes.

Hydrolysis

This is the most common degradation pathway since water plays an important role in many processes especially in solution but also in solid systems where it maybe present albeit at low concentrations. Hydrolysis occurs via a nucleophilic attack of the water molecule on labile bonds with susceptibility dependent on the bond type and decreasing from lactam > ester > amide > imine. This can be influenced by pH if the molecule is ionizable with maximum instability in the ionized form, since it has the greatest solubility and therefore exposure. This leads to a change in hydrolysis reaction rate with pH with the shape of the pH/hydrolysis curve related to the underlying chemical processes. If the solvent is not water, solvolysis is also possible if the solvent and compound react.

Oxidation

Oxidation is an environmental phenomenon requiring oxygen (or an oxidizing agent), light, and trace metals capable of catalyzing the reaction. If molecular oxygen is involved, the reaction is generally rapid and termed "auto-oxidation." Chemically, oxidation is classed as a loss of electrons, which requires an electron acceptor, or oxidizing agent, which could be, for example, iron undergoing a ferric (Fe^{3+}) to ferrous (Fe^{2+}) change. Oxidation reactions generally involve free radical chain reactions, and the initial free radical may arise through thermal or photolytic bond cleavage or a redox process involving a trace metal ion. Once formed the radical can then be propagated, catalyzed by the metal ions present, until a suitable chemical inhibitor (antioxidant) or termination reaction intervenes. Oxidation reactions usually produce highly colored degradation products, which can be detected by eye before chemical detection is possible. Many drugs undergo oxidation; for example, adrenaline produces adrenochrome, which is intensely pink, and degradation is initiated by free radicals induced by light and further catalyzed by multivalent metal ions.

Photolysis

If the compound absorbs light, it is absorbing energy with the potential to break or rearrange bonds, produce light emission such as fluorescence or phosphorescence, or increase temperature. Light energy is inversely proportional to wavelength, therefore UV light (220–370 nm) with the shortest wavelength has the highest energy. Photodegradation is therefore dependent on the wavelength of the light and also its intensity. Most degradation occurs through UV light, which is present in sunlight (290–1750 nm) and also artificial lighting such as fluorescent tubes (320–380 nm). Prevention of photodegradation is achieved by suitable light opaque packaging such as foil wraps or amber glass.

Reaction Kinetics

Any chemical reaction is controlled by reactant concentrations. Therefore for a hydrolysis reaction it is possible to write the simple equation:

$$[C] + [H_2O] \rightarrow [degradant]$$

where [C] is the drug's concentration and $[H_2O]$ the water concentration. There are therefore two concentration terms present, a second-order reaction, but the water concentration can be considered constant relative to the drug since it is normally present in large excess, and the reaction can be simplified to a pseudo–first order.

$$[C] \rightarrow [degradant]$$

Mathematically this can be described by a monoexponential equation as follows:

$$\ln [C] = \ln[C_o] - Kt$$

where $[C_o]$ is the initial concentration, K is the reaction rate constant, and t is the elapsed time. This is a linear equation, and determination of [C] at various time intervals permit the calculation of K from the slope of the resulting line (Fig. 5). A suitable acceptable level of degradation is 95%, therefore $C/C_o = 0.95$, $\ln 0.95 = -0.051$, thus time to 95% degradation $= -0.051/K$. Knowledge of the reaction constant therefore permits calculation of the time required to reach a particular level of degradation. This is only applicable if the degradation obeys first-order kinetics, and it is important to verify that these assumptions are fully applicable.

Temperature

Since degradation is a chemical reaction it is influenced by the temperature (i.e., storage conditions) at which the reaction is conducted. An increase in temperature produces an increase in reaction rate with generally a 10°C rise producing a two- to fivefold increase

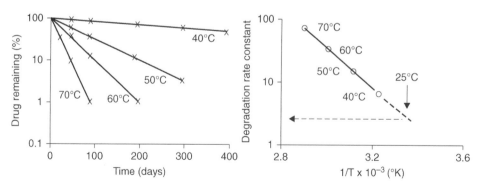

Figure 5 Stability testing and shelf life determination. A degradation study is conducted to determine the rate constant of degradation at various accelerated conditions, in this case, temperature. Note that degradation measurements should be tailored to the rate of degradation, and only sufficient measurements to determine the rate constant are required. The various rate constants can then be plotted using an Arrhenius plot, which can be extrapolated to determine shelf life at lower storage temperatures, for example, 25°C or 4°C.

in reaction rate. The Arrhenius relationship, which links temperature and reaction rate, is described by:

$$\ln K = \ln A - \left(\frac{E_a}{RT}\right)$$

where T is the temperature ($^{\circ}$K), R the gas constant, E_a the reaction's activation energy, A the frequency factor, and K the reaction rate constant. A plot of the ln K determined at various temperatures against the reciprocal of absolute temperature provides a straight line. Determination of this relationship allows the reaction rate constant to be determined at any temperature, and from this it is possible to calculate the time taken to reach a predetermined level of degradation.

Stability Testing

The above information indicates that a range of factors affect drug stability, and it is important within preformulation to test these and define storage and handling parameters that permit development studies. It is also important to provide sufficient information to allow a submission to regulatory authorities should the drug progress. A key factor in stability is time, and it is important to initiate these studies as timely as possible. Accelerated studies are normally conducted in an attempt to speed up time by deliberately stressing the compound through elevated temperatures and utilizing the relationships above to calculate stability at the proposed storage temperature. One other feature is the container and closure system employed. If the effect of humidity is under examination, then a sealed glass container, which prevents water vapor ingress, may provide a very different result to a polymeric container where water vapor and oxygen transmission rates maybe appreciable, especially over prolonged time periods.

Initial Studies

Initial studies are directed at quickly determining suitable handling and storage parameters, see Table 3, and a range of conditions usually accelerated will be tested possibly in combination with analytical development studies. This dual approach determines stability and ensures that degradation products will be detected by the analytical method. For solutions a quick accelerated approach is to autoclave at terminal sterilization conditions of 121°C for 15 minutes. If the solution survives and Arrhenius conditions apply, then stability for 15 minutes at 121°C translates to stability at 21°C of between 5 days and 50 years. This information will also guide future longer-term studies, since testing at reduced temperature (4°C) may not be warranted if adequate stability exists under ambient conditions and vice versa. Since a large number of parameters can influence stability, these can be examined either using a structured approach or statistically using a factorial approach. The latter is outside the scope of this chapter but can provide useful information related to the interaction of the various stability parameters.

Regulatory Stability

If the compound looks as though it may progress beyond development, regulatory-compliant stability studies will be required for the API. The conditions are detailed in

Table 3 Stability Study Test Conditions

Initial test studies

State	Condition	Test conditions
Solid	Temperature	4°C
		25°C/60% RH or 30°C/65% RH[a]
		40°C/75% RH[a]
		50°C
Solution	Humidity	Variable humidity at main storage temperature
	Processing	Ball milling or compression
	Temperature	4°C, 25°C, or 30°C; 40°C, 50°C, or 121°C
	PH	1, 3, 5, 7, 9, and 11 at 25°C and elevated temperature
	Oxidation	Solution sparged with oxygen or containing H_2O_2
	Photolysis	Light source producing outdoor daylight as defined by ISO 10977 (1993)[a]

Regulatory[a]

Study	Storage conditions	Minimum duration at submission
General conditions		
Accelerated	40°C ± 2°C/75% RH ± 5% RH	6 mo
Intermediate	30°C ± 2°C/65% RH ± 5% RH	6 mo
Long term	25°C ± 2°C/60% RH ± 5% RH or same as intermediate	12 mo
Drugs intended for refrigerated storage		
Accelerated	25°C ± 2°C/60% RH ± 5% RH	6 mo
Long term	5°C ± 3°C	12 mo
Drugs intended for frozen storage		
Long term	−20°C ± 5°C	12 mo

Test time points recommended for above: 0, 3, 6, 9, 12, 18, 24, 36, 48, and 60 mo

[a]Conditions specified by ICH for stability testing.

published guidelines (20), and permit accelerated and real-time data to be presented. However, there are requirements that the material is in its final container during the test and that three batches, which have been manufactured at close to final production levels, are tested to ensure consistency. In addition, long-term testing at the proposed storage conditions should be for a minimum of one year or the proposed shelf life of the API. The pass specification for these studies will be the final specification for the API, including all appropriate quality parameters.

Excipient Compatibility

Preformulation excipient compatibility studies can be performed to screen potential formulation mixtures. These can be guided by the information obtained on the solid properties, which may indicate a particular formulation approach, that is, tablet or capsule is favored. A broad range of excipients should be tested such as diluents (lactose, microcrystalline cellulose, and dibasic calcium phosphate), disintegrants (maize starch, modified starch, and polyvinyl pyrrolidone), lubricants (magnesium stearate and stearic acid) and glidants (colloidal silica). The current accepted technique is to mix the compound and excipient together in a 50:50 ratio and examine the mix using DSC over a temperature range that encompasses thermal changes due to both the drug and excipient. If the resulting trace contains new thermal events or gross changes to existing events, this is indicative of an interaction. This may warrant further investigation using accelerated stability testing approaches.

CONCLUSIONS

Preformulation is an important stage in drug development either for a program as a whole or for individual candidate compounds. Since the current development paradigm is to collect key decision-making information as quickly as possible through virtual or high-throughput systems, the boundary between preformulation, development, and even drug discovery is not precise. High-throughput systems are now available and will be increasingly employed in preformulation studies to permit early development decisions with concomitant commercial advantages. Preformulation should therefore maximize the information available while minimizing the resource expenditure and time taken. However, it is a staged process that starts by gathering basic information on a candidate drug, and utilization of that information will be linked to other discovery/development stages, and preformulation therefore cannot occur in isolation. For example, it interacts with preclinical pharmacology to provide suitable diluents for testing, medicinal chemistry to optimize molecular properties for absorption or solubility, and formulation to identify suitable excipients. However, during this it should always be to the fore that if development is successful and the drug proceeds to a marketed product, the final contribution will be an acceptable specification for the API that can be traced back to the original discovery with no postmarketing issues.

REFERENCES

1. Bauer J, Spanton S, Henry R, et al. Ritonavir: an extraordinary example of conformational polymorphism. Pharm Res 2001; 18(6):859–866.
2. Wells JI. Pharmaceutical Preformulation—The Physicochemical Properties of Drug Substances. In: Rubinstein MH, ed. Pharmaceutical Technology. Chichester: Ellis Horwood Ltd, 1988:225.
3. Carstensen JT. Pharmaceutical Preformulation. Boca Raton: CRC Press, 1998:305.
4. Crommelin DJA, Sindelar RD. Pharmaceutical Biotechnology. 2nd ed. London: Taylor Francis, 2002:423.
5. McNally EJ, Hastedt JE. Protein Formulation and Delivery. In: Swarbrick J, Series ed. Drugs and the Pharmaceutical Sciences, Vol 175, 2nd ed. New York: Marcel Dekker, 2008:351.
6. Guarino RA. New Drug Approval Process—The Global Challenge. In: Swarbrick J, Series ed. Drugs and the Pharmaceutical Sciences, Vol 100, 3rd ed. New York: Marcel Dekker, 2000:471.
7. Nusim S. Active Pharmaceutical Ingredients—Development, Manufacture and Regulation. In: Swarbrick J, Series ed. Drugs and the Pharmaceutical Sciences. Vol 151. New York: Marcel Dekker, 2005.
8. Hirsch CA, Messenger RJ, Brannon JL. Fenoprofen—drug form selection and pre-formulation stability studies. J Pharma Sci 1978; 67(2):231–236.
9. Manly CJ, Louise-May S, Hammer JD. The impact of informatics and computational chemistry on synthesis and screening. Drug Discov Today 2001; 6(21):1101–1110.
10. Tetko IV. Computing chemistry on the web. Drug Discov Today 2005; 10(22):1497–1500.

11. Pehourcq F, Jarry C, Bannwarth B. Potential of immobilized artificial membrane chromatography for lipophilicity determination of arylpropionic acid nonsteroidal anti-inflammatory drugs. J Pharm Biomed Anal 2003; 33(2):137–144.

12. Hou T, Wang J. Structure—ADME relationship: still a long way to go? Expert Opin Drug Metab Toxicol 2008; 4(6):759–770.

13. Bevan CD, Lloyd RS. A high-throughput screening method for the determination of aqueous drug solubility using laser nephelometry in microtiter plates. Anal Chem 2000; 72(8):1781–1787.

14. Wong KS, Kenseth J, Strasburg R. Validation and long-term assessment of an approach for the high throughput determination of lipophilicity (log P-OW) values using multiplexed, absorbance-based capillary electrophoresis. J Pharm Sci 2004; 93(4):916–931.

15. Llinas A, Box KJ, Burley JC, et al. A new method for the reproducible generation of polymorphs: two forms of sulindac with very different solubilities. J Appl Crystallogr 2007; 40:379–381.

16. Dehring KA, Workman HL, Miller KD, et al. Automated robotic liquid handling/laser-based nephelometry system for high throughput measurement of kinetic aqueous solubility. J Pharm Biomed Anal 2004; 36(3):447–456.

17. Rao RN, Nagaraju V. An overview of the recent trends in development of HPLC methods for determination of impurities in drugs. J Pharm Biomed Anal 2003; 33(3):335–377.

18. Qiu FH, Norwood DL. Identification of pharmaceutical impurities. J Liq Chromatogr Relat Technol 2007; 30(5–8):877–935.

19. Snyder LR, Kirkland JJ, Glajch JL. Practical HPLC Method Development. 2nd ed. New York: John Wiley and Sons, 1997.

20. Anon. International Conference on Harmonisation, 2008 [cited May 2008]. Available at: http://ich.org.

21. Denyer SP, Baird RM. Guide to microbiological control in pharmaceuticals. In: Rubinstein MH, ed. Ellis Horwood Series in Pharmaceutical Technology. New York: Ellis Horwood, 1990.

22. Aguiar AJ, Krc J Jr., Kinkel AW, et al. Effect of polymorphism on absorption of chloramphenicol from chloramphenicol palmitate. J Pharm Sci 1967; 56(7):847–853.

23. Huang LF, Tong WQ. Impact of solid state properties on developability assessment of drug candidates. Adv Drug Deliv Rev 2004; 56(3):321–334.

24. Carstensen JT. Advanced Pharmaceutical Solids. In: Swarbrick J, Series ed. Drugs and the Pharmaceutical Sciences. Vol 110. New York: Marcel Dekker, 2001:518.

25. Byrn S, Pfieffer R, Ganey M, et al. Pharmaceutical solids—a strategic approach to regulatory considerations. Pharm Res 1995; 12(7):945–954.

26. Serajuddin ATM. Salt formation to improve drug solubility. Adv Drug Deliv Rev 2007; 59 (7):603–616.

27. Paulekuhn GS, Dressman JB, Saal C. Trends in active pharmaceutical ingredient salt selection based on analysis of the Orange Book Database. J Med Chem 2007; 50(26):6665–6672.

28. Brittain HG. Physical Characterisation of Pharmaceutical Solids. In: Swarbrick J, Series ed. Drugs and the Pharmaceutical Sciences. Vol 70, 1st ed. New York: Marcel Dekker, 1995:424.

29. Singhal D, Curatolo W. Drug polymorphism and dosage form design: a practical perspective. Adv Drug Deliv Rev 2004; 56(3):335–347.

30. Devilliers MM, Vanderwatt JG, Lotter AP. Kinetic study of the solid-state photolytic degradation of 2 polymorphic forms of furosemide. Int J Pharm 1992; 88(1–3):275–283.

31. Zhang GGZ, Law D, Schmitt EA, et al. Phase transformation considerations during process development and manufacture of solid oral dosage forms. Adv Drug Deliv Rev 2004; 56 (3):371–390.

32. Yu L. Amorphous pharmaceutical solids: preparation, characterization and stabilization. Adv Drug Deliv Rev 2001; 48(1):27–42.

33. Rabel SR, Jona JA, Maurin MB. Applications of modulated differential scanning calorimetry in preformulation studies. J Pharm Biomed Anal 1999; 21(2):339–345.

34. Craig DQM, Reading M. Thermal Analysis of Pharmaceuticals. 1st ed. Boca Raton: CRC Press, 2007:416.

35. Tumer YTA, Roberts CJ, Davies MC. Scanning probe microscopy in the field of drug delivery. Advanced Drug Delivery Reviews 2007; 59:1453–1473.

36. Morissette SL, Soukasene S, Levinson D, et al. Elucidation of crystal form diversity of the HIV protease inhibitor ritonavir by high-throughput crystallization. Proc Natl Acad Sci U S A 2003; 100(5):2180–2184.

37. Price SL. The computational prediction of pharmaceutical crystal structures and polymorphism. Adv Drug Deliv Rev 2004; 56(3):301–319.

38. Beyer T, Day GM, Price SL. The prediction, morphology, and mechanical properties of the polymorphs of paracetamol. J Am Chem Soc 2001; 123(21):5086–5094.

39. Hickey AJ, Concessio NM. Descriptors of irregular particle morphology and powder properties. Adv Drug Deliv Rev 1997; 26(1):29–40.

40. Liu R. Introduction. In: Liu R, ed. Water-Insoluble Drug Formulation. CRC Press: Boca Raton, 2008:1–4.

41. Chen Y, Qi X, Liu R. Prediction of solubility. In: Liu R, ed. Water-Insoluble Drug Formulation. CRC Press: Boca Raton, 2008:23–59.

42. Sangster J. Octanol-water partition coefficients: fundamentals and physical chemistry. In: Fogg P, ed. Series in Solution Chemistry. Vol 2. Chichester: John Wiley and Sons, 1997:170.

43. Lipinski CA, Lombardo F, Dominy BW, et al. Experimental and computational approaches to estimate solubility and permeability in drug discovery and development settings. Adv Drug Deliv Rev 1997; 23(1–3):p. 3–25.

44. Wilson CG, Washignton N. Physiological Pharmaceutics: Biological Barriers to Drug Absorption. 2nd ed. Chichester: Ellis Horwood, 2001.

45. Artursson P, Palm K, Luthman K. Caco-2 monolayers in experimental and theoretical predictions of drug transport. Adv Drug Deliv Rev 2001; 46(1–3):27–43.

46. Shah P, Jogani V, Bagchi T, et al. Role of Caco-2 cell monolayers in prediction of intestinal drug absorption. Biotechnol Prog 2006; 22(1):186–198.

11

Disperse Systems

Wandee Rungseevijitprapa
Faculty of Pharmaceutical Sciences, Ubon Ratchathani University, Ubon Ratchathani, Thailand

Florence Siepmann and Juergen Siepmann
Department of Pharmaceutical Technology, College of Pharmacy, Université Lille Nord de France, Lille, France

Ornlaksana Paeratakul
Faculty of Pharmacy, Srinakharinwirot University, Nakhon Nayok, Thailand

INTRODUCTION

A disperse system is defined as a heterogeneous, two-phase system in which the internal (dispersed, discontinuous) phase is distributed or dispersed within the continuous (external) phase or vehicle. Various pharmaceutical systems are included in this definition, the internal and external phases being gases, liquids, or solids. Disperse systems are also important in other fields of application, for example, processing and manufacturing of household and industrial products such as cosmetics, foods, and paints.

This chapter describes the basic principles involved in the development of disperse systems. Emphasis is laid on systems that are of particular pharmaceutical interest, namely, suspensions, emulsions, and colloids. Theoretical concepts, preparation techniques, and methods used to characterize and stabilize disperse systems are presented. The term "particle" is used in its broadest sense, including gases, liquids, solids, molecules, and aggregates.

Classification

Disperse systems can be classified in various ways. Classification based on the physical state of the two constituent phases is presented in Table 1. The dispersed phase and the dispersion medium can be solids, liquids, or gases. Pharmaceutically most important are suspensions, emulsions, and aerosols. Suspensions and emulsions are described in detail in sections "Suspensions" and "Emulsions"; pharmaceutical aerosols are treated in volume 2, chapter 5. A suspension is a solid-liquid dispersion, for example, a solid drug that is dispersed within a liquid being a poor solvent for the drug. An emulsion is a liquid-liquid

Table 1 Classification Scheme of Disperse Systems on the Basis of the Physical State of the Dispersed Phase and the Dispersion Medium

Dispersed phase	Dispersion medium		
	Solid	Liquid	Gas
Solid	Solid suspension (zinc oxide paste, toothpaste)	Suspension (tetracycline oral suspension USP, bentonite magma NF)	Solid aerosol (epinephrine bitartrate inhalation aerosol USP)
Liquid	Solid emulsion (hydrophilic petrolatum USP)	Emulsion (mineral oil emulsion USP)	Liquid aerosol (nasal sprays, fog)
Gas	Solid foam (foamed plastics)	Foam (rectal and topical foams)	None

Pharmaceuticals and other examples are given in brackets.
Abbreviations: USP, United States Pharmacopoeia.

Table 2 Classification Scheme of Disperse Systems on the Basis of the Particle Size of the Dispersed Phase

Category	Range of particle size	Characteristics	Examples
Molecular dispersion	<1.0 nm	Particles invisible by electron microscopy; pass through semipermeable membranes; generally rapid diffusion	Oxygen molecules, potassium and chloride ions dissolved in water
Colloidal dispersion	1.0 nm–1.0 µm	Particles not resolved by ordinary microscope but visible by electron microscopy; pass through filter paper but not through semipermeable membranes; generally slow diffusion	Colloidal silver sols, surfactant micelles in an aqueous phase, latexes and pseudolatexes
Coarse dispersion	>1.0 µm	Particles visible by ordinary microscopy; do not pass through normal filter paper or semipermeable membranes	Pharmaceutical emulsions and suspensions

dispersion in which the two phases are either completely immiscible or saturated with each other. In the case of aerosols, either a liquid (e.g., drug solution) or a solid (e.g., fine drug particles) are dispersed within a gaseous phase. As evident, there is no disperse system in which both phases are gases.

Another classification scheme is based on the size of the dispersed particles within the dispersion medium (Table 2). The particles of the dispersed phase may vary considerably in size, from large particles visible to the naked eye, down to particles in the colloidal size range, and particles of atomic and molecular dimensions. Generally, three classes are distinguished: molecular, colloidal, and coarse dispersions. Molecular dispersions are homogeneous in character and form true solutions. Colloidal dispersions are intermediate in size between true solutions and coarse dispersions. The term "colloidal" is usually applied to systems in which the particle size of the dispersed phase is in the range of 1 to 1000 nm and the dispersion medium is a liquid. Nanoparticles distributed within a liquid and aqueous polymer dispersions for pharmaceutical coating applications are examples of colloidal systems. Colloidal dispersions are described in more detail in section "Colloids and Colloidal Dispersions." Dispersions containing larger dispersed phases, usually 10 to 50 μm in size, are referred to as "coarse dispersions," which include most pharmaceutical suspensions and emulsions.

The defined size ranges and limits are somewhat arbitrary since there are no specific boundaries between the categories. The transition of size ranges, either from molecular dispersions to colloids or from colloids to coarse dispersions, is very gradual. For example, an emulsion may exhibit colloidal properties, and yet the average droplet size may be larger than 1 μm. This is due to the fact that most disperse systems are heterogeneous with respect to their particle size (1).

In colloid science, colloidal systems are commonly classified as being lyophilic or lyophobic, based on the interaction between the dispersed phase and the dispersion medium. In lyophilic dispersions, there is a considerable affinity between the two constituent phases (e.g., hydrophilic polymers in water, polystyrene in benzene). The more restrictive terms "hydrophilic" and "oleophilic"can be used when the external phase is water and a nonpolar liquid, respectively. In contrast, in lyophobic systems there is little attraction between the two phases (e.g., aqueous dispersions of sulfur). If the dispersion medium is water, the term "hydrophobic" can be used. Resulting from the high affinity between the dispersed phase and the dispersion medium, lyophilic systems often form spontaneously and are considered as being thermodynamically stable. On the other hand, lyophobic systems generally do not form spontaneously and are intrinsically unstable.

The number of the constituent phases of a disperse system can be higher than two. Many commercial multiphase pharmaceutical products cannot be categorized easily and should be classified as complex disperse systems. Examples include various types of multiple emulsions and suspensions in which solid particles are dispersed within an emulsion base. These complexities influence the physicochemical properties of the system, which, in turn, determine the overall characteristics of the dosage forms with which the formulators are concerned.

Disperse systems can also be classified on the basis of their aggregation behavior as molecular or micellar (association) systems. Molecular dispersions are composed of single macromolecules distributed uniformly within the medium, for example, protein and polymer solutions. In micellar systems, the units of the dispersed phase consist of several molecules, which arrange themselves to form aggregates, such as surfactant micelles in aqueous solutions.

Pharmaceutical Applications

Disperse systems have found a wide variety of applications in pharmacy (1). Liquid dispersions, such as emulsions and suspensions, have the advantage to be easily swallowed and flexibly dosed compared with solid dosage forms. Patient compliance is generally better, particularly in the case of infants, children, and elderly (patient compliance). In addition, the small particle size of the drug present in disperse systems results in a large specific surface area. This leads to a higher rate of drug dissolution and possibly a superior bioavailability compared with solid dosage forms containing larger drug particles (2–6). This can be of major importance in the case of poorly soluble drugs.

A suspension dosage form is often selected if the drug is insoluble in aqueous vehicles at the dosage required and/or when the attempts to solubilize the drug through the use of cosolvents, surfactants, and other solubilizing agents would compromise the stability or the safety of the product or, in the case of oral administration, its organoleptic properties (7–10). The bitter or unpleasant tastes of dissolved drug molecules can often be improved by the selection of an insoluble form of the drug.

Colloidal systems have been used extensively in pharmacy, and their applications have grown rapidly over the last decades. Colloids have been employed in nuclear medicine as diagnostic and therapeutic aids (e.g., colloidal ^{198}Au, ^{99m}Tc, and sulfur); as adjuvants enhancing the immune effect of various agents (e.g., toxins adsorbed onto a colloidal carrier); and as anticancer agents (e.g., colloidal copper) (11). Certain drugs show improved therapeutic effects when formulated in a colloidal state (12). Colloidal silver chloride, silver iodide, and silver protein are effective germicides and do not cause irritation that is characteristic of ionic silver salts. More advanced applications of colloids include a variety of drug delivery systems, the development of polypeptide chemo-therapeutic agents, and the utilization of colloidal systems as pharmaceutical excipients, product components, vehicles, and carriers. Colloidal drug delivery systems, administered topically, orally, parenterally, or by inhalation, have been prepared for the purposes of drug targeting, controlled release, and/or protection of the drugs (13–17). Certain naturally occurring plant macromolecules are capable of existing in the colloidal state and have been used for medical purposes; for example, hydroxyethyl starch (HES) has been used widely as plasma extender. Aqueous polymer dispersions (latexes and pseudolatexes) based on cellulosic and acrylic polymers have replaced organic solvent-based systems in a wide range of pharmaceutical coatings and controlled-release technologies (18,19).

Patient acceptance is probably the most important reason why emulsions are popular oral and topical dosage forms. Oils and drugs having an objectionable taste or texture can be made more palatable for oral administration by formulating into emulsions (20–25). As a result, mineral oil-based laxatives, oil-soluble vitamins, vegetable oils, high-fat nutritive preparations for enteral feeding, and certain drugs such as valproic acid are formulated frequently in an oil-in-water (o/w) emulsion form. With topically applied emulsions, the formulation scientist can control the viscosity, appearance, and degree of greasiness of cosmetic and dermatologic products. o/w emulsions are most useful as water-washable bases, whereas water-in-oil (w/o) emulsions are used widely for the treatment of dry skin and emollient applications to provide an occlusive effect. Semisolid preparations, such as ointments and creams, represent the dispersions of liquids in solids, which are used topically. Emulsions are also employed in many other clinical applications as radiopaque emulsions and parenteral emulsions and in blood replacement therapy (26–33).

Solid dispersions are disperse systems in which both phases, the dispersed phase as well as the dispersion medium, are in the solid state. The drug can for example be present in the form of very fine particles or molecules distributed within an inert water-soluble carrier. This type of system is frequently used to enhance the dissolution rate and oral absorption of poorly water-soluble drugs (1,34–36). Several techniques have been used to prepare such solid dispersions. The drug may be dissolved in the molten carrier. After cooling, a mixture of drug and carrier or a solid solution (molecular dispersion) of the drug in the carrier results. Another method is to dissolve the drug and the carrier in a suitable organic solvent, followed by evaporation of the solvent and subsequent coprecipitation of the drug and carrier.

A solid or a liquid aerosol can be defined as a solid-gas or liquid-gas disperse system (37,38). The main purpose of this dosage form is to deliver the drug to body surfaces/cavities, such as nasal passages or the respiratory tract (for details, the reader is referred to chap. 5, "Delivery of Drugs by the Pulmonary Route," vol. 2). Pharmaceutical dosage forms include aerosol sprays, inhalations, and insufflations. Another type of the dispersion involving gas is the foam product, in which air or a propellant is emulsified within a liquid phase. Such preparations containing drugs (e.g., antibiotics or steroids) are often used topically. Foams containing spermicides are used for topical application within the vagina. Others have also been used widely for cosmetic purposes.

From a technical point of view, disperse systems are often involved in various steps of pharmaceutical manufacturing processes. The principles of colloid science govern many practices and operations in industrial pharmacy, such as particle size reduction (e.g., milling of pharmaceuticals), coating of pharmaceutical solids/solid dosage forms, microencapsulation, solubilization, and complexation of drugs. Solutions of water-soluble polymers act as viscosity-imparting agents, thus permitting the improvement of the physical stability of emulsions and suspensions. Organic polymer solutions or aqueous polymer dispersions are used as coating materials for solid dosage forms to achieve controlled drug release, to improve chemical stability, and to provide taste masking, moisture protection, and/or the identification of the product (39–42). Dispersions of surfactants provide a means of enhancing the solubility of a drug via micellar solubilization.

FUNDAMENTAL PROPERTIES

Particle Properties

The most significant characteristics of a dispersion are the size and shape of the dispersed particles. Both properties depend largely on the chemical and physical nature of the dispersed phase and on the method used to prepare the dispersion. The mean particle diameter as well as the particle size distribution of the dispersed phase have a profound effect on the properties of the dosage forms, such as product appearance, settling rate, drug solubility, resuspendability, and stability. Clinically important, the particle size can affect the drug release from the dosage forms that are administered orally, parenterally, rectally, and topically. Thus, these parameters have to be taken into account when formulating pharmaceutical products with good physical stability and reproducible bioavailability. This section discusses the basic principles of micromeritics, the science and technology of small particles. Further information on the techniques and equipment currently used in the determination of particle size can be found in the section "Particle Size Analysis."

Particle Shape

Insoluble particles of drugs or pharmaceutical excipients obtained from various sources and manufacturing processes are seldom uniform spheres even after size reduction and classification. For example, precipitation and mechanical comminution generally produce randomly shaped particles, unless the solids possess pronounced crystal habits or the solids being ground possess strongly developed cleavage planes. Primary particles may exist in various shapes, ranging from simple to irregular geometries. Their aggregation behavior produces an even greater variety of shapes and structures. The terminology and definitions of different particle shapes have been described previously (43). Most common shapes found with pharmaceutical solids are spheres, cylinders, rods, needles, and various crystalline shapes.

Emulsification processes produce spherical droplets of the internal phase to minimize the interfacial area between the two phases. For example, the particles of true latexes are spherical because they are typically prepared by emulsion polymerization, and the polymerization of solubilized monomer is initiated inside the spherical, swollen surfactant micelles (44). Polymeric particles of pseudolatexes prepared from preformed polymers by either solvent evaporation or inverse emulsification processes are also spherical, or near spherical, for analogous reasons. Various pharmaceutical excipients exhibit characteristic particle morphologies determined by their molecular structure and the arrangement of the molecules. Some clay particles have platelike structures possessing straight edges and hexagonal angles, for example, bentonite and kaolin, while other clays may have lath-shaped or rod-shaped particles.

Characterization of the particle shape is generally described by the deviation from sphericity, as in the case of ellipsoids, where the ratio of the two radii is the measure of deviation. The surface and volume are important properties affected by the overall shape of a particle. A more complicated relationship for particle characterization was described by Heywood who introduced shape coefficients, such as surface and volume coefficients, and elongation and flatness ratios (45).

The information on particle shape is particularly important for the understanding of the behavior of suspensions during storage. The particle shape of the suspended particles (suspensoids) may have an impact on the packing of sediment (e.g., packing density and settling characteristics), and thus product's resuspendability and stability. Packing density is defined as the weight to volume ratio of the sediment at equilibrium. Goodarznia and Sutherland (46) reported that the deviations from spherical shape and/or size uniformity can affect the packing density of suspensions containing cubes and spheroids. A wide particle size distribution often results in a high-density suspension, whereas widely differing particle shapes (e.g., plates, needles, filaments, and prisms) often produce low-density slurries. Symmetrical barrel-shaped particles of calcium carbonate were found to produce stable suspensions without caking upon storage, while asymmetric needle-shaped particles formed a tenacious sediment cake, which could not be easily redispersed (47). Also the viscosity of colloidal dispersions is affected by the shape of the dispersed phases. Spherocolloids form dispersions of relatively low viscosity, while systems containing linear particles are generally more viscous. The relationship of particle shape and viscosity reflects the degree of solvation of the particles. In a good solvent, a colloidal particle unrolls and exposes its maximum surface area due to an extensive interaction between the dispersed phase and the dispersion medium. In contrast, in a poor solvent, the particle tends to coil up to assume a spherical shape, and the viscosity drops accordingly. Properties such as flow, sedimentation, and osmotic pressure are also affected by the changes in the particle shape of colloids.

Particle Size and Size Distribution

The particle size and size distribution of the dispersed phase represent a very important part of the knowledge required for a thorough understanding of any disperse systems. The particle size can significantly affect the absorption behavior of a drug (5,6,48,49). Certain types of dosage forms require specific size ranges; for example, suspension aerosols delivering drugs into the respiratory tract should contain particles in the order of 0.5 to 5 μm and no particles larger than 10 μm.

The size of a spherical particle is readily expressed in terms of its diameter. With asymmetric particles, an equivalent spherical diameter is used to relate the size of the particle to the diameter of a perfect sphere having the same surface area (surface diameter, d_s), the same volume (volume diameter, d_v), or the same observed area in its most stable plane (projected diameter, d_p) (12). The size may also be expressed using the Stokes' diameter, d_{st}, which describes an equivalent sphere undergoing sedimentation at the same rate as the sample particle. Obviously, the type of diameter reflects the method and equipment employed in determining the particle size. Since any collection of particles is usually polydisperse (as opposed to a monodisperse sample in which particles are fairly uniform in size), it is necessary to know not only the mean size of the particles, but also the particle size distribution.

The particle size data can be presented by graphical and digital methods. When the number or weight of particles lying within a certain size range is plotted against the size range or mean particle size, a bar graph (histogram) or a frequency distribution curve is obtained (12). Alternatively, the cumulative percentage over or under a particular size can be plotted against the particle size. This results in a typical sigmoidal curve called cumulative frequency plot. From these data, the mean particle size, standard deviation, and the extent of polydispersity may be determined.

Various theoretical distribution functions have been proposed, such as normal or Gaussian distribution and the lognormal distribution. The simplest case is described by the normal distribution equation with a specific mean value and standard deviation. However, for most pharmaceutical disperse systems, the normal equation is usually not appropriate and the lognormal equation is commonly applied. For example, the lognormal distributions are often used to describe the particle size distributions of ground drug powders (43,50).

Special attention must be paid to the interpretation of particle size data presented in terms of either *weight* or *number* of particles. Particle weight data may be more useful in sedimentation studies, whereas number data are of particular value in surface-related phenomena such as dissolution. Values on the basis of number can be collected by a counting technique such as microscopy, while values based on weight are usually obtained by sedimentation or sieving methods. Conversion of the estimates from a number distribution to a weight distribution, or vice versa, is also possible using adequate mathematical approaches, for example, the Hatch–Choate equations.

Surface Properties and Interfacial Phenomena

One of the most obvious properties of a disperse system is the vast interfacial area that exists between the dispersed phase and the dispersion medium (51–53). When considering the surface and interfacial properties of the dispersed particles, two factors must be taken into account: the first relates to an increase in the surface free energy as the particle size is reduced and the specific surface increased; the second deals with the presence of an electrical charge on the particle surface. This section covers the basic theoretical concepts related to interfacial phenomena and the characteristics of colloids, which are fundamental to an understanding of the behavior of any disperse systems having larger dispersed phases (for further details on surfactants the reader is referred to chap. 12, "Surfactant Systems").

The Interface

An interface is defined as a boundary between two phases. The solid-liquid and the liquid-liquid interfaces are of primary interest in suspensions and emulsions, respectively. Other types of interfaces such as the liquid-gas (foams) or solid-gas interfaces also play a major role in certain pharmaceutical dosage forms, for example, aerosols.

A large surface area of the dispersed particles is associated with a high surface free energy that renders the system thermodynamically unstable. The surface free energy, ΔG, can be calculated from the total surface area, ΔA, as follows:

$$\Delta G = \gamma_{SL} \cdot \Delta A \quad \text{or} \quad \Delta G = \gamma_{LL} \cdot \Delta A \tag{1}$$

where γ_{SL} and γ_{LL} are the interfacial tensions between the solid particles and the liquid medium and the liquid and liquid mediums, respectively.

Very small dispersed particles are highly energetic. To approach a stable state, they tend to regroup themselves to reduce the surface free energy of the system. An equilibrium will be reached when $\Delta G = 0$. This condition may be accomplished either by a reduction of the interfacial tension or by a decrease of the total surface area.

Particle Interactions

The interactions between similar particles, dissimilar particles, and the dispersion medium constitute a complex but essential part of dispersion technology. Such interparticle interactions include both attractive and repulsive forces. These forces depend upon the nature, size, and orientation of the species as well as on the distance of separation between and among the particles of the dispersed phase and the dispersion medium, respectively. The balance between these forces determines the overall characteristics of the system.

The particles in a disperse system, with liquid or gas being the dispersion medium, are thermally mobile and occasionally collide as a result of the Brownian motion. As the particles approach one another, both attractive and repulsive forces are operative. If the attractive forces prevail, agglomerates result, indicating an instability in the system. If repulsive forces dominate, a homogeneously dispersed or stable dispersion remains.

Various types of attractive interactions are operating: (*i*) dipole-dipole or Keesom orientation forces, (*ii*) dipole-induced dipole or Debye induction forces, (*iii*) induced dipole-induced dipole or London dispersion forces, and (*iv*) electrostatic forces between charged particles. The strongest forces are the electrostatic interactions between charged particles. These forces, either attractive or repulsive, are effective over a relatively long range and dependent on the ionic charge and size of the particle. Forces that are weaker and effective over a shorter distance include other types of electrostatic forces such as ion-dipole, ion-induced dipole, and (*i*) to (*iii*). The group of these last three forces is often referred to as van der Waals forces, which result from the interaction of electromagnetic dipoles within the particles. They produce a short-range type of interaction, varying inversely with r^6; where r is the interparticle distance. Even though they are relatively weak, the van der Waals forces coupled with hydrogen bond interactions are significant factors describing the behavior of most nonionic compounds in liquids and other dispersion media. These various types of attractive interparticulate forces can lead to the instabilities of disperse systems described in section "Instabilities and Stabilization Concepts."

Electrical Properties of the Interfaces

Most insoluble materials, either solids or liquids, develop a surface charge when dispersed within an aqueous medium. These surface charges of particles may arise from several mechanisms. For example, the ionization of functional groups present at the surface of the particle, such as carboxylic acid or amine groups, can be involved. The charge is then dependent on the extent of ionization and is a function of the pH of the dispersion medium. Furthermore, surface charges can be developed due to the adsorption or desorption of protons. A variety of colloidal systems (e.g., polymers, metal oxides) fall into this group. For example, the surface hydroxyl groups of aluminum hydroxide gel can adsorb protons and become positively charged or may donate protons to become negatively charged. An important property of such systems is the point of zero charge (PZC), which represents the pH at which the net surface charge is zero. More general, surface charges of dispersed particles may be caused by preferential adsorption of specific ions onto the surface. Surface charges can also be introduced by ionic surfactants. For example, oil globules in an o/w emulsion exhibit a surface charge if anionic or cationic surface-active agents are used. The surfactant molecules are oriented at the oil-water interface so that the charged hydrophilic groups are directed toward the water phase. Ion deficiencies in the crystal lattice or interior of the particles may also cause surface charges. Many mineral clays exhibit a negative surface charge because of isomorphic substitution; for example, an Al^{3+} ion occupies a site that is usually occupied by a Si^{4+} ion, resulting in a deficit of charge. Similarly, antacid magaldrate exhibits a positive surface charge: Mg^{2+} ions in the crystal lattice are partially substituted by Al^{3+} ions.

When a charged particle is dispersed within a dispersion medium containing dissolved cations and anions, the surface charges of the particle interact with the dissolved ions in solution. For a detailed description of the occurring phenomena, the reader is referred to the literature (12). Roughly, the electric distribution at the interface is equivalent to a double layer of charge, a first layer being tightly bound, and a second layer that is more diffusive. The ζ-potential is defined as the potential at the shear plane (interface separating layers that move with the particle from layers that do not move with the particle) and can be regarded as the "apparent" or "active" charge of the particle.

Derjaguin, Landau, Verwey, and Overbeek developed a theory giving insight into the energy of interaction between suspended particles (54–56). This theory is thus often referred to as the DLVO theory. It relates the stability of a disperse system to the electrolyte content in the continuous phase and provides an insight into the factors responsible for controlling the rate at which particles in disperse systems come into contact or aggregate. The process of aggregation subsequently accelerates particle sedimentation and affects redispersibility of the disperse systems. In general, the DLVO theory is applicable to pharmaceutical dosage forms (57–59) such as colloids, suspensions, and o/w emulsions. In the case of w/o systems, it must be applied with extreme caution. Figure 1 shows a typical total potential energy curve for the interaction of two charged particles (same sign) as a function of interparticle distance: the total potential energy of interaction V_{total} is the sum of the attractive potential energy V_A and the electrostatic repulsive energy V_R:

$$V_{total} = V_A + V_R \tag{2}$$

The maximum and minimum energy states are illustrated. At small distances, the van der Waals energy is greater than the repulsion energy. If the maximum is too small, two interacting particles may reach the primary minimum, and at this state of close approach the depth of the energy minimum can mean that escape is unlikely. Subsequent irreversible changes in the system might then occur, for example, sintering in suspensions or coalescence in emulsions. When the maximum in V_{total} is sufficiently high, the two particles do not reach the stage of being in close contact. To gain information about the stability of a disperse system, it is important to compare the total energy of the particles with their kinetic energy, kT (where k is the Boltzmann constant and T is the absolute temperature). The value of the maximum in V_{total} necessary to prevent the irreversible contact of particles is considered to be about 10 to 20 kT, which corresponds to a ζ-potential of approximately 50 mV (44). If the secondary minimum is deep enough

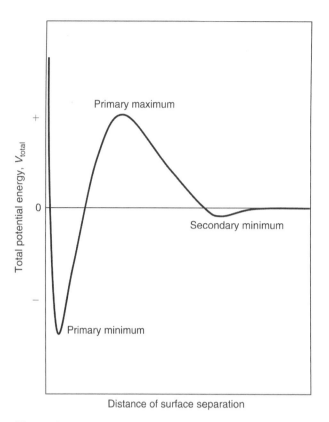

Figure 1 Schematic form of the curve of total potential energy (V_{total}) against distance of surface separation (H) for interaction between two particles, with $V_{\text{total}} = V_A + V_R$.

(about 5 kT or more), the particles might associate to form a cluster, which is loose and reversible, called a floc or floccule. Such flocculation in the secondary minimum, however, does not occur with small colloidal particles since the energy minimum is of the same order as the thermal energy of the particles, and the aggregation is easily reversed by Brownian motion.

According to the DLVO theory, disperse systems become unstable whenever their kinetic energy is sufficient to overcome the primary maximum. Thus, the instability of disperse systems increases when decreasing the height of this energy barrier and when increasing the kinetic energy of the particles. The reduction of the primary maximum can result from the addition of substances, which (*i*) neutralize the surface particle charge or cause the loss of the hydration layer; (*ii*) compress the electric double layer; and/or (*iii*) cause adsorbed species (e.g., surfactants) to desorb from the particle surface. The primary factor determining the thickness of the electric double layer is the potential energy drop-off. The potential gradient strongly depends on the concentration and charge of any electrolyte present in the dispersion medium. In water at room temperature, the thickness of the electric double layer ranges from 1 to 1000 Å, depending on the concentration of ions in the bulk phase. Increasing electrolyte concentrations lead to compressed double layers (decreasing double layer thicknesses). Thus, the particles can approach each other more closely, and the attractive forces become more important. The concentration of foreign electrolytes required to cause flocculation decreases as the valence of the coagulating ion increases. For example, less Al^{3+} ions are required to flocculate a suspension than Na^+ ions. This has been observed in many instances and is known as Schulze–Hardy rule (12). It has been shown that the quantity of electrolyte required to cause flocculation decreases by a factor of 10 when a monovalent electrolyte, for example, Na^+, is replaced by a divalent electrolyte, for example, Mg^{2+}. Furthermore, the efficiency of electrolytes to precipitate a dispersion depends on how extensively the electrolytes are hydrated. The Hofmeister or lyotropic series arranges ions in the order of increasing hydration and increasing efficiency in causing the instability. For example, the series for monovalent cations is $Cs^+ < Rb^+ < NH_4^+ < K^+ < Na^+ < Li^+$, and for divalent ions, $Ba^{2+} < Sr^{2+} < Ca^{2+} < Mg^{2+}$.

Wetting

The wetting process is a primary concern particularly in the preparation of a liquid disperse system in which the internal phase is a solid (suspension). A solid material to be suspended must first be separated into single particles, and the particles must be individually wetted by the dispersion medium to achieve a homogeneous distribution of the internal phase. Upon wetting, the air at the solid surface is replaced by the liquid medium. Obviously, the tendency of a solid to be wetted by a liquid is primarily determined by the interaction between the three phases. Experimentally, the degree of wetting of a powder can be evaluated by observing the contact angle, θ, which is defined by the boundaries of the solid surface and the tangent to the curvature of the liquid drop. The contact angle results from an equilibrium involving three interfacial tensions: those acting at the interfaces liquid-gas, solid-liquid, and solid-gas. A contact angle of $0°$ indicates an extensive interaction between the solid and the liquid phase. Thus, the solid is completely wetted by the liquid. Partial wetting occurs when the contact angles are between $0°$ and $90°$. In contrast, contact angles greater than $90°$ are classified as nonwetting situations in which the liquid cannot spread over the solid surface spontaneously. If the angle is close to $180°$, the solid substance is called "unwettable" by the liquid.

Hydrophilic substances are readily wetted by water or other polar liquids because of the good interfacial interaction resulting in small contact angles (Fig. 2). Once dispersed, they may significantly increase the viscosity of the liquid system. On the other hand, hydrophobic substances repel water but can easily be wetted by nonpolar liquids. They usually do not alter the viscosity of aqueous systems. In pharmaceutical dosage forms, aqueous vehicles or hydroalcoholic mixtures are often used. Thus, proper wetting of hydrophobic drugs is a necessary first step when preparing suspensions. Hydrophobic materials are often extremely difficult to disperse owing to poor wetting or presence of entrained air pockets, minute quantities of grease, and other contaminants. The powder may just float on the surface of the liquid, despite its higher density. Fine powders are particularly susceptible to this effect, and they may fail to become wetted even when mechanically forced below the surface of the suspending medium. To overcome this problem, to improve the wetting characteristics of hydrophobic drug powders, often

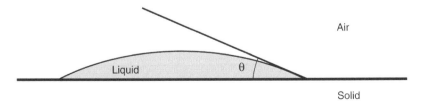

Figure 2 Scheme of a drop of liquid placed on a flat, solid surface: θ denotes the contact angle.

anionic or nonionic surfactants are used. These substances decrease the solid-liquid interfacial tension, thus facilitating the wetting process. The mechanism of surfactant action involves the preferential adsorption of the hydrophobic part of the surfactant onto the hydrophobic surface of the particle. The polar part of the surfactant is directed toward the aqueous medium.

Different experimental methods have been developed to provide a measure for the efficiency of a wetting agent. For example, narrow lyophobic troughs can be used, in which one end holds the powder while a solution of a wetting agent is placed in the other end. The rate of penetration is observed and measured as the degree of wettability. Another technique involves measuring the relative ability of solutions of different wetting agents to carry a drug powder through a gauze when the solutions are dropped onto the gauze supporting a powder. Good wetting agents are able to carry greater amounts of powder through the gauze than poor wetting agents. Also for nonaqueous systems, different methods have been developed to compare the efficiency of wetting agents (e.g., for certain lanolin derivatives). In the paint industry two techniques are often used that could also be applied to pharmaceutical systems: the so-called wet and flow point methods. In the first case, the amount of vehicle required to wet a known amount of powder is measured, whereas in the second case, the amount of vehicle needed to prepare a pourable system is measured.

Adsorption

Adsorption is the tendency of atoms, molecules, ions, etc. to locate at a particular surface/ interface in a concentration that is different from the concentrations in the surrounding bulk media. The adsorption process occurs as a result of the unequal distribution of the forces at the interfaces. The adsorbing species may be gases, solvents, or solutes, and the interfaces may be solid-solid, solid-liquid, solid-gas, liquid-liquid, or liquid-gas interfaces. Adsorption is termed "positive" if the concentration of adsorbed species at the interface is greater than that in the bulk, and "negative" when the opposite is true. According to the nature of interaction, adsorption can be divided into two main classes: (*i*) physical adsorption or physisorption, where the forces and processes are reversible, nonspecific, and of relatively low energy; and (*ii*) chemisorption, where the forces and processes of adsorption are specific, irreversible, and of higher energy.

Of special interest in liquid dispersions are the surface-active agents that tend to accumulate at air-liquid, liquid-liquid, and/or solid-liquid interfaces. Surfactants can arrange themselves to form a coherent film surrounding the dispersed droplets (in emulsions) or suspended particles (in suspensions). This process is an oriented physical adsorption. Adsorption at the interface tends to increase with increasing thermodynamic activity of the surfactant in solution, until a complete monolayer is formed at the interface, or until the active sites are saturated with surfactant molecules. Also a multilayer of adsorbed surfactant molecules may occur, resulting in more complex adsorption isotherms.

Adsorption of species onto a particle surface is responsible for many resultant properties of the system. The adsorption of surfactants alters the properties at the interface and promotes wetting of the dispersed phase in suspensions. The reduction of the interfacial tension can effectively decrease the resulting surface free energy and hence the tendency for coalescence or aggregation. Thus, the formation and stabilization of the disperse systems can be significantly facilitated. An additional effect promoting stability is the presence of a surface charge, which causes electrostatic repulsion between adjacent particles. The adsorption of ionic surfactants generally increases the charge density on the surface of the dispersed particles, thus improving the stability of the dispersion.

Protective colloids or polymeric materials can be adsorbed onto the surface of the dispersed phase. Polymer adsorption can be accomplished simply by adding a solution of adsorbable polymeric species into a slurry of the dispersed particles. Then, adequate time required for the system to equilibrate and complete the interaction between the adsorbent and the adsorbate must be provided. The mode of adsorption strongly depends on the number of sites and functional groups of the polymer chains available for the interaction with the particle surface. Most nonelectrolyte polymers promote steric stabilization, which is generally due to either entropic stabilization or osmotic repulsion (44). The entropic stabilization arises when two opposing adsorbed polymer layers of adjacent particles overlap, resulting in compression and interpenetration of their chain segments. The restriction of the movements of the polymer chains in the overlap region leads to a negative entropy change. Thus, the reverse process of disentanglement of the two adsorbed layers occurs and is energetically more favorable. This mechanism predominates when the concentration of polymer in the adsorbed layer is low. The osmotic repulsion is operative in cases where more polymer segments are involved and become crowded in the overlap regions. The increase in polymer concentration within these areas causes a local increase in osmotic pressure and results in an influx of water. This influx pushes the particles apart.

Instabilities and Stabilization Concepts

The content uniformity and long-term stability of a pharmaceutical product are required for a consistent and accurate dosing. Aggregation of dispersed particles and resulting instabilities such as flocculation, sedimentation (in suspensions), or creaming and coalescence (in emulsions) often represent major challenges in formulating pharmaceutical disperse systems.

Instabilities

As discussed above, an instability of a dispersion may result from the tendency of the system to reduce its surface free energy, ΔG. Unfortunately, the terminology used in the literature to describe the occurring phenomena is not uniform. "Flocculation" is generally understood as a process in which particles are allowed to come together and form loosely bound clusters, having an open type of structure. Unlike "coalescence," the total surface area is not reduced during the flocculation process. Deflocculation is the opposite, that is, breakdown of clusters into individual particles. Some authors differentiate between the terms "aggregates" and "agglomerates." They say that in "aggregates" the particles are more strongly bound than in flocculates, thus, these systems are more difficult to redisperse. The term agglomerates is then used as a general expression covering both "flocculates" and "aggregates." Other authors use the terms aggregates and agglomerates as synonyms. In the case of coalescence, the total surface area of the particles is reduced (for a more detailed description of the instabilities of emulsions and suspensions, the reader is referred to sections "Suspensions" and "Emulsions," respectively).

Although disperse systems are thermodynamically unstable, certain systems can remain "stable" over a prolonged period of time. Thermodynamically driven changes to a lower energy state may be reversible or irreversible. The type and kinetics of these changes determine the usefulness of a product, as indicated, for example, by its shelf life. A disperse system remains stable as long as the repulsive forces are sufficiently strong to outweigh the van der Waals and/or other attractive forces. These repulsive forces are generally acquired through one or more of the following mechanisms: (*i*) electrostatic repulsion, which arises from the presence of an ionic charge on the surface of the dispersed particles and (*ii*) steric repulsion, which arises from the presence of uncharged molecules on the surface of the particles.

Stabilization by Electrostatic Repulsion

The electrostatic stabilization of disperse systems can be described by the DLVO theory (as discussed earlier in the chapter). The electrostatic repulsive forces can prevent the dispersed particles having surface charges of the same sign from approaching each other, thus stabilizing the dispersion against interparticle attraction or coagulation. As long as the height of the potential energy barrier, V_{max}, exceeds the kinetic energy, the approaching particles do not come sufficiently close to each other to establish important attractive forces (van der Waals forces), but move away from each other due to steric or electrostatic effects. A net positive potential energy of about 20 kT is usually sufficient to keep the particles apart, rendering the dispersion stable. At $T = 298°K$, this equals to 1×10^{-12} erg or 1×10^{-5} J. Correspondingly, moderate physical stability is achieved when the ξ-potential is between ±30 and ±60 mV, and good to excellent physical stability is achieved when the ξ-potential is between ±60 and ±100 mV. However, when the size of the dispersed particles exceeds 1 μm and the density is greater than 1.0 g/cm³, the effect of the ξ-potential becomes less significant.

Ionic solids with surface layers containing the ionic species in near-proper stoichiometric balance and most water-insoluble organic compounds have relatively low surface charge densities. They may adsorb ionic, equally charged surfactants from solutions, which increases their surface charge densities and the magnitude of their ξ-potentials, resulting in an enhanced electrostatic stabilizing effect. In suspensions, the addition of ions that are adsorbed onto the surface of the dispersed particles generally creates strong repulsion forces between suspended particles and stabilizes the system. In contrast, the addition of water-miscible solvents (e.g., alcohols, glycerin, or propylene glycol) to aqueous dispersions can lower the dielectric constant of the medium. This results in a reduction of the thickness of the electric double layer and the magnitude of the potential energy barrier. Thus, the addition of these solvents tends to cause instability or makes the system more sensitive to coagulation.

Stabilization by Steric Repulsion

When a strongly hydrated hydrophilic polymer is adsorbed onto the surface of a hydrophobic solid particle surrounded by an aqueous medium, the affinity of the polymer for water can exceed the attractive forces between the suspended particles. For example, a hydrophilic polymer such as gelatin can increase the strength of the protective hydration layer formed around the dispersed particles. Water-soluble polymers, whose adsorption stabilizes dispersions and protects them against coagulation, are also called "protective colloids." The hydrated, protective shell becomes an integral part of the particles' surface. Adsorption of nonionic polymers (e.g., gums or water-soluble cellulosic derivatives) or surfactants (e.g., polysorbate 80) of sufficient chain length can create steric hindrance between adjacent particles. A polymer can be adsorbed in the forms of loops, tails, and trains. Parts of the long-chain molecules are adsorbed onto the surface of the particles (e.g., trains), whereas other parts extend into the bulk liquid (e.g., tails) (60). Some molecules are adsorbed onto the solid surfaces in the form of loops projecting into the aqueous phase rather than lying flat against the solid substrate. The stabilizing efficiency of the adsorbed macromolecules depends on the presence of sufficiently long tails and/or loops. The adsorbed species usually form multi- rather than monomolecular films at the interface.

Two mechanisms of steric stabilization can be distinguished: (*i*) entropic stabilization and (*ii*) osmotic repulsion. Entropic stabilization arises when two opposing adsorbed polymer layers of adjacent particles overlap, resulting in compression and interpenetration of their chain segments. The restriction of the movements of the polymer chains in the overlap region leads to a negative entropy change. Thus, the reverse process of disentanglement of the two adsorbed layers occurs and is energetically more favorable. This mechanism predominates when the concentration of polymer in the adsorbed layer is low. The osmotic repulsion mechanism is operative in cases where more polymer segments are involved and become crowded in the overlap regions. The increase in polymer concentration within these areas causes a local increase in osmotic pressure and results in an influx of water. This influx pushes the particles apart. Figure 3 illustrates two particles with a hydrated stabilizing layer of thickness δ. The volume of the overlapping region (V_{ov}) can be calculated as follows (61):

$$V_{OV} = \frac{2\pi}{3} \left(\delta - \frac{H}{2} \right)^2 \left(3a + 2\delta + \frac{H}{2} \right) \tag{3}$$

The difference between chemical potential in the overlap volume (μ_H) and the potential when the particles are at an infinite distance apart (μ_∞) is a measure of the repulsive force, an osmotic force, caused by the increased concentration of the polymer chains in the region of overlap:

$$\mu_H - \mu_\infty = -\pi_E V_1 \tag{4}$$

where V_1 is the partial molal volume of solvent. By analogy, with osmotic pressure relationships μ_E can be expressed as:

$$\pi_E = RTBc^2 \tag{5}$$

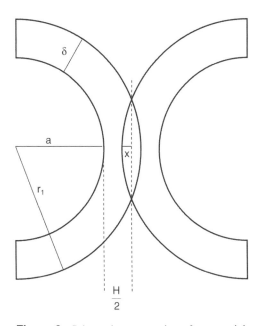

Figure 3 Schematic presentation of two particles of radius a with a hydrated stabilizing layer of thickness δ approach to a distance H between the particle surfaces, $r_1 = (a + \delta)$, and x is the distance between the surface and the line bisecting the volume of overlap. *Source*: From Ref. 61.

where B is the second virial coefficient. The free energy of mixing is

$$\Delta G_m = 2 \int_0^{V_{OV}} \pi_E dV = 2\pi_E V_{OV} \tag{6}$$

and therefore,

$$\Delta G_m = 2\pi_E \frac{2\pi}{3} \left(\delta - \frac{H}{2}\right)^2 \left(3a + 2\delta + \frac{H}{2}\right) \tag{7}$$

When substituting for μ_E and using $R = kN_A$, where k is the Boltzmann constant, the following relationship can be derived:

$$\frac{\Delta G_m}{kT} = \frac{4\pi}{3} B N_A c^2 \left(\delta - \frac{H}{2}\right)^2 \left(3a + 2\delta + \frac{H}{2}\right) \tag{8}$$

with c denoting the polymer concentration in the hydrated layer and N_A being the Avogadro constant.

Steric stabilization is particularly useful and widely applied during emulsification processes. One major advantage compared with electrostatic stabilization is the relative insensitivity toward added electrolytes. An auxiliary effect promoting dispersion stability is the significant viscosity increase of the dispersion medium.

Rheological Properties

Rheology is the study of flow and deformation of materials under the influence of external forces. It involves the viscosity characteristics of powders, liquids, and. Rheological studies are also important in the industrial manufacture and applications of plastic materials, lubricating materials, coatings, inks, adhesives, and food products. Flow properties of pharmaceutical disperse systems can be of particular importance, especially for topical products. Such systems often exhibit rather complex rheological properties, and pharmaceutical scientists have made several fundamental investigations in this area (62–68).

Newton's Law and Newtonian Flow

To characterize rheological behavior of materials, some basic terms need to be defined first. Consider a liquid material that is subjected to a shearing force. The liquid is assumed to consist of a series of parallel layers with the surface area A, the bottom layer being fixed (Fig. 4). When a force is applied on the top layer, the top plane moves at a constant velocity, whereas each lower layer moves with a velocity directly proportional to its distance from the stationary bottom layer. The velocity gradient (dv/dr, the difference in velocity, dv, between the top and bottom planes of liquid separated by the distance, dr) is also called the rate of shear, G:

$$G = \frac{dv}{dr} \tag{9}$$

The force per unit area, F'/A, required to cause flow is called the shear stress (F):

$$F = \frac{F'}{A} \tag{10}$$

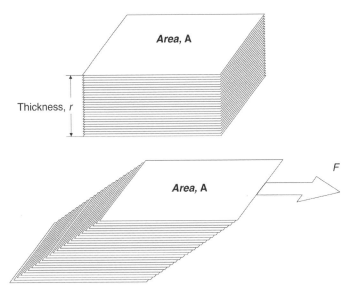

Figure 4 Model of a liquid material that is subjected to a shearing force. The liquid is assumed to consist of a series of parallel layers, the bottom layer being fixed.

The rate of shear, G, is directly proportional to the shear stress, F; and the relationship can be expressed as follows:

$$\frac{F'}{A} = \eta \frac{dv}{dr} \quad \text{or} \quad \eta = \frac{F}{G} \tag{11}$$

where η is the coefficient of viscosity, or viscosity.

A plot of F versus G yields a rheogram or a flow curve. Flow curves are usually plotted on a log-log scale to include the many decades of shear rate and the measured shear stress or viscosity. The higher the viscosity of a liquid, the greater the shear stress required to produce a certain rate of shear. Dividing the shear stress by the shear rate at each point results in a viscosity curve (or a viscosity profile), which describes the relationship between the viscosity and shear rate. The unit of viscosity is poise, which is the shearing force required to produce a velocity of 1 cm/sec between two parallel planes of liquid, each 1 cm^2 in area and separated by a distance of 1 cm. The most often used unit is centipoise, or cp (equivalent to 0.01 poise). Another term, "fluidity," ϕ, is defined as the reciprocal of viscosity:

$$\phi = \frac{1}{\eta} \tag{12}$$

In addition, the United States Pharmacopoeia (USP) includes the explanation of kinematic viscosity [units in stoke (s) and centistoke (cs)], defined as the absolute viscosity divided by the density of the liquid at a definite temperature, ρ:

$$\text{kinematic viscosity} = \frac{\eta}{\rho} \tag{13}$$

For simple Newtonian fluids (e.g., pure water), a plot of rate of shear against shear stress gives a straight line, thus the slope (η) is constant (Fig. 5A, curve A) (69). In other words, the viscosity is constant, neither depending on the shear rate nor on time. However, most pharmaceutical disperse systems rarely exhibit simple Newtonian flow, and their viscosity is not constant but changes as a function of shear rate and/or time. The rheological properties of such systems cannot be defined simply in terms of only one value. These non–Newtonian phenomena are either time independent or time dependent. In the first case, the systems can be classified as pseudoplastic, plastic, or dilatant, and in the second case as thixotropic or rheopective.

Pseudoplastic Flow

Many fluids show a decrease in viscosity with increasing shear rate. This behavior is referred to as "shear thinning," which means that the resistance of the material to flow decreases and the energy required to sustain flow at high shear rates is reduced. These materials are called "pseudoplastic" (Fig. 5A,B, curves B). At rest, the material forms a network structure, which may be an agglomerate of many molecules attracted to each other or an entangled network of polymer chains. Under shear, this structure is broken

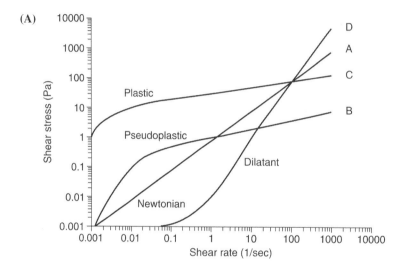

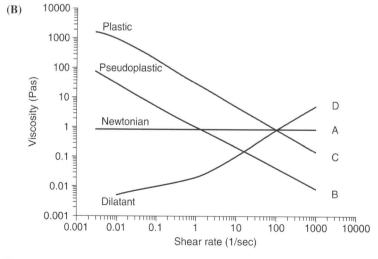

Figure 5 Newtonian and non–Newtonian behaviors as a function of shear rate: (**A**) flow profile; (**B**) viscosity profile. *Source*: From Ref. 69.

down, resulting in a shear thinning behavior. With linear polymers, it is speculated that the axes of such molecules become more oriented in the direction of flow as shear stress is increased. Pseudoplastic flow can be found in emulsions, suspensions, as well as various pharmaceutical thickening agents, for example, polymer solutions.

Plastic Flow

Plastic fluids are Newtonian or pseudoplastic liquids, which exhibit a "yield value" (Fig. 5A,B, curves C). At rest, they behave like a solid because of their interparticle association. The external force has to overcome these attractive forces between the particles and disrupt the structure. Beyond this point, the material changes its behavior from that of a solid to that of a liquid. The viscosity can then either be a constant (ideal Bingham liquid) or a function of the shear rate. In the latter case, the viscosity can initially decrease and then become a constant (real Bingham liquid) or continuously decrease as in the case of a pseudoplastic liquid (Casson liquid). Plastic flow is often observed in flocculated suspensions.

Dilatant Flow

In some cases, the viscosity increases with increasing shear rate. The system appears to become more structured and more viscous with increasing shear stress. This flow behavior is called "dilatant" (Fig. 5A,B, curves D). Examples include pastes containing plasticizers, ionic polymers, suspensions with high solids content, highly pigmented systems, and quicksand.

Thixotropy and Rheopexy

Thixotropy is a phenomenon that occurs frequently in dispersed systems. It is defined as a reversible, time-dependent decrease in viscosity at a constant shear rate. Generally, a dispersion that shows an isothermal gel–sol–gel transformation is a thixotropic material. The mechanism of thixotropy is the breakdown and re-forming of the gel structure.

An example for a rheogram of a thixotropic material is given in Figure 6 (12). Here, the rate of shear, G, is plotted as a function of the shear stress, F. Because of the time dependence of the viscosity, a hysteresis loop results: The upcurve (early times) is not

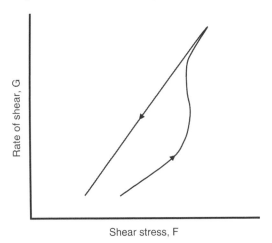

Figure 6 Flow curves of a system exhibiting thixotropy.

identical with the down-curve (late times). The upcurve shows the rate of shear when increasing the shear stress, whereas the downcurve shows the rate of shear when subsequently decreasing the shear stress. As the shear rate decreases, the structure rebuilds, and viscosity is restored to its original value. If the recovery is fast, such as in many water-based systems, the downcurve is superimposed on the upcurve. If the rearrangement is slow, such as in many organic solvent-based systems, it may take longer for the fluid to regain its initial properties after shearing, and therefore the downcurve will be above the upcurve. The hysteresis area between the upcurve and the downcurve defines the energy required to break down the network structure of the material; its dimensions are energy/volume.

If, in contrast, the viscosity increases with time while the material is being sheared and recovers to its original viscosity when allowed to rest, the material is called "rheopective." In this case, the downcurve is positioned below the upcurve.

FORMULATION ADDITIVES

Surfactants

According to the colloid scientist Winsor, surfactants are defined as "compounds that possess in the same molecule distinct regions of hydrophilic and lipophilic character." For example, in the oleate ion, there is an alkyl chain that is basically hydrophobic (lipophilic tail) and a COO^- headgroup that is hydrophilic (lipophobic). Being amphiphilic in nature, surfactants have the ability to modify the interface between various phases (70). Their effects on the interface are the result of their ability to orient themselves in accordance with the polarities of the two opposing phases. The polar part can be expected to be oriented toward the more polar (hydrophilic, aqueous) phase, whereas the nonpolar tails can be expected to be oriented toward the nonpolar (lipophilic, oil) phase (the reader is referred to chap. 12, "Surfactant Systems" for more details).

Surfactants are useful in formulating a wide variety of disperse systems. They are required not only during manufacture but also for maintaining an acceptable physical stability of these thermodynamically unstable systems. Besides the stabilizing efficiency, the criteria influencing the selection of surfactants for pharmaceutical or cosmetic products include safety, odor, color, and purity.

When the variation of any colligative property of a surfactant in aqueous solution is examined, two types of behavior are apparent. At low concentrations, properties approximate those to be expected from ideal behavior. However, at a concentration value that is characteristic for a given surfactant system (so-called critical micelle concentration, CMC), an abrupt deviation from such behavior is observed. At concentrations above the CMC, molecular aggregates termed "micelles" are formed. By increasing the concentration of the surfactant, depending on the chemical and physical nature of the molecule, structural changes to a more orderly state than micellar structure in the molecular assembly of amphiphiles occur. These are, generally, hexagonal, cubic, and lamellar liquid crystalline structures, and their occurrence relates mostly to the concentration of the surfactant in the system. Liquid crystals have been known for more than a century and have been formulated as parts of many creams, lotions, and cosmetic products.

Surfactants can be classified according to their functionality and their natures of hydrophilic and hydrophobic portions. A typical functional scheme was developed in the Personal Care Products Council (CTFA) (*Cosmetic Ingredient Handbook*) by creating six functional categories for surfactants: (*i*) cleansing agents, (*ii*) emulsifying agents, (*iii*) foam boosters, (*iv*) hydrotropes, (*v*) solubilizing agents, and (*vi*) suspending agents. Another means for classification is based on the nature of the hydrophobic portions of surfactants. Such a classification would create groups on the basis of the presence of hydrophobes derived from paraffinic, olefinic, aromatic, cycloaliphatic, or heterocyclic hydrophobes. This type of classification is of particular interest in comparing the surfactants' characteristics with regard to their physiological effects related to the origin of the lipophilic constituents.

The most useful and widely accepted classification is based on the nature of the *hydrophilic* headgroups. This classification system has universal acceptance and has been found to be practical throughout the surfactant industry. This approach creates four large groups of surfactant structures: (*i*) anionics, (*ii*) cationics, (*iii*) amphoterics (zwitterionics), and (iv) nonionics. Anionic surfactants carry negative charges and include a large group of surfactants used in pharmaceutical products, such as soaps, sulfates, and sulfonates. Soaps can be prepared in situ by a reaction between a fatty acid and an alkali. Cationic surfactants, carrying positively charged headgroups, are of special pharmaceutical interest since they often possess antimicrobial activity. Examples include quaternary ammonium compounds and cetyltrimethylammonium bromide. Cationic surfactants should not be used in the same formulation with anionic surfactants because they will interact. Amphoteric surfactants possess both positive and negative charges in their structures and include substances like lecithin, *N*-dodecyl-*N*,*N*-dimethylglycine. Nonionic surfactants are not dissociated and, thus, are not charged. Unlike the anionic and cationic types, they are not susceptible to pH changes and to the presence of electrolytes. *N*-alkyl poly(oxyethylene) surfactants, of the general formula $CH_3(CH_2)_n(OCH_2CH_2)_mOH$, for which *n* is often between 10 and 18 and *m* between 6 and 60, are good examples for nonionic surfactants.

Particularly useful is the physical classification of surfactants based on the hydrophile-lipophile balance (HLB) system, established by Griffin (71,72). Sixty years ago, he introduced an empirical scale of HLB values for a variety of *nonionic* surfactants. Griffin's original concept defined the HLB value as the percentage (by weight) of the hydrophile divided by 5 to yield more manageable values:

$$HLB = \frac{\text{wt\% hydrophile}}{5} \qquad (14)$$

Griffin studied primarily ethylene oxide (EO) adducts and routinely substituted "% EO" for "% hydrophile." Since that time, the HLB system has become very popular, especially to characterize emulsifying agents (the reader is referred to section "Formulation and Preparation Techniques for Emulsions" for a more detailed discussion of the use of the HLB system for the identification of adequate emulsifiers and combinations thereof).

Also, finely divided solid particles that are wetted to some degree by both oil and water can act as emulsifying agents. This results from the fact that they can form a particulate film around dispersed droplets, preventing coalescence. Powders that are wetted preferentially by water form o/w emulsions, whereas those more easily wetted by oil form w/o emulsions. The compounds most frequently used in pharmacy are colloidal clays, such as bentonite (aluminum silicate) and Veegum (magnesium aluminum silicate). These compounds tend to be adsorbed at the interface, and also increase the viscosity of the aqueous phase. They are frequently used in conjunction with a surfactant for external purposes, such as lotions or creams.

The common concentration of a surfactant used in a formulation varies from 0.05% to 0.5% and depends on the surfactant type and the solids content of the dispersion. In practice, very often combinations of surfactants rather than single agents are used to prepare and stabilize disperse systems. The combination of a more hydrophilic surfactant with a more hydrophobic surfactant leads to the formation of a complex film at the interface. A good example for such surfactant pair is the Tween-Span system of Atlas-ICI (73).

Protective Colloids and Viscosity-Imparting Agents

Protective colloids can be divided into synthetic and natural materials. Table 3 classifies the pharmaceutical gums, thickeners, and other hydrophilic polymers according to their origins (74). Protective colloids of natural origin, such as gelatin, acacia, and tragacanth, have been used for years as emulsifying agents (75,76). Gelatin and serum albumin are preferred protective colloids for stabilizing parenteral suspensions because of their biocompatibility. These two polymers, as well as casein, dextrin, and plant gums, can be metabolized in the human body. Dispersing a natural gum within water yields a thick, viscous liquid called "mucilages." They are used primarily to aid in suspending insoluble

Table 3 Classification of Protective Colloids (Gums, Thickeners, and Polymers) According to Their Origins

Classification		Origin	Products
Natural	Plant	Tree and shrub exudates	Karaya gum Tragacanth gum Gum acacia
		Seed extracts	Guar gum Locust bean gum Psyllium seed Quince seed
		Seaweed extracts	Carrageenan Alginates Agar
		Tree extracts	Larch gum
		Fruit extracts	Pectins
		Grains and roots	Starches
	Microbial	Exocellular polysaccharides	Xanthan gum Dextran
	Animal	Milk protein	Casein
		Skin and bones	Gelatin Keratin
		Insect secretion	Shellac

Modified natural	Plant	Wood pulp and cotton	Cellulose derivatives:
			  methylcellulose, sodium
			  carboxymethylcellulose

		Seed extracts	Guar derivatives
Synthetic		Petroleum based	Acrylic acid polymers Polyacrylamides Alkylene/alkylene oxide polymers
Inorganic		Clays	Smectite hydrophilic and organoclays
		Amorphous silicon dioxide	Hydrated silica Fumed silica

Source: From Ref. 74.

substances within liquids because their colloidal character and viscosity can help to prevent sedimentation. However, the drawbacks of these mucilages include their sensitivity to pH changes, addition of electrolytes, and/or heat, which produce an adverse effect on the viscosity. Mucilages of vegetable gums are prone to microbial decomposition and show appreciable decrease in viscosity upon storage.

Besides these naturally derived protective colloids, several synthetic, water-soluble substances are widely used at appropriate concentrations as mucilage substitutes, suspending agents, emulsifying agents, and/or viscosity-imparting agents. Synthetic cellulose derivatives include sodium carboxymethylcellulose, hydroxypropylcellulose, hydroxypropylmethylcellulose, and methylcellulose. The resulting viscosity depends on the concentration and specification (e.g., molecular weight) of the polymers. Many of these substances are used as protective colloids at low concentrations (<0.1%) and as viscosity builders at relatively high concentrations (>0.1%). Since these agents do not reduce the surface and interfacial tension significantly, it is often advantageous to use them in combination with surfactants. Unlike many natural polymers, cellulose derivatives and most synthetic protective colloids are not biotransformed. When administered orally, they are not absorbed, but excreted intact.

When polymeric substances and hydrophilic colloids are used as suspending agents, it is recommended that appropriate tests are performed to show that the agent does not interfere with the drug and does not modify the resulting therapeutic effect. With regard to the raw material selection, the protective colloids may be chosen according to their abilities to aid in stabilizing a dispersion as well as other factors, such as costs, toxicity, and resistance to chemical and/or microbial attack. Although many natural substances are nontoxic and relatively inexpensive, they do often show considerable batch-to-batch variations and relatively high risks for microbial contamination.

pH-Controlling Agents

A properly formulated disperse system should exhibit an acceptable physical stability over a wide range of pH values. If a specific pH is required, the system can be maintained at the desired pH value using an adequate buffer. This is especially important for drugs that possess ionizable acidic or basic groups for which the pH of the vehicle often influences their stabilities and/or solubilities. However, these buffering salts or electrolytes must be used with extreme caution since small changes in electrolyte concentration can alter the surface charge of the dispersed phase and, thus, affect the overall stability of the system. Osmotically active salts (e.g., sodium chloride) and/or stabilizers (e.g., disodium edetate) may be replaced by organic nonelectrolytes, such as dextrose, mannitol, or sorbitol, to avoid possible destabilization. Adjustments in osmolarity or tonicity are generally required when preparing ophthalmic or injectable disperse systems.

For suspensions primarily stabilized by a *polymeric* material, it is important to carefully consider the optimal pH value of the product since certain polymer properties, especially the rheological behavior, can strongly depend on the pH of the system. For example, the viscosity of hydrophilic colloids, such as xanthan gums and colloidal microcrystalline cellulose, is known to be somewhat pH dependent. Most disperse systems are stable over a pH range of 4 to 10, but may flocculate under extreme pH conditions. Therefore, each dispersion should be examined for its pH stability over an adequate storage period. Any changes in the pH values could be indicative of a potential instability problem.

Preservatives

Preservation against microbial growth is an important aspect for disperse systems, not only with respect to the primary microbiological contamination but also in terms of the physical and chemical integrity of the system (77). Aqueous liquid products are prone to microbial contamination because water in combination with excipients derived from natural sources (e.g., polypeptides, carbohydrates) serves as an excellent medium for the growth of microorganisms. Besides the pathogenic hazards, microbial contamination can result in discoloration or cracking (separation into two bulk phases) of the products. The evolution of carbon dioxide gas may result in the explosion of containers. Colloidal dispersions and systems prepared by a controlled flocculation may become unstable and deflocculate because of a decrease in the ξ-potential in the absence of adequate preservation.

The types of microorganisms found in various products are *Pseudomonas* species (including *Pseudomonas aeruginosa*), *Salmonella* species, *Staphylococcus aureus*, and *Escherichia coli*. The USP and other pharmacopoeias recommend certain classes of products to be tested for specified microbial contaminants, e.g., natural plant, animal, and some mineral products for the absence of *Salmonella* species, suspensions for the absence of *E. coli*, as well as topically administered products for the absence of *P. aeruginosa* and *S. aureus*. Emulsions are particularly susceptible to contamination by fungi and yeasts. Consumer use may also result in the introduction of microorganisms. For aqueous-based products, it is therefore mandatory to include a preservative in the formulation to provide further assurance that the product retains its pharmaceutically acceptable characteristics until the patient uses it.

Substances that have been used as preservatives for disperse systems include chlorocresol, chlorobutanol, benzoates, phenylmercuric nitrate, parabens, and others (78,79). The use of cationic antimicrobial agents, such as quaternary ammonium compounds (e.g., benzalkonium chloride), is contraindicated in many cases because they may be inactivated by other formulation components and/or they may alter the charge of the dispersed phase. Clay suspensions and gels should be adequately preserved with nonionic antimicrobial preservatives. The use of preservatives is generally limited to products that are not intended for parenteral use. Intravenous injectable preparations should be prepared according to stringent sterile conditions from pyrogen-free raw materials, and normally, be terminally sterilized, for example, by autoclaving.

In emulsions, partitioning of the incorporated preservative can occur between the aqueous and the oil phase. A lipophilic preservative may pass into the oil phase so that a significant portion is removed from the aqueous phase. Since it is the latter in which microorganisms tend to grow, the use of water-soluble preservatives can be more effective, especially for o/w emulsions. For most emulsion systems, the esters of *p*-hydroxybenzoic acid (parabens) appear to be the most satisfactory. Since microorganisms can also reside within the oil phase, it is further recommended that a pair of preservatives having different oil and water solubilities are used to ensure appropriate concentrations in both phases.

The major criteria for the selection of an appropriate preservative include (*i*) efficiency against a wide spectrum of microorganisms, (*ii*) stability (shelf life), (*iii*) toxicity, (*iv*) sensitizing effects, (*v*) compatibility with other ingredients in the dosage form, and (*vi*) taste and odor. Other specific factors to be considered may include the application site (e.g., external, ophthalmic, parenteral), pH of the dispersion medium, solubility in the vehicle, partitioning into an oil phase (in emulsions), and adsorption onto the solid phase (in suspensions) or the packaging materials (80). Finally, the establishment of microbiological standards for raw materials and strict adherence to the Good Manufacturing Practice (GMP) protocols during industrial-scale production can efficiently reduce the severity of the contamination problem.

Antioxidants

Many pharmaceutical products undergo oxidative deterioration upon storage because the therapeutic ingredients or adjuvants oxidize in the presence of atmospheric oxygen. Vitamins, essential oils, and almost all fats and oils can be oxidized readily. The decomposition can be particularly significant in disperse systems, such as emulsions, because of the large area of interfacial contact and because the manufacturing process may introduce air into the product. Many drugs commonly incorporated into emulsions are subjected to autoxidation and subsequent decomposition. Traces of oxidation products are undesirable as they are generally easily noticed by their smell and/or taste. The term "autoxidation" is used when the ingredient(s) in the product react(s) with oxygen without drastic external interference. Series of autoxidative reactions involve the initiation step or the formation of a free radical, the propagation step where the free radical is regenerated and reacts with more oxygen, followed by the termination step as the free radicals react with each other, resulting in the inactive products.

Antioxidants are classified into three main groups. The first group, comprising the true antioxidants, probably inhibits oxidation by reacting with free radicals, thus blocking the chain reaction. Examples include tocopherols, alkyl gallates, butylated hydroxyanisole (BHA), and butylated hydroxytoluene (BHT). They are commonly used at concentrations ranging from 0.001% to 0.1%. The second group, comprising the reducing agents, has a lower redox potential than the drug or other substances that it should protect and is therefore more readily oxidized. They may also react with free radicals. Examples are ascorbic and isoascorbic acids and the potassium or sodium salts of sulfurous acid. The latter group, such as sodium metabisulfite, has been reported to produce sensitivity reactions. The third group comprises the antioxidant synergists, including sequestering and chelating agents, which possess little antioxidant effect themselves but enhance the action of a true antioxidant by reacting with heavy metal ions that catalyze oxidation. The synergist class includes citric acid, tartaric acid, disodium edetate, and lecithin.

The selection of an appropriate antioxidant depends on factors such as stability, toxicity, efficiency, odor, taste, compatibility with other ingredients, and distribution phenomena between the two phases. Antioxidants that give protection primarily in the aqueous phase include sodium metabisulfite, ascorbic acid, thioglycerol, and cysteine hydrochloride. Oil-soluble antioxidants include lecithin, propyl gallate, ascorbyl palmitate, and BHT. Vitamin E has also been used, but its virtue as a natural antioxidant has been the subject of some controversy (the reader is referred to the chap. "Chemical Kinetics and Drug Stability" for more details).

SUSPENSIONS

A suspension is defined as a disperse system where the dispersed phase is in the solid state, whereas the dispersion medium is in the liquid state. For example, the internal phase (suspensoid, suspended phase) can be uniformly distributed throughout the suspending medium (suspending vehicle) in which it exhibits a minimum degree of solubility. The internal phase consists of a homogeneous or heterogeneous distribution of solid particles having a specific range of size. Coarse suspensions contain suspended particles, which are larger than about 1 μm, with the practical upper limit of about 75 μm. The particle diameter of most good pharmaceutical suspensions lies between 1 and 50 μm. When one or more of the ingredients constituting the internal phase are pharmaceutically useful and/ or pharmacologically active, the system is called a pharmaceutical suspension.

Suspensions have several advantages as a dosage form. They allow the development of a liquid product containing an appropriate quantity of the active ingredient in a reasonable volume. Resistance to hydrolysis and oxidation is generally good in suspensions when compared with that in respective aqueous solutions. In such a case, a suspension would insure chemical stability while permitting liquid therapy. Suspensions can also be used for taste masking. A disagreeable taste of certain drugs when given in the form of a solution can be overcome when administered as undissolved particles in an oral suspension (reduced surface area for interaction with taste receptors in the mouth). A number of chemical derivatives of many poor-tasting drugs, such as chloramphenicol, have been specifically developed for their insolubility in a desired vehicle for the purpose of preparing a palatable liquid dosage form.

On the other hand, there are a number of disadvantages of suspensions, which should be noted. The content uniformity and dosage accuracy of suspensions are unlikely to compare favorably with that obtainable by the use of tablets, capsules, or solutions. Sedimentation and compaction of sediment, so-called caking, frequently cause problems that are not always easy to solve. In addition, the product is liquid and relatively bulky compared with solid dosage forms. These properties are disadvantageous for both pharmacists and patients. However, the above-mentioned advantages can, under certain circumstances, outweigh the disadvantages of this type of dosage forms.

Sedimentation and Stokes' Law

The control of sedimentation is required to ensure a sufficient and uniform dosage. Sedimentation behavior of a disperse system depends largely on the motion of the particles, which may be thermally or gravitationally induced. If a suspended particle is sufficiently small in size, the thermal forces will dominate the gravitational forces and the particle will follow a random motion owing to molecular bombardment, called "Brownian motion." The distance moved or displacement, D_i, is given by:

$$D_i^2 = \frac{RTt}{3N\pi\eta r} \tag{15}$$

where R is the universal gas constant, T the absolute temperature, t the time, N the Avogadro's number, η the viscosity, and r the particle radius. Note that the displacement, D_i, decreases with increasing radius of the particle, r. For any given system, one can define a "no sedimentation diameter" (NSD), a value below which the Brownian motion will be sufficient to keep particles from sedimentation. The value of NSD obviously depends on the density and viscosity of the respective system.

On increasing the radius of the suspended particles, Brownian motion becomes less important and sedimentation becomes more dominant. These larger particles therefore settle gradually under gravitational forces. The basic equation describing the sedimentation of spherical, monodisperse particles in a suspension is the so-called Stokes' law. It states that the velocity of sedimentation, v, can be calculated as follows:

$$v = \frac{2gr^2(\rho_1 - \rho_2)}{9\eta} = \frac{gd^2(\rho_1 - \rho_2)}{18\eta} \tag{16}$$

where g is the acceleration caused by gravity, r denotes the particle radius; d is the particle diameter; ρ_1 and ρ_2 represent the densities of the particle and dispersion medium, respectively; and η is the viscosity of the medium.

The settling velocity is proportional to the second power of the particle radius or particle diameter. It is apparent that agglomerates and flocculates settle more rapidly than individual particles. Since both gravity and buoyancy are operating simultaneously on the particle, either upward movements or downward movements result. Suspensions generally undergo sedimentation upon storage, while emulsions may exhibit either upward creaming (o/w type) or downward creaming (w/o type). The determining factor is the difference in the densities of the internal and the external phases.

Stokes' law is rigorously applicable only for the ideal situation in which uniform and perfectly spherical particles in a very dilute suspension settle without turbulence, interparticle collisions, and without chemical/physical attraction or affinity for the dispersion medium (81). Obviously, the equation does not apply precisely to common pharmaceutical suspensions in which the above-mentioned assumptions are most often not completely fulfilled. However, the basic concept of the equation does provide a valid indication of the many important factors controlling the rate of particle sedimentation and, therefore, a guideline for possible adjustments that can be made to a suspension formulation.

Since the sedimentation rate increases with increasing particle size, it is apparent that particle size reduction is beneficial to the stability of suspensions. However, one should avoid reducing the particles to an extreme degree of fineness since very fine particles have the tendency to form compact cakes upon storage. The rate of sedimentation may also be appreciably reduced by increasing the viscosity of the continuous phase. But this can only be achieved within a practical limit. From Stokes' law, it can also be seen that if the density difference of both phases is eliminated, sedimentation can be entirely prevented. However, it is seldom, if ever possible, to increase the vehicle density above about 1.3. In addition, a product having a too high viscosity is not desirable because of its poor pourability and difficulty of redispersion. A wide variety of suspending agents are available. Some excipients, such as cellulose derivatives, have a pronounced effect on the viscosity, but hardly any on density. Others, such as sorbitol, can modify both density and viscosity.

Generally, the physical stability of a pharmaceutical suspension can be appropriately adjusted by an alteration in the dispersed phase rather than by significant modifications in the dispersion medium. These adjustments mainly are concerned with particle size, uniformity of particle size, and separation of the particles so that they are not likely to become larger or to form a solid cake upon standing.

Flocculation and Deflocculation Phenomena

The ζ-potential is a measurable indication for the apparent particle charge in the dispersion medium. When its value is relatively high, the repulsive forces usually exceed the attractive forces. Accordingly, the particles are individually dispersed and said to be "deflocculated." Thus, each particle settles separately, and the rate of sedimentation is relatively small. The settling particles have plenty of time to pack tightly by falling over one another to form an impacted bed. The sedimentation volume of such a system is low, and the sediment is often difficult to redisperse. The supernatant remains cloudy even when settling is apparent.

Controlled flocculation is the intentional formation of loose agglomerates of particles held together by comparatively weak bonding forces. This can, for example, be achieved by the addition of a preferentially adsorbed ion whose charge is opposite in sign to that of the ζ-potential-determining ions. Thus, the apparent active charge of the particles is progressively lowered. At a certain concentration of the added ion, the forces of repulsion are sufficiently small, so that the forces of attraction start to dominate. Under these conditions, the particles may approach each other closely and form loose agglomerates, termed "flocs," "flocculates," or "floccules" ("flocculated" system). When compared with the deflocculated particles, the flocs settle rapidly and form a higher sedimentation volume. The loose structure permits the flocculates to break up easily and distribute uniformly with only a small degree of agitation. Controlled flocculated systems usually develop a *clear* supernatant solution above the loose sediment. Thus, they might look less uniform upon standing, even though they provide easy redispersion and better dose uniformity than many other types of suspensions.

Flocculating agents can be simple electrolytes that are capable to reduce the ζ-potential of suspended charged particles. Examples include small concentrations (0.01–1%) of monovalent ions (e.g., sodium chloride, potassium chloride) and di- or trivalent ions (e.g., calcium salts, alums, sulfates, citrates, or phosphates) (12,82,83). These salts are often used jointly in the formulations as pH buffers and flocculating agents. But controlled flocculation of suspensions can also be achieved by the addition of polymeric colloids or alteration of the pH of the preparation.

A caking diagram, as described by Martin and Bustamante (12, pp. 477–511), shows the flocculation of a bismuth subnitrate suspension by means of the flocculating agent monobasic potassium phosphate. The addition of the negatively charged phosphate ions to the suspended drug particles causes the positive ζ-potential to decrease. Upon further phosphate addition, the ζ-potential falls to zero and then becomes negative. Microscopic examination reveals that maximum flocculation occurs and persists until the ζ-potential becomes sufficiently negative for deflocculation. The onset of flocculation coincides with the maximum sedimentation volume determined.

The controlled flocculation method may be used in conjunction with the addition of a polymeric material to form a *structured* vehicle. After the formation of the flocs, an aqueous solution of polymeric material, usually negatively charged, such as carboxymethylcellulose or carbopol, is added. The concentration employed depends on the consistency desired for the suspension, which also relates to the size and density of the dispersed phase. Care must be taken to ensure the absence of any incompatibility between the flocculating agent and the polymer used for the formation of the structured vehicle.

When formulating a deflocculated system, a number of materials may be used as dispersion aids. Deflocculating agents include polymerized organic salts of sulfonic acid of both types, alkyl–aryl and aryl–alkyl, which can alter the surface charge of the particles by physical adsorption. Unlike surfactants, these agents do not lower surface and interfacial tension appreciably; hence, they have little or no tendency to create foam or wet particles. Most defloculants are not generally considered as safe for internal use; lecithin is an example for an acceptable dispersant for parenteral products.

Crystal Growth and Polymorphism

The growth in time of unprotected, slightly soluble drug particles and the resultant changes in their particle size distribution in suspension have been reviewed by several researchers (85–90). The crystal growth in disperse systems may be attributed to one or more of the following mechanisms: Ostwald ripening, temperature changes, and polymorphic transformations.

Ostwald ripening is the growth of large particles at the expense of smaller ones, as a result of a difference in the solubility of the particles of varying sizes. The surface free energy of small particles is greater than that of large particles. Therefore, small particles can be appreciably more soluble than larger ones. A concentration gradient results, with higher drug concentrations in the surrounding of small particles and lower drug concentrations in the surrounding of large particles. Thus, according to Fick's law of diffusion the dissolved particle molecules diffuse from the environment of the smaller particles to the environment of the larger particles. The resulting increase in the concentration in the surrounding of the large particles leads to crystallization and particle growth. Thus, small particles become smaller, whereas large particles become larger upon storage. Small fluctuations in temperature can accelerate this effect. Small particles dissolve to a greater extent when the temperature increases, and the dissolved particle molecules recrystallize on the surface of existing larger particles when the temperature drops. The suspension becomes coarser, the mean particle size spectrum shifts to higher values. This effect can be expressed by the following relationship:

$$\log \frac{S}{S_0} = \frac{k}{2.303r} \tag{17}$$

where S is the initial solubility rate of small particles; S_0 is the solubility rate of large particles at equilibrium; r is the particle radius in cm; and k is a constant that includes surface tension, temperature, molar volume, and thermodynamic terms ($k = 1.21 \times 10^{-6}$). Thus, it can be seen that the increase in solubility rate of a 0.2-μm particle is 13%, 1% for a 2-μm particle, and negligible for particles of 20 μm and larger.

Crystal growth due to temperature fluctuations during storage is of importance especially when the suspensions are subjected to temperature cycling of 20°C or more. These effects depend on the magnitude of temperature change, the time interval, and the effect of temperature on the drug's solubility and subsequent recrystallization process. At each crystal contact point, there exists a thin layer of supersaturated solution that facilitates crystal growth. The type of inherent crystal form is determined by the factors governing the rate of crystal growth. The degree of supersaturation is dependent on the rate of cooling, the extent and degree of agitation, and the size and number of nuclei available for the particle nucleation. Other factors include pH, solvent effects, and the impurities present.

As crystal growth generally increases with an increase in particle solubility, the excipients that tend to increase the particle solubility should be kept to a minimum. Many pharmaceutical gums can adsorb onto the surfaces of drug crystals and, thus, can be used to inhibit the crystal growth. In a dilute suspension, crystal growth increases with the degree of agitation because the mass transfer in the bulk fluid is increased (convectional transport). If sedimentation occurs, the local increase in particle concentration decreases the mean free diffusion path of the solute molecules and may, thus, promote the particle growth.

Polymorphism refers to the different internal crystal structures of a chemically identical compound. Drugs may undergo a change from one metastable polymorphic form to a more stable polymorphic form. Also, the crystal *habit* might change because of the degree of solvation or hydration. The formation of distinct new crystalline entities during storage is possible. For example, an originally anhydrous drug in a suspension may rapidly or slowly form a hydrate. These various forms may exhibit different solubilities, melting points, and X-ray diffraction patterns. When preparing suspensions using precipitation methods, the solvent and the rate of cooling are important factors determining the type of polymorph(s) obtained.

Various drugs are known to exist in different polymorphic forms (e.g., cortisone and prednisolone). The rate of conversion from a metastable into the stable form is an important criterion to be considered with respect to the shelf life of a pharmaceutical product. Polymorphic changes have also been observed during the manufacture of steroid suspensions. When steroid powders are subjected to dry heat sterilization, subsequent rehydration of anhydrous steroid in the presence of an aqueous vehicle results in the formation of large, needlelike crystals. A similar effect may be produced by subjecting finished suspensions to moist heat sterilization in an autoclave.

Higuchi showed that crystal growth may also arise when the more energetic *amorphous* form of a drug exhibits significantly greater solubility in water than the corresponding *crystalline* forms (85). In addition, size reduction by crushing and grinding can produce particles whose different surfaces exhibit high or low dissolution rates. This effect can be correlated to differences in the free surface energy introduced during comminution.

To prevent crystal growth and possible changes in the particle size distribution, one or more of the following procedures and techniques may be employed (8,90): (*i*) selection of particles with a narrow size range; (*ii*) selection of a more stable crystalline form of the drug; (*iii*) avoidance of the use of high-energy milling during particle size reduction; (*iv*) incorporation of a wetting agent (e.g., surfactant) and/or a protective colloid (e.g., cellulose derivatives forming film barriers around the particles); (*v*) increase of the viscosity of the vehicle to retard particle dissolution and subsequent crystal growth; and (*vi*) avoidance of temperature extremes during storage.

Pharmaceutical Suspensions

During the preparation of physically stable pharmaceutical suspensions, a number of formulation components can be incorporated to maintain the solid particles in the dispersed state. These substances can be classified as: (*i*) components of the suspending system, including wetting agents, dispersants, or deflocculating/flocculating agents; and (*ii*) components of the suspending vehicle (external phase), including pH-controlled agents/buffers, osmotic agents, coloring/flavoring agents, preservatives, and liquid vehicles. The components of each category are individually selected for their use in the preparation of orally, topically, or parenterally administered suspensions.

Orally administered suspensions, containing a wide class of active ingredients (e.g., antibiotics, antacids, radiopaque agents) are of major commercial importance. The solids content of an oral suspension may vary considerably. For example, antibiotic preparations may contain 125 to 500 mg solid drug per 5 mL, or a teaspoonful dose, while a drop concentrate may provide the same amount of drug in only 1 to 2 mL dose. Antacid or radiopaque suspensions also contain relatively high amounts of suspended material for oral administration. The suspending vehicle can, for example, be a syrup, sorbitol solution, or gum-thickened water with added artificial sweeteners. Also, taste and mouthfeel are important considerations when formulating oral suspensions.

Many antibiotic drugs are unstable in the presence of an aqueous vehicle and, therefore, are frequently supplied as dry powder mixtures for reconstitution at the time of dispensing. Generally, this type of product is either a powder mixture or a completely/ partially granulated product, which upon dilution and agitation with a specified quantity of vehicle (e.g., water) results in the formation of a suspension suitable for administration (91). The preparation is typically designated in the USP by a title of the form "... For Oral Suspension," whereas the ready-to-use suspension preparations are simply designated as

"... Oral Suspension." The dry-mix products often contain drugs, colorants, flavorants, sweeteners (e.g., sucrose or sodium saccharin), stabilizing agents (e.g., citric acid, sodium citrate), suspending agents (e.g., guar gum, xanthan gum, methylcellulose), and preservatives (e.g., parabens, sodium benzoate).

The formulation of oral *sustained-release* suspensions has shown only a limited success because of the difficulty in maintaining the stability of sustained-release particles when present in liquid systems. Different formulation approaches have been proposed, for instance, on the basis of coated beads, drug-impregnated wax matrices, micro-encapsulation techniques, and ion-exchange resins (92–94). The combination of an ion-exchange resin complex with particle coating has resulted in a commercial product, the so-called Pennkinetic system. By this technique, ionic drugs are complexed with ion-exchange resins, and the drug-resin complex particles are then treated with an impregnating polymer such as polyethylene glycol 4000, followed by coating with a sustaining polymer such as ethylcellulose (95,96). In liquid suspension (the dispersion medium being free of ions that could replace drug ions in the resin complex), the drug remains adsorbed to the resin. However, upon swallowing ions from the gastrointestinal (GI) tract, liquid can penetrate into the particles and replace the drug ions, which subsequently diffuse out of the system (at a controlled rate). Drug release from these systems depends on the type of drug-resin complex, on the ionic environment (e.g., pH and electrolyte concentration within the GI tract), as well as on the properties of the resin. Most ion-exchange resins currently employed in sustained-release products contain sulfonic acid groups that exchange cationic drugs with amine groups. An example is hydrocodone polistirex [Tussionex® Pennkinetic Extended-Release Suspension (Pennwalt, Philadelphia, Pennsylvania, U.S.A.)].

Topical suspensions are intended to be applied externally. Shake lotion and calamine lotion are good examples of historical products in this class. Because safety and toxicity are dealt with in terms of dermatological acceptability, many useful new suspending agents have been introduced in topical formulations. The protective action and cosmetic properties of topical lotions usually require the use of high concentrations of disperse phase.

In contrast, *parenteral* suspensions have relatively low solids contents, usually between 0.5% and 5%, with the exception of insoluble forms of penicillin in which concentrations of the antibiotic may exceed 30%. These sterile preparations are designed, for instance, for intramuscular, intradermal, intralesional, intra-articular, or subcutaneous injection. Syringeability is an important factor to be taken into consideration with injectable dosage forms. The viscosity of a parenteral suspension should be sufficiently low to allow for an easy injection. Common suspending vehicles include preserved isotonic saline solution or a parenterally acceptable vegetable oil. Ophthalmic and otic suspensions that are instilled into the eye/ear must also be prepared in a sterile manner. The vehicles are essentially isotonic and aqueous in composition.

Methods of Evaluating Suspensions

Suspensions are generally evaluated with respect to their particle size, electrokinetic properties (ζ-potential), and rheological characteristics. A detailed discussion of the methods/techniques and relevant instrumentation used is given in section "Characterization of disperse systems." However, a number of evaluating methods that are *specific for suspensions*, such as the determination of the sedimentation volume, redispersibility, and specific gravity measurements, are treated in this section.

The sedimentation volume F of a pharmaceutical suspension can be measured using simple graduated cylinders (100–1000 mL). It is defined as the ratio of the equilibrium volume of sediment, V_u, to the total volume of the suspension, V_o.

$$F = \frac{V_u}{V_o} \qquad (18)$$

The value of F ranges between 0 and 1, and increases as the volume of suspension, which appears occupied by the sediment, increases. For example, if 100 mL of a well-shaken test formulation is placed in a graduate cylinder and the final height of the sediment is at the 20-mL line, then F is 0.2. It is normally found that the greater the value of F, the more stable the product. When $F = 1$, no sediment is apparent and caking is absent; and the suspension is considered aesthetically pleasing. This method of evaluation is quite useful in determining the physical stability of suspensions. It can be used to determine the settling rates of flocculated and deflocculated suspensions by making periodic measurement of the sedimentation height. Tingstad (97) indicated that a flocculated suspension, which settles to a level that is 90% of the initial suspension height ($F = 0.9$) and no further, is probably satisfactory.

The degree of flocculation, β, is defined as the ratio of the sedimentation volume of the flocculated suspension, F, to the sedimentation volume of the suspension when deflocculated, F_∞. It is expressed as:

$$\beta = \frac{F}{F_\infty} \qquad (19)$$

The degree of flocculation, therefore, is an expression of the increased sediment volume resulting from flocculation. For example, if β has a value of 5.0, this means that the volume of sediment in the flocculated system is five times that in the deflocculated state. As the value of β approaches unity, the degree of flocculation decreases.

Great care must be taken when using very narrow cylinders, because "wall effects" might become significant, affecting the observed settling rate and/or ultimate sedimentation volume of the investigated suspensions. Cylinders with very small diameters tend to slow down sedimentation because of adhesive forces acting between the container's inner surface and the suspended particles.

If a pharmaceutical suspension produces a sediment upon storage, it is essential that the latter is readily dispersible so that dose uniformity is always assured. The degree of shaking required to achieve this should be minimal. Various redispersibility tests have been proposed. For example, the suspension is placed in a 100-mL cylinder, which after storage and sedimentation is rotated through 360° at 20 rpm. The endpoint is taken when the inside of the base of the cylinder is clear of sediment. The ultimate test of redispersibility is the uniformity of the drug dose delivered from a product, from the first to the last volumetric dose, using one or more standard shaking conditions.

EMULSIONS

An emulsion is a two-phase system consisting of at least two immiscible liquids (or two liquids that are saturated with each other), one of which is dispersed as globules (internal or dispersed phase) within the other liquid phase (external or continuous phase), generally stabilized by an emulsifying agent (12,98). Emulsions have been widely used in many areas of application, including the petroleum industry (99), agriculture (100,101), food technologies (102–108), pharmaceutics (109–115), and cosmetics (116–120). Very frequently, emulsions are used in cosmetic products as topical vehicles for dermal application since they have a high patient/consumer acceptance. Pharmaceutical emulsions are also used internally for the administration of drugs and diagnostic agents. Emulsions discussed in this chapter include macroemulsions, multiple emulsions, microemulsions, liposomes, and a special emulsion type, in situ-forming microparticle (ISM) systems.

Types of Emulsions

Macroemulsions

On the basis of the nature of the dispersed phase and the dispersion medium, two types of macroemulsions can be distinguished: (*i*) If the continuous phase is an *aqueous* solution, and the dispersed phase an oil, the system is called an o/w emulsion. Such an o/w emulsion is generally formed if the aqueous phase constitutes more than 45% of the total weight, and if a hydrophilic emulsifier is used. (*ii*) Conversely, if the aqueous phase is dispersed within the oil, the system is called a w/o emulsion. w/o emulsions are generally formed when the aqueous phase constitutes less than 45% of the total weight and if a lipophilic emulsifier is used. Generally, o/w emulsions are more popular than w/o emulsions in the pharmaceutical field, especially when they are designed for oral administration. In the cosmetic industries, lotions or creams are either of the o/w or w/o type, depending on their applications. o/w emulsions are most useful as water-washable drug bases and for general cosmetic purposes, while w/o emulsions are employed more widely for the treatment of dry skin and emollient applications. It is important for a pharmacist to know the type of emulsion since it can significantly affect its properties and performance. There are several methods to determine the emulsion type, as summarized in Table 4 (121).

Multiple Emulsions

Multiple emulsions are more complex systems (25,122,123). If a simple emulsion is further dispersed within another continuous phase, a triple emulsion is obtained, which can again be dispersed within a further continuous phase, etc. Figure 7 shows as an example the two preparation steps for a water-in-oil-in-water (w/o/w) emulsion: In the first step, an aqueous phase is added to an oily phase containing a lipophilic surfactant.

Table 4 Methods to Determine the Type of a Macroemulsion (w/o or o/w)

Test	Method/observation
Phase dilution test	Place two emulsion droplets on a glass slide and add a droplet of one component to each emulsion droplet, stir, and observe under a microscope. This test is based on the principle that an emulsion can only be diluted with the liquid that constitutes the continuous phase
Dye solubility test	A colored dye soluble in only one component is added to the emulsion. If the color spreads throughout the whole emulsion, the phase in which the dye is soluble is the continuous phase.
Conductivity test	Immerse a pair of electrodes connected to an external electric source in the emulsion. If the external phase is water-containing electrolytes, a current passes through the emulsion. If the oil is the continuous phase, the emulsion fails to carry the current

Abbreviations: W/O, water in oil; o/w, oil in water.

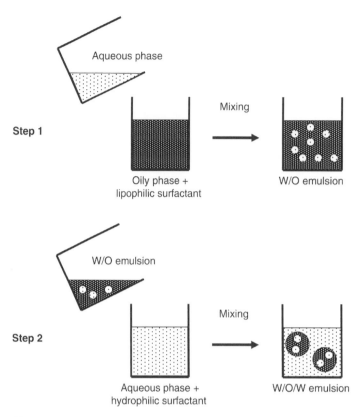

Figure 7 Schematic presentation of a two-step preparation procedure used to obtain a water-in-oil-in-water (w/o/w) emulsion.

Upon mixing, a w/o emulsion is formed. In the second step, this w/o emulsion is poured into a second aqueous phase containing a hydrophilic surfactant. Upon mixing, the multiple w/o/w emulsion is formed.

   Multiple emulsions can be end products or serve as intermediate products, for instance, during the preparation of drug-loaded microparticles (124–126). The use of multiple emulsions, such as w/o/w, o/w/o, w/o/o, and w/o/o/o emulsions, can, for example, help to reduce drug loss into an outer aqueous phase and, thus, increase the resulting drug encapsulation efficiency.

Microemulsion

Already in the early 1940s, Hoar and Schulman introduced the concept of microemulsions (127). However, the term "microemulsion" was only proposed in 1959 (128). Since then it has been redefined on various occasions. In 1981, Danielsson and Lindman (129) defined a microemulsion as "a system of water, oil, and amphiphile, which is a single optically isotropic and thermodynamically stable liquid solution." A three-phase diagram illustrating the area of existence of microemulsions is presented in Figure 8 (130). The phase equilibria, structures, applications, and chemical reactions of microemulsion have been reviewed by Sjöblom et al. (131). In contrast to macroemulsions, microemulsions are optically transparent, isotropic, and thermodynamically stable (132,133). Microemulsions have been subject of various investigations, because their unique properties

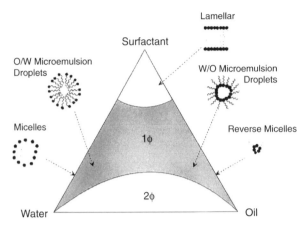

Figure 8 A hypothetical pseudoternary phase diagram of an oil/surfactant/water system with emphasis on microemulsion and emulsion phases. Within the phase diagram, existence fields are shown where conventional micelles, reverse micelles, or water-in-oil (w/o) microemulsions and oil-in-water (o/w) microemulsions are formed along with the bicontinuous microemulsions. At very high surfactant concentrations two-phase systems are observed. *Source*: From Ref. 130.

allow for a wide range of potential practical applications (134–139). However, there is still substantial controversy concerning the exact nature of these systems and the appropriateness of the terminology. Terms such as "transparent emulsions," "micellar solutions," "solubilized systems," and "swollen micelles" have all been applied to the same or similar systems. Nonetheless, emulsions and microemulsions may be differentiated on the basis of particle size: microemulsions contain particles in the nanometer size range (typically 10–100 nm), whereas conventional emulsions (or "macroemulsions" or "coarse emulsions") contain particles in the micrometer range.

Liposomes

Liposomes are vesicular lipid systems of a diameter ranging between 50 nm and a few µm. They are composed of membrane-like, lipid layers surrounding aqueous compartments. The lipid layers consist of phospholipids, making liposomes biocompatible and biodegradable. The phospholipids have a hydrophilic head and a lipophilic tail. Different preparation methods for liposomes have been described by Vemuri et al. (140), leading to different types of vesicular structures (Fig. 9) (141). Nowadays, liposomes are widely used for drug delivery and drug targeting (142–147).

In Situ-Forming Microparticle Systems

The ISM systems were first introduced by Bodmeier and coworkers (148–152). They are included in this chapter as special disperse systems because these formulations are based on o/o or o/w emulsions. Being liquids, the ISM systems can easily be injected intramuscularly or subcutaneously and subsequently form microparticles within the human body upon contact with physiological fluids. The ISM system is composed of a drug and biodegradable polymer, which are codissolved in a water-miscible, biocompatible solvent. This solution is emulsified into an external phase, either oily or aqueous, containing an emulsion stabilizer to form o/o or o/w emulsions. Upon contact with aqueous physiological fluids, the polymer solvent dissipates, leading to polymer

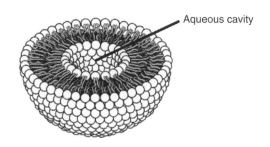

LIPOSOME MODEL

Denomination	Large unilamellar vesicles LUV	Multi- or Oligolamellar vesicles MLV/OLV	Small unilamellar vesicles SUV
Diameter (Nm)	80–1000	100–4000	20–80

Figure 9 Different types of vesicular structures of liposomes. *Source*: From Ref. 141.

solidification and hardening of the emulsion droplets. Thus, the microparticle formation occurs in situ. The resulting microparticles are regular in shape, and their formation is reproducible. Furthermore, drug release can be prolonged and controlled during desired periods of time (153–155). The major advantages of this new technology over implants and the classical solvent evaporation method to prepare microparticles are the ease of preparation and the avoidance of surgical insertion or removal of empty remnants.

Formulation and Preparation Techniques for Emulsions

The preparation techniques for emulsions can be divided into laboratory-scale productions and large-scale productions. Details on the latter are given in the section "Manufacturing and Equipment" of this chapter. Each method requires that energy be introduced into the system by trituration, homogenization, agitation, or heat. The production of satisfactory stable emulsions requires adequate formulations and preparation techniques. Griffin et al. (72) has suggested that the formulator first determines the physical and chemical characteristics of the drug, which include the (*i*) structure formula, (*ii*) melting point, (*iii*) solubilities in different media, (*iv*) stability, (*v*) dose, and (*vi*) specific chemical incompatibilities. This information is essential for the selection of the appropriate type of emulsion. Then, the required emulsifying agent(s) and its (their) concentration(s) should be identified. The choice of materials to be used largely depends on the purpose for which the emulsion is designed.

Phase to Volume Ratio

The ratio of "volume of disperse phase" to "volume of the dispersion medium" greatly influences the characteristics of an emulsion. The choice of the phase to volume ratio depends on a number of factors, including the requested consistency. It is generally difficult to formulate emulsions containing less than about 25% of disperse phase because of their susceptibility to severe creaming or sedimentation problems. However, a combination of proper emulsifying agents and suitable processing technology makes it possible to prepare emulsions with only 10% disperse phase without considerable stability problems. Conversely, products containing a high percentage of disperse phase (more than about 70%) are likely to exhibit phase inversion (the disperse phase becomes the dispersion medium).

Emulsifying Agents

Emulsions are thermodynamically unstable systems. However, using appropriate emulsifying agents (emulsifiers) to decrease the interfacial tension, the stability of these systems can be significantly increased. A satisfactory emulsifier should (*i*) have a reasonable balance between its hydrophilic and hydrophobic groups; (*ii*) produce a stable emulsion (both initially and during storage); (*iii*) be stable itself; (*iv*) be chemically inert; (*v*) be nontoxic and cause no irritation upon application; (*vi*) be odorless, tasteless, and colorless; and (*vii*) be inexpensive. The following three groups of emulsifying agents can be distinguished:

1. Surfactants, which are adsorbed at oil-water interfaces to form monomolecular films and reduce the interfacial tension.
2. Natural macromolecular materials, which form multimolecular films around the disperse droplets of o/w emulsions. They are frequently called auxiliary emulsifying agents and have the desirable effect to increase the viscosity of the dispersion medium. However, they often suffer from the disadvantages of being subject to hydrolysis and sensitive to variations in pH.
3. Very finely dispersed solids, which are adsorbed at the liquid-liquid interfaces, forming films of particles around the dispersed globules. Certain powders can very effectively stabilize against coalescence. The solid's particle size must be very small compared with the emulsion droplet size and must exhibit an appropriate angle of contact at the three-phase (oil/water/solid) boundary (156).

The selection of a suitable emulsifying agent and its appropriate concentration are matters of experience and of trial and error. It is not necessary to use emulsifier amounts above the required quantities to produce complete interfacial films, unless an increase in the viscosity of the dispersion medium is intended. Reducing the interfacial tension makes emulsification easy, but does not by itself prevent coalescence of the particles and resultant phase separation. Frequently, combinations of two or more emulsifying agents are used (1) to (*i*) adequately reduce the interfacial tension, (*ii*) produce a sufficiently rigid interfacial film, and (*iii*) achieve the most suitable viscosity of the external phase. Care must be taken to ensure the compatibility between the different emulsifiers. For example, charged emulsifying agents of opposite sign are likely to interact and coagulate when combined.

As described in section "Formulation Additives," surfactants can be classified using the HLB system established by Griffin. This system provides a scale of surfactant hydrophilicity (HLB value range from 0 to 20; 20 corresponding to the highest possible hydrophilicity) that simplifies emulsifier selection and blending. In Table 5 the HLB values of some pharmaceutically relevant surfactants are listed. Surfactants with a low HLB value (<6) tend to provide stable w/o emulsions; those with a high HLB value (>8) tend to stabilize o/w emulsions. Table 6 gives an overview on the classical use of surfactants in the preparation of pharmaceutical dosage forms depending on their HLB value. The HLB values required for the emulsification of commonly used oils and waxes in pharmaceutical applications are given in Table 7 (157). To obtain a desired HLB value, lipophilic and hydrophilic surfactants can also be mixed. The following equation allows for the calculation of the resulting HLB value of a mixture of two surfactants (A and B):

$$\text{HLB (blend)} = f \times \text{HLB(A)} + (1 - f) \times \text{HLB(B)} \tag{20}$$

Table 5 HLB Values of Surfactants Commonly Used in Pharmaceutical Products

Surfactant	HLB
Nonionic	
Sorbitan monolaurate (Span 20)	8.6
Sorbitan monopalmitate (Span 40)	6.7
Sorbitan monostearate (Span 60)	4.7
Sorbitan monooleate (Span 80)	4.3
Sorbitan trioleate (Span 85)	1.8
Polyoxyethylene (20) sorbitan monolaurate (Tween 20)	16.7
Polyoxyethylene (20) sorbitan monopalmitate (Tween 40)	15.6
Polyoxyethylene (20) sorbitan monostearate (Tween 60)	14.9
Polyoxyethylene (20) sorbitan monooleate (Tween 80)	15.0
Polyoxyethylene-polyoxypropylene block copolymers (pluronics or Poloxamers)	29.0
Amphoteric	
Lecithin (from egg yolk or soybean)	7–10
Hydrogenated lecithin	7–10
Anionic	
Sodium dodecyl sulfate	40.0
Bile salts	20–25

Abbreviation: HLB, hydrophile–lipophile balance.

Table 6 Relationship Between the Use of Surfactants in the Preparation of Pharmaceutical Dosage Forms, Their Dispersibility in Water and Their HLB Values

HLB	Dispersibility in water	Suitable application
1–4	Nil	
3–6	Poor	w/o Emulsifier
6–8	Milky dispersion on agitation	Wetting agent
8–10	Stable milky dispersion	Wetting agent; o/w emulsifier
10–13	Translucent to clear dispersion	o/w emulsifier
>13	Clear solution	o/w emulsifier; solubilizing agent

Abbreviations: HLB, hydrophile–lipophile balance; w/o, water in oil; o/w, oil in water.

Table 7 Required HLB Values for the Emulsification of Oils and Waxes Commonly Used in Pharmaceutical Applications

Compound	HLB	Compound	HLB
o/w emulsions			
Isostearic acid	15–16	Ethyl benzoate	13
Linoleic acid	16	Isopropyl myristate	12
Oleic acid	17	Isopropyl palmitate	12
Ricinoleic acid	16	Kerosene	12
Cetyl alcohol	16	Lanolin anhydrous	12
Stearyl alcohol	15–16	Mineral oil, aromatic	12
Tridecyl alcohol	14	Mineral oil, paraffinic	10
Beeswax	9	Mink oil	9
Carbon tetrachloride	16	Paraffin wax	10
Carnauba wax	15	Petrolatum	7–8
Castor oil	14	Pine oil	16
Cacao butter	6	Rapeseed oil	7
Corn oil	8	Safflower oil	7
Cottonseed oil	6	Soybean oil	6
w/o emulsion			
Mineral oil	6	Stearyl alcohol	7

Abbreviations: HLB, hydrophile–lipophile balance; o/w, oil in water; w/o, water in oil.
Source: From Ref. 157.

where f is the fraction of the surfactant A in the binary mixture. For example, a blend of 30% Span 80 (HLB = 4.3) and 70% Tween 80 (HLB = 15) has an overall HLB value: HLB = $(0.3 \times 4.3) + (0.7 \times 15) = 11.8$.

Viscosity-Imparting Agents

The viscosity of an emulsion can be of crucial importance for its stability, especially the viscosity of the external phase. A high viscosity reduces creaming and the tendency of particles to coalescence, resulting in phase separation. Examples of widely used viscosity-imparting agents include alginates, bentonite, carboxymethyl cellulose, polyvinyl pyrrolidone, hydroxy propyl cellulose, and carbomer.

Emulsification Techniques

Techniques of emulsification of pharmaceutical products have been reviewed by Zografi (53), Block (24), and Freitas et al. (158). The location of the emulsifier, the method of incorporation of the phases, the rates of addition, the temperature of each phase, and the rate of cooling after mixing of the phases can considerably affect the average droplet size, size distribution, viscosity, and stability of the final emulsion. Roughly, four emulsification methods can be distinguished:

1. Addition of the internal phase to the external phase, while subjecting the system to shear or fracture.
2. Phase inversion technique: The external phase is added to the internal phase. For example, if an o/w emulsion is to be prepared, the aqueous phase is added to the oil phase. First, a w/o emulsion is formed. At the so-called inversion point, the addition of more water results in the inversion of the emulsion system

and the formation of an o/w emulsion. The phase inversion technique generally allows for the formation of small droplets with only minimal mechanical action and attendant heat. A classical example is the so-called dry gum technique, which is a phase inversion technique with hydrophilic colloids being part of the formulation. First, the dry hydrocolloid (e.g., acacia, tragacanth, methyl cellulose) is dispersed within the oil phase. Then, water is added until the phase inversion occurs, resulting in the formation of an o/w emulsion.

3. Mixing both phases upon separate heating of each phase. This method is frequently used for the preparation of creams.
4. Alternate addition of the two phases (in small portions) to the emulsifying agent. This technique is especially suitable for the preparation of food emulsions.

Emulsion Stability

Types of Instability

Four major phenomena are associated with the physical instability of emulsions: flocculation, creaming, coalescence, and breaking (Fig. 10) (159–161). *Flocculation* is best defined as the association of particles within an emulsion to form large aggregates, which can easily be redispersed upon shaking (see also section "Flocculation and Deflocculation Phenomena"). Flocculation is generally regarded as a precursor to the irreversible process of coalescence. It differs from coalescence primarily by the fact that the interfacial film and individual droplets remain intact. The reversibility of flocculation depends mainly on the strength of the interaction between the droplets and on the phase to volume ratio. The relationship between droplet deformation, surfactant transfer, and interfacial rheology for emulsion stability has been discussed by Evanov et al. (162). *Creaming* occurs when the disperse droplets or floccules separate from the disperse medium under the influence of gravitational force. Generally, a creamed emulsion can be restored to its original state by gentle agitation. According to Stokes' law, the direction in which the droplets move depends on the relative values of the densities of the two phases. Furthermore, larger droplets cream more rapidly than smaller droplets. Reducing the droplet sizes and thickening the continuous phase can minimize the rate of creaming. *Coalescence* is a much more serious type of instability. It occurs when the mechanical or electrical barrier is insufficient to prevent the formation of progressively larger droplets

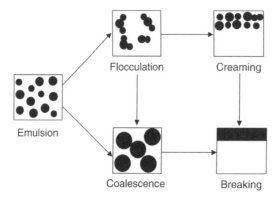

Figure 10 Schematic illustration of the different types of instability of emulsions.

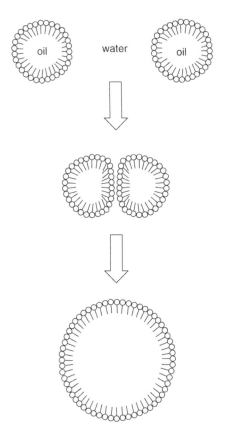

—○   surfactant molecule

Figure 11   Schematic presentation of flocculation and coalescence of emulsion droplets.

(Fig. 11) (159), which can finally lead to the *breaking* of the emulsion (complete phase separation). Coalescence might be avoided by the formation of thick interfacial films consisting of macromolecules or particulate solids.

Stress Tests

The primary objective when studying the stability of emulsions is to predict the shelf life of these systems under ambient storage conditions. The challenge of stability assessment studies under ambient storage conditions is that they last for long periods. To overcome this restriction, different types of stress tests and stress conditions have been proposed to provide the basis for the prediction of the stability of an emulsion under ambient conditions. These methods can be very valuable; however, it should always be kept in mind that changes occurring under stress conditions must not necessarily occur under ambient conditions. Great care must be taken that the accelerated conditions do not introduce new mechanisms of instability, especially those bearing little relationship to what happens at long term under ambient conditions. Stress conditions used for the evaluation of the stability of emulsions include thermal stress and gravitational stress.

Thermal stress   The Arrhenius equation states that a 10°C increase in temperature doubles the rate of most chemical reactions. However, this approach is generally only useful to predict a product's shelf life if the instability of the emulsion is due to a chemical degradation process. Furthermore, this degradation must be identical in mechanism at the investigated temperatures. Thus, the instability of emulsion systems seldom obeys the Arrhenius equation. Emulsion systems are often more complex; their instability might include phenomena such as (*i*) temperature-dependent solubilities and phase distributions of emulsifiers; (*ii*) degradation reactions occurring only at higher temperatures; (*iii*) temperature-induced phase changes, resulting in composition changes and altered rheological behavior; and (*iv*) structural deformations and reformations, which may markedly vary with temperature (159). It is generally considered reasonable to use the time for destabilization at 40°C multiplied by 4 to give an estimate shelf life at room temperature (141). In addition, *low* temperature may as well cause instabilities, for example, because of the precipitation of emulsifiers.

Gravitational stress. Gravitational stress such as centrifugation may accelerate phase separation. Although this technique has been considered in a casual manner in the evaluation of emulsion stability, prediction of emulsion shelf lives based on this method has not been investigated in much detail until the use of ultracentrifuges (156). Becher (121) indicates that centrifugation at 3750 rpm in a 10-cm radius centrifuge for a period of five hours is equivalent to the effect of gravity for about one year. In general, centrifugation is a useful tool to predict the emulsion shelf life; however, the technique may not be suitable for very viscous or semisolid products.

Evaluation of Emulsion Stability

The most useful parameters commonly measured to assess the effect of stress conditions on emulsions include (*i*) the occurrence/absence of phase separation, (*ii*) the rheological properties of the system, (*iii*) the electrical properties of the emulsion, and (*iv*) the particle size distribution.

Phase separation An estimation of whether phase separation occurs or not may be obtained visually. In general, creaming, flocculation, and coalescence take place before phase separation becomes visible, thus, rendering quantitative evaluations difficult. Accelerating the separation process by centrifugation, followed by an appropriate analysis of the specimens may be useful to quantitatively determine this process. Details on the mechanisms of creaming and phase separation as well as on some advances in the monitoring techniques have been reviewed by Robins (163).

Rheological properties The rheology of an emulsion can serve as an important indicator when determining the system's stability. Any variation in droplet size distribution, degree of flocculation, or phase separation frequently results in viscosity changes. Since most emulsions are non-Newtonian, the cone-plate-type device should be used to determine their viscosity rather than the capillary viscometer.

Electrical properties Also, the surface charge and ζ-potential (measure of the apparent, active charge) of emulsified droplets can be a very useful indicator for the stability of the system, because electrostatic repulsion can significantly contribute to the avoidance of flocculation and coalescence (see also section "Instabilities and Stabilization Concepts"). In addition, the conductivity of the emulsion can provide very valuable information, in particular when measured at different heights of the storage cell and at different times points (164–167).

Particle size distribution The best evaluation of an emulsion's stability is probably to measure its particle size distribution. A number of methods are available for droplet size determination (see section "Particle Size Analysis"). Optical microscopy, although a time-consuming technique, is a direct means of particle size measurement of droplets greater than 1 μm. Laser light scattering, diffraction, and transmission methods have become standard techniques for a routine determination of the particle size (168,169).

COLLOIDS AND COLLOIDAL DISPERSIONS

A colloid is defined as a system consisting of discrete particles in the size range of 1 nm to 1 μm, distributed within a continuous phase (170). On the basis of the interaction of particles, molecules, or ions of the disperse phase with molecules of the dispersion medium, colloidal systems can be classified as being lyophilic or lyophobic. In lyophilic systems, the disperse phase molecules are dissolved within the continuous phase and in the colloidal size range, or spontaneously form aggregates in the colloidal size range (association systems). In lyophobic systems, the disperse phase is very poorly soluble or insoluble in the continuous phase. During the last several decades, the use of colloids in the pharmaceutical sciences has gained considerable attention. These systems have been investigated primarily for site-specific drug delivery, for controlled drug delivery, and also for the enhancement of the dissolution rate/bioavailability of poorly water-soluble drugs. Applications of colloidal materials for the preparation of pharmaceutical dosage forms are listed in Table 8 (11). In this section, two types of colloidal systems, namely, drug-free aqueous colloidal polymeric dispersions (latexes and pseudolatexes) and drug-loaded nanoparticles will be discussed.

Latexes and Pseudolatexes

An aqueous colloidal polymeric dispersion is by definition a two-phase system comprising a disperse phase and a dispersion medium. The disperse phase consists of spherical polymer particles, usually with an average diameter of 200 to 300 nm. According to their method of preparation, aqueous colloidal polymer dispersions can be divided into two categories: (true) latexes and pseudolatexes. True latexes are prepared by controlled polymerization of emulsified monomer droplets in aqueous solutions, whereas pseudolatexes are prepared starting from already polymerized macromolecules using different emulsification techniques.

To prepare (*true*) *latexes*, the monomers are emulsified in water under stirring and addition of emulsifiers, which help to stabilize the monomer droplets. The molecular weight of the polymer molecules in the resultant latex can be controlled by the concentration and decomposition rate of added polymerization initiators. The residual monomer content can be reduced by optimizing the polymerization conditions and can also later be eliminated, for instance, by steam distillation.

For the preparation of *pseudolatexes*, the following three methods are commonly used (44):

1. Direct emulsification: A solution of the polymer within a volatile, water-immiscible organic solvent (or mixture of solvents), or a polymer melt is emulsified within a surfactant-containing aqueous phase. If used, the organic solvent is then removed by steam distillation to obtain the pseudolatexes.
2. Inverse emulsification: A solution of the polymer within a volatile, water-immiscible organic solvent (or mixture of solvents), or a polymer melt is

Table 8 Examples of Colloidal Materials Used for the Preparation of Pharmaceutical Dosage Forms

Colloidal material	Application
Acacia	Emulsifier, microcapsule wall material, suspending agent
Alginic acid	Microcapsule wall material, viscosity-imparting agent, disintegrant, binder
Bentonite	Stabilizer, gelling agent, suspending agent, viscosity-imparting agent
Calcium carbonate	Diluent
Carbomer	Emulsifier, gelling agent, suspending agent
Carboxymethyl cellulose	Emusifier, gelling agent, suspending agent, disintegrant, binder
Cellulose	Binder, disintegrant, filler
Cellulose acetate phthalate	Enteric coating material
Dextrin	Stabilizer, viscosity-imparting agent, adhesive agent, binder, plasticizer
Ethylcellulose	Viscosity-imparting agent, microcapsule wall material, binder
Gelatin	Microcapsule wall material, suspending agent, binder, coating material
Guar gum	Viscosity-imparting agent, stabilizer, binder
Hydroxypropyl cellulose	Viscosity-imparting agent, microcapsule wall material, granulating agent
Methyl cellulose	Emulsifier, viscosity-imparting agent, gelling agent, suspending agent, binder, disintegrant
Poloxamer 188	Emulsifier, stabilizing agent, gelling agent
Polyethylene glycols	Gelling agents, coating materials, lubricants, plasticizers
Polymethacrylates	Film coating materials, binders
Silicon dioxide	Lubricant for capsules and tablets, viscosity-imparting agent, adsorbent
Starch	Binder, disintegrant
Tragacanth	Emulsifier, viscosity-imparting agent, suspending agent

Source: From Ref. 11.

compounded with a long-chain fatty acid (e.g., oleic acid) using conventional rubber-mixing equipment and mixed slowly with a dilute aqueous phase to give a w/o emulsion, which then inverts into an o/w emulsion upon further addition of the aqueous phase. If used, the organic solvent is then removed by steam distillation to obtain the pseudolatexes (171,172).

3. Self-emulsification: The polymer molecules are modified chemically by the introduction of basic (e.g., amino) or acidic (e.g., carboxyl) groups in such concentrations and locations that the polymer undergoes self-emulsification (without the addition of surfactants) after dispersion into an acidic or basic solution.

Latexes and pseudolatexes are widely used for the coating of solid pharmaceutical dosage forms such as tablets, capsules, and pellets (40,41). The major advantage compared with conventional coating techniques is the avoidance of hazardous, toxic, and/ or explosive organic solvents.

Nanoparticles

As indicated by the name, nanoparticles are colloidal particles in the size range of 1 to 1000 nm. The term "nanoparticles" encompasses both nanocapsules and nanospheres. Nanocapsules have a core-shell structure (reservoir systems), while nanospheres are one-block devices (matrix systems). Analogous to the above-described latexes and pseudolatexes (which are spherical, drug-free, aqueous, polymeric, nanoparticulate dispersions with a narrow size distribution), the techniques used to prepare polymeric nanoparticles can be classified into two groups. Either the nanoparticles are prepared from preformed polymers or via various polymerization reactions of lipophilic and/or hydrophilic monomers. The choice of a particular preparation method and of a suitable polymer mainly depends on the physicochemical properties of the drug, the desired release patterns, the therapeutic goal, the route of administration, the biodegradability/biocompatibility of the carrier material, and the regulatory aspects. From a technological point of view, the ideal preparation method can provide high drug loadings, high encapsulation efficiencies, and high product yields and is easily upscalable.

Nanoparticles Based on Water-Insoluble Polymers

To prepare nanoparticles, which are based on water-insoluble polymers, a solution of the polymer in an organic solvent can be emulsified within an aqueous phase. This o/w emulsion is then homogenized under high shear with an appropriate homogenization equipment (e.g., microfluidizer, sonication) prior to the precipitation of the polymer to further reduce the particle size of the internal organic phase into the colloidal size range (173–177). The high-pressure emulsification–solvent evaporation method is limited to water-insoluble drugs. Unless specific binding exists, water-soluble drugs are difficult to be encapsulated because of partitioning into the external aqueous phase during emulsification and the significant surface area of the interface "organic solvent-water." The particle size of the solidified nanoparticles is determined by the size of the emulsified polymer-drug-solvent droplets and hence depends on the homogenization equipment. Nanoparticles have been prepared with conventional laboratory homogenizers (11) by ultrasonication (174–176) or by microfluidization (176). With the microfluidizer, the particle size decreases with increasing operating pressure and increasing number of cycles (176). The particle size of the nanoparticles is also affected by the type of surfactant and surfactant concentration, the viscosity of the organic polymer solution, and the phase ratio of the internal to the aqueous phase (176,178).

A similar technique, the so-called spontaneous emulsification solvent diffusion method is derived from the solvent injection method to prepare liposomes (179). Niwa et al. (180) used a mixed solvent system of methylene chloride and acetone to prepare poly (lactic-co-glycolic acid) (PLGA) nanoparticles. The addition of the water-miscible solvent, acetone, results in the formation of particles in the submicron range; this is not possible with only the water-immiscible organic solvent. The addition of acetone decreases the interfacial tension between the organic and the aqueous phase and, in addition, results in the perturbation of the droplet interface because of the rapid diffusion of acetone into the aqueous phase.

Nanocapsules based on poly(lactic acid) (PLA), PLA-copolymers or poly (ε-caprolactone) can be prepared by an "interfacial polymer deposition" (181–184). A solution of the polymer, the drug and a water-immiscible oil in a water-miscible solvent such as acetone is added to an external aqueous phase. This technique results in nanocapsules with a core-shell structure. The drug must have a high solubility in the oil-solvent mixture to obtain nanoparticles with high drug loadings.

An interesting modification of the solvent evaporation method is based on a salting-out effect (185–190): An aqueous phase saturated with an electrolyte or nonelectrolyte is added to a solution of the polymer and drug in a water-miscible organic solvent (e.g., acetone) under agitation until an o/w emulsion is formed. Saturation of the aqueous phase reduces the miscibility of acetone and water by a salting-out process and allows for the formation of an o/w emulsion under these conditions of the otherwise miscible phases. The major advantages of the salting-out method include the avoidance of chlorinated solvents and surfactants commonly used for the conventional solvent evaporation method.

Nanoparticles Based on Hydrophilic Polymers

Nanoparticles based on hydrophilic polymers (e.g., albumin, chitosan, gelatin, or carbohydrates) can be prepared by w/o emulsification techniques. This process has initially been developed for the preparation of albumin microspheres (191–194). However, the use of high shear homogenization equipment or ultrasonication allows for the formation of emulsions in the nanometer size range. Basically, an aqueous polymer solution is emulsified into an external, water-immiscible phase, such as an oil or organic solvent followed by homogenization. The polymer droplets solidify on removal of water. Insoluble nanoparticles can be obtained by further hardening/insolubilizing the polymer via chemical cross-linking, using aldehydes or other cross-linking agents, or via denaturation at elevated temperatures. To obtain high encapsulation efficiencies, the drug must be insoluble in the external phase. Gelatin nanoparticles have been prepared by emulsifying a concentrated gelatin solution (30%) into hydrogenated castor oil (containing appropriate emulsifying agents) at a temperature above the gelation temperature of the gelatin solution (195). The w/o emulsion is then cooled to gel the aqueous gelatin droplets. Chitosan is one of the few naturally derived polysaccharides with basic functional groups. Since it is only soluble in acidic media, chitosan micro- or nanoparticles can be prepared by emulsifying aqueous solutions of chitosan in acetic acid into an external oil phase (196). Furthermore, chitosan and sodium alginate form gels with counterions such as tripolyphosphate or calcium chloride. Nanoparticles can thus be prepared by emulsifying an aqueous polysaccharide solution into the oil phase followed by emulsification of an aqueous solution of the counterion solution.

The drawbacks of the w/o emulsification method include the use of large amounts of oils as the external phase, which must be removed by washing with organic solvents, thermal instability of certain drugs, possible interactions of the cross-linking agent with the drug, and (as in the case of all nanoparticles prepared by emulsification techniques) a fairly broad particle size distribution.

Gelatin- and albumin-based nanoparticles can also be prepared via the desolvation of the dissolved macromolecules upon addition of either salts (e.g., sodium sulfate or ammonium sulfate) or ethanol (197–200). This is, in principle, similar to a simple coacervation method. The particles can then be insolubilized via cross-linking, using aldehydes. These phase separation methods avoid the use of oils as the external phase.

Alginate-based nanoparticles can be prepared by the addition of calcium chloride to a sodium alginate solution (201). This so-called microgel can be cross-linked with the oppositely charged polymer poly(L-lysine) to form nanospheres. This technique is based on the gelation of sodium alginate with Ca ions, however, at much lower concentrations than normally used for gel formation. Again, since only one phase is used, high drug loadings are difficult to obtain unless specific binding of the drug to the anionic polymeric carrier occurs.

PARENTERAL DISPERSE SYSTEMS

During the past 30 years, there have been significant developments of parenteral disperse formulations. The use of parenteral emulsions can overcome the problems of low aqueous solubility and hydrolytic instability of many drugs (202,203). Such formulations can avoid the use of conventional cosolvent systems and the undesirable effects caused by precipitation of drugs at the injection site. Recent developments of parenteral disperse formulations have the potential to provide sustained release and targeting of drugs (204–207).

Parenteral Emulsions

In addition to the general requirements for parenteral products (e.g., sterility, nontoxicity, and stability), particular attention must be paid to the droplet size and surface charge of parenteral emulsions (208), since these parameters can directly affect both toxicity and stability.

Particle Size

The British Pharmacopoeia states that the diameter of emulsion globules for intravenous administration may not exceed 5 μm. Emulsion globules larger than 4 to 6 μm are known to increase the incidence of emboli and may cause changes in blood pressure (29,208). However, lipid particles larger than 7.5 μm have been reported to deform and pass through the pulmonary vasculature without difficulty (209). In general, emulsions that contain globules of 200 to 500 nm in size tend to be most physically stable. Smaller-sized emulsions are utilized by the body more rapidly than the larger-sized ones (208).

Surface Charge

A reduction in the electrical charge is known to increase the flocculation and coalescence rate. A sufficiently high ζ-potential (absolute value) ensures stable emulsions via electrostatic repulsion of adjacent droplets. The selection of suitable surfactants can help to optimize the droplet surface charges and, thus, to enhance emulsion stability. Lipid particles with either positive or negative surface charges are more stable and are more rapidly cleared from the bloodstream than neutral particles (210,211).

Ingredients

Oils Among many investigated oils, soy oil, middle-chain triglycertides (MCT), safflower oil, and cottonseed oils seem to be suitable to form the oil phase because of the low incidence of toxic reactions (212). Obviously, purity is a crucial parameter in the case of parenteral application. Undesirable contaminants such as pigments or oxidative decomposition products must be minimized.

Emulsifiers Natural lecithin is one of the most widely used emulsifiers because it is metabolized in the body. However, type I allergic reaction to soybean lecithin emulsified in lipid solutions has been observed (213). Among the synthetic emulsifying agents, block copolymers of polyoxyethylene-polyoxypropylene (poloxamer) have gained increasing interest for parenteral emulsions. Other examples of emulsifiers commonly found in parenteral formulations are listed in Table 9.

Additives Additives are used to adjust the tonicity and pH of emulsions and/or to increase emulsion stability. For instance, glycerol is a commonly used agent to adjust the osmolarity of parenteral emulsions. The pH of the emulsion should be adjusted close to the physiological pH by adding aqueous solutions of NaOH or HCl. Tocopherols and oleic acid may be added as antioxidants and stabilizers, respectively. Some commercially available fat emulsions and their compositions are listed in Table 10.

Table 9 Most Commonly Used Emulsifiers in Parenteral Emulsions

Emulsifiers	Concentration range
Egg lecithin	1–3% w/w
Soybean lecithin	1–3% w/w
Phosphatidylcholine	~50%
Polysorbate 80: PEG-PE	no data
Ethylene glycol ether	no data
Glycerol/propylene glycol	30–70% w/w individually
Glyceryl fatty acid esters	3% w/w
Poloxamer 188, 238, 338 (pluronic F68, 88, 108)	1.5–10%
Poloxamer 401 (pluronic L121)	5%
Polysorbate 80	0.4% w/w

Source: From Ref. 208.

Table 10 Compositions of Some Commercially Available Fat Emulsions

Trade name (company)	Oil phase	Emulsifier	Other components
Intralipid (Kabi-Vitrum)	Soybean oil 10–20%	Lecithin 1.2%	Glycerol 2.5%
Lipofundins (Braun)	Soybean oil 10–20%	Soybean lecithin 0.75–1.2%	Xylitol 5%
Lipofundins (Braun)	Cottonseed oil 10%	Soybean lecithin 0.75%	Sorbitol 5%
Liposyn (Abbott)	Safflower oil 10–20%	Lecithin 1.2%	Glycerol 2.5%
Travemulsion (Travenol)	Soybean protein 10–20%	Lecithin 1.2%	Glycerol 2.5%

Source: From Ref. 159.

Sterilization

Autoclaving can be used for the sterilization of parenteral emulsions, provided the required sterilization conditions do not lead to significant product degradation and/or physical instability. Alternatively, parenteral emulsions might be sterilized by filtration, if the emulsion globules can pass through the filter. For thermolabile products and/or products that cannot be filtered, terminal γ-irradiation may be useful. However, restrictions to utilize γ-sterilization differ from country to country, and in some cases, changes in the product might be caused. Most desirable in terms of stability is aseptic processing in clean rooms, but this is associated with a certain risk of contamination of the final product.

Parenteral Suspensions

Parenteral suspensions consist of a solid phase, which is dispersed within a liquid phase. The requirements for and limitations to prepare parenteral suspensions include microbiological controls, ingredient allowances, and mechanical flow properties (214–216). Excipients used in parenteral suspensions should be nonpyrogenic, nontoxic, and chemically inert. Flocculating and wetting agents are important ingredients to maintain product stability and good mechanical properties. Water for injection is the most widely used solvent in parenteral formulations. Nonaqueous solvents might be used to increase the solubility of certain compounds and/or the stability of the system. Examples for nonaqueous solvents used in parenteral products include polyethylene glycols, glycerin, and ethanol (217).

Because of particle sizes in the micrometer range, parenteral suspensions are generally limited to either subcutaneous or intramuscular routes of administration. However, ultrafine suspensions can be prepared by high-pressure homogenization (218). The particle size obtained by using this technique can be in the 100- to 500-nm range, thus allowing for intravenous administration (219).

CHARACTERIZATION OF DISPERSE SYSTEMS

Particle Size Analysis

The particle size is a major characteristic of a disperse system. Particle size measurements allow for the detection of potential particle aggregation and/or crystal growth. Particle size distribution data are often employed as fundamental quality control standards for pharmaceutical disperse systems. A broad particle size distribution is known to promote uneven settling in suspensions and coalescence in emulsions.

Various techniques and equipments are available for the measurement of the particle size, shape, and volume. These include, for example, microscopy, sieve analysis, sedimentation methods, photon correlation spectroscopy (PCS), and the Coulter Counter or other electrical sensing devices. The specific surface area of original drug powders can also be assessed using gas adsorption or gas permeability techniques. It should be noted that most of the particle size measurements are not truly direct methods. As the different types of equipments are based on different physical principles and simplifications/assumptions, the obtained particle sizes may not always be directly comparable between the various methods.

Microscopy

Microscopic or optical methods range in complexity and costs from a simple laboratory microscope to refined pieces of automated equipment. The microscope provides a *direct* observation of the sample and allows for the determination of particle diameters. An ordinary microscope generally measures the particle size in the range of 0.2 to about 100 μm. A diluted or undiluted sample (e.g., an emulsion or suspension) is mounted on a slide or ruled cell and placed on a mechanical stage. The microscope eyepiece is fitted with a micrometer or a graticule with which the linear dimension of the particles may be estimated. The field might be photographed or projected onto a screen to ease the process of particle measurements. Electronic scanners and video-recording equipment have been developed to avoid the necessity of measuring particles by visual observation.

To obtain a value for the dimensions of an irregular particle, several approaches of measurements can be used: Martin's diameter (defined as the length of a line that bisects the particle image); Feret's diameter (or end-to-end measurement, defined as the distance between two tangents on opposite sides of the particle parallel to some fixed direction); and the projected area diameter (defined as the diameter of a circle having the same area as that of the particle observed perpendicular to the surface on which the particle rests). With any technique, a sufficiently large number of particles must be measured to obtain a statistically reliable value.

A major advantage of optical methods is the possibility to obtain also information on the particle *shape* and potential presence of particle aggregations, including the degree and character of the aggregation. A disadvantage is that the diameter is obtained from only two (of the three) dimensions of the particle, for example, length and width; no information on the thickness or depth is available. The large number of particles that must be measured (in general 300–500) to obtain a good estimation of the distribution renders the method rather slow and tedious.

Electron microscopes provide high resolutions and allow visualization of particle sizes below the limit of resolution of an optical microscope. The radiation source is a beam of high-energy electrons having wavelengths in the region of 0.1 Å. With current instrumentation, this results in smallest distances of approximately 5 Å by which two objects are separated and remain distinguishable. Scanning electron microscopy (SEM) finds wide application in the field of pharmaceutical technology followed by transmission electron microscopy (TEM) (220–222).

Sieve Analysis

Sieve analysis, based either on the vibratory or the suction principle, uses a series of standard sieves calibrated by the National Bureau of Standards. The method is generally used for screening coarse particles down to a size of 44 µm (no. 325 sieve). However, sieves produced by photoetching and electroforming techniques are available with apertures from 90 down to 5 µm.

A typical testing procedure involves several steps. First, the selected number and size of sieves are stacked upon one another, with the largest openings being at the top of the stack, and beneath a pan to collect the particles finer than the smallest sieve. The known amount of powder to be analyzed is then placed on the top sieve and the set is vibrated in a mechanical device for a predetermined time period. The results are obtained by weighing the amount of material retained on each sieve and on the collecting pan. The suction method uses one sieve at a time and examines the amount retained on the screen. In both methods, the data are expressed as frequency or cumulative frequency plots, respectively.

Sieving errors can arise from a number of variables, including the sieve loading as well as the duration and intensity of agitation (223). Sieving can also cause attrition and, thus, size reduction of granular materials. Standard sieving protocols must be employed to ensure reproducible particle size distributions between different batches of raw materials.

Sedimentation Method

This method is based on Stokes' law (see section "Sedimentation and Stokes' Law"). Practical techniques include simple sedimentation methods such as the Andreason pipette and the Cahn sedimentation balance. The Andreason pipette involves measuring the percentage of solids that settle with time in a graduated sedimentation vessel. Samples are withdrawn from the bottom of the vessel using a pipette, and the amount of solids is determined by drying and weighing. The Cahn sedimentation balance electronically records the amount of disperse powder settling out as a function of time. One advantage of this method is that the mass of particles is recorded continuously. Both methods are appropriate when the particle size is generally larger than 5 µm. If particles smaller than 5 µm are to be evaluated, a centrifugal method is often employed to speed up the data collection, by overcoming the effects of convection and diffusion. The method involves a photosedimentation device in which the light transmittance is measured through a cell filled with a dispersion of interest. An ultracentrifuge can also be used in such cases to increase the sedimentation rate of colloidal particles.

Coulter Counter and Electrical Sensing Devices

Counters, such as the Coulter Counter, determine the number of particles in a known volume of an electrolyte solution. The device employs the electrolyte displacement method and measures the equivalent spherical volume diameter, d_v. This type of equipment is used primarily to obtain the particle size distribution of the sample. It measures the change in an electrical sensing zone, which occurs when a particle passes through an orifice positioned between two electrodes. The dispersion is drawn through a small orifice that has an electrode on either side. The disperse particles interfere with the current flow, causing the resistance to change. The resistance changes are related to the particle volumes and, when amplified as voltage pulses, may be counted. The instrument is capable of counting particles at a rate of approximately 4000 per second, and so both gross counts and particle size distributions are obtained in a relatively short period of time. Electronic pulse counters are also useful in studying particle growth, dissolution, and particulate contamination. Examples are the Coulter Counter and the Electrozone Counter. Coulter Electronics also manufactures a submicron particle-sizing instrument, the Coulter Model N4, for analyzing particles in the size range of 0.003 to 0.3 μm. The instrument also provides molecular weights and diffusion coefficients.

Light Scattering

The quasi-elastic light-scattering technique (QELS), also called PCS, is based on the principle of light scattering and can be employed to determine the mean particle diameter and size distribution (polydispersity). Light scattering shows the Faraday–Tyndall effect and can be used for the determination of the molecular weight, size, and shape of colloidal particles. Scattering may be described in terms of the turbidity, τ, the fractional decrease in intensity due to scattering as the incident light passes through a solution. When the particle is asymmetric, the intensity of scattered light varies with the angle of observation, thus permitting an estimation of the shape and size of the particle. However, caution should be exercised (224). Light scattering has been used to study proteins, synthetic polymers, association colloids, and lyophobic sols.

Racey et al. (225,226) applied QELS, which uses laser light to determine diffusion coefficients and particle sizes as the Stokes' diameters. It consists of a laser light source, a temperature-controlled sample compartment, and a photomultiplier to detect the scattered light at a certain angle (usually 90°). QELS has been used in the examination of heparin aggregates in commercial preparations. The method is applicable for measuring particle sizes ranging from 5 nm to approximately 3 μm. In this size range, the particles exhibit Brownian motion, as a result of collisions with the molecules of surrounding liquid medium, which causes the fluctuation in the intensity of scattered light. PCS, however, cannot characterize systems having broadly distributed particles. This restriction might be overcome by combining sedimentation field-flow fractionation and QELS, which presents a detailed record of the particle size at each size interval.

Hydrodynamic Chromatography

This method is used particularly for colloids. A colloidal dispersion is forced through a long column packed with nonporous beads with an approximate radius of 10 μm. Particles of different particle size travel with different speeds around the beads and are, thus, collected in different-sized fractions.

Determination of Electrical Properties

The movement of a charged particle with respect to an adjacent liquid phase is the basic principle underlying two electrokinetic phenomena: electrophoresis and electroosmosis.

Electrophoresis involves the movement of a charged particle through a liquid under the influence of an applied potential difference. A sample is placed in an electrophoresis cell, usually a horizontal tube of circular cross section fitted with two electrodes. When a known potential is applied across the electrodes, the particles migrate to the oppositely charged electrode. The direct current voltage applied needs to be adjusted to obtain a particle velocity that is neither too fast nor too slow. It is also important that the measurement is taken reasonably quickly to avoid sedimentation in the cell. Prior to each measurement, the apparatus should be calibrated with particles of known ζ-potential, such as rabbit erythrocytes.

The velocity of particle migration, v, across the field is a function of the surface charge or ζ-potential, and is observed visually by means of an ultramicroscope equipped with a calibrated eyepiece and a scale. The movement is measured by timing the individual particles over a certain distance; and the results of approximately 10 to 15 timing measurements are then averaged. From the measured particle velocity, the electrophoretic mobility (defined as v/E, where E is the potential gradient) can be calculated.

Electroosmosis is essentially based on the opposite principle: In this case, the particles are rendered immobile by forming a capillary or a porous plug. The liquid now moves through this plug or membrane, across which a potential is applied. The rate of liquid flow through the plug is determined under standardized conditions.

The determination of the ζ-potential of particles in a disperse system provides useful information concerning the sign and magnitude of the charge and its effect on the stability of the system (see section "Surface Properties and Interfacial Phenomena") (59,227–229). It can be of value in the development of pharmaceutical suspensions, particularly if the controlled aggregation approach is used. The use of the ζ-potential to evaluate the electrophoretic properties of other dosage forms, such as liposomes and microcapsules, has also been reported (230,231).

A number of semiautomated or fully automated instruments are currently used for studying the electrokinetic properties. These include the electrophoretic mass transport analyzer (Zeta Potential Analyzer, Micrometrics Instrument Corp., Norcross, Georgia, U.S.), the streaming current detector (Hydroscan, Leeds and Northrup Corporation, Philadelphia, Pennsylvania, U.S.), the electrokinetic sonic amplitude device (Matec Instruments, Northborough, Massachusetts, U.S.), and the instruments that determine the ζ-potential by measuring the electrophoretic mobility of the disperse particles in a charged electric field (Zeta Reader, Komline-Sanderson, Peapack, New Jersey, U.S.; Zeta Meter, Laser Zee Meter, Pen Kem, Bedford Hills, New York, U.S.). The first three devices are suitable for determining the average ζ-potential of coarse suspensions in systems having high solids contents, whereas the latter three are more useful for the measurement of colloidal particles in diluted systems.

Rheological Measurements

Rheological evaluations can be simple or complex, depending on the nature of the product. They feature an important quality control of all disperse systems. For example, the adequacy of hydration and quality control of the gums used as viscosity-imparting agents in the products is best confirmed by a rheological test. These natural or synthetic gums are polymers of varying molecular weights from batch to batch, which directly affect the product's viscosity. In addition, the degree of dispersion, particle size, and size distribution influence the viscosity and dispersion consistency. Also, formulation additives, such as sweeteners, surfactants, and flocculating agents influence the rheological properties of the dispersions. Viscosity characteristics of a suspension may be altered not only by the vehicle used but also by the solids content. Increasing amounts of solid particles lead to increased viscosities of the disperse system. The viscosity of lyophobic dispersions is not much higher than that of the original liquid because of minimal interaction between the internal and external phases. The viscosity of lyophilic systems, especially polymer solutions, is much higher because of the interaction between the two phases. As a result of this interaction, dispersions possessing both Newtonian and non–Newtonian properties are formed. Highly viscous or rigid gels can be formed at higher polymer concentrations.

A wide variety of viscometers (ranging from simple to sophisticated) have been designed to evaluate the rheological properties of various disperse systems. It is important to select a suitable viscometer, one that is adapted to the viscosity ranges encountered in a given application. The instrument should provide the required rheological data over the desired range of shear, time under shear, and temperature. Viscometers are classified into those that operate at a single shear rate and those that allow more than one rate of shear to be examined. The simplest qualitative measurement of viscosity may be obtained by bubble, cup, falling ball, falling rod, and capillary viscometers. These simple devices provide a one-point measurement and are widely used for Newtonian fluids and dilute solutions. The glass capillary Cannon-Fenske, Ubbelohde, and Ostwald viscometers are the most popular instruments based on this method.

Many rheometers are based on the principle to rotate the sample and to measure its response to the applied stress by a variety of sensors. The advantages of rotational viscometers are that the shear rate can be varied over a wide range, and that continuous measurements at a given shear rate or shear stress can be made for extended periods of time, allowing for the evaluation of time- and/or shear-dependent properties. Viscometers of this type are routinely used in many pharmaceutical laboratories. Simple rotational viscometers are the Stormer viscometer, the ICI viscometer, and the Brookfield viscometer. A Brookfield viscometer with the helipath attachment is a valuable piece of rheological equipment for measuring the settling behavior and structure of pharmaceutical suspensions. The instrument consists of a slowly rotating T-bar spindle, which is descended into an undisturbed sample. The dial reading of the viscometer measures the resistance to flow that the spindle encounters from the structure at various levels in the sediment. Recording rheograms at various time intervals (under standardized conditions) gives a description of the suspension and its physical stability. The technique is most useful for viscous suspensions with high solid contents, which develop sufficient shear stress for the measurements. The instrument is also suitable for characterizing flocculated systems. To simulate the situation illustrated in Figure 4, coaxial-cylinder viscometers have been designed in which the plates are bent to form cylindrical surfaces, one of which is stationary and the other is rotating. There are two types of concentric cylinder viscometers, namely, the Searle system and the Couette system. In the Couette type, the material is contained in an annular gap between the inner cylindrical bob or spindle and the outer concentric cylindrical cup. In the Stormer viscometer or the more advanced Haake Rotovisco, the cup is stationary. Cone and plate and parallel-plate rheometers are designed to handle small-quantity samples, from about 0.2 to 5 mL. The plate may be stationary while the cone is rotating or vice versa. The angle between the cone and the plate has to be extremely small, usually 0.1° to 3°. Since the sample size is very small, this method is very sensitive to sample drying and temperature changes. Another disadvantage of this method is the loss of material due to slinging from the gap and sample heating, especially at high shear rates.

Temperature and Gravitational Stress Tests

Disperse systems can be subjected to cyclic temperature testing, for example, to conditions of repeated freezing and thawing (e.g., $-5°C-+40°C$ in 24 hours) or exposing them to elevated temperatures ($>40°C$) for short periods of storage to test for the physical stability. The value of such stress test procedure may be questionable since the exposure to elevated temperatures often results in a drastic change in the drug's solubility. Significant amounts of drug may go into solution and reprecipitate upon subsequent cooling. Most suspension systems contain surfactants and protective colloids to prevent crystal growth, and thus, inducing crystal growth during stress testing may be of limited value. The use of stressful aging tests, however, has one advantage. If a given suspension is able to withstand exposure to extreme temperatures, it is likely that the product will show good physical stability during prolonged storage at ambient temperature. On the other hand, failure of any preparations to meet such stringent testing procedures should not be considered a bar to further testing, since many marketed pharmaceutical suspensions would have been rejected from further consideration on this basis alone. The use of stress tests to study the stability of *emulsions* has been described in section "Emulsion Stability."

MANUFACTURING AND EQUIPMENT

The preparation of satisfactory disperse systems consists of three main steps: preparing the internal phase in the proper size range, dispersing the internal phase in the dispersion medium, and finally, stabilizing the resultant product. These three steps may be realized sequentially; however, in many cases (e.g., emulsions) they are performed simultaneously.

Suspensions can be prepared by either dispersing finely divided powders in an appropriate vehicle or by causing precipitation within the vehicle. For most pharmaceutical preparations, the proper size of the internal phase is obtained by a mechanical breakdown of the solid material. One of the most rapid, convenient, and inexpensive methods of producing fine drug powders of about 10 to 50 μm in size is micropulverization. Micropulverizers are high-speed, attrition or impact mills, which are efficient in reducing powders to the size acceptable for most oral and topical suspensions. For finer particles, fluid energy grinding, sometimes referred to as jet milling or micronizing, is quite effective. By this process, the shearing action of high-velocity compressed air streams on the particles in a confined chamber produces the desired ultrafine or micronized particles. The particles are accelerated to high velocities by the sonic and supersonic velocity of turbulent air streams and collide with each other, resulting in fragmentation and size reduction. These micronized drugs are often employed in parenteral and ophthalmic preparations. Particles of very small dimension may also be produced by spray-drying techniques (232). Other equipments for particle size reduction include colloid mills, ball mills, ultrasonic generators, or homogenizers.

The precipitation (condensation, aggregation) method is more complex and has been used to create particles of suitable size by permitting the atoms or molecules of the material to gather together. In this process, the material is dissolved in a suitable solvent, then a miscible nonsolvent is added, and a precipitate is formed. For example, fine sulfur particles can be obtained when water (nonsolvent) is added into an alcoholic solution of sulfur. Suspensions can be prepared by controlled crystallization wherein a supersaturated solution is cooled rapidly with constant agitation to obtain a large number of small, uniform drug crystals. Microcrystals can also be conveniently produced by bubbling liquid nitrogen through a saturated solution of solute prior to solvent freezing. Other methods for obtaining fine particles are based on phase changes, such as sublimation and pH adjustment. Shock cooling methods can offer a possible solution to the electrostatic charge problems associated with dry particle milling. Chemical reactions can also be used for certain pharmaceutical preparations, for example, white lotion.

The second step is to disperse the particles within the dispersion medium. In emulsions, this step is accomplished at the same time as particle reduction occurs (section "Formulation and Preparation Techniques for Emulsions" gives more details on the commonly applied techniques to obtain pharmaceutically relevant emulsions). Surfactants are usually added to promote both particle size reduction and uniform dispersion. Suspensions may be prepared by dispersing the particles resulting from the mechanical breakdown process, along with an addition of a surfactant to aid the wetting process. Alternatively, both size reduction and dispersion processes can take place simultaneously in a manner similar to that for emulsions. Homogenization is normally required when various other additives are incorporated. On a laboratory scale, an ultrasonic generator may be used, whereas a colloid mill is more suitable for an industrial-scale production. The most important techniques to prepare *nanoparticles* are described in the section "Nanoparticles."

For the production of emulsions at a large scale, the oil and water phases are often heated separately. When waxes are present, both phases are generally heated to a temperature above the highest melting point of any component present. One phase is then pumped into the tank containing the second phase with constant agitation throughout the time of addition. After cooling, the product is once again homogenized and then packaged. Semisolid preparations, such as creams and ointments, are prepared using appropriate mixing machinery. Often, the dispersion step is carried out with colloid mills or homogenizers at elevated temperatures to reduce the viscosity of waxy constituents. On a small scale, a mortar and pestle may be used. Once a satisfactory R&D laboratory-scale formulation has been developed, the production process needs to be scaled up, resulting in challenges encountered during mixing and dispersion that are not observed at a small scale (233,234).

REFERENCES

1. Nairn JG. Disperse systems. In: Swarbrick J, Boylan JC, eds. Encyclopedia of Pharmaceutical Technology. Vol 4. New York: Marcel Dekker, 1992:107–120.
2. Patel RB, Patel UR, Roggle MC, et al. Bioavailability of hydrochlorothiazide from tablets and suspensions. J Pharm Sci 1984; 73:359–365.
3. Stout PJ, Howard SA, Mauger JW. Dissolution of pharmaceutical suspensions. In: Swarbrick J, Boylan JC, eds. Encyclopedia of Pharmaceutical Technology. Vol 4. New York: Marcel Dekker, 1992:169–192.
4. Donovan MD, Flanagan DR. Bioavailability of disperse dosage form. In: Lieberman HA, Rieger MM, Banker GS, eds. Pharmaceutical Dosage Forms: Disperse Systems. Vol 1, 2nd ed. New York: Marcel Dekker, 1996:315–376.
5. Mauger JW, Howard SA, Amin K. Dissolution profiles for finely divided drug suspensions. J Pharm Sci 1983; 72:190–193.

6. Hirano K, Yamada H. Studies on the absorption of practically water-insoluble drugs following injection VI: subcutaneous absorption from aqueous suspensions in rats. J Pharm Sci 1982; 71:500–505.

7. Nash RA. Pharmaceutical suspensions. In: Lieberman HA, Rieger MM, Banker GS, eds. Pharmaceutical Dosage Forms: Disperse Systems. Vol 1. New York: Marcel Dekker, 1988:151–198.

8. Patel NK, Kennon L, Levinson RS. Pharmaceutical suspensions. In: Lachman L, Lieberman HA, Kanig JL, eds. The Theory and Practice of Industrial Pharmacy. 3rd ed. Philadelphia: Lea & Febiger, 1986:479–501.

9. Swarbrick J. Coarse dispersions. In: Gennaro AR, ed. Remington: The Science and Practice of Pharmacy. 19th ed. Pennsylvania: Mack Publishing Co., 1995:278–291.

10. Falkiewicz MJ. Theory of suspensions. In: Lieberman HA, Rieger MM, Banker GS, eds. Pharmaceutical Dosage Forms: Disperse Systems. Vol 1. New York: Marcel Dekker, 1988: 13–48.

11. Burgess DJ. Colloids and colloid drug delivery systems. In: Swarbrick J, Boylan JC, eds. Encyclopedia of Pharmaceutical Technology. Vol 3. New York: Marcel Dekker, 1990: 31–64.

12. Martin A, Bustamante P, eds. Physical Pharmacy. 4th ed. Philadelphia: Lippincott Williams & Wilkins, 1993:82–84, 98, 393–422, 423–452, 477–511.

13. Alonso MJ. Nanoparticulate drug carrier technology. In: Cohen S, Bernstein H, eds. Microparticulate Systems for the Delivery of Proteins and Vaccines. New York: Marcel Dekker, 1996:203–242.

14. Bodmeier R, Maincent P. Polymeric dispersions as drug carriers. In: Lieberman HA, Rieger MM, Banker GS, eds. Pharmaceutical Dosage Forms: Disperse Systems. Vol 3, 2nd ed. New York: Marcel Dekker, 1998:87–128.

15. Jaeghere F, Doelker E, Gurny R. Nanoparticles. In: Mathiowitz E, ed. Encyclopedia of Controlled Drug Delivery. Vol 2. New York: John Wiley & Sons, 1999:641–664.

16. Torchilin VP, ed. Nanoparticulates as Drug Carriers. London: Imperial College Press, 2006.

17. Müller RH, Böhm BHL. Nanosuspensions. In:Müller RH, Benita S, Böhm BHL, eds. Emulsions and Nanosuspensions for the Formulation of Poorly Soluble Drugs. Stuttgart: Medpharm Scientific Publishers, 1998:149–174.

18. McGinity JW, Felton L, eds. Aqueous Polymeric Coatings for Pharmaceutical Dosage Forms. 3rd ed. New York: Informa Healthcare, 2008.

19. Wang J, Ghebre-Sellassie I. Aqueous polymer dispersions as film formers. In: Lieberman HA, Rieger MM, Banker GS, eds. Pharmaceutical Dosage Forms: Disperse Systems. Vol 3, 2nd ed. New York: Marcel Dekker, 1998:129–161.

20. Idson B. Pharmaceutical emulsions. In: Lieberman HA, Rieger MM, Banker GS, eds. Pharmaceutical Dosage Forms: Disperse Systems. Vol 1. New York: Marcel Dekker, 1988:199–244.

21. Eccleston GM. Emulsions. In: Swarbrick J, Boylan JC, eds. Encyclopedia of Pharmaceutical Technology. Vol 5. New York: Marcel Dekker, 1992:137–188.

22. Mulley BA. Medicinal emulsions. In: Lissant KJ, ed. Emulsions and Emulsion Technology, Part I: Surfactant Science Series. Vol 6. New York: Marcel Dekker, 1974:291–350.

23. Rieger MM. Emulsions. In: Lachman L, Lieberman HA, Kanig JL, eds. The Theory and Practice of Industrial Pharmacy. 3rd ed. Philadelphia: Lea & Febiger, 1986:502–532.

24. Block LH. Pharmaceutical emulsions and microemulsions. In: Lieberman HA, Rieger MM, Banker GS, eds. Pharmaceutical Dosage Forms: Disperse Systems. Vol 2. New York: Marcel Dekker, 1996:47–110.

25. Garti N. Double emulsions-scope, limitations and new achievements. Colloids Surf A: Physicochem Eng Asp 1997; 123–124:233–246.

26. Klang SH, Parnas M, Benita S. Emulsions as drug carriers – possibilities, limitations and future perspectives. In: Müller RH, Benita S, Böhm BHL, eds. Emulsions and Nano-suspensions for the Formulation of Poorly Soluble Drugs. Stuttgart: Medpharm Scientific Publishers, 1998:31–78.

27. Lundberg B. Preparation of drug-carrier emulsions stabilized with phosphatidylcholine-surfactant mixtures. J Pharm Sci 1994; 83:72–75.
28. Bluhm DP, Summers RS, Lowes MMJ, et al. Lipid emulsion content and vitamin A stability in TPN admixtures. Int J Pharm 1991; 68:277–280.
29. Boyett JB, Davis CW. Injectable emulsions and suspensions. In: Lieberman HA, Rieger MM, Banker GS, eds. Pharmaceutical Dosage Forms: Disperse Systems. Vol 2. New York: Marcel Dekker, 1989:379–416.
30. Breen PJ, Wasan DT, Kim Y-H, et al. Emulsions and emulsion stability. In:Sjöblom J, ed. Emulsions and Emulsion Stability, Surfactant Science Series. Vol 61. New York: Marcel Dekker, 1996:237–286.
31. Parnham MJ. Safety and tolerability of intravenously administered phospholipids and emulsions. In: Müller RH, Benita S, Böhm BHL, eds. Emulsions and Nanosuspensions for the Formulation of Poorly Soluble Drugs. Stuttgart: Medpharm Scientific Publishers, 1998: 131–140.
32. Rosoff M. Specialized pharmaceutical emulsions. In: Lieberman HA, Rieger MM, Banker GS, eds. Pharmaceutical Dosage Forms: Disperse Systems. Vol 3, 2nd ed. New York: Marcel Dekker, 1998:1–42.
33. Westesen K, Wehler T. Physicochemical characterization of a model intravenous oil-in-water emulsion. J Pharm Sci 1992; 81:777–786.
34. Leuner C, Dressman J. Improving drug solubility for oral delivery using solid dispersions. Eur J Pharm Biopharm 2000; 50:47–60.
35. Urbanetz NA. Stabilization of solid dispersions of nimodipine and polyethylene glycol 2000. Eur J Pharm Sci 2006; 28:67–76.
36. Li P, Zhao L. Developing early formulations: practice and perspective. Int J Pharm 2007; 341:1–19.
37. Sciarra JJ. Aerosols. In: Gennaro AR, ed. Remington: The Science and Practice of Pharmacy. 19th ed. Pennsylvania: Mack Publishing Co., 1995:1676–1692.
38. Clarke MJ, Tobyn MJ, Staniforth TN. Physicochemical factors governing the performance of nedocromil sodium as a dry powder aerosol. J Pharm Sci 2000; 89:1160–1169.
39. Bando H, McGinity JW. Relationship between drug dissolution and leaching of plasticizer for pellets coated with an aqueous Eudragit® S100:L100 dispersion. Int J Pharm 2006; 323:11–17.
40. Siepmann F, Hoffmann A, Leclercq B, et al. How to adjust desired drug release patterns from ethylcellulose-coated dosage forms. J Control Release 2007; 119:182–189.
41. Siepmann F, Muschert S, Leclercq B, et al. How to improve the storage stability of aqueous polymeric film coatings. J Control Release 2008; 126:26–33.
42. Siepmann F, Siepmann J, Walther M, et al. Polymer blends for controlled release coatings. J Control Release 2008; 125:1–15.
43. Allen T. Particle size measurement. In: Williams JC, ed. The Powder Technology Series. London: Chapman and Hall, 1975.
44. Vanderhoff JW, El-Aasser MS. Theory of colloids. In: Lieberman HA, Rieger MM, Banker GS, eds. Pharmaceutical Dosage Forms: Disperse Systems. Vol 1, 2nd ed. New York: Marcel Dekker, 1996:91–152.
45. Heywood H. Symposium on particle size analysis. Inst Chem Eng Suppl 1947; 25:14–24.
46. Goodarznia I, Sutherland DN. Floc simulation: effects of particle size and shape. Chem Eng Sci 1975; 30:407–412.
47. Heyd A, Dhabhar D. Particle shape effect on caking of coarse granulated antacid suspensions. Drug Cosmet Ind 1979; 125:42–45.
48. Bisrat M, Nyström C. Physicochemical aspects of drug release. VIII. The relation between particle size and surface specific dissolution rate in agitated suspensions. Int J Pharm 1988; 47:223–231.
49. Jinno J, Kamada N, Miyake M, et al. Effect of particle size reduction on dissolution and oral absorption of a poorly water-soluble drug, cilostazol, in beagle dogs. J Control Release 2006; 111:56–64.

50. McNamara DP, Vieira ML, Crison JR. Dissolution of pharmaceuticals in simple and complex systems. In: Amidon GL, Lee PI, Topp EM, eds. Transport Processes in Pharmaceutical Systems. New York: Marcel Dekker, 2000:109–146.

51. Hiemenz PC. Principles of Colloid and Surface Chemistry. 2nd ed. New York: Marcel Dekker, 1986.

52. Handa T, Maitani Y, Miyazima K, et al. Interfacial phenomena. In: Swarbrick J, Boylan JC, eds. Encyclopedia of Pharmaceutical Technology. Vol 8. New York: Marcel Dekker, 1993:131–174.

53. Zografi G. Interfacial phenomena. In: Gennaro AR, ed. Remington: The Science and Practice of Pharmacy. 19th ed. Pennsylvania: Mack Publishing Co., 1995:241–251.

54. Verwey EJW, Overbeek JTHG. Theory of the Stability of Lyophobic Colloids. Amsterdam: Elsevier, 1948.

55. Derjaguin B, Landau L. Theory of the stability of strongly charged lyophobic sols and adhesion of strongly charged particles in solution of electrolytes Acta Phys Chim USSR 1941; 14:633–662.

56. Derjaguin B, Landau L. The theory of stability of highly charged lyophobic sols and coalescence of highly charged particles in electrolyte solutions, J Exp Theor Physics USSR 1941; 11:802–821.

57. Matthews BA, Rhodes CT. Use of the Derjaguin, Landau, Verwey and Overbeek theory to interpret pharmaceutical suspension stability. J Pharm Sci 1970; 59:521–525.

58. Kayes JB. Pharmaceutical suspensions: Relation between zeta potential, sedimentation volume and suspension stability. J Pharm Pharmacol 1977; 29:199–204.

59. Delgado A, Gallardo V, Parrera A, et al. A study of the electrokinetic and stability properties of nitrofurantoin suspensions. II: Flocculation and redispersion properties as compared with theoretical interaction energy curves. J Pharm Sci 1990; 79:709–718.

60. Tadros TF. Polymeric surfactants: Stabilization of emulsions and dispersions. In: Desmond Goddard E, Gruber JV, eds. Principles of Polymer Science and Technology in Cosmetics and Personal Care. New York: Marcel Dekker, 1999:73–112.

61. Florence AT, Attwood D. Physicochemical Principles of Pharmacy. 4th ed. London: Pharmaceutical Press, 2006.

62. Meyer RJ, Cohen L. Rheology of natural and synthetic hydrophilic polymer solutions and related to suspending ability. J Soc Cosmet Chem 1959; 10:1–11.

63. Sherman P. The flow properties of emulsions. J Pharm Pharmacol 1964; 16:1–25.

64. Carstensen JT. Theory of Pharmaceutical Systems, Heterogeneous Systems. Vol 2. New York: Academic Press, 1973:1–89.

65. Deem DE. Rheology of dispersed systems. In: Lieberman HA, Rieger MM, Banker GS, eds. Pharmaceutical Dosage Forms: Disperse Systems. Vol 1. New York: Marcel Dekker, 1988:367–514.

66. Ramadan MA, Tawashi R. Effect of surface geometry and morphic features on the flow characteristics of microsphere suspensions. J Pharm Sci 1990; 79:929–933.

67. Miner PE. Emulsion rheology: creams and lotions. In: Laba D, ed. Rheological Properties of Cosmetics and Toiletries. New York: Marcel Dekker, 1993:313–370.

68. Vaughan CD. Predicting stability in rheologically modified systems. In: Laba D, ed. Rheological Properties of Cosmetics and Toiletries. New York: Marcel Dekker, 1993:371–401.

69. Naé HN. Introduction to rheology. In: Laba D, ed. Rheological Properties of Cosmetics and Toiletries. New York: Marcel Dekker, 1993:9–33.

70. Rieger MM. Surfactants. In: Lieberman HA, Rieger MM, Banker GS, eds. Pharmaceutical Dosage Forms: Disperse Systems. Vol 1, 2nd ed. New York: Marcel Dekker, 1996:211–286.

71. Griffin WC. Classification of surface-active agents by "HLB". J Soc Cosmet Chem 1949; 1:311–326.

72. Griffin WC. Emulsions. In: Kirk RE, Othmer DF, eds. Encyclopedia of Chemical Technology. Vol 5. New York: Interscience, 1950:692–718.

73. Atlas Booklet. A Guide to Formulation of Industrial Emulsions with Atlas Surfactants. Wilmington: Atlas Powder Co., 1953.

74. Clarke MT. Rheological additives. In: Laba D, ed. Rheological Properties of Cosmetics and Toiletries. New York: Marcel Dekker, 1993:55–152.

75. Zatz JL, Berry JJ, Alderman DA. Viscosity-imparting agents in disperse systems. In: Lieberman HA, Rieger MM, Banker GS, eds. Pharmaceutical Dosage Forms: Disperse Systems. Vol 2. New York: Marcel Dekker, 1989:171–204.

76. Ranucci JA, Silverstein IB. Polymeric pharmaceutical excipients. In: Lieberman HA, Rieger MM, Banker GS, eds. Pharmaceutical Dosage Forms: Disperse Systems. Vol 3, 2nd ed. New York: Marcel Dekker, 1998:243–289.

77. Anger CB, Rupp D, Lo P, et al. Preservation of dispersed systems. In: Lieberman HA, Rieger MM, Banker GS, eds. Pharmaceutical Dosage Forms: Disperse Systems. Vol 1, 2nd ed. New York: Marcel Dekker, 1996:377–435.

78. Haag TE, Loncrini DF. Esters of para-hydroxybenzoic acid. In: Kabara JJ, ed. Cosmetic and Drug Preservation. New York: Marcel Dekker, 1984:63–77.

79. Hugo WB. Phenols as preservatives for pharmaceutical and cosmetic products. In: Kabara JJ, ed. Cosmetic and Drug Preservation. New York: Marcel Dekker, 1984:109–113.

80. McCarthy TJ. Formulated factors affecting the activity of preservatives. In: Kabara JJ, ed. Cosmetic and Drug Preservation. New York: Marcel Dekker, 1984:359–388.

81. Alexander KS, Azizi J, Dollimore D, et al. Interpretation of the hindered settling of calcium carbonate suspensions in terms of permeability. J Pharm Sci 1990; 79:401–406.

82. Jones RDC, Matthews BA, Rhodes CT. Physical stability of sulfaguanidine suspensions. J Pharm Sci 1970; 59:518–520.

83. Zatz JL, Schnitzer L, Sarpotdar P. Flocculation of sulfamerazine suspensions by a cationic polymer. J Pharm Sci 1979; 68:1491–1494.

84. Jeffrey GC, Ottewill RH. Reversible aggregation. Part I: Reversible flocculation monitored by turbidity measurements. Colloid Polym Sci 1988; 266:173–179.

85. Higuchi T. Some physical chemical aspects of suspension formulation. J Am Pharm Assoc Sci Ed 1958; 47:657–660.

86. Frederick KJ. Performance and problems of pharmaceutical suspensions. J Pharm Sci 1961; 50:531–535.

87. Matthews BA. The use of the Coulter counter in emulsion and suspension studies. Can J Pharm Sci 1971; 6:29–34.

88. Carless JE. Dissolution and crystal growth in aqueous suspension of cortisone acetate. J Pharm Pharmacol 1968; 10:630–639.

89. Young SA, Buckton G. Particle growth in aqueous suspensions: the influence of surface energy and polarity. Int J Pharm 1990; 60:235–241.

90. Shah NB, Sheth BB. Effect of polymers on dissolution from drug suspensions. J Pharm Sci 1976; 65:1618–1623.

91. Ofner III CM, Schnaare RL, Schwartz JB. Reconstitutable suspensions. In: Lieberman HA, Rieger MM, Banker GS, eds. Pharmaceutical Dosage Forms: Disperse Systems. Vol 2. New York: Marcel Dekker, 1989:317–334.

92. Bodmeier R, Paeratakul O. Suspensions and dispersible dosage forms of multiparticulates. In: Ghebre-Sellassie I, ed. Multiparticulate Oral Drug Delivery. New York: Marcel Dekker, 1994:143–157.

93. Kawashima Y, Iwamoto T, Niwa T, et al. Preparation and characterization of a new controlled release ibuprofen suspension for improving suspendability. Int J Pharm 1991; 75:25–36.

94. Sjöqvist R, Graffner C, Ekman I, et al. In vivo validation of the release rate and palatability of remoxipride-modified release suspension. Pharm Res 1993; 10:1020–1026.

95. Raghunathan Y. Pennwalt Corporation. U.S. patent 4,221,778, 1980.

96. Raghunathan Y, Amsel L, Hinsvark O, et al. Sustained-release drug delivery system I: coated ion-exchange resin system for phenylpropanolamine and other drugs. J Pharm Sci 1981; 70:379–384.

97. Tingstad JE. Physical stability testing of pharmaceuticals. J Pharm Sci 1964; 53:955–962.

98. Tadros TF, Vincent B. Emulsion stability. In: Becher P, ed. Encyclopedia of Emulsion Technology. Vol 1. New York: Dekker, 1983:129–285.

99. Mikula J, Munoz VA. Characterization of emulsions and suspensions in the petroleum industry using cryo-SEM and CLSM. Colloids Surf A: Physicochem Eng Asp 2000; 174:23–36.

100. Ju Z, Duan Y, Ju Z. Plant oil emulsion modifies internal atmosphere, delays fruit ripening and inhibits internal browning in Chinese pears. Postharvest Biol Technol 2000; 20:243–250.

101. Sela Y, Magdassi S, Garti N. Release of markers from the inner water phase of W/O/W emulsions stabilized by silicone based polymeric surfactants. J Control Release 1995; 33:1–12.

102. Rousseau D. Fat crystals and emulsion stability-a review. Food Res Intern 2000; 33:3–14.

103. Heinzelmann K, Franke K. Using freezing and drying techniques of emulsions for the microencapsulation of fish oil to improve oxidation stability. Colloids Surf B Biointerfaces 1999; 12:223–229.

104. Paquin P. Technological properties of high pressure homogenizers: the effect of fat globules, milk proteins and polysaccharides. Int Dairy J 1999; 9:329–335.

105. Joscelyne SM, Traegardh G. Food emulsions using membrane emulsification: conditions for producing small droplets. J Food Eng 1999; 39:59–64.

106. Goff HD. Colloidal aspects of ice cream-A review. Int Dairy J 1997; 7:363–373.

107. McClements DJ. Advances in the application of ultrasound in food analysis and processing. Trends Food Sci Technol 1995; 6:293–299.

108. Peressini D, Sensidoni A, de Cindio B. Rheological characterization of traditional and light mayonnaises. J Food Eng 1998; 35:409–417.

109. Adolph M. Lipid emulsions in parenteral nutrition. Ann Nutr Metab 1999; 43:1–13.

110. Ding S. Recent developments in ophthalmic drug delivery. Pharm Sci Technol Today 1998; 1:328–335.

111. Gogos CA, Kalfarentzos F. Total parenteral nutrition and immune system activity: a review. Nutrition 1995; 11:339–344.

112. Okochi H, Nakano M. Preparation and evaluation of W/O/W type emulsions containing vancomycin. Adv Drug Deliv Rev 2000; 45:5–26.

113. Nielloud F, Marti-Mestres G, Laget JP, et al. Emulsion formulations: study of the influence of parameters with experimental designs. Drug Dev Ind Pharm 1996; 22:159–166.

114. Suitthimeathegorn O, Turton JA, Mizuuchi H, et al. Intramuscular absorption and biodistribution of dexamethasone from non-aqueous emulsions in the rat. Int J Pharm 2007; 331:204–210.

115. Suitthimeathegorn O, Jaitely V, Florence AT. Novel anhydrous emulsions: Formulation as controlled release vehicles. Int J Pharm 2005; 298:367–371.

116. Gallarate M, Carlotti ME, Trotta M, et al. On the stability of ascorbic acid in emulsified systems for topical and cosmetic use. Int J Pharm 1999; 188:233–241.

117. Gallegos C, Franco JM. Rheology of food, cosmetics and pharmaceuticals. Curr Opin Colloid Interface Sci 1999; 4:288–293.

118. Miller D, Wiener EM, Turowski A, et al. O/W emulsions for cosmetics products stabilized by alkyl phosphates rheology and storage tests. Colloids Surf A: Physicochem Eng Aspects 1999; 152:155–160.

119. Clark R. Cosmetic emulsions. In: Hibbott HW, ed. Handbook of Cosmetic Science. New York: Pergamon Press, 1963:175–204.

120. Barry BW. Dermatological Formulations. New York: Marcel Dekker, 1983:296–350.

121. Becher P. Testing of emulsion properties. In: Emulsions Theory and Practice. 2nd ed. New York: Reinhold Publ. Co., 1957:381–429.

122. Couvreur P, Blanco-Prieto MJ, Puisieux F, et al. Multiple emulsion technology for the design of microspheres containing peptides and olegopeptides. Adv Drug Deliv Rev 1997; 28:85–96.

123. Garti N, Aserin A. Double emulsions stabilized by macromolecular surfactants. Adv Colloid Interfaces Sci 1996; 65:37–69.

124. Herrmann J, Bodmeier R. Biodegradable somatostatin acetate containing microspheres prepared by various aqueous and non-aqueous solvent evaporation method. Eur J Pharm Biopharm 1998; 45:75–82.

125. O'Donnell PB, McGinity JW. Preparation of microspheres by the solvent evaporation technique. Adv Drug Deliv Rev 1997; 28:25–42.

126. Hombreiro-Pérez M, Siepmann J, Zinutti C, et al. Non-degradable microparticles containing a hydrophilic and/or a lipophilic drug: preparation, characterization and drug release modeling. J Control Release 2003; 88:413–428.

127. Hoar TP, Schulman JH. Transparent water-in-oil dispersions: the oleophatic hydro-micelle. Nature 1943; 152:102–103.

128. Schulman JH, Stoeckenius W, Prince LM. Mechanism of formation and structure of micro emulsions by electron microscopy. J Phys Chem 1959; 63:1677–1680.

129. Danielsson I, Lindman B. The definition of a microemulsion. Colloids Surf 1981; 3:391–392.

130. Lawrence MJ, Rees GD. Microemulsion-based media as novel drug delivery systems. Adv Drug Deliv Rev 2000; 45:89–121.

131. Sjöblom J, Lindberg R, Friberg SE. Microemulsions-phase equilibria characterization, structures, applications and chemical reactions. Adv Colloid Interface Sci 1996; 65:125–287.

132. Bhargava HN, Narurkar A, Lieb LM. Using microemulsions for drug delivery. Pharm Tech 1987; 11:46–54.

133. Wennerström H, Söderman O, Olsson U, et al. Macroemulsions versus microemulsions. Colloids Surf A: Physicochem Eng Asp 1997; (123–124):13–26.

134. Ritschel WA. Microemulsions for improved peptide absorption from the gastrointestinal tract. Methods Find Exp Clin Pharmacol 1991; 13:205–220.

135. Haße A, Keipert S. Development and characterization of microemulsions for ocular application. Eur J Pharm Biopharm 1997; 43:179–183.

136. Charro MB, Vilas GI, Méndez JB, et al. Delivery of a hydrophilic solute through the skin from novel microemulsion systems. Eur J Pharm Biopharm 1997; 43:37–42.

137. Sintov AC, Brandys-Sitton R. Facilitated skin penetration of lidocaine: combination of a short-term iontophoresis and microemulsion formulation. Int J Pharm 2006; 316:58–67.

138. Graf A, Ablinger E, Peters S, et al. Microemulsions containing lecithin and sugar-based surfactants: nanoparticle templates for delivery of proteins and peptides. Int J Pharm 2008; 350:351–360.

139. Nornoo AO, Osborne DW, Chow DSL. Cremophor-free intravenous microemulsions for paclitaxel. I: Formulation, cytotoxicity and hemolysis. Int J Pharm 2008; 349:108–116.

140. Vemuri S, Rhodes CT. Preparation and characterization of liposomes as therapeutic delivery systems: a review. Pharm Acta Helv 1995; 70:95–111.

141. Bochot A, Couvreur P, Fattal E. Intravitreal administration of antisense oligonucleotides: potential of liposomal delivery. Prog Retin Eye Res 2000; 19:131–147.

142. Nastruzzi C, Cortesi R, Esposito E, et al. Liposomes as carriers for DNA PNA hybrids. J Control Release 2000; 68:237–249.

143. Welz C, Neuhuber W, Schreier H, et al. Nuclear gene targeting using negatively charged liposomes. Int J Pharm 2000; 196:251–252.

144. Mader C, Küpcü S, Sleytr UB, et al. S-layer-coated liposomes as a versatile system for entrapping and binding target molecules. Biochim Biophys Acta Biomembr 2000; 1463:142–150.

145. Zaru M, Mourtas S, Klepetsanis P, et al. Liposomes for drug delivery to the lungs by nebulization. Eur J Pharm Biopharm 2007; 67:655–666.

146. Al-Jamal WT, Kostarelos K. Construction of nanoscale multicompartment liposomes for combinatory drug delivery. Int J Pharm 2007; 331:182–185.

147. Foged C, Nielsen HM, Frokjaer S. Liposomes for phospholipase A2 triggered siRNA release: preparation and in vitro test. Int J Pharm 2007; 331:160–166.

148. Bodmeier R. Multiphase system. Int patent application WO 98/55100, 1998.

149. Im-Emsap W, Brazeau GA, Simpkins JW, et al. Sustained drug delivery of 17-β estradiol from injectable biodegradable in situ forming microparticles (ISM) system. AAPS PharmSci Supplement 2(4), AAPS Annual Meeting Abstracts, 2000.

150. Im-Emsap W, Bodmeier R. In vitro drug release from in situ forming microparticles (ISM)-Systems with dispersed drug. AAPS PharmSci Supplement 2(4), AAPS Annual Meeting Abstracts, 2000.

151. Kranz H, Brazeau GA, Napaporn J, et al. Myotoxicity studies of injectable biodegradable in-situ forming drug delivery systems. Int J Pharm 2001; 212:11–18.

152. Rungseevijitprapa W, Brazeau GA, Simkins JW, et al. Myotoxicity studies of O/W-in situ forming microparticle systems. Eur J Pharm Biopharm 2008; 69:126–133.

153. Luan X, Bodmeier R. Influence of the poly(lactide-co-glycolide) type on the leuprolide release from in situ forming microparticle systems. J Control Release 2006; 110:266–272.

154. Luan X, Bodmeier R. In situ forming microparticle system for controlled delivery of leuprolide acetate: influence of the formulation and processing parameters. Eur J Pharm Biopharm 2006; 27:143–149.

155. Kranz H, Bodmeier R. A novel in situ forming drug delivery system for controlled parenteral drug delivery. Int J Pharm 2007; 332:107–114.

156. Friberg SE, Quencer LS, Hilton ML. Theory of emulsions. In: Lieberman HA, Rieger MM, Banker GS, eds. Pharmaceutical Dosage Forms: Disperse Systems. Vol 1, 2nd ed. New York: Marcel Dekker, 1996:53–90.

157. Shinoda K, Kunieda H. Phase properties of emulsions: PIT and HLB. In: Becher P, ed. Encyclopedia of Emulsion Technology. Vol 1. New York: Marcel Dekker, 1983:337–368.

158. Freitas S, Merkle HP, Gander B. Microencapsulation by solvent extraction/evaporation: reviewing the state of the art of microsphere preparation process technology. J Control Release 2005; 102:313–332.

159. Garti N, Aserin A. Pharmaceutical Emulsions, Double emulsions and microemulsions. In: Benita S, ed. Microencapsulation-Methods an Industrial Applications. New York: Marcel Dekker, 1996:411–534.

160. Florence AT, Whitehill D. The formulation and stability of multiple emulsions. Int J Pharm 1982; 11:277–308.

161. Florence AT, Whitehill D. Some features of breakdown in water-in-oil-in-water multiple emulsions. J Colloid Interface Sci 1982; 79:243–256.

162. Ivanov IB, Danov KD, Kralchevsky PA. Flocculation and coalescence of micron-size emulsion droplets. Colloids Surf A: Physicochem Eng Asp 1999; 152:161–168.

163. Robins MM. Emulsions-creaming phenomena. Curr Opin Colloid Interface Sci 2000; 5: 265–272.

164. Bury M, Gerhards J, Erni W. Monitoring sedimentation processes by conductivity measurements. Int J Pharm 1991; 76:207–217.

165. Bury M, Gerhards J, Erni W, et al. Application of a new method based on conductivity measurements to determine the creaming stability of O/W emulsions. Int J Pharm 1995; 124:183–194.

166. Al-Malah KI, Azzam MOJ, Omari RM. Emulsifying properties of BSA in different vegetable oil emulsions using conductivity technique. Food Hydrocolloids 2000; 14:485–490.

167. Babick F, Hinze F, Ripperger S. Dependence of ultrasonic attenuation on the material properties. Colloids Surf A: Physicochem Eng Asp 2000; 172:33–46.

168. Black DL, McQuay MQ, Bonin MP. Laser-based techniques for particle-size measurement: a review of sizing methods and their industrial applications. Prog Energy Combust Sci 1996; 22:267–306.

169. de Boer AH, Gjaltema D, Hagedoorn P, et al. Characterization of inhalation aerosols: a critical evaluation of cascade impactor analysis and laser diffraction technique. Int J Pharm 2002; 249:219–231.

170. Dikinson E, Stainsby G. Colloids in Food. New York: Applied Sci Publ, 1982.

171. Chang RK, Hsiao C, Robinson JR. A review of aqueous coating techniques and preliminary data on release from a theophylline product. Pharm Technol 1987; 11:56–68.

172. Moore KL. Physicochemical properties of Opadry®, Coateric®, and Surelease®. In Mcginity JW, ed. Aqueous Polymeric Coatings for Pharmaceutical Dosage Forms. New York: Dekker, 1989:303–315.

173. Gurny R, Peppas NA, Harrington DD, et al. Development of biodegradable and injectable latices for controlled release of potent drugs. Drug Dev Ind Pharm 1981; 7:1–25.

174. Krause HJ, Schwarz A, Rohdewald P. Polylactic acid nanoparticles, a colloidal drug delivery system for lipophilic drugs. Int J Pharm 1985; 27:145–155.

175. Koosha F, Müller RH, Davis SS, et al. The surface chemical structure of poly (β-hydroxybutyrate) microparticles produced by solvent evaporation process. J Control Release 1989; 9:149–157.

176. Bodmeier R, Chen H. Indomethacin polymeric nanosuspensions prepared by microfluidization. J Control Release 1990; 12:223–233.

177. Yang J, Park SB, Yoon HG, et al. Preparation of poly-caprolactone nanoparticles containing magnetite for magnetic drug carrier. Int J Pharm 2006; 324:185–190.

178. Scholes PD, Coombes AGA, Illum L, et al. The preparation of sub-200 nm poly (lactide-co-glycolide) microspheres for site-specific drug delivery. J Control Release 1993; 25: 145–153.

179. Batzri S, Korn ED. Single bilayer liposomes prepared without sonication. Biochim Biophys Acta 1973; 443:629–634.

180. Niwa T, Takeuchi H, Hino T, et al. Preparations of biodegradable nanospheres of water-soluble and insoluble drugs with d,l-lactide/glycolide copolymer by a novel spontaneous emulsification solvent diffusion method, and the drug release behavior. J Control Release 1993; 25:89–98.

181. Fessi H, Puisieux F, Devissaguet JP. Procédé de préparation de systÉmes colloidaux dispersibles d'une substance, sous forme de nanocapsules. European patent 274 961, 1987.

182. Ammoury N, Fessi H, Devissaguet JP, et al. Effect on cerebral blood flow of orally administered indomethacin-loaded poly (isobutylcyanoacrylate) and poly(d,l-lactide) nanocapsules. J Pharm Pharmacol 1990; 42:558–561.

183. Ammoury N, Fessi H, Devissaguet JP, et al. Jejunal absorption, pharmacological activity, and pharmacokinetic evaluation of indomethacin-loaded poly(d,l-lactide) and poly(isobutyl-cyanoacrylate) nanocapsules in rats. Pharm Res 1991; 8:101–105.

184. Ammoury N, Fessi H, Devissaguet JP, et al. In vitro release kinetic pattern of indomethacin from poly (d,l-lactide) nanocapsules. J Pharm Sci 1990; 79:763–767.

185. Bindschaedler C, Gurny R, Doelker E. Process for preparing a powder of water-insoluble polymer which can be redispersed in a liquid phase, the resulting powder and utilization thereof. Swiss patent 1497/88, 1988.

186. Ibrahim H, Bindschaedler C, Doelker E, et al. Concept and development of ophthalmic pseudo-latices triggered by pH. Int J Pharm 1991; 77:211–219.

187. Ibrahim H, Bindschaedler C, Doelker E, et al. Aqueous nanodispersions prepared by a salting-out process. Int J Pharm 1992; 87:239–246.

188. Allemann E, Gurny R, Doelker E. Preparation of aqueous polymeric nanodispersions by a reversible salting-out process, influence of process parameters on particle size. Int J Pharm 1992; 87:247–253.

189. Allemann E, Leroux JC, Gurny R, et al. In vitro extended-release properties of drug loaded poly (dl-lactic acid) nanoparticles produced by a salting-out procedure. Pharm Res 1993; 10:1732–1737.

190. Allemann E, Doelker E, Gurny R. Drug loaded poly (lactic acid) nanoparticles produced by a reversible salting-out process: purification of an injectable dosage form. Eur J Pharm Biopharm 1992; 39:13–18.

191. Ekman B, Sjöholm I. Incorporation of macromolecules in microparticles: Preparation and characteristics. Biochemistry 1976; 15:5115–5120.

192. Yapel AF Jr. Albumin microspheres: heat and chemical stabilization. In: Widder KJ, Green R, eds. Methods in Enzymology. Part A: Drug and Enzyme Targeting. Orlando: Academic Press, 1985:3–18.

193. Longo WE, Goldberg EP. Hydrophilic albumin microspheres. In: Widder KJ, Green R, eds. Methods in Enzymology. Part A: Drug and Enzyme Targeting. Orlando: Academic Press, 1985:18–26.

194. Tomlinson E, Burger JJ. Incorporation of water-soluble drugs in albumin microspheres. In: Widder KJ, Green R, eds. Methods in Enzymology. Part A: Drug and Enzyme Targeting. Orlando: Academic Press, 1985:27–43.

195. Yoshioka T, Hashida M, Muranishi S, et al. Specific delivery of mitomycin C to the liver, spleen, and lung: nano- and microspherical carriers of gelatin. Int J Pharm 1981; 8:131–141.

196. Hassan EE, Parish RC, Gallo JM. Optimized formulation of magnetic microspheres containing the anticancer agent, oxantrazole. Pharm Res 1992; 9:390–397.

197. Marty JJ, Oppenheim RC, Speiser P. Nanoparticles-a new colloidal drug delivery system. Pharm Acta Helv 1978; 53:17–22.

198. El-Samaligy M, Rohdewald P. Triamcinolone diacetate nanoparticles, a sustained release drug delivery system suitable for parenteral administration. Pharm Acta Helv 1982; 57:201.

199. El-Samaligy M, Rohdewald P. Reconstituted collagen nanoparticles, a novel drug carrier delivery system. J Pharm Pharmacol 1983; 35:537–539.

200. Oppenheim RC. Solid colloidal drug delivery systems: nanoparticles. Int J Pharm 1981; 8:217–234.

201. Rajanorivony M, Vauthier C, Couarraze G, et al. Development of a new drug carrier made from alginate. J Pharm Sci 1993; 82:912–917.

202. Perkins WR, Ahmad I, Li X, et al. Novel therapeutic nano-particles (lipocores): trapping poorly water soluble compounds. Int J Pharm 2000; 200:27–39.

203. Driscoll DF, Bacon MN, Bistrian BR. Physicochemical stability of two types of intravenous lipid emulsion as total nutrient admixtures. JPEN J Parenter Enteral Nutr 2000; 24:15–22.

204. Yoo HS, Oh JE, Lee KH, et al. Biodegradable nanoparticles containing doxorubicin-PLGA conjugate for sustained release. Pharm Res 1999; 16:1114–1118.

205. Müller RH, Mäder K, Gohla S. Solid lipid nanoparticles (SLN) for controlled drug delivery—A review of the state of the art. Eur J Pharm Biopharm 2000; 50:161–177.

206. Harnisch S, Müller RH. Adsorption kinetics of plasma proteins on oil-in-water emulsions for parenteral nutrition. Eur J Pharm Biopharm 2000; 49:41–46.

207. Constantinides PP, Lambert KJ, Tustian AK, et al. Formulation development and antitumor activity of a filter-sterilizable emulsion of paclitaxel. Pharm Res 2000; 17:175–182.

208. Floyd AG. Top ten considerations in the development of parenteral emulsions. Pharm Sci Technol Today 1999; 2:134–143.

209. Koster VS, Kuks PFM, Langer R, et al. Particle size in parenteral fat emulsions, what are the true limitations? Int J Pharm 1996; 134:235–238.

210. Chansiri G, Lyons RT, Patel MV, et al. Effect of surface charge on the stability of oil/water emulsions during steam sterilization. J Pharm Sci 1999; 88:454–458.

211. Labhasetwar V, Song C, Humphrey W, et al. Arterial uptake of biodegradable nanoparticles: effect of surface modifications. J Pharm Sci 1998; 87:1229–1234.

212. Jumaa M, Müller BW. The effect of oil components and homogenization conditions on the physicochemical properties and stability of parenteral fat emulsions. Int J Pharm 1998; 163:81–89.

213. Kawano Y, Noma T. Inhibition by lecithin-bound iodine (LBI) of inducible allergen-specific T lymphocytes' responses in allergic diseases. Int J Immunopharmacol 1996; 18:241–249.

214. Na GC, Stevens HJ, Yuan BO, et al. Physical stability of ethyl diatrizoate nanocrystalline suspension in steam sterilization. Pharm Res 1999; 16:569–574.

215. Westesen K, Siekmann B. Investigation of the gel formation of phospholipid-stabilized solid lipid nanoparticles. Int J Pharm 1997; 151:35–45.

216. Mewis J. Flow behaviour of concentrated suspensions: predictions and measurements. Int J Miner Process 1996; 44–45:17–27.

217. Spiegel AJ, Noseworthy MM. Use of nonaqueous solvents in parenteral products. J Pharm Sci 1963; 52:917–927.

218. Müller RH, Peters K. Nanosuspensions for the formulation of poorly soluble drugs I. Preparation by a size-reduction technique. Int J Pharm 1998; 160:229–237.

219. Peters K, Leitzke S, Diederichs JE, et al. Preparation of a clofazimine nanosuspension for intravenous use and evaluation of its therapeutic efficacy in murine Mycobacterium avium infection. J Antimicrob Chemother 2000; 45:77–83.

220. Schmidt PC. Secondary electron microscopy in pharmaceutical technology. In: Swarbrick J, Boylan JC, eds. Encyclopedia of Pharmaceutical Technology. Vol 19. New York: Marcel Dekker, 2000:311–356.

221. Hooton JC, German CS, Davies MC, et al. A comparison of morphology and surface energy characteristics of sulfathiazole polymorphs based upon single particle studies. Eur J Pharm Sci 2006; 28:315–324.

222. Attama AA, Schicke BC, Paepenmueller T, et al. Solid lipid nanodispersions containing mixed lipid core and a polar heterolipid: characterization. Eur J Pharm Biopharm 2007; 67:48–57.

223. Mullin JW. Sieving of pharmaceuticals. In: Swarbrick J, Boylan JC, eds. Encyclopedia of Pharmaceutical Technology. Vol 14. New York: Marcel Dekker, 1996:63–86.

224. Keck CM, Müller RH. Size analysis of submicron particles by laser diffractometry—90% of the published measurements are false. Int J Pharm 2008; 355:150–163.

225. Racey TJ, Rochon P, Awang DVC, et al. Aggregation of commercial heparin samples in storage. J Pharm Sci 1987; 76:314–318.

226. Racey TJ, Rochon P, Mori F, et al. Examination of a possible role of dermatan sulfate in the aggregation of commercial heparin samples. J Pharm Sci 1989; 78:214–218.

227. Kayes JB. Pharmaceutical suspensions: microelectrophoretic properties. J Pharm Pharmacol 1977; 29:163–168.

228. Gallardo V, Zurita L, Ontiveros A, et al. Interfacial properties of barium sulfate suspensions. Implications in their stability. J Pharm Sci 2000; 89:1134–1142.

229. Thode K, Müller RH, Kresse M. Two-time window and multiangle photon correlation spectroscopy size and zeta potential analysis—highly sensitive rapid assay for dispersion stability. J Pharm Sci 2000; 89:1317–1324.

230. Crommelin DJA. Influence of lipid composition and ionic strength on the physical stability of liposomes. J Pharm Sci 1984; 73:1559–1563.

231. Takenaka H, Kawashima Y, Lin SY. Electrophoretic properties of sulfamethoxazole microcapsules and gelatin-acacia coacervates. J Pharm Sci 1981; 70:302–305.

232. Killeen MJ. Spray drying and spray congealing of pharmaceuticals. In: Swarbrick J, Boylan JC, eds. Encyclopedia of Pharmaceutical Technology. Vol 14. New York: Marcel Dekker, 1996:207–222.

233. Block LH. Scale-up of disperse systems: theoretical and practical aspects. In: Lieberman HA, Rieger MM, Banker GS, eds. Pharmaceutical Dosage Forms: Disperse Systems. Vol 3, 2nd ed. New York: Marcel Dekker, 1998:363–394.

234. Nash RA. Validation of disperse systems. In: Lieberman HA, Rieger MM, Banker GS, eds. Pharmaceutical Dosage Forms: Disperse Systems. Vol 3, 2nd ed. New York: Marcel Dekker, 1998:473–512.

12
Surfactants

David Attwood

School of Pharmacy and Pharmaceutical Sciences, University of Manchester, Manchester, U.K.

INTRODUCTION

Compounds in which there is a clear separation between lyophilic (solvent-liking) and lyophobic (solvent-hating) regions of the molecule are referred to as *amphiphilic* or *amphipathic* compounds or *amphiphiles*. When, as with most pharmaceutical systems, the solvent is water, we refer to hydrophilic and hydrophobic regions, respectively. Note, of course, that a polar group will act as a lyophilic group in a polar solvent such as water, but as a lyophobic group in a nonpolar solvent such as heptane. The dual nature of these compounds leads to their accumulation at interfaces in such a way as to remove the hydrophobic group from the aqueous environment, with a consequent reduction of surface or interfacial tension, hence their alternative description as *surface-active agents* or simply as *surfactants*. The adsorption at the various interfaces between solids, liquids, and gases results in changes in the nature of the interface, which are of considerable importance in pharmacy. In this chapter, the various characteristic properties of surfactants, which arise as a consequence of their amphiphilic nature, will be examined, with particular emphasis on the role of surfactants in reducing interfacial tension, so facilitating the formation of emulsions and microemulsions; adsorbing onto solid surfaces with implications for the wetting of the particle, its dissolution in solution and enhancement of the stability of suspensions; and the formation of micelles capable of solubilizing water-insoluble drugs.

CLASSIFICATION OF SURFACTANTS

The primary classification of surfactants is according to the nature of the hydrophilic (or head) group, which can be anionic, cationic, zwitterionic, or nonionic; the hydrophobic portions of surfactants are usually saturated or unsaturated hydrocarbon chains or, less commonly, heterocyclic or aromatic ring systems. Typical examples are illustrated in Table 1.

Table 1   Classification of Surfactants

Anionic

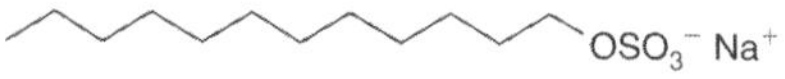

Alkyl sulfate 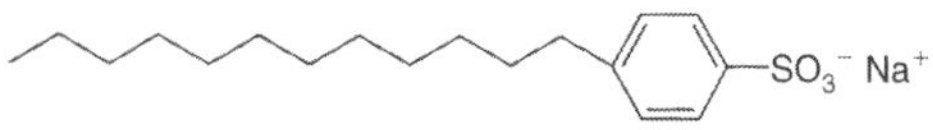   Alkylbenzene sulfonate

Cationic

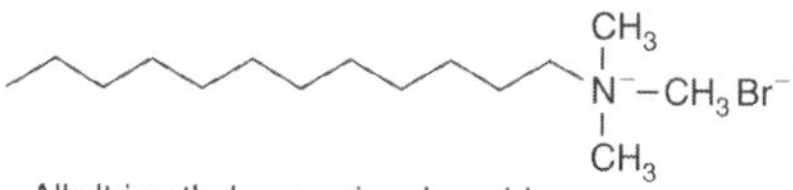

Alkyltrimethylammonium bromide 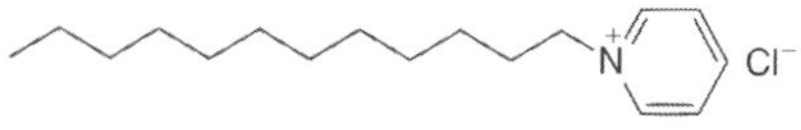   Alkylpyridinium chloride

Zwitterionic

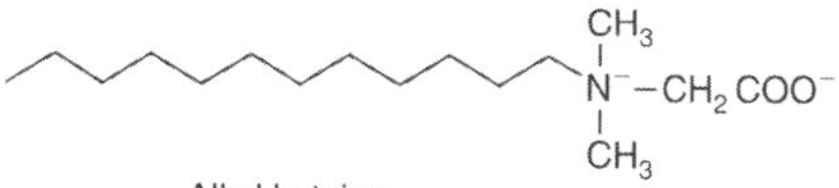

Alkyl betaine 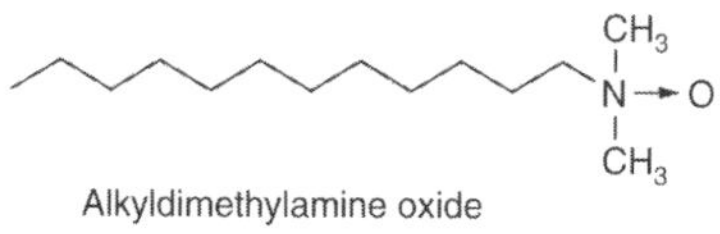   Alkyldimethylamine oxide

Nonionic

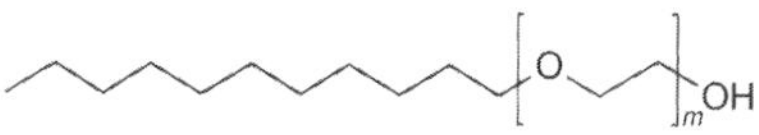

Alcohol ethoxylate 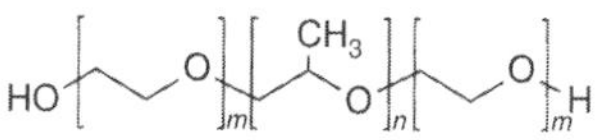   Polyoxyethylene–polyoxypropylene–polyoxyethylene
                                                 block copolymer

Anionic Surfactants

The most commonly encountered anionic surfactants have carboxylate, sulfate, sulfonate, and phosphate polar groups in combination with counterions such as sodium and potassium (for water solubility) or calcium and magnesium (for oil solubility). Sodium and potassium salts of carboxylic acids derived from animal fats or vegetable oils are generically referred to as soaps and constitute the largest single type of surfactant. Linear alkylbenzene sulfonates are commonly used in household detergents and a variety of industrial applications. A commonly used surfactant for pharmaceutical application is sodium lauryl sulfate, which is a mixture of sodium alkyl sulfates, the chief of which is sodium dodecyl sulfate (SDS), $C_{12}H_{25}SO_4^-$ Na^+. It is very soluble in water and is used pharmaceutically as a preoperative skin cleaner, having bacteriostatic action against gram-positive bacteria, and also in medicated shampoos. It is a component of emulsifying wax. An alkyl sulfonate useful for the preparation of water-in-oil microemulsions is 1,4-bis(2-ethylhexyl) sodium sulfosuccinate (Aerosol OT, AOT, docusate sodium USP).

Cationic Surfactants

In the most common cationic surfactants, the charge is carried on a nitrogen atom as, for example, with amine and quaternary ammonium surfactants. The latter compounds retain this charge over the whole pH range, whereas the amine-based compounds function as surfactants in the protonated state only, and therefore cannot be used at high pH. The quaternary ammonium and pyridinium cationic surfactants are important pharmaceutically because of their bactericidal activity against a wide range of gram-positive and some gram-negative organisms. They may be used on the skin, especially in the cleaning of wounds. Aqueous solutions are used for cleaning contaminated utensils.

Cetrimide BP consists mainly of tetradecyltrimethylammonium bromide, together with smaller amounts of dodecyl- and hexadecyltrimethylammonium bromides. Solutions containing 0.1% to 1.0% of cetrimide are used for cleaning the skin, wounds and burns, contaminated vessels, polythene tubing and catheters, and for storage of sterilized surgical instruments. Solutions of cetrimide are also used in shampoos to remove scales in seborrhoea. In the form of emulsifying wax, cetrimide is used as an emulsifying agent for producing oil-in-water creams suitable for the incorporation of cationic and nonionic medicaments (anionic medicaments would, of course, be incompatible with this cationic surfactant). Benzalkonium chloride is a mixture of alkylbenzyldimethylammonium chlorides of the general formula $[C_6H_5CH_2N(CH_3)_2R]Cl$, where R represents a mixture of the alkyls from C_8H_{17} to $C_{18}H_{37}$. In dilute solution (1 in 1000 to 1 in 2000), it may be used for the preoperative disinfection of skin and mucous membranes, for application to burns and wounds, and for cleaning polythene and nylon tubing and catheters. Benzalkonium chloride is also used as a preservative for eyedrops and is a permitted vehicle for the preparation of certain eyedrops.

Nonionic Surfactants

Nonionic surfactants are, from a toxicological point of view, generally regarded as the most suitable for pharmaceutical formulation (1). By far the most common nonionic surfactants are those with a poly(oxyethylene) chain as the polar head group. In principle, it is possible to ethoxylate any material containing an active hydrogen, but the most commonly used starting materials are fatty alcohols, alkylphenols, fatty acids, and fatty amines.

Poly(oxyethylene) Alkyl Ethers (Macrogols)

The poly(oxyethylene) alkyl ethers (macrogols) are a series of poly(oxyethylene) glycol ethers of linear fatty alcohols with structural formula $CH_3(CH_2)_n(OCH_2CH_2)_mOH$. Alkyl chain lengths ($n + 1$) are usually 12 (lauryl, dodecyl), 14 (myristyl, tetradecyl), 16 (cetyl, hexadecyl), or 18 (stearyl, octadecyl), and the number of ethylene oxide groups (m) typically ranges between 10 and 60. Commercially produced polyethylene alkyl ethers are mixtures with a narrow range of chain lengths, for example, cetomacrogol has n equal to 15 or 17 and m between 20 and 24. Cetomacrogol is a water-soluble substance used in the form of cetomacrogol emulsifying wax in the preparation of oil-in-water emulsions, and also as a solubilizing agent for volatile oils. Other macrogol ethers are commercially available as the Brij series, for example, Brij 30 [poly(oxyethylene) (4) lauryl ether, $C_{12}H_{35}(OCH_2CH_2)_4OH$], Brij 72 [poly(oxyethylene) (2) stearyl ether, $C_{18}H_{37}(OCH_2CH_2)_2OH$], and Brij 97 [poly(oxyethylene) (10) oleyl ether, $C_{18}H_{35}(OCH_2CH_2)_{10}OH$]. Cremophor EL is a polyoxyethylated castor oil containing approximately 35 oxyethylene groups to each triglyceride unit. It is used as a solubilizing agent in the preparation of intravenous anesthetics and other products. Polyoxyethylated hydrogenated castor oils are also commercially available, the most common being Cremophor RH40 with approximately 40 ethylene oxide units.

Sorbitan Esters and Polysorbates

This subgroup of nonionic surfactants has polyhydroxyl (polyol) polar groups and includes the sorbitan esters, alkyl glucosides, sucrose esters, and polyglycerol esters. Widely used examples of this group are the fatty acid esters of sorbitan and the corresponding ethoxylated sorbitans or polysorbates (Tweens). The commercial sorbitan esters (marketed under the trade name Spans) are mixtures of the partial esters of sorbitol

Table 2 Structures and HLB Values of Selected Sorbitan Esters

Sorbitan monoesters: $R^1 = R^2 = OH$; $R^3 = R$
Sorbitan triesters: $R^1 = R^2 = R^3 = R$

Chemical name	Commercial name	R	HLB
Sorbitan monolaurate	Span 20	$C_{11}H_{23}COO$	8.6
Sorbitan monopalmitate	Span 40	$C_{15}H_{31}COO$	6.7
Sorbitan monostearate	Span 60	$C_{17}H_{35}COO$	4.7
Sorbitan tristearate	Span 65	$C_{17}H_{35}COO$	2.1
Sorbitan monooleate	Span 80	$C_{17}H_{33}COO$	4.3
Sorbitan trioleate	Span 85	$C_{17}H_{33}COO$	1.8

Abbreviation: HLB, hydrophile-lipophile balance.

and its mono- and di-anhydrides with oleic acid (Table 2). They are generally insoluble in water and are used as water-in-oil emulsifiers and wetting agents. They are also commonly used as emulsifying agents in topical creams, emulsions, and ointments.

Commercial polysorbates (Tweens) are complex mixtures of partial esters of sorbitol and its mono- and di-anhydrides condensed with an approximate number of moles of ethylene oxide; Table 3 lists the compositions of the commonly used polysorbates. The polysorbates are miscible with water and are used as emulsifying agents for oil-in-water emulsions. They may also be used as solubilizing agents, for example, for oil-soluble vitamins, and as wetting agents in the preparation of suspensions.

Block Copolymers

The molecular structure of nonionic surfactants composed of an alkyl chain, and an oxyethylene group may be abbreviated to C_nE_m, and these simple nonionic surfactants may therefore be regarded as AB block copolymers. ABA triblock copolymers with the general structure $E_mP_nE_m$, where the hydrophobic block is oxypropylene P [$OCH_2CH(CH_3)$], are referred to as poloxamers and are commercially available under the trade names Pluronics (BASF-Wyandotte) and Synperonics (Uniqema). The convention for naming these compounds is to use a number, the first two digits of which, when multiplied by 100, correspond to the approximate average molecular weight of the poly(oxypropylene) block, and the third digit, when multiplied by 10, corresponds to the percentage by weight of the poly(oxyethylene) block. For example, the poly(oxypropylene) block of poloxamer 188 has a molecular weight of approximately 1800, and about 80% by weight of the molecule is poly(oxypropylene). The nomenclature originally proposed BASF-Wyandotte and now also adopted by Uniqema for the Synperonic series indicates the physical state by a letter (F, P, or L, denoting solid, paste, or liquid,

Table 3 Structures and HLB Values of Selected Polyoxyethylene Sorbitan Esters

Polyoxyethylene sorbitan monoester

Polyoxyethylene sorbitan triester

Chemical name[a]	Commercial name	R	HLB
Polyoxyethylene (20) sorbitan monolaurate	Polysorbate (Tween) 20	$C_{11}H_{23}$	16.7
Polyoxyethylene (20) sorbitan monopalmitate	Polysorbate (Tween) 40	$C_{15}H_{31}$	15.6
Polyoxyethylene (20) sorbitan monostearate	Polysorbate (Tween) 60	$C_{17}H_{35}$	14.9
Polyoxyethylene (20) sorbitan tristearate	Polysorbate (Tween) 65	$C_{17}H_{35}$	10.5
Polyoxyethylene (20) sorbitan monooleate	Polysorbate (Tween) 80	$C_{17}H_{33}$	15.0
Polyoxyethylene (20) sorbitan trioleate	Polysorbate (Tween) 85	$C_{17}H_{33}$	11.0

[a] $w + x + y + z = 20$.
Abbreviation: HLB, hydrophile-lipophile balance.

respectively), followed by a two- or three-digit number. The last digit of this number is the same as that for the equivalent poloxamer and is approximately one-tenth of the weight percentage of poly(oxyethylene); the first one (or two digits in a three-digit number) multiplied by 300 gives a rough estimate of the molecular weight of the hydrophobe. So, for example, Pluronic F68 is a solid, the molecular weight of the hydrophobe is approximately 1800, and the poly(oxyethylene) content is approximately 80% of the molecule by weight. A grid was developed by BASF to interrelate the

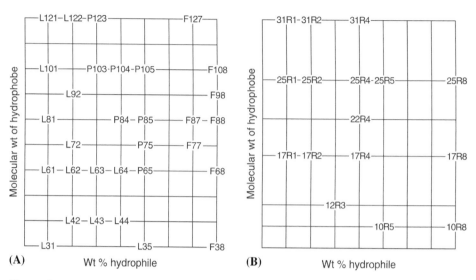

Figure 1 The Pluronic grid for (**A**) the poly(oxyethylene)-poly(oxypropylene)-poly(oxyethylene) [Pluronic series] and (**B**) the poly(oxypropylene)-poly(oxyethylene)-poly(oxypropylene) [Pluronic R series] of block copolymers.

properties of the Pluronics (Fig. 1A). The relationship between the Pluronic (and Synperonic) and poloxamer nomenclatures is shown in Table 4, which also gives the approximate composition of each copolymer.

Included in Table 4 are examples of block copolymers of poly(oxyethylene) and poly(oxypropylene) with the general formula $P_nE_mP_n$ (meroxapols). The nomenclature for these "reverse" block copolymers uses three digits, the first two [approximately one-hundredth of the molecular weight of the poly(oxypropylene) block] separated from the third [approximately one-tenth of the weight percentage of poly(oxyethylene) in the molecule] by the letter R. For example, 25R4 contains 40% by weight of poly(oxyethylene), and the total molecular weight of the poly(oxypropylene) blocks is approximately 2500. The properties of the Pluronic R series are interrelated using the grid shown in Figure 1B.

The poloxamers are water soluble and, as might be expected from their amphiphilic structure, also surface active. Many of the $E_mP_nE_m$ series form micelles, the properties of which have been reviewed by several authors (2,3).

Poloxamers are used as emulsifying agents for intravenous fat emulsions, as solubilizing agents to maintain clarity in elixirs and syrups, and as wetting agents for antibacterials. They may also be used in ointment or suppository bases and as tablet binders or coaters.

HLB System

For pharmaceutical applications of nonionic surfactants, particularly in the formulation of emulsions, it is useful to express their amphiphilic nature in terms of the balance between the hydrophobic and hydrophilic portions of the molecule. An empirical scale of hydrophile-lipophile balance (HLB) numbers was devised by Griffin at the end of the 1940s, with values ranging from 0 to 20 on an arbitrary scale (Fig. 2). At the higher end of the scale (HLB > 8), the surfactants are hydrophilic and act as solubilizing agents,

Table 4 Nomenclature of $E_mP_nE_m$ and $P_nE_mP_n$[a] Block Copolymers

Poloxamer	Pluronic	Mol. wt. of P block	Chain length, n	Weight percent of E block	Chain length, m	Average mol. wt. of copolymer
188	F68	1750	30	80	80	8750
217	F77	2050	35	70	54	6835
237	F87	2250	39	70	60	7500
238	F88	2250	39	80	102	11250
288	F98	2750	47	80	125	13750
338	F108	3250	56	80	148	16250
407	F127	4000	69	70	106	13335
105	L35	5950	103	50	68	11900
123	L43	1200	21	30	6	1715
124	L44	1200	21	40	9	2000
181	L61	1750	30	10	2	1945
182	L62	1750	30	20	5	2190
183	L63	1750	30	30	9	2500
184	L64	1750	30	40	13	2915
212	L72	2050	35	20	6	2565
231	L81	2250	39	10	3	2500
282	L92	2750	47	20	8	3440
331	L101	3250	56	10	4	3610
401	L121	4000	69	10	5	4445
402	L122	4000	69	20	11	5000
185	P65	1750	30	50	20	3500
235	P85	2250	39	50	27	4600
333	P103	3250	56	30	16	4645
334	P104	3250	56	40	25	5415
335	P105	3250	56	50	37	6500
403	P123	4000	69	30	19	5715
171[a]	17R1	1410	–	10	–	1565
252[a]	25R2	2100	–	20	–	2625
258[a]	25R8	2100	–	80	–	10500
311[a]	31R1	2450	–	10	–	2720

detergents, and emulsifiers for oil-in-water emulsions. Oil-soluble surfactants with a low HLB act as emulsifiers for water-in-oil emulsions. Typically, the polysorbate (Tween) surfactants have HLB values in the range 9.6 to 16.7; the sorbitan ester (Span) surfactants have HLB values in the lower range of 1.8 to 8.6 (Tables 2 and 3).

There are several methods for estimating the HLB, depending on the molecular structure. The HLB of polyhydric alcohol fatty acid esters such as glyceryl monostearate may be obtained from

$$HLB = 20\left(1 - \frac{S}{A}\right) \tag{1}$$

where S is the saponification number of the ester, and A is the acid number of the fatty acid. The HLB of polysorbate 20 (Tween 20) calculated using this formula is 16.7, with $S = 45.5$ and $A = 276$. For those materials for which it is not possible to obtain

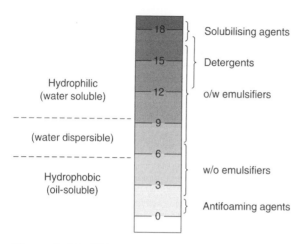

Figure 2 The HLB scale and its application in formulation. *Abbreviation*: HLB, hydrophile-lipophile balance.

saponification numbers, for example, beeswax and lanolin derivatives, the HLB is calculated from

$$HLB = (E + P)/5 \qquad (2)$$

where E is the percentage by weight of oxyethylene chains, and P is the percentage by weight of polyhydric alcohol groups (glycerol or sorbitol) in the molecule. If the hydrophile consists only of oxyethylene groups (CH_2CH_2O, mol. wt. = 44), a simpler version of the equation is

$$HLB = \frac{E}{5} \qquad (3)$$

giving the upper end of the scale (20) for polyoxyethylene glycol itself.

HLB values can also be calculated using group contributions (group numbers) for the constituent groups of the surfactant (see Table 5 for common examples) using

$$HLB = \Sigma(\text{hydrophilic group numbers}) - \Sigma(\text{lipophilic group numbers}) + 7 \qquad (4)$$

Table 5 HLB Group Numbers for Hydrophilic and Lipophilic Groups

Hydrophilic groups	Group number	Lipophilic groups	Group number	Derived groups	Group number
$-SO_4-Na^+$	+ 38.7	$-CH-$	−0.475	$-(OCH_2CH_2)-$	+ 0.33
$-COO-K^+$	+ 21.1	$-CH_2-$	−0.475	$-(OCH_2CH_2CH_2)-$	− 0.15
$-COO-Na^+$	+ 19.1	$-CH_3$	−0.475		
$-SO_3-Na^+$	+ 11.0	$=CH-$	−0.475		
N (tertiary amine)	+ 9.4	$-CF_2-$	−0.870		
Ester (sorbitan ring)	+ 6.8	$-CF_3$	−0.870		
Ester (free)	+ 2.4				
$-COOH$	+ 2.1				
$-OH$ (free)	+ 1.9				
$-O$ (ether group)	+ 1.3				
$-OH$ (sorbitan ring)	+ 0.5				

Abbreviation: HLB, hydrophile-lipophile balance.

In formulations where a mixture of surfactants is used, the resultant HLB of the mixture is calculated assuming that the HLB of a mixture of two surfactants containing fraction f of A and $(1 - f)$ of B is an algebraic mean of the two HLB numbers.

$$\text{HLB}_{\text{mixture}} = f\text{HLB}_A + (1 - f)\text{HLB}_B \tag{5}$$

In practice, required HLB values of the oil phases of emulsions are used in the selection of suitable surfactants or surfactant mixtures. These are the optimum HLB numbers required to produce stable emulsions of a variety of oils.

Zwitterionic and Amphoteric Surfactants

These types of surfactants possess polar head groups, which on ionization may impart both positive and negative charges. The positive charge is almost always carried by an ammonium group, and the negative charge is often a carboxylate. If the ammonium group is quaternary, the molecule will exist as a zwitterion over a wide pH range, since the quaternary ammonium group will be permanently charged. If not, the molecule will behave as a true amphoteric surfactant, that is, the molecule will change from net cationic to zwitterionic, and finally to net anionic as the pH is increased; such surfactants will only therefore be zwitterionic over a certain range of pH, which depends on the pK_a values of each charge group. At the isoelectric point, both charged groups will be fully ionized, and the molecule will have properties similar to those of nonionic surfactants. As the pH shifts away from the isoelectric point, the molecule will gradually assume the properties of either a cationic or anionic surfactant. Common examples are N-alkyl derivatives of simple amino acids, such as glycine (NH_2CH_2COOH), aminopropionic acid ($NH_2CH_2CH_2COOH$), and betaine (($CH_3)_2NCH_2COOH$) (Table 1).

Surface-Active Drugs

A wide variety of drugs have also been reported to be surface active (1), this surface activity being a consequence of the amphiphilic nature of the drugs. The hydrophobic portions of the drug molecules are usually more complex than those of typical surface-active agents being composed of aromatic or heterocyclic ring systems. Examples include the tranquillizers, such as chlorpromazine (CPZ), which are based on the large tricyclic phenothiazine ring system; the antidepressant drugs, such as imipramine, which also possess tricyclic ring systems; and the antihistamines, such as diphenhydramine, which are based on a diphenylmethane group. Representative examples are illustrated in Table 6. The physicochemical properties of the amphiphilic drugs are discussed in section "Micelle Formation in Aqueous Solution."

SURFACE AND INTERFACIAL PROPERTIES

Surface and Interfacial Tension

The surface tension of a liquid is a consequence of the attractive forces between the molecules of the liquid originating from the short-range forces of attraction existing between the molecules. The molecules located in the bulk of the liquid are subject to equal attractive forces acting in all directions; there is, however, an imbalance of attractive forces acting on the molecules at the surface because of the much smaller number of molecules in the vapor phase than in the bulk. As a consequence, there is a net

Table 6 Examples of Surface-Active Drugs

Antidepressants

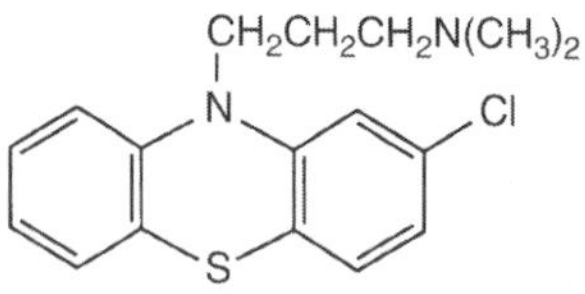

Chlorpromazine

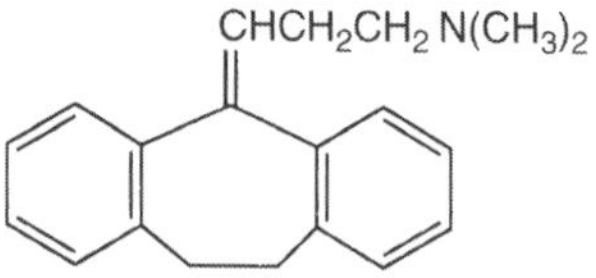

Amitriptyline

Antihistamines

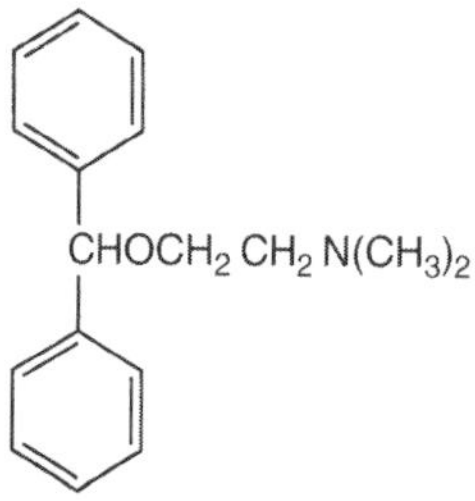

Diphenhydramine

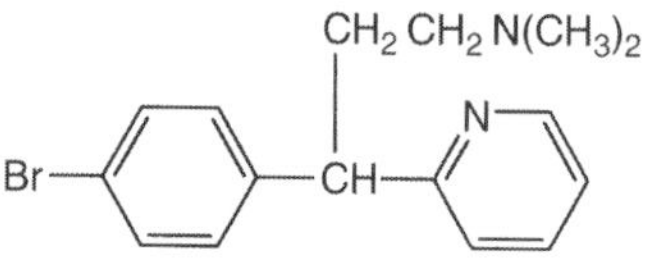

Brompheniramine

Anticholinergic drugs

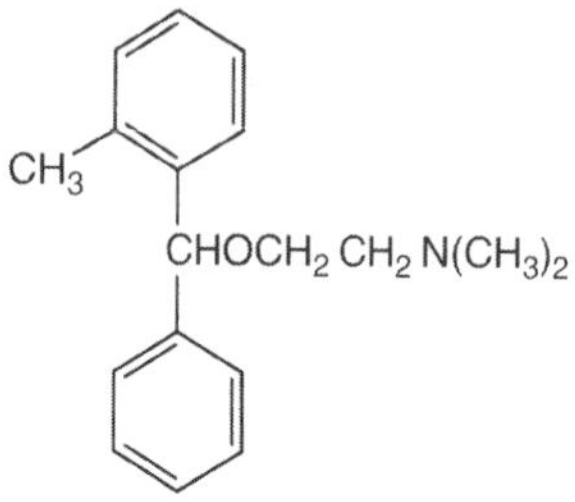

Local anaesthetics

Orphenadrine

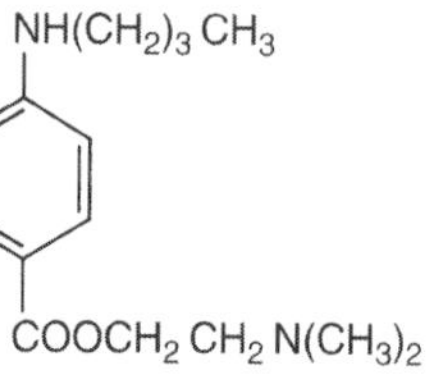

Tetracaine

inward pull on the surface, which tends to diminish the surface area. It is for this reason, of course, that droplets of liquids and bubbles of gas assume a spherical shape. The contraction of the surface is spontaneous, that is, it is accompanied by a decrease in free energy. The contracted surface thus represents a minimum free-energy state, and any attempt to expand the surface must involve an increase in the free energy. The surface tension (and surface free energy) is the work required to increase the area of a surface isothermally and reversibly by a unit amount.

A similar imbalance of attractive forces exists at the interface between two immiscible liquids. The value of the interfacial tension is generally between that of the surface tensions of the two liquids involved, except where there is interaction between them, as for example, in the case of the octanol-water interface where the interfacial tension is considerably lower than the surface tension of octanol because of hydrogen bonding between these two liquids.

The *surface free energy* of a liquid is defined as the work, w, required to increase the surface area A by 1 m^2

$$w = \gamma \Delta A \qquad (6)$$

where ΔA is the increase in the surface area. γ is also referred to as *surface tension* and in this context is defined as the force acting at right angles to a line 1 m in length along the surface. Surface free energy and surface tension are numerically equal. The surface tension is usually expressed in units of mN/m; surface free energy is more usually expressed in energy units as mJ/m^2. The two units are of course equal (J = Nm).

The ability of amphiphilic molecules to reduce the surface or interfacial tension is a direct consequence of their dual structure; in simple terms, their location at the liquid surface is a means by which the hydrophobic region of the molecule can "escape" from the hostile aqueous environment by protruding into the vapor phase above. Similarly, adsorption at the interface between nonaqueous solutions occurs in such a way that the hydrophobic group is in solution in the nonaqueous phase, leaving the hydrophilic group in contact with the aqueous solution. As a result of adsorption of the amphiphile at the surface, some of the water molecules at the surface are replaced by nonpolar groups. The attractive forces between these groups and the water molecules, or between the groups themselves, are less than those existing between the water molecules. The contracting power of the surface is thus reduced and so is the surface tension.

Surface Tension Reduction and Spontaneous Emulsification

Intrusion of surface-active molecules at the interface between two immiscible liquids leads to a reduction of interfacial tension. In some cases, the interfacial tension between two liquids may be reduced to such a low level that spontaneous emulsification of the two immiscible liquids is observed. These low interfacial tensions are of relevance in an understanding of the formation and stabilization of emulsions. In the formation of microemulsions, however, very low interfacial tensions are required (4). Microemulsions by definition have droplet sizes of less than about 200 nm (hence their transparency), and consequently, there is a very large interface between oil and water. An important characteristic of these formulations is their thermodynamic stability, and this can only be achieved if the interfacial tension is so low that the positive interfacial energy (given by γA_{int} where A_{int} is the interfacial area) can be compensated by the negative free energy of mixing ΔG_{m}. An estimate of the interfacial tension required can be obtained as follows: ΔG_{m} is given by $-T \Delta S_{\text{m}}$ where T is the temperature and ΔS_{m} is the entropy of mixing, which is of the same approximate magnitude as the Boltzmann constant k_{B}. Hence $k_{\text{B}} T = 4\pi r^2 \gamma$, and for a droplet radius, r, of about 10 nm, an interfacial tension of 0.03 mN/m would be required. To reduce the interfacial tension between oil and water (typically about 50 mN/m) to this level, it is usually necessary to include a cosurfactant in the formulation, as it is usually not possible to achieve such a low value using a single surfactant. The importance of the cosurfactant is illustrated in the following example given by Overbeek (5). The interfacial tension between cyclohexane and water is approximately 42 mN/m in the absence of any surfactant. This can be reduced to about 2 mN/m by the addition of increasing amounts of SDS, but further reduction does not occur because the cyclohexane-water interface becomes saturated with SDS, and any additional SDS forms micelles (as discussed in sect. "Gibbs Adsorption Equation") in the aqueous solution (Fig. 3). When 20% pentanol is added to the cyclohexane/water system in the absence of SDS, the interfacial tension is reduced to 10 mN/m. The pentanol,

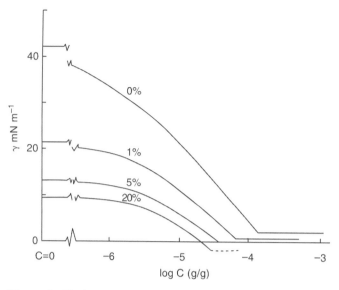

Figure 3 The interfacial tension, γ, between solutions of sodium dodecylsulfate of concentration C in aqueous 0.30 M NaCl and solutions of n-pentanol in cyclohexane with the percentage concentration indicated. *Source*: From Ref. 5.

although not generally considered to be a surfactant, is nevertheless amphiphilic (a short hydrophobic chain and a terminal hydrophilic –OH) and has the ability to act as a cosurfactant, causing an appreciable lowering of the interfacial tension between the cyclohexane and water. It is now theoretically possible by the addition of SDS to achieve a "negative" interfacial tension at SDS concentrations below the concentration at which it forms micelles as seen in Figure 3, thus facilitating the formation of a microemulsion.

Gibbs Adsorption Equation

The Gibbs adsorption equation enables the extent of adsorption at a liquid surface to be estimated from surface tension data. In considering adsorption of soluble amphiphiles, it is important to note that an equilibrium is established between the surfactant molecules at the surface or interface and those remaining in the bulk of the solution, with a continuous interchange of molecules between the two sites. In developing this expression, it is necessary to imagine the interface as a mathematical plane between the two phases. This is clearly an unrealistic model because of the finite thickness of the interfacial layer and the influence of this layer on the properties of the solution in its immediate vicinity; nevertheless, this simplistic model permits a thermodynamic treatment of the adsorption process [see, e.g., (6) for details].

The form of the Gibbs equation applicable to the adsorption of a nonionic surfactant at the surface of an aqueous solution of concentration c is

$$\Gamma_2 = \frac{-1}{RT}\frac{d\gamma}{d\ln c} = \frac{-c}{RT}\frac{d\gamma}{dc} \tag{7}$$

where R is the gas constant (8.314 J/mol K) and Γ_2 is the amount of surfactant in the surface phase in excess of that in the bulk (the surface excess concentration). For ionic surfactants, the derivation becomes more complex since consideration must be taken of the adsorption of both surfactant ion and counterion. The general form of the Gibbs equation is then written

$$\Gamma_2 = -\frac{1}{xRT}\frac{d\gamma}{d\ln c} = -\frac{1}{xRT}\frac{d\gamma}{2.303d\log c} \tag{8}$$

where x has a numerical value varying from 1 (for ionic surfactants in dilute solution or in the presence of excess electrolyte) to 2 (in concentrated solution). The surface excess concentration can then, in principle, be derived from the gradient of a plot of surface tension as a function of log c. Examination of such plots for solutions of surfactants (Fig. 3) shows a gradual change in gradient with increase in surfactant concentration until saturation of the interfacial layer, at which point the gradient becomes zero (or almost zero). The surfactant concentration at this inflection point is the *critical micelle concentration* (CMC) and corresponds to the first formation of *micelles* in the solution (see sect. "Micellization"). By taking the limiting gradient of the surface tension–log c plot at concentrations immediately below the CMC, it is possible to estimate the area A occupied by each molecule in the interfacial layer, and hence gain an indication of the ordering of molecules in the surfactant monolayer, from

$$A = 1/N_A\Gamma_2 \tag{9}$$

where N_A is the Avogadro constant.

An interesting effect arises if the surfactant solution contains highly surface-active impurities. The presence of these impurities leads to a minimum, often very pronounced, in the surface tension–log c plot at the CMC. The surface-active impurity is preferentially adsorbed at the interface, causing a greater lowering than the surfactant itself. When micelles form in the solution, however, the impurities become solubilized in the micelles, and hence desorb from the surface, thus causing the surface tension to increase.

Insoluble Monolayers at the Air-Water Interface

Many water-insoluble amphiphiles, such as long chain fatty acids, will form monolayers on the water surface when spread on the surface using a suitable volatile solvent. These molecules will orientate on the surface in a similar manner to the soluble amphiphiles discussed in the earlier section, but there is an important difference between monolayers formed by water-soluble and water-insoluble amphiphiles. Monolayers of the latter contain all the molecules spread on the surface; there is no equilibrium between molecules in the surface and those in the bulk of the solution as there is with monolayers of soluble surfactants because of the low aqueous solubility of the surfactant. As a consequence, the number of molecules per unit area of surface, and hence the surface area A per molecule, is generally known directly without recourse to the Gibbs equation. Changes in the packing of the molecules resulting from a change in the surface area of the film are usually determined from surface pressure/surface area isotherms, which are plots of the change in surface pressure, π of the film, that is, the difference between the surface tension of the clean surface γ_0 and that of the film-covered surface, γ_m, as a function of the area available to each molecule on the aqueous subphase surface. The measurement is usually carried out under a pseudoequilibrium condition, by continuously compressing the monolayer while monitoring the surface pressure, though one can obtain equilibrium values by compressing the monolayer on a point-to-point basis.

The most widely used method to measure the surface pressure during monolayer compression uses the Langmuir trough (Fig. 4). Essentially, the apparatus consists of a shallow trough with waxed or Teflon sides (nonwetting), along which a nonwetting

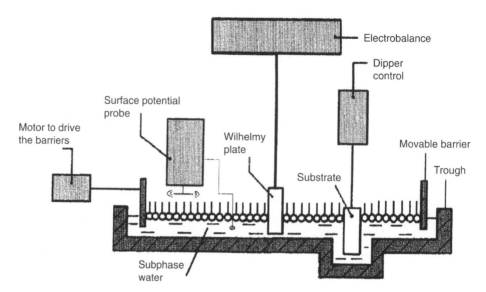

Figure 4 Schematic representation of a Langmuir trough that uses a Wilhelmy plate attached to an electrobalance for measuring surface pressure. Also shown is the dipper employed for transferring LB films onto a solid substrate and a probe for measuring the surface potential. *Abbreviation*: LB, Langmuir/Blodgett. *Source*: From Ref. 15.

barrier may be mechanically moved. In use, the trough is filled completely so as to build up a meniscus above the level of the sides. The surface is swept clean with the moveable barrier and any surface impurities removed. The film-forming material is dissolved in a suitable volatile solvent and an accurately measured amount, usually about 0.01 mL of this solution, is carefully injected onto the surface. The solvent evaporates and leaves a uniformly spread film, which is contained entirely within a well-defined surface area.

There are two techniques for measuring the surface pressure during compression: the Langmuir balance and the Wilhelmy plate. The first one is essentially a differential measurement, in which a clean water or aqueous surface is separated from the surface covered with the monolayer by a float connected to the conventional balance that measures the force acting on the float. In the second method (depicted in Fig. 4), the surface tension of the film-covered surface is measured directly using a Wilhelmy plate partially immersed in the subphase and attached to a sensitive electrobalance. One important drawback of the Wilhelmy plate as a method of measuring surface tension of the film is the change in contact angle when the plate is covered with monolayer material. This problem may be obviated by using a paper Wilhelmy plate for measuring surface pressure as suggested by Gaines (7). Such plates, made of high-quality filter or chromatography paper, are always wet when in contact with the aqueous subphase in the Langmuir trough, so the contact angle of the subphase liquid on the plate surfaces is always zero. This feature enables the plate to be used reliably in both the compression and expansion of a monolayer, and permits accurate automatic control of surface pressure. Such control is particularly important when the monolayer must be held at constant surface pressure while some other measurement, such as the surface potential, is made. The surface film balance has been the principal instrument for manipulating and examining floating monolayers since its invention by Pockels over a century ago. Over that time there have been steady improvements in precision and convenience culminating with the introduction of computer control and data collection in recent years.

Other methods of measuring surface tension during film compression, in addition to the Wilhelmy and Langmuir methods described above, include monitoring the diffraction of a laser light from the surface capillary waves generated by the small periodic mechanical disturbances of the air-water interface (8). In this latter work, the change in surface tension was measured by investigating the dependence of the spatial separation, that is, diffraction of the laser light striking at these capillary waves, and from the frequency of the disturbance.

Sources of experimental error during surface pressure measurements have been discussed by Pethica (9). These include impurities in the monolayer material under study, impurities in subphase water, solubility of the monolayer material, drifts in the surface pressure–measuring system, change in water level by evaporation, leakage through the barrier, and change in surface density of monolayer material by spreading of different amounts or excess materials.

In addition to the floating monolayers discussed earlier, there has been considerable interest in probing the structure of films, both mono- and multilayer, transferred from the water surface onto solid substrates, the *Langmuir/Blodgett (LB) films*. When only a single LB monolayer is required, the deposition is performed by raising a hydrophilic substrate upward through the monolayer-covered surface; when further layers are to be deposited, the first layer may be formed by upward motion on a hydrophilic substrate or by downward motion on a hydrophobic substrate. A comprehensive account of the structures of LB films has been presented by Schwartz (10), and their significance and applications have been reviewed (11,12).

Types of Monolayers

Monolayers are two-dimensional systems that can be classified into three main types, which in some ways resemble the solid, liquid, and gaseous states of three-dimensional matter. The general appearance of the three types of film is illustrated in Figure 5.

Solid or condensed films are formed by, for example, long chain fatty acids. At high surface areas, the strong cohesion between the hydrocarbon chains maintains the film molecules in small clusters on the surface. The surface pressure remains low during compression, until these molecules become tightly packed, at which point there is a rapid rise in surface pressure. The extrapolated limiting surface area for fatty acids such as stearic and palmitic is about 0.20 nm^2, very close to the cross-sectional area of the

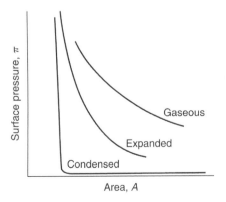

Figure 5 Diagrammatic representation of the surface pressure, π, versus area per molecule, A, plots for three main types of insoluble monolayer.

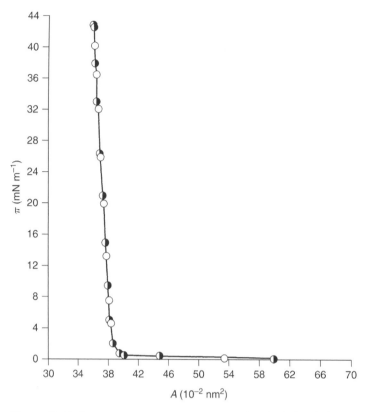

Figure 6 Surface pressure, π, versus area per molecule, A, for cholesterol, which shows a typical condensed monolayer. *Source*: From Ref. 13.

compounds in the bulk crystal as determined by X-ray diffraction. This type of film is also evident in π-A curves of cholesterol (Fig. 6) (13). Simultaneous electron micrographs of the film-covered surface have confirmed the presence of cholesterol clusters or islands, which gradually pack more tightly at greater pressures, until eventually becoming continuous as the molecules come into close contact. On further compression, monolayer collapse occurs. The extrapolated limiting surface area of 0.39 nm^2 is very close to the cross-sectional area of a cholesterol ring system calculated from molecular models, indicating a vertical orientation of the cholesterol molecules in the highly compressed monolayer.

Gaseous monolayers resemble the gaseous state of three-dimensional matter in that the molecules move around in the film, remaining a sufficiently large distance apart so as to exert very little force on each other. There is a gradual change in the surface pressure on compression rather than the abrupt change observed on compression of condensed films. It is thought that the molecules in these types of monolayers lie along the surface, and this is certainly so with those dibasic esters with terminal polar groups that anchor the molecules flat on the surface. Steroids in which the polar groups are distributed about the molecule also tend to form gaseous films for similar reasons.

Liquid or expanded monolayers represent intermediate states between gaseous and condensed films. Although the π-A plots are quite steeply curved, extrapolation to a limiting surface area yields a value that is usually significantly greater than the cross-sectional area from molecular models. Films of this type tend to be formed by molecules

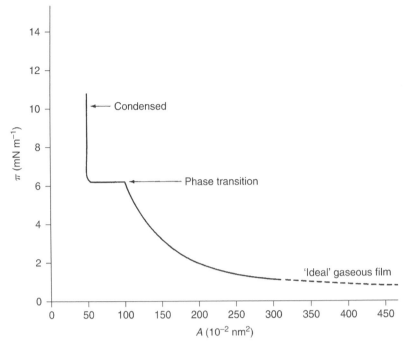

Figure 7 Surface pressure, π, versus area per molecule for β-estradiol diacetate showing a transition from a gaseous to a condensed film on compression. *Source*: From Ref. 14.

in which close packing into condensed films is prohibited by bulky side chains or the presence of an unsaturated double or triple bond. In the latter case, the effect is more pronounced for *cis*- than for *trans*-isomers.

Transition Between Monolayer States

Many simple molecules, rather than exhibiting behavior exclusively characteristic of one monolayer state, show transitions between one state and another as the film is compressed. Estradiol diacetate, for example (Fig. 7), shows typical gaseous behavior at a large area per molecule, and in this state the molecules are thought to be lying along the surface, as might be expected from the location of the hydrophilic groups on the molecule. As compression is applied, the molecules are gradually pressed closer together until at a molecular surface area of approximately 0.96 nm^2, the molecules begin to stand upright. The film then undergoes a gradual transition to a condensed film as the proportion of upright molecules increases with further compression, until at approximately 0.38 nm^2, the film is totally in the condensed form (14).

Factors Influencing Monolayer Type

Many factors influence the type of monolayer formed including both external factors such as temperature and modifications to the molecular structure (15). Figure 8 shows changes in monolayer type as the length of the alkyl chain is increased from lauric acid (*n*-dodecanoic acid) to stearic acid (*n*-octadecanoic acid). Lauric acid represents the minimum alkyl chain length for the formation of monolayers; shorter chain length compounds have sufficient aqueous solubility to cause loss of monolayer and resultant

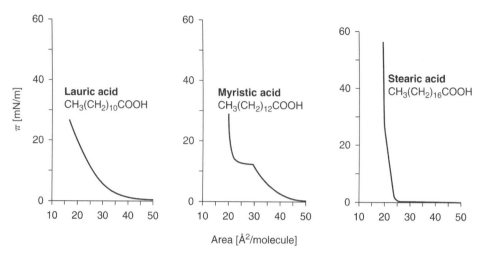

Figure 8 Surface pressure-*A* isotherms of lauric acid, myristic acid, and stearic acid spread on 10^{-3} M HCl aqueous subphase at 20°C, showing changes in the nature of the isotherm caused by increasing length of the hydrophobic chain. *Source*: From Ref. 15.

decrease in monolayer area. Lauric acid forms slightly soluble, gaseous monolayers; the addition of two more carbon atoms causes myristic acid (*n*-tetradecanoic acid) to exhibit a condensed gaseous phase region as well as an expanded phase, and further increase in the hydrocarbon chain length results in the additional formation of the solid phase. Replacement of the hydrogen atoms of the alkyl chain with a halogen such as fluorine also affects the type of monolayer. Monolayers containing fluorocarbon chains are more stable than those formed from their hydrocarbon counterparts and, because the fluorocarbon chain is more hydrophobic than a hydrocarbon chain, compounds with shorter chains are able to form insoluble monolayers. Similarly, changes in the polarity, size, and shape of the head group can influence the arrangements of the hydrocarbon chains and hence the monolayer structure, as illustrated by early studies with alcohols, esters, amides, amines, and nitriles.

Mono-, di-, and trivalent ions present in the aqueous subphase play a critical role in determining the stability of monolayers (16,17). The complexation of metal ions with the acid head group of fatty acids generally causes the surface pressure–area isotherm to be more condensed (18). Divalent metal ions interact with the –COOH group in different ways, depending on their electronegativity (19,20); metal ions with higher electro-negativity interact with the –COOH group covalently and those with lower electro-negativity interact electrostatically. Such interactions affect the packing behavior of the alkyl chains (21).

Changing the subphase pH influences the characteristics of isotherms of amphiphiles possessing ionizable head groups, such as –COOH or –NH$_2$, when the pH change is such as to cause changes in the ionization of the molecules. In general, there is a shift in the π-A curves toward lower molecular areas in comparison to the isotherm recorded for uncharged molecules (22).

Phase transitions in surface pressure–area isotherms are strongly influenced by the subphase temperature. Figure 9 shows more expanded films and a corresponding decrease in collapse pressure as the temperature was increased over the range 22°C to 42°C for several sorbitan esters (Spans) (23).

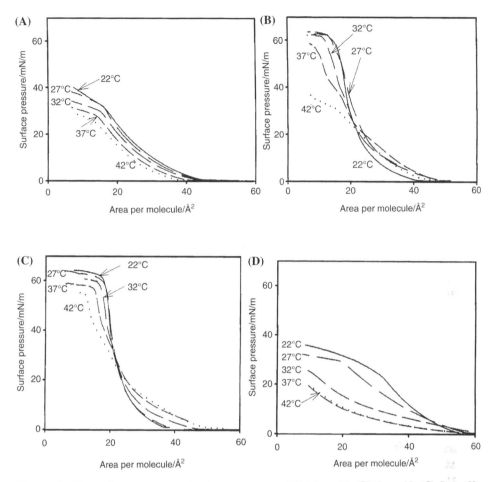

Figure 9 The surface pressure–molecular area curves of (**A**) Span 20, (**B**) Span 40, (**C**) Span 60, and (**D**) Span 80 in the temperature range 22°C to 42°C. *Source*: From Ref. 23.

The Structures of Monolayers in Different Phases

Recently developed techniques that have proved invaluable in the study of both floating and LB monolayers include X-ray diffraction and reflection, neutron reflection, infrared and Raman spectroscopy, electron diffraction, and scanning probe microscopy methods. Two highly sensitive imaging techniques, namely fluorescence microscopy (24,25) and Brewster angle microscopy (BAM) (26,27), have proved invaluable in investigating the morphology of condensed phase domains formed after the main phase transition in the two-phase coexistence region of Langmuir monolayers. In fluorescence microscopy, an insoluble fluorescent amphiphilic marker is added to the monolayer material, the solubility of which depends on the ordering of the phases; the more ordered the monolayer phase, the lower is its solubility. Consequently, when two phases coexist in the monolayer, the contrast arises from the varied solubility of the probe in the two phases. Figure 10 shows fluorescence microscopy images for a model lipid matrix, composed of binary mixture 7:1 mol/mol of DPPC (dipalmitoylphosphatidyl choline) and DPPG (dipalmitoylphosphatidyl glycerol) (28). The images show the first appearance of domain structures near the phase transition at 7 mN/m similar to pure phospholipid monolayers. Upon compression, the domains grow in size, and above 16mN/m, a progressive blurring

(A)

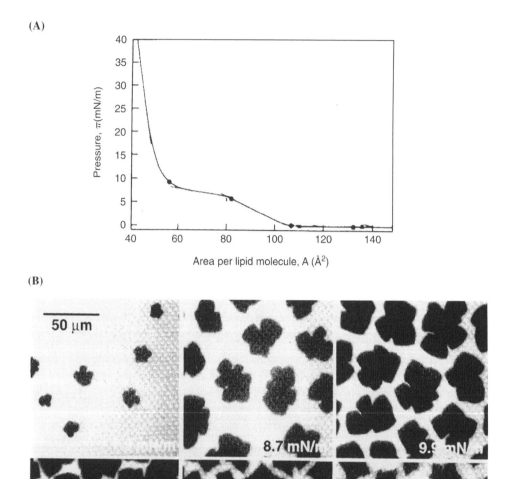

(B)

Figure 10 (**A**) Surface pressure-area isotherms of monolayers of lipid mixtures of DPPC and DPPG with a DPPC:DPPG molar ratio of 7:1 on 120 mM NaCl (**B**) fluorescence micrographs at increasing surface pressures as indicated. *Abbreviations*: DPPC, dipalmitoylphosphatidyl-choline; DPPG, dipalmitoylphosphatidyl-glycerol. *Source*: From Ref. 28.

of the domain boundaries occurs. A perceived disadvantage of the fluorescence technique is the requirement for the addition of fluorescent probes, which can possibly modify the monolayer properties. The advantage of BAM is that no probe molecules or other intervention in the system is necessary. BAM is based on the fact that at the Brewster angle of incidence, a parallel, polarized laser beam has a zero reflectance. The presence of a condensed monolayer phase leads to a change in the refractive index and, thus, to a measurable change in reflectivity. By introducing an analyzer in the reflected beam path, not only the shape of the condensed phase domains but also their inner texture can be visualized.

Atomic force microscopy (AFM) has proved a useful technique for the visualization of structures coexisting in monolayers deposited on solid substrates. For example, Flanders et al. (29) have used this technique to probe the submicrometer phase structure in palmitic acid (PA) monolayers containing the 25 peptide amino terminus of lung surfactant protein B (SP-B$_{1-25}$). In the AFM images illustrated in Figure 11, the light-gray regions, which are topographically higher than those represented by dark gray, were assigned to the more upright liquid condensed (LC) phase, and the darker regions to the liquid expanded (LE) phase. Figure 11A shows elliptically shaped LE domains roughly 10 μm in diameter coexisting with an expansive sheet of LC phase in monolayers containing 5 wt% SP-B$_{1-25}$. Within the boundaries of the LE phase are seen micrometer-sized domains of approximately the same height as the sheetlike LC phase. Increase in the SP-B$_{1-25}$ content to 10 wt% (Fig. 11B) causes an apparent breakup of the sheetlike structure of the LC phase, the LE phase then existing as a sheetlike domain that covers

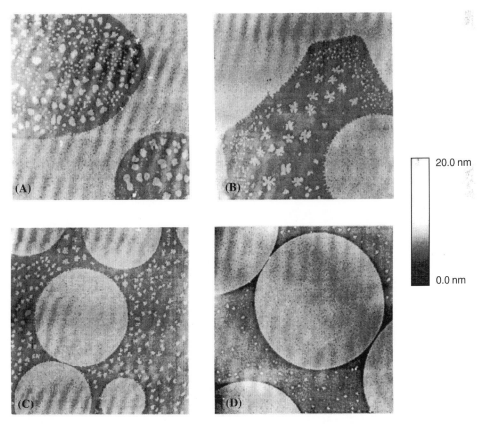

Figure 11 AFM images of monolayers of PA and the 25 peptide amino terminus of lung surfactant protein B (SP-B$_{1-25}$) that were deposited at a surface pressure of 15 mN/m onto mica substrates. Dark gray denotes regions of LE phase. Light gray denotes regions of LC phase. The scale bar applies to each of the four images. Monolayers contain concentrations of SP-B$_{1-25}$ of (**A**) 5 wt%: elliptical LE regions coexist amid an expanse of LC phase; (**B**) 10 wt%, (**C**) 15 wt%, (**D**) 20 wt%: circular LC regions coexist amid an expanse of LE phase. *Abbreviations*: AFM, atomic force microscopy; PA, palmitic acid; LE, liquid expanded; LC, liquid condensed. *Source*: From Ref. 29.

more than one-third of the area of the image. This image shows a wide distribution of LC domain shapes and sizes and the presence of clover-shaped LC domains roughly 5 μm in dimension existing amid the sheetlike LE region far from the boundaries of the large LC regions. AFM images at SP-B$_{1-25}$ contents of 15 and 20 wt% (Fig. 11C,D) show the existence of a broad, sheetlike domain of LE phase in which LC domains of various shapes and sizes coexist, including clover-shaped LC domains. The LC domains are seen to become circular (approximately 20 μm diameter) with uniformly smooth boundaries. The phase distribution dependence on SP-B$_{1-25}$ concentration suggests that the peptide induces disorder in the monolayer.

Peng et al. (30) and Dynarowicz-Łatka et al. (15) have presented detailed overviews of these experimental techniques. The application of AFM in the study of ordered monolayers has been reviewed (31,32), and Vollhardt (33) has discussed the use of fluorescent microscopy and BAM in elucidating the molecular organization of condensed monolayers. These developments have led to major advances in an understanding of both Langmuir and LB films, sometimes confirming ideas that had emerged on the basis of earlier macroscopic measurements, but often revealing new and hitherto unsuspected detail.

Monolayers as Cell Membrane Models

Phospholipid monolayers provide useful models for studying drug-lipid interactions. Hidalgo et al. (34) have shown interesting differences in the interaction of the phenothiazine drugs trifluoperazine (TFP) and chlorpromazine (CPZ) with the anionic glycerophospholipid dipalmitoylphosphatidylglycerol (DPPG). The surface pressure isotherms in Figure 12 show that incorporation of CPZ expands the monolayer, and an additional phase transition appears at higher drug concentrations; at high surface pressures there is little increase in area, suggesting that this drug is being excluded from the interface. TFP also expands the monolayer, although there is no appearance of an additional phase transition, the increase in area per molecule is noted even at high surface pressures indicating that this drug remains in the monolayer. The considerable expansion of the monolayer observed even at relatively low drug/phospholipid ratios for both systems suggests that phospholipid molecules not in immediate contact with the drug are affected by incorporation of the drug into the monolayer. This "cooperative effect," which is thought to be a consequence of either a significant reorientation and different packing of the DPPG molecules or a change in their hydration state, may explain why drugs such as these with relatively nonspecific effects on the membrane are highly effective at very low concentrations.

Cholesterol monolayers are also used to model drug-membrane interactions. Figure 13 shows the surface pressure-area isotherms for equimolar mixtures of valinomycin (a cyclic peptide), which orientates horizontally at the air-solution interface to give an expanded film, and cholesterol, which orientates vertically to give a solid film (35). The shape of the mixed isotherm at low and intermediate pressures is similar to that of valinomycin, while the behavior at high surface pressures is similar to that of cholesterol, suggesting that the valinomycin has been squeezed out of the mixed film. The position of the mixed curve to the left of the calculated average curve suggests some form of interaction between the components, which condenses the mixed film.

Surfactant Monolayers at the Liquid-Liquid Interface

It is of interest to study the properties of surfactant monolayers at the oil-water interface because of the key role of such interfacial monolayers in the emulsification process. The

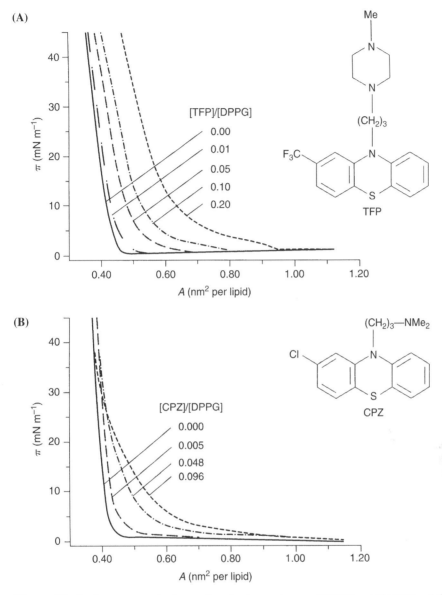

Figure 12 Surface pressure isotherms for mixed monolayers of DPPG and (**A**) TFP and (**B**) CPZ for a range of drug/phospholipid molar ratios. *Abbreviations*: DPPG, dipalmitoylphosphatidyl-glycerol; TFP, trifluoperazine; CPZ, chlorpromazine. *Source*: From Ref. 34.

interactions of the hydrophobic components of the surfactant molecules and the oil phase at the closely packed state of the monolayers can provide an insight on how they act on emulsion stability by influencing the preferred curvature of the surfactant layer and hence the droplet size. However, the preparation and study of monolayers at the liquid-liquid interface is difficult and, compared to numerous studies of monolayers at the air-water interface, there are relatively few direct investigations of liquid-liquid interfacial monolayers. One of the difficulties in forming such monolayers is the limited number of compounds that are insoluble in both polar and nonpolar solvents. Some surfactants, for

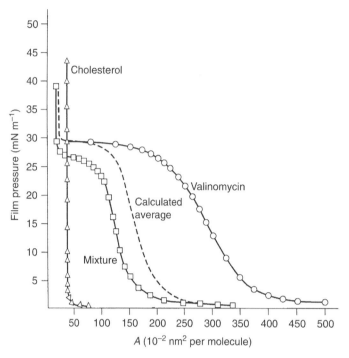

Figure 13 Surface pressure–area isotherms for cholesterol, valinomycin, and an equimolar mixture of the two. *Source*: From Ref. 35.

example, distribute into both liquids and give ultralow interfacial tension of the order of μN/m, causing difficulty in obtaining phase equilibrium and accurate interfacial tension values. There are also experimental difficulties in studying the properties of monolayers at the liquid-liquid interface. Several innovative techniques have been reported for the formation and compression of insoluble films at this interface. The technique usually employed to form the film involves the initial formation of the monolayer by spreading out the compound on the surface of the denser phase and then the addition of a lower-density phase by carefully pouring it on the top of the monolayer. Ghaicha et al. (36) have designed a modified Langmuir trough allowing the interface to be compressed between the water and oil phases. These authors found that, in contrast to the air-water interface, the monolayers at the oil-water interface were more expanded at low surface pressures, suggesting greatly reduced van der Waals forces of interaction between the hydrocarbon chains of the surfactant molecules resulting in expansion of the monolayers. In a closely packed state, however, the monolayers appeared to be condensed with extrapolated values of molecular area significantly lower than expected values from molecular modeling, suggesting a partial loss of surfactant molecules from the interface due to their dissolution into the oil phase.

The structural features of the interfacial monolayers have been examined using a range of experimental techniques including neutron reflectivity (37) and X-ray scattering (38); theoretical treatments of the thermodynamics of adsorption at the liquid-liquid interface have been given by Aratono and Takanori (39). For a detailed review of the study and properties of these systems, the reader is directed to the review by Lowy (40).

ADSORPTION OF SURFACTANTS ONTO SOLIDS
FROM AQUEOUS SOLUTION

Adsorption from a dilute solution onto the walls of a container or onto particulate matter present in suspension may involve specific chemical interaction between the adsorbate and adsorbent (chemisorption). The most common interactions of this type include an ion-exchange process in which the counterions of the substrate are replaced by surfactant ions of similar charge, hydrogen bond formation between adsorbate molecule and substrate, and an ion-pairing interaction in which surfactant ions are adsorbed onto oppositely charged sites unoccupied by counterions. Alternatively, the interaction may be less specific as in adsorption through weak van der Waals forces between the adsorbent and adsorbate molecules. Frequently, more than one mechanism may be involved in the adsorption process, for example, the charged groups of the adsorbate may undergo chemical interaction while the remainder of the molecule is adsorbed by van der Waals attraction.

The physicochemical nature of the adsorbent can have profound effects on the rate and capacity for adsorption. The most important property affecting adsorption is the surface area of the adsorbent. The extent of adsorption is directly proportional to the specific surface area; the more finely divided or the more porous the solid, the greater its adsorption capacity. Particular adsorbents have affinities for particular adsorbates for a wide variety of reasons. The surfaces of adsorbent clays such as bentonite, attapulgite, and kaolin carry cation-exchange sites, and such clays have strong affinities for protonated compounds, which they adsorb by an ion-exchange process. In many cases, different parts of the surface of the same adsorbent have different affinities for different types of adsorbents. There is evidence, for example, that anionic materials are adsorbed on the cationic edge of kaolin particles, while cationics are adsorbed on the cleavage surface of the particles that are negatively charged. The adsorptive capacity of a particular adsorbent often depends on the source from which it was prepared and also on its pretreatment.

The orientation of the surfactant at the solid surface depends on the nature of both the surfactant and the surface, and may be generalized in the following way. For adsorption of surfactants from dilute solution (below the CMC) onto hydrophobic surfaces in systems where the interaction with the surface plays only a minor role, the surfactants adsorb with their hydrophobic moiety in contact with the surface and their hydrophilic moiety extending into the solution, very much as in adsorption at the air-water interface. As a result, a hydrophilic surface is created. On very polar surfaces, the surfactants adsorb with their polar moiety in contact with the surface and their hydrophobic chains protruding into the solution. This orientation, however, creates a hydrophobic surface, which will in turn adsorb further surfactant molecules to form a bilayer; this may happen with the adsorption of ionic surfactants onto oppositely charged surfaces. Under certain conditions, when the attraction between the hydrocarbon chains is stronger than the interaction of the surfactant head groups and the surface, micellar structures may be formed at the surface as discussed below.

Experimental Study of Adsorption

The simplest, most widely used, method for determining the amount of surfactant adsorbed from aqueous solution is the depletion method, that is, the difference in surfactant concentration in the liquid phase is measured before and after contact with the surface. The solid is usually removed by centrifugation or filtration before analysis of the solution by a suitable analytical technique such as potentiometric titration, spectrophotometry, high performance liquid chromatography (HPLC), or fluorimetry. Dynamic light scattering (41) and surface tension (42) techniques have also been used for this purpose (for surfactant concentrations below the CMC). The data from such measurements are generally plotted in the form of adsorption isotherms, that is, as plots of adsorption against the equilibrium concentration of the solution. The appearance of these plots depends on the charge characteristics of the surfactant and the solid adsorbent.

Empirical Data Treatment

The Langmuir equation has been widely used in the interpretation of adsorption data for nonionic surfactants:

$$\frac{n_2^s}{n^s} = \frac{bc}{1 + bc} \tag{10}$$

where n_2^s is the number of moles of solute adsorbed per gram of adsorbent, n^s is the number of moles of adsorption sites per gram, c is the concentration of the surfactant in solution at equilibrium, and b is a constant related to the adsorption-free energy that governs the partition of the solute between the surface and the bulk solution. Rearrangement into a linear form gives

$$\frac{c}{n_2^s} = \frac{1}{n^s b} + \frac{c}{n^s} \tag{11}$$

from which it is seen that a plot of c/n_2^s against c should be linear with a gradient $1/n^s$ and an intercept $1/n^s b$, permitting the evaluation of the Langmuir constants. The Langmuir equation is based on the assumption of monolayer formation, negligible solute-solute or solute-solvent in either solution or surface layer, equal molecular cross-sectional areas of surfactant and solvent, and the presence of a homogeneous adsorbent. Despite the rather unrealistic nature of these assumptions, this equation has proved satisfactory in modeling the adsorption of a large number of systems.

Another empirical equation, often applied to characterize adsorption data that does not fit the Langmuir equation, for example, where there is evidence of multilayer formation, is the Freundlich equation. The Freundlich equation is generally written in the form

$$x/m = ac^{1/n} \tag{12}$$

where a and n are constants, the form $1/n$ being used to emphasize that c is raised to a power less than unity. $1/n$ is a dimensionless parameter and is related to the intensity of adsorption. Equation 12 can be written in a linear form by taking logarithms of both sides, giving

$$\log(x/m) = \log a + (1/n) \log c \tag{13}$$

A plot of log (x/m) against log c should be linear, with an intercept of log a and gradient of $1/n$.

Adsorption Isotherms for Nonionic and Ionic Surfactants

Adsorption of Nonionic Surfactants

Figure 14 shows typical plots for the adsorption (moles of solute adsorbed per gram of adsorbent) against the equilibrium molar concentration of surfactant for a homologous series of octylphenyl polyether alcohols (commercially known by the trade name Triton)

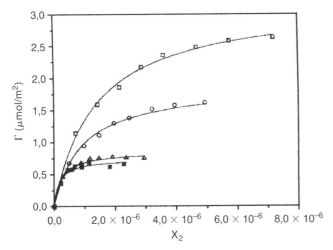

Figure 14 Adsorption isotherms of ($\square$) $C_8PhE_{9.5}$; ($\bigcirc$) C_8PhE_{16}; (Δ) C_8PhE_{30}; (*) C_8PhE_{40} on polystyrene latex. Langmuir fitting (—). *Source*: From Ref. 43.

of the type C_8PhE_m (where Ph = phenyl) with ethylene oxide chain lengths m of 9.5, 16, 30, and 40, onto polystyrene particles (43). Isotherms of similar appearance have been reported, for example, for the adsorption of polyoxyethylated nonylphenols onto carbon (44) and polyoxyethylated nonionic surfactants onto graphitized carbon black (Graphon) (45). A common feature of the plots is a well-defined plateau signifying a saturation of the surface, which is reached at concentrations just below the CMC of the surfactants. Figure 14 shows a decrease in adsorption on the negatively charged polystyrene lattices as the number of ethylene oxide chains increases, indicating the existence of a repulsive interaction energy between these chains in this series of surfactants with a fixed hydrocarbon chain length (octylbenzene). A fairly flat orientation of the surfactant on the surface was suggested from these results.

The influence of the alkyl chain length on absorption onto Graphon particles is illustrated in Figure 15 for a homologous series of C_nE_m nonionics with hexaoxyethylene ($m = 6$) chains and alkyl chains of lengths n between 6 and 12 (45). Graphon has only a few hydrophilic sites, and the results shown in Figure 15 clearly illustrate the increased adsorption associated with increased hydrophobic interaction between the alkyl chains and the surface.

Several generalizations may be drawn from the reported investigations on the adsorption of nonionic surfactants. Adsorption isotherms at different pH or ionic strengths were found to be almost identical, indicating the absence of any important electrical contribution to the adsorption-free energy (43). The saturation coverage on each polymer surface decreases with increase in the oxyethylene chain length, and the surfactant packing at maximum coverage becomes less dense as the hydrophilic character of the surface increases. Even though hydrophobic interaction is the most important contribution to adsorption, there is evidence that interaction of the ethylene oxide groups with the surface influences the conformation of the adsorbed surfactant (43,46–48). The adsorption of nonionic surfactants increases with temperature because of a decrease in surfactant solubility (49).

Figure 14 shows successful fitting of the data for the adsorption of a series of Tritons onto polystyrene lattices to the Langmuir equation. A similar satisfactory fitting to

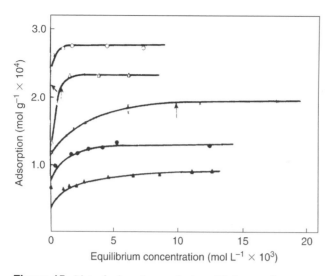

Figure 15 Plot of adsorption against equilibrium surfactant concentration at 25°C for (●) C_6E_6, (x) C_8E_6, (Δ) $C_{10}E_6$, (○)$C_{12}E_6$, and (▲) hexaoxyethylene glycol. Arrows indicate CMC values. *Abbreviation*: CMC, critical micelle concentration. *Source*: From Ref. 45.

this equation was reported by Romero-Cano et al. for the adsorption of Triton X-100 ($C_8PhE_{9.5}$) onto polystyrene particles with different functionalities (50).

Adsorption of Ionic Surfactants

The adsorption of ionic surfactants onto nonpolar or hydrophobic surfaces or surfaces with the same charge as the surfactant generally results in Langmuirian isotherms similar to those for nonionic surfactants. The maximum amount adsorbed generally increases with increase in the length of the alkyl chain.

The adsorption isotherm, however, becomes more complex for the adsorption of an ionic surfactant onto an oppositely signed charged surface. The influence of any surface group on the adsorbent, on the form of the isotherm, was shown in early work by Connor and Ottewill (51) in a study of the adsorption of hexadecyltrimethylammonium bromide onto polystyrene and polystyrene latex particles. Langmuirian isotherms were observed for the adsorption onto the polystyrene sample without surface charge (Fig. 16), whereas S-shaped isotherms were reported for adsorption of the same surfactant onto the polystyrene latex, which had surface carboxyl and hydroxyl groups. The S-shaped isotherms are thought to reflect three distinct modes of adsorption. At low surfactant concentrations, the ionic surfactant adsorbs onto the charged sites on the solid surface with the alkyl chains lying flat on the surface. As the concentration is increased, there is a well-defined "knee," following which a slow increase in adsorption occurs because of hydrophobic interaction between vacant sites on the surface and the alkyl chains. As the CMC of the surfactant in solution is approached, lateral association of the alkyl chains on the particle surface occurs and a plateau is reached. Evidence for the occurrence of lateral interactions between the alkyl chains was presented by Fuerstenau and coworkers (52) in a study of the adsorption of alkyl ammonium ions onto quartz. It was concluded by these workers that once the adsorbed ions reached a certain critical concentration at the interface (well below the CMC), they begin to associate into two-dimensional patches of ions, which they termed "hemimicelles." The forces responsible for this association at the

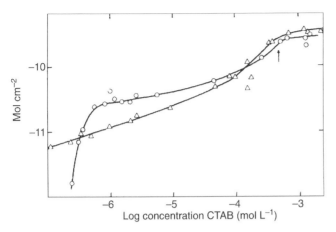

Figure 16 Adsorption isotherms for hexadecyltrimethylammonium ions on (Δ) polystyrene and ($\bigcirc$) polystyrene latex particles (carboxyl and hydroxyl groups) at pH 8.0 in 10^{-3} M KBr solution. $\uparrow$ CMC value. *Abbreviation*: CMC, critical micelle concentration. *Source*: From Ref. 51.

surface were assumed to be the same as those operating in the bulk, except that coulombic attraction for the surface adsorption sites aided the association. The amounts adsorbed at the knee and the final plateau depend on the pH and ionic strength of the adsorption medium. An increase in the ionic strength causes a decrease in the concentration at which the surface association process occurs, and a corresponding decrease in the area per molecule at maximum adsorption. The adsorption at the knee is also modified by changing the pH, confirming that electrostatic effects are involved at this step.

Information on the orientation/conformation of the adsorbed molecules has been obtained from a range of techniques. For example, small-angle neutron scattering (53,54) and small-angle X-ray scattering (55) have been used to calculate the segment density profile, time-resolved techniques such as ellipsometry and reflectometry have provided insights into dynamic aspects of adsorption and desorption of surfactant molecules (56,57); neutron reflectivity is sensitive to changes in the net layer thickness and the amount of surfactant adsorbed (58,59). Nuclear magnetic resonance (NMR) techniques can also be used for adsorption studies because of differences in NMR spectra between free and adsorbed surfactant, which allow quantification of the amount adsorbed (60).

Although empirical models such as the ones based on the Langmuir equation often give an approximation to the adsorption isotherms for nonionic surfactants, more complex theories that account for structural details and interactions among different components in the system are required to model adsorption of ionic surfactants. A comprehensive review of recent theoretical treatments of adsorption, which also includes a discussion of the modeling of the kinetics of surfactant adsorption at solid-liquid interfaces, has been presented by Martín-Rodriguez and Jódar-Reyes (61).

Applications and Consequences of Adsorption in Pharmaceutical Formulation

Examples of adsorption onto solid surfaces are found in many aspects of drug formulation, some of which, for example, the adsorption of surfactants and polymers in the stabilization of suspensions, will be considered elsewhere in this book. An interesting approach to the improvement of the dissolution rate of poorly water-soluble drugs is to adsorb very small amounts of surfactant onto the drug surface. For example, the adsorption of Pluronic F127 onto the surface of the hydrophobic drug phenylbutazone significantly increased its dissolution rate when compared with that of untreated material (62).

As discussed in section "Surface Active Drugs," a large number of drugs are amphiphilic and are readily adsorbed at solid surfaces, such as the surfaces of containers or tubing, or onto suspended particles in solution. Adsorption isotherms are generally Langmuirian when the adsorbent is uncharged as, for example, with the adsorption of sulfonamides (63), barbiturates (64), phenothiazines (65), and antidepressants (66) onto carbon black. In the limited number of adsorption studies in which the adsorbent was charged, departure from Langmuirian behavior was reported (67,68).

Abe et al. (69) reported Freundlich isotherms for the adsorption of local anesthetics onto activated carbon, with good correlation between the Freundlich adsorption constant, $1/n$ (related to the extent of adsorption), and the molecular weight of the local anesthetics, signifying an increase in adsorption as the molecules became more hydrophobic.

As might be anticipated, pH has a marked effect on the adsorption of ionizable amphiphilic drugs, mainly through its effect on ionization and solubility of the drug. Solubility is an important factor affecting adsorption; as a general rule, the extent of adsorption of a solute is inversely proportional to its solubility in the solvent from which adsorption occurs (Lundelius' rule). For simple molecules, adsorption increases as the ionization of the drug is suppressed (and therefore its solubility decreased), the extent of adsorption reaching a maximum when the drug is completely unionized. This effect is well illustrated for the sorption of benzocaine onto nylon 6 powder, which shows a good fit of the sorption data by the drug dissociation curve (70). For amphoteric compounds, adsorption is at a maximum at the isoelectric point, that is, when the compound bears a net charge of zero.

In general, pH and solubility effects act in concert, since the unionized form of most drugs in aqueous solution has a low solubility. Of the two effects, the solubility effect is usually the stronger. Thus, in the adsorption of hyoscine and atropine on magnesium trisilicate, it was noted (71) that hyoscine, although in its completely unionized form, was less strongly adsorbed than atropine, which at the pH of the experiment was 50% ionized. The reason for this apparently anomalous result is clear when the solubilities of the two bases are considered. Hyoscine base is freely soluble (1 in 9.5 parts of water at 15°C) compared with atropine base (1 in 400 parts of water at 20°C). Even when 50% ionized, atropine is less soluble than hyoscine and consequently more strongly adsorbed.

Unfortunately, in addition to the beneficial use of surfactants in the preparation of formulations, problems can arise as a result of inadvertent adsorption occurring both in the manufacture and storage of the product and in its subsequent usage. Problems can result from the adsorption of medicaments by adsorbents such as antacids, which may be taken simultaneously by the patient or, in some cases, may be present in the same formulation. Problems also arise from the adsorption of medicaments onto the container walls. Containers for medicaments, whether glass or plastic, may adsorb a significant quantity of the drug, bacteriostatic or fungistatic agents present in the formulation, and thereby affect the potency and possibly the stability of the product. The problem is particularly significant where the drug is highly surface active and present in low concentration. With plastic containers, the process is often referred to as sorption rather than adsorption, since it often involves significant penetration of the drug into the polymer matrix. Plastics are a large and varied group of materials, and various additives, such as plasticizers, fillers, and stabilizers often modify their properties. Such additives may have a pronounced effect on the sorption characteristics of the plastics. The sorption of the fungistatic agent, sorbic acid, from aqueous solution by plastic cellulose acetate and cellulose triacetate shows an appreciable pH dependence; the sorption declining to zero in the vicinity of the point of maximum ionization of the sorbic acid (72). The sorption of local anesthetics by polyamide and polyethylene depends on the kind of plastic, the reaction conditions, and the chemical structure of the drugs. As with sorbic acid, significant sorption was only observed when the drugs were in their unionized forms (73).

MICELLIZATION

Micelle Formation in Aqueous Solution

As the concentration of surfactants in aqueous solution is increased, a concentration is reached when the surface tension reaches an almost constant value (see sect. "Surface and Interfacial Tension"). Similar abrupt changes in other physical properties of the solution such as the osmotic pressure, conductivity, and light-scattering intensity are noted (Fig. 17). The concentration at which such inflections occur is the CMC and is attributable to the self-association of the amphiphile into small aggregates called micelles. At the CMC, there is a change from a solution containing single surfactant molecules or ions (monomers) to one at higher concentrations containing monomers and micelles in equilibrium. As the surfactant concentration is increased above the CMC, the monomer concentration remains at the CMC value, the additional surfactant appearing in micellar form. It is important to note that the change in physical properties at the CMC occurs over a narrow concentration range rather than at a precise point, but generally it becomes more well-defined with increase in micelle size. The CMC value measured for a particular surfactant may be dependent on the physical property that is measured, particularly for small micelles, and there are systematic differences between the various techniques for determining the CMC (74), depending, for example, on whether the technique is sensitive to changes in monomer concentration (as in surface tension techniques) or micelle concentration (as in light scattering).

The primary reason for micelle formation, as with all spontaneous processes, is the attainment of a state of minimum free energy. At low concentration, amphiphiles can achieve an adequate decrease in the overall free energy of the system by accumulation at the surface or interface, in such a way as to remove the hydrophobic group from the

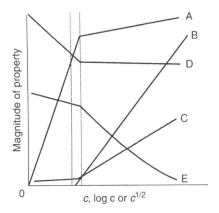

Figure 17 Solution properties of an ionic surfactant as a function of concentration, c. (**A**) osmotic pressure (against c); (**B**) solubility of a water-insoluble solubilizate (against c); (**C**) intensity of light scattered by the solution (against c); (**D**) surface tension (against log c); (**E**) molar conductivity (against $\sqrt{c}$).

aqueous environment. As the concentration is increased, this method of free energy reduction becomes inadequate, and the monomers form into micelles. The hydrophobic groups form the core of the micelle and so are shielded from the water. The free energy change of a system is dependent on changes in both the entropy, ΔS, and enthalpy, ΔH; that is, $\Delta G = \Delta H - T\Delta S$. For a micellar system at normal temperatures, the entropy term is by far the most important in determining the free energy changes ($T\Delta S$ constitutes approximately 90–95% of the ΔG value). Micelle formation entails the transfer of a hydrocarbon chain from an aqueous to a nonaqueous environment (the interior of the micelle). Water may be thought of as a mixture of structured (or ice-like) regions and free water molecules. A nonpolar molecule or portion of a molecule tends to seek out the more ice-like regions within the water, which contain open structures into which the nonpolar molecules may fit without breaking hydrogen bonds or otherwise disturbing the surrounding ice-like material. In solution, therefore, hydrophobic molecules tend always to be surrounded by structured water, and it is the changes in the water structure around the nonpolar groups that play an important role in the formation of bonds between the nonpolar molecules—the so-called *hydrophobic bonds*. When the nonpolar groups approach each other, until they are in contact, there will be a decrease in the total number of water molecules in contact with the nonpolar groups. The formation of the hydrophobic bond in this way is thus equivalent to the partial removal of hydrocarbon from an aqueous environment and a consequent loss of the ice-like structuring surrounding the hydrophobic molecules. The increase in entropy and decrease in free energy, which accompany the loss of structuring, make the formation of the hydrophobic bond an energetically favorable process. There is much experimental evidence to support this explanation for the decrease in ΔG: the enthalpy of micelle formation becomes more negative as the temperature is increased as a consequence of a concomitant reduction in water structure; NMR measurements indicate an increase in the mobility of water protons at the onset of micellization, and the addition of urea, a water-structure-breaking compound, to surfactant solutions leads to an increase in CMC, again indicating the role of water structure in the micellization process. It has been suggested that an additional contributory factor to free energy decrease on micellization arises from an increase in internal freedom of the hydrocarbon chains when the hydrophobic chains are transferred from the aqueous environment, where their motion is restrained by the hydrogen-bonded water molecules, to the "liquid-like" interior of the micelle—a process that will be accompanied by an increase in entropy.

Micelles are in dynamic equilibrium with each other and with the molecularly dispersed amphiphiles present in solutions and should not be thought of as "frozen" objects. It is this fact that distinguishes micellar solutions from other types of colloidal solutions, and the difference is emphasized by referring to micelle-forming compounds as *association colloids*. Micelles undergo various spontaneous processes occurring on a time scale ranging from seconds to nanoseconds. The two most important processes are the intermicellar exchanges, through which monomers are exchanged between micelles, and the micelle formation and breakup. The kinetics of micelle formation and breakup have been examined using chemical relaxation techniques, essentially the ultrasonic absorption, temperature-jump, and pressure-jump methods (including the shock-tube method) (75,76). The results have shown the existence of two relaxation processes that have been attributed to the intermicellar surfactant exchange (fast process with relaxation times typically of the order of nanoseconds) and to the micelle formation and breakup (slow process with relaxation times in the millisecond range). The quantitative analysis of the experimental chemical relaxation data using expressions derived by Aniansson and Wall (77) permitted the determination of the first values of the rate constants for the surfactant entry (association or incorporation) into, and exit (dissociation) from, micelles. A detailed review of the kinetics of micellization and related processes has been presented by Zana (78).

Association Models

Micelle formation is generally discussed in terms of either a phase separation model or a mass action model, although many more realistic, and necessarily more complex, models have been proposed [(see, e.g., the review by Maeda (79)].

In the phase separation model, the CMC is assumed to represent the saturation concentration of the unassociated molecules, and the micelles are regarded as a distinct phase, which separates out at the CMC. Addition of surfactants above the CMC consequently affects the concentration of micelles but not the monomer concentration. Although the phase separation model is particularly simple for the interpretation of experimental observations, it is important to note important differences between micellar systems and conventional macroscopic phases. The micelle is not a macroscopic phase but a small system consisting of several tens or hundreds of molecules and, because of geometrical and electrostatic constraints, cannot grow indefinitely into a macroscopic phase with curved interfaces.

In the mass action approach, the micelle and associated monomers are assumed to be in an association-dissociation equilibrium to which the law of mass action may be applied. The aggregation process leading to the formation of a cationic micelle M^{p+} from N surfactant ions D^+ and $(N-p)$ firmly held counterions X^- is then described in its simplest form by

$$ND^+ + (N-p)X^- \leftrightarrows M^{p+} \tag{14}$$

An equilibrium constant K_m may be written in the usual way:

$$K_m = \frac{[M^{p+}]}{[D^+]^N [X^-]^{N-p}} \tag{15}$$

where concentrations (denoted by square brackets) rather than activity coefficients have been used for each of the component species. The analogous equation for the equilibrium constant for the formation of nonionic micelles is of a simpler form, since counterion terms and charges need not be considered

$$K_m = \frac{[M]}{[D]^N} \tag{16}$$

Equations 15 and 16 are important in that they can be used to predict the variation of both monomers and micelles with total solution concentration. Figure 18 shows the fraction of added surfactant that goes into the micelle as a function of the total surfactant concentration for different aggregation numbers N (average numbers of surfactant molecules per micelle). It is clear from this figure that the inflection point at the CMC becomes more abrupt with increase in N, and for very high aggregation numbers, the two theoretical approaches are similar, both predicting a sudden stepwise change at the CMC. More complex versions of the mass action model have been proposed, for example, the Burchfield and Woolley mass action model of association (80), which is based on the Guggenheim equations for the activity coefficients of mixed electrolyte solutions, and have been successfully applied in the modeling of micellar association.

Actual micelles are not all of the same size as assumed in the mass action model, and it is more realistic, but impractical for anything but very small micelles, to consider micelle

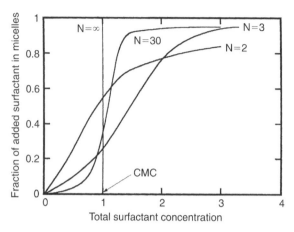

Figure 18 The fraction of added surfactant that forms micelles as a function of the total surfactant concentration for different aggregation numbers, N, as indicated.

growth in terms of a stepwise addition of monomers in a *multiple equilibrium* model, each step in the growth being associated with its own individual equilibrium constant. The distribution of aggregate sizes in a typical micellar system is bimodal with one peak in the region of the monomers, and possibly including some dimers and trimers, the other peak being in the region of the mean aggregation number. The half-width of this second micellar region is, of course, a measure of the polydispersity of the system. In the multiple equilibrium model, micellization is regarded as a multistep process involving a series of equilibria

$$A_1 + A_1 \xleftrightarrow{K_2} A_2$$

$$A_1 + A_2 \xleftrightarrow{K_3} A_3$$

$$A_1 + A_3 \xleftrightarrow{K_4} A_4 \qquad\qquad (17)$$

$$\cdots\cdots\cdots\cdots\cdots$$

$$A_1 + A_{N-1} \xleftrightarrow{K_N} A_N$$

which, in theory, could result in a wide range of micelle sizes in solution. Each of the steps represented in the above equation will be associated with a particular equilibrium constant K_N. It is the particular dependence of K_N on N that defines the type of association.

The fact that, within the limitation of experimental technique, most micellar systems would appear reasonably monodisperse suggests a specific relationship between K_N and N in which during the early stages of the growth of the micelles, K_N increases with N (cooperativity) and then eventually decreases (anticooperativity) so that the K_N against N plot shows a maximum at the mean micellar size. This type of self-association, which leads to the formation of aggregates of uniform size, is termed "closed association" and may be rationalized in terms of the factors that promote and inhibit the growth of aggregates. As discussed earlier, the impetus for micelle formation derives mainly from the entropic changes accompanying the transfer of hydrocarbon from an aqueous environment to the micelle interior. It is readily shown that the efficiency of shielding the hydrocarbon group from water, as monomer is added to the micelle, increases with micelle size. On the basis of hydrophobic interaction alone, an increase in K_N with N would be expected. The factor that is responsible for the subsequent decrease in K_N and which limits the micelle size arises from the progressive increase in the density of the head groups at the micelle surface as the micelle size increases. In the case of nonionic surfactants, this increased density results in an increased crowding at the surface, and with ionic surfactants, in increased charge repulsion between head groups.

The manner in which K_N varies with aggregate size defines the association pattern. In a typical micellar system, the K_N values in the intermediate region between the initial monomer peak and the peak representing the micelle are thought to be of insignificant magnitude. There are, however, a limited number of amphiphilic systems in which this is not so, and several empirical relationships between K_N and N have been considered to model the open or continuous association of such systems. For example, early work in defining models to describe open association focused on the self-association of cationic dyes such as methylene blue, which could be successfully described using a stepwise association model in which all the equilibrium constants were assumed to be of equal value, that is, $K_2 = K_3 = K_4 = K_N = K$. (81). In later work by Attwood and coworkers (82–84), cooperative and anti-cooperative models have been used to describe the self-association of amphiphilic drugs. These include, for example, a cooperative model in which K_N increases with N according to

$$K_N = K(N - 1)/N \qquad N \geq 2 \tag{18}$$

that is, $K_2 = K/2$, $K_3 = 2K/3$ and so on, where K is a global equilibrium constant; anti-cooperative models such as

$$K_N = KN/(N - 1) \tag{19}$$

which are mildly anti-cooperative, and

$$K_N = K/N \tag{20}$$

in which the equilibrium constants decrease rapidly with increase in aggregate size.

Association of Amphiphilic Drugs

The type of association exhibited by a particular amphiphilic drug is particularly important because of the relatively low drug concentrations present in vivo following administration. In open association, there is a tendency for aggregates to form in very dilute solution and increase in size with increasing concentration, often leading to a high degree of polydispersity of aggregate sizes. As a consequence, it is not unreasonable to assume that the biological activity of the drug might be affected due to decreased transport rates or decreased ability of the associated molecules to pass through biological barriers. In closed association, micelles are formed at a CMC, which for these ionic molecules is much higher than that normally encountered in vivo following administration of the drug. It is possible, however, that accumulation of drug molecules in certain sites in the body may cause a localized high concentration, resulting in aggregation and consequent changes in biological activity. Consequently, it is equally important to characterize the micellar properties of drugs with a closed association pattern. The biological and pharmaceutical implications of drug association have been reviewed (1).

Mukerjee (85,86) identified several aspects of molecular structure that are thought to be influential in determining the association pattern of hydrophobic solutes. Features that are seen to be requirements for a micellar mode of association are a high degree of molecular flexibility and a clear separation of charge, creating distinct polar and nonpolar ends. Rigid aromatic or heteroaromatic ring or fused ring structures with no identifiable polar or nonpolar regions, such as the cationic dyes and the purines and pyrimidines associate by a face-to-face stacking in a continuous association pattern. Amphiphilic drugs represent an interesting intermediate group of compounds between these two extremes. Although the hydrophobic groups of most drugs are aromatic, they may have a high degree of flexibility in some cases, and as a consequence, these drugs may resemble typical surfactants in their association behavior. Flexibility of the hydrophobic group as in, for example, the large number of drugs with a diphenylmethane structure, such as diphenhydramine and orphenadrine (Table 6), is conducive to closed or micellar association. The application of static light-scattering techniques to aqueous solutions of these drugs has yielded aggregation numbers that are typically in the region 9 to 12 in the absence of added electrolyte (87). Association commences at a well-defined CMC, and can be modeled using mass action theory. However, when the phenyl rings are linked together to form a more rigid moiety, as for example in drugs with tricyclic hydrophobic ring systems, there is often a change to a continuous (or open) association pattern characterized by the lack of an inflection in the concentration dependence of the static light-scattering intensity (88,89).

However, although a lack of flexibility of the hydrophobic moiety is a necessary criterion for continuous association, it is clearly not the only structural requirement, since many rigid, planar, tricyclic drug molecules have been shown to exhibit inflections in their solution properties at well-defined critical concentrations. This group of drugs, which includes the tricyclic antidepressants and the phenothiazine tranquillizers, differs from the cationic dyes in that their charge is generally localized at a terminal group of a relatively long side chain rather than being delocalized in the ring system as is common with dye molecules. The association pattern in water and dilute electrolyte is complex, with discontinuities in solution properties at several critical concentrations (90). Evidence from a variety of experimental techniques indicates limited association in dilute solution leading to the formation of a stable aggregate at the first critical concentration. NMR studies of the changes in the chemical shifts of aromatic protons and carbon atoms over a wide concentration range have suggested an offset, concave-to- convex vertical stacking of the molecules within these aggregates, with the alkyl side chains on alternate sides of the stack (91) as illustrated in Figure 19. The association of several phenothiazines in the presence of high concentrations of added electrolyte (0.2–0.8 mol/kg sodium chloride) has been described by an association scheme in which a primary unit of three to four monomers is formed below the critical concentration by a continuous association process and grows with increasing solution concentration by the stepwise addition of monomers (92).

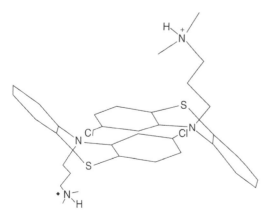

Figure 19 Schematic representation of the stacking of two molecules of chlorpromazine. *Source*: From Ref. 91.

More detailed accounts of the relationship between the molecular structure of the drug molecule, particularly that of its hydrophobic group, and the mode of association in aqueous solution are given in reviews by Attwood (82–84).

Micelle Structure

The Critical Packing Parameter

The shape of the micelle formed by a particular surfactant is influenced to a large extent by the geometry of the surfactant molecule, as can be seen by a consideration of the packing of space-filling models of the surfactants. If the micelle is regarded as a sphere with a core composed of the hydrocarbon chains of the constituent molecules, then the maximum radius must approximate to that of the fully extended alkyl chain. Exceeding this value would create a void in the micelle center or require that some of the molecules would not be anchored at the micelle surface; neither are feasible options. On this premise, it is a simple matter to characterize the limiting conditions for the formation of spherical micelles in terms of the molecular characteristics of the constituent surfactant molecules. The aggregation number N can be expressed as the ratio between the volume of the micelle core V_{mic} and the volume v of one chain, that is, $N = V_{mic}/v = 4\pi r_{mic}^3/3v$, where r_{mic} is the radius of the micelle. In addition, the aggregation number can be expressed as the ratio between the surface area of the micelle A_{mic} and the cross-sectional area a of the surfactant head group, that is, $N = A_{mic}/a = 4\pi r_{mic}^2/a$. Equating these two expressions for N gives $v/r_{mic}a = 1/3$, and since r_{mic} cannot exceed the extended length l_c of the surfactant alkyl chain, $v/(l_c a) \leq 1/3$. The dimensionless parameter $v/(l_c a)$ is called the *critical packing parameter* (CPP) and is useful when considering the structure of the aggregate that will be formed in solution by a given amphiphile as illustrated in Figure 20.

Surfactants composed of a single hydrophobic chain and a simple ionic or large nonionic head group have a CPP $\leq 1/3$ and form spherical micelles. It is easily seen that if v is doubled by adding a second alkyl chain, then the value of CPP will exceed $1/3$ and nonspherical structures such as bilayers (CPP ≈ 1) will form in solution, from which vesicles are formed (see sect. "Lamellar Phase"). One important factor not considered in this simple geometrical model is the interaction between the head groups in the aggregate. The "effective" cross-sectional area of the surfactant molecule is strongly influenced by the interaction forces between adjacent head groups in the micelle surface. These forces are decreased by addition of electrolyte leading to a decrease in a, an increase in the CPP, and a change in the shape of the aggregate, as discussed below.

In nonaqueous media, reversed (or inverted) micelles may form in which the hydrophilic charge groups form the micellar core shielded from the nonaqueous environment by the hydrophobic chains; such structures are generally formed when CPP > 1 (Fig. 20).

Ionic Micelles

Ionic micelles of low aggregation number have a CPP < 1/3 and consequently adopt a spherical or near-spherical shape at concentrations not too far removed from the CMC. The hydrophobic part of the amphiphile is located in the core or the micelle and is surrounded by a concentric shell of hydrophilic head groups referred to as the *Stern layer* (Fig. 21), which contains $(1-\alpha)N$ counterions, where α is the degree of ionization. For most ionic micelles, the degree of ionization α is between 0.2 and 0.3; that is, 70% to 80% of the counterions may be considered to be bound to the micelles. The outer surface of the Stern layer is the shear surface of the micelle, and the core and the Stern layer together constitute what is termed the "kinetic micelle." Surrounding the Stern layer is a diffuse

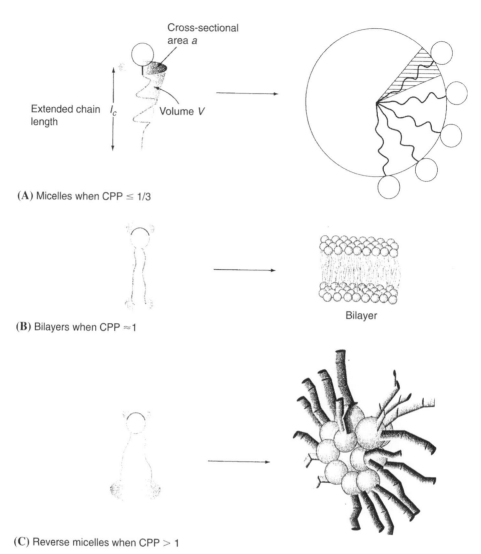

(A) Micelles when CPP ≤ 1/3

(B) Bilayers when CPP ≈1

Bilayer

(C) Reverse micelles when CPP > 1

Figure 20 The critical packing parameter, CPP $= v/(l_c\ a)$ and its influence on the type of aggregates formed by surfactants in solution.

layer called the *Gouy-Chapman electrical double layer* that contains the αN counterions required to neutralize the charge on the kinetic micelle. The thickness of the double layer is dependent on the ionic strength of the solution and is greatly compressed in the presence of electrolyte.

Nonionic Micelles

Nonionic micelles have a hydrophobic core surrounded by a shell of oxyethylene chains, which is often termed the "palisade layer" or "corona" (Fig. 22). This layer is capable of mechanically entrapping a considerable number of water molecules, as well as those that are hydrogen bonded to the oxyethylene chains. Micelles of nonionic surfactants tend, as a consequence, to be highly hydrated. The outer surface of the palisade layer forms the shear surface; that is, the hydrating molecules form part of the kinetic micelle.

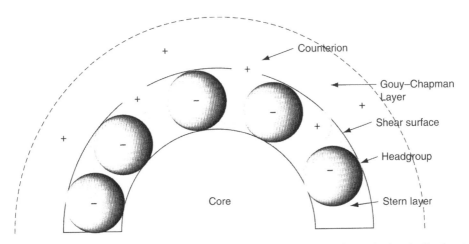

Figure 21 Diagrammatic representation of a partial cross section of an anionic micelle showing charged layers.

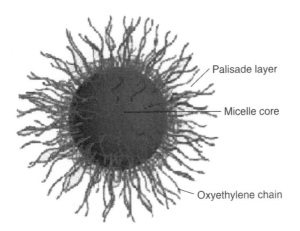

Figure 22 Diagrammatic representation of the cross section of a nonionic micelle.

As discussed in section "Nonionic Surfactants" AB block copolymers, where A is a hydrophilic block (usually oxyethylene) and B is a hydrophobic block, have a similar architecture to C_nE_m nonionic surfactants (where C is an alkyl chain and E is an oxyethylene group) and form a similar type of core-shell micelle. In contrast, ABA triblock copolymers such as the poloxamers ($E_mP_nE_m$ where the hydrophobic block is oxypropylene P) form micelles in which the hydrophobic block is looped in the core (Fig. 23), effectively halving the diameter of the core compared with an AB diblock of identical hydrophobic chain length. As a result, the core volume (proportional to radius^3) of an AB diblock is approximately eight times (2^3) that of the equivalent ABA triblock, with consequences for the relative solubilization capacities of these block copolymers as discussed in section "Solubilization." In addition, triblock copolymers have CMCs approximately two orders of magnitude higher than the equivalent diblock copolymers. The effect is as expected and originates in the lower entropy of the triblock chains constrained by two block junctions in the core-fringe interface of the micelle compared with only one constraint for the diblock chain.

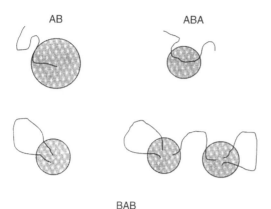

Figure 23 Schematic representation of chain conformations in micelles formed from AB diblock and ABA and BAB triblock copolymers.

Micelles formed by BAB triblock copolymers in dilute solution have their E blocks looped in the micelle corona (Fig. 23). As concentration is increased, transient bridging by chains with hydrophobic end blocks leads to molecular and micellar clusters.

Factors Influencing Micelle Properties

The CMC of surfactants, whether ionic or nonionic, is determined by the overall hydrophobicity of the surfactant molecule; changes in molecular structure that lead to an increased hydrophobicity will cause a decrease of the CMC and, conversely, changes that increase the hydrophilicity will increase the CMC. The CMC of surfactants that have hydrophobic groups constructed from hydrocarbon chains decreases with increase in the length of this chain, and for compounds with identical polar head groups, this relationship is expressed by the linear equation:

$$\log \text{CMC} = A - Bn$$

where n is the number of carbon atoms in the chain and A and B are constants for a homologous series. A corresponding increase in micellar size with increase in hydrocarbon chain length is also observed.

In general, nonionic surfactants have much lower CMC values and higher aggregation numbers than their ionic counterparts with similar hydrocarbon chains, mainly because the micellization process for such compounds does not involve any electrical work. The CMCs of the polyoxyethylated nonionic surfactants are increased when the poly(oxyethylene) chain length is increased as a consequence of the increased hydrophilicity.

The counterion associated with the charged group of ionic surfactants has a significant effect on the micellar properties, particularly on the micelle size. There is an increase in micelle size for a particular cationic surfactant as the counterion is changed according to the series $Cl^- < Br^- < I^-$, and for a particular anionic surfactant according to $Na^+ < K^+ < Cs^+$. Generally, the more weakly hydrated a counterion, the larger the micelles formed by the surfactant. This is because the weakly hydrated ions can be adsorbed more readily in the micellar surface and so decrease the charge repulsion between the polar groups. A lower CMC and larger micelles are observed with organic counterions, such as maleates, than with inorganic ions.

Addition of electrolytes to ionic surfactants decreases the CMC and increases the micellar size; electrolyte has very little effect on nonionic surfactants as might be expected. The effect is simply explained in terms of a reduction in the magnitude of the forces of repulsion between the charged head groups in the micelle and a consequent decrease in the electrical work of micellization.

Shape Transitions

On the simple assumption that the micelle radius is limited by the maximum extension of the alkyl chain, it is possible, using density values for the relevant hydrocarbons, to estimate maximum aggregation numbers consistent with the existence of spherical micelles as a function of alkyl chain length for both ionic and nonionic surfactants (93) and so gain an insight into the probable micelle shape. Eisenberg and coworkers stressed the importance of taking into account such differences in morphology, that is, whether micelle is spherical or cylindrical, when optimizing drug delivery vehicles (94).

As discussed above, the size and shape of block copolymers depend on the block architecture. Comparison of the aggregation numbers, N, of AB diblock and ABA triblock copolymers at a given B-block length shows a ratio of N (diblock) to N (triblock) of approximately 8. Looping in the core of the ABA copolymers effectively halves the maximum length of their core chains and thereby the maximum possible radius of the core. The value of N (diblock) to N (triblock) $\approx$ 8 simply reflects this geometric restriction. Cylindrical diblock copolymer micelles are favored if the E blocks are short (leading to high-association numbers) and the hydrophobic blocks are short (placing a low ceiling on the radius of a spherical micelle). Careful choice of the relative hydrophilic and hydrophobic block lengths of diblock copolymers can result in the formation of wormlike micelles, as for example, occurs with the diblock copolymers $E_{11}B_8$ (95), $E_{13}B_{10}$ (96), $E_{17}B_{12}$ (B = oxybutylene) (97), and $E_{17}S_8$ (S denotes an oxyphenylethylene unit from polymerization of styrene oxide) (98). Wormlike micelles are of interest from a formulation point of view because of their high solubilization capacities for poorly water-soluble drugs, as will be discussed in section "Solubilization."

Factors such as concentration, temperature, and electrolyte can have an appreciable influence on micelle shape, often leading to a change of micelle shape from spherical to more asymmetrical form. The CPP of nonionic surfactants increases progressively with increasing temperature, suggesting closer packing of head groups at the micelle surface at higher temperatures, attributable to a decrease in the hydration of the oxyethylene chains as water becomes a poorer solvent for poly(oxyethylene) with increase of temperature. As a consequence, the aggregation number increases, and there is often a transition from spherical to cylindrical micelles when the radius of the core exceeds the stretched length of the hydrophobic block. Further increase of temperature results in increased turbidity of the solution at a well-defined temperature referred to as the *cloud point* and phase separation into one surfactant-rich and one surfactant-poor solution. The process is reversible, clarity being restored on cooling. Similar transitions from spherical to cylindrical micelles are noted with block copolymers, the most widely investigated being the poloxamers $E_{27}P_{39}E_{27}$ (P85) and $E_{21}P_{47}E_{21}$ (P94) (2). Similarly, a dramatic increase of micelle size is observed with a series of EB diblock copolymers as the temperature is raised above onset temperatures of approximately 15°C, 20°C, and 30°C for, respectively, $E_{17}B_{12}$, $E_{13}B_{10}$, and $E_{11}B_8$ in dilute aqueous solution (96). Spherical to asymmetrical micelle transitions are frequently observed on increasing the concentration in solutions of both ionic and nonionic surfactants. For example, flexible, rodlike aggregates of cetyltrimethylammonium chloride are observed at a concentration of approximately

0.15 M (99,100). The nature of the head group can have an appreciable effect on the extent to which the micelle grows. With the alkyl sulfates, for example, growth is negligible with Li^+ counterions, moderate with Na^+, but very pronounced with K^+ or Cs^+. Even more dramatic growth, occurring at low concentration, is observed when the surfactant counterions are organic. In general, micelle growth with increasing concentration is very pronounced for nonionic surfactants with poly(oxyethylene) chain lengths of 4 to 6 oxyethylene units, and almost negligible when the chain length is >8 units. In sufficiently high electrolyte concentration, the reduction of head group interaction at the surface of ionic micelles allows significant growth of the micelles such that spherical micelles can no longer form, and a transition to rodlike micelles occurs. For example, such a transition in solutions of SDS at concentrations well above the CMC is noted when the concentration of added sodium chloride exceeds 0.45 M (101).

SOLUBILIZATION

As discussed above, the micellar core is essentially a paraffin-like region and as such provides a reservoir in which lipophilic molecules may dissolve. The process whereby poorly water-soluble substances are brought into solution by incorporation into micelles is termed "solubilization" and has for many years been studied as a method of improving the water solubility of poorly soluble drug candidates, particularly in formulations intended for oral or parenteral administration [see review by Attwood and Florence (1)].

Site of Solubilization

The site of solubilization within the micelle is closely related to the chemical nature of the solubilizate (Fig. 24). It is generally accepted that nonpolar solubilizates (e.g., aliphatic

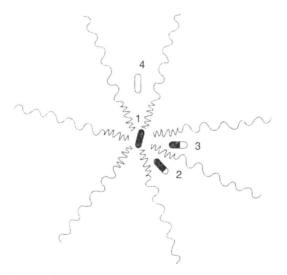

Figure 24 Schematic representation of sites of solubilization depending on the hydrophobicity of the solubilizate. Completely water-insoluble hydrophobic molecules are incorporated in the micelle core (*case 1*); water-soluble molecules may be solubilized in the polyoxyethylene shell of a nonionic micelle (*case 4*); solubilizates with intermediate hydrophobicities (*cases 2 and 3*) are incorporated in the micelle with the hydrophobic region (*black*) in the core and the hydrophilic region (*white*) at the micelle-water interface.

hydrocarbons) are dissolved in the hydrocarbon core of ionic and nonionic micelles. Water-insoluble compounds containing polar groups are oriented with the polar group at the core-surface interface of the micelle, and the hydrophobic group buried inside the hydrocarbon core of the micelle. In addition, solubilization in nonionic polyoxyethylated surfactants and block copolymers can occur in the poly(oxyethylene) shell (corona or palisade layer), which surrounds the core.

Except for very water-insoluble compounds, solubilization in micellar solutions of surfactants can be regarded as a partition phenomenon, similar to that of octanol/water partitioning. A direct relationship between the lipophilicity of the solubilizate, expressed by the partition coefficient between octanol and water, $P_{octanol}$, and its partitioning between micelles and the aqueous phase, P_m, has been noted for the solubilization of substituted barbituric acids by poly(oxyethylene) stearates (102), substituted benzoic acids by polysorbate 20 (103,104), and of several steroids by polyoxyethylated nonionic surfactants (105). An exhaustive survey of data for the solubilization of some 64 drugs by bile salt micelles revealed linear relationships between log P_m and log $P_{octanol}$ for each of seven bile salts examined (106). An important factor influencing water solubility, and hence micelle/water partitioning, is the ionization state of the drug if this is a weak electrolyte such as indomethacin. Although from a formulation viewpoint, the solubility of a particular drug in the surfactant solution is often of more importance than its location within the components of the solution, such information is of interest if a more detailed analysis of the solubilization process is required. In such cases, consideration must be given to the state of ionization of the drug in these systems when interpreting the data.

Preparation of Solubilized Systems

The method of preparation of the solubilized system can have a significant influence on the solubilization capacity (107). The simplest and most commonly used method of incorporation of the drug is the so-called "shake-flask" method in which excess solid drug is equilibrated with the micellar solution, and unsolubilized drug subsequently removed by filtration or centrifugation. Larger amounts of drug can often be solubilized by comixing the drug and copolymer at elevated temperature (typically about 60°C) and adding the resultant intimate mixture to water or buffer to form the solubilized micellar solution; a method often referred to as "melt loading." Other methods, including dialysis, solvent evaporation, and cosolvent evaporation methods, involve the use of nonaqueous solvents to dissolve the drug and copolymer. In the dialysis method, drug and copolymer are dissolved in a water-miscible organic solvent followed by dialysis against water until the organic phase is replaced with water. In the solvent evaporation method, the drug and copolymer are dissolved in volatile organic solvents that are allowed to evaporate at room temperature; the resultant dried drug/copolymer film is then pulverized and dispersed in water. Alternatively, a micellar solution is formed by adding water slowly to a solution of drug and polymer in a water-miscible organic solvent (cosolvent) and removing the organic solvent by evaporation (cosolvent evaporation method). In a variation of this method, an oil-in-water emulsion is formed by mixing the organic solvent containing dissolved drug with an aqueous solution of the copolymer; the volatile solvent is then allowed to evaporate leaving the solubilized micellar solution.

Influence of Micelle Structure on Solubilization Capacity

Nonionic surfactants, rather than ionic surfactants, are generally considered to be more suitable for pharmaceutical usage, not only because of their lower toxicity but also because the poly(oxyethylene) shell can confer stealth properties to the micelle, allowing them to avoid uptake by macrophages of the reticular endothelial system, so prolonging their lifetime in the blood circulation. Moreover, a low CMC confers stability to the micelles on dilution, allowing them to circulate in the blood stream for sufficient time to accumulate at tumor sites after intravenous injection, by the enhanced permeability and retention (EPR) effect. Despite these potential advantages, however, micellar solubilization finds comparatively little current commercial application as a means of enhancing the uptake into solution of drug candidates, except for very potent drugs such as testosterone, because of the low solubilization capacity of those micellar systems that have received regulatory approval for pharmaceutical use.

Many studies have focused on the elucidation of structural features of the surfactant molecule that affect solubilization capacity, with the aim of designing more effective micelles for the solubilization of poorly soluble drugs. In cases where the solubilizate is located within the core or deep within the micelle structure, the solubilization capacity increases with increase in alkyl chain length as might be expected. Table 7 clearly shows an increase in solubilizing capacity of a series of polysorbates for selected barbiturates as the alkyl chain length is increased from C_{12} (Polysorbate 20) to C_{18} (Polysorbate 80) (102).

Similar effects have been noted for the solubilization of barbiturates in poly(oxyethylene) surfactants with the general structure $CH_3(CH_2)_n(OCH_2CH_2)_mOH$ with increasing alkyl chain length, n (108). There is a limit, however, to the improvement of solubilizing capacity caused by increase in alkyl chain length in this way; an increase in n from 16 to 22, although producing larger micelles, does not result in a corresponding increase in solubilization (109). For solubilizates incorporated in the micelle core, it might be expected that solubilization capacity would decrease with increase in ethylene oxide block length, because of a concomitant decrease in micelle size. Table 8, which shows the solubilization capacity of a series of $C_{16}E_m$ polyoxyethylated nonionic surfactants for several steroidal drugs (110), illustrates this effect, and also highlights one of the problems associated with the interpretation of solubilization data. Although this table shows a decrease in the aggregation number with increase in the hydrophilic chain length and a corresponding decrease in the number of steroid molecules solubilized per micelle, there is in fact an increase in the total amount solubilized per mole of surfactant (number of steroid molecules per micelle × number of micelles per mole) because of the increasing number of micelles.

Table 7 Solubilizing Capacity of Polysorbates for the Barbiturates at 30°C

Drug	Surfactant	Solubility (mg drug per g surfactant)
Phenobarbital	Polysorbate 20	55
	Polysorbate 40	61
	Polysorbate 60	63
	Polysorbate 80	66
Amobarbital	Polysorbate 20	32
	Polysorbate 40	38
	Polysorbate 80	40
Secobarbital	Polysorbate 20	111
	Polysorbate 80	144

Source: From Ref. 102.

Table 8 Micellar Solubilization Parameters for Steroids in n-alkyl Polyoxyethylene Surfactants C_nE_m (where n = alkyl chain length and m = polyoxyethylene chain length) at 25°C

Surfactant	Aggregation number	Micelles per mole ($\times 10^{-21}$)	Steroid molecules per micelle			
			Hydro-cortisone	Dexa-methasone	Testo-sterone	Proge-sterone
$C_{16}E_{17}$	99	6.1	9.1	6.7	6.0	5.6
$C_{16}E_{32}$	56	10.8	7.6	5.3	4.6	4.3
$C_{16}E_{44}$	39	15.4	5.8	4.2	3.6	3.3
$C_{16}E_{63}$	25	24.1	4.0	3.3	2.4	2.3

Source: From Ref. 110.

Similar results were observed in a study of the solubilization of the poorly water-soluble mydriatic drug tropicamide by a series of poloxamers (111). There was an increase in solubilization with increase in the oxyethylene content of the poloxamer when the data were expressed as moles of tropicamide per mole of poloxamer, but when expressed as the moles of drug solubilized per ethylene oxide unit of the poloxamer, however, the solubilization capacity decreased with increasing ethylene oxide chain length. Again, the reason for this decrease is that the micellar size per ethylene oxide equivalent decreases with increasing length of the ethylene oxide chain.

Design of Micelles with High Solubilization Capacity

It is probably with the amphiphilic block copolymers, and particularly those with poly(oxyethylene) as the hydrophilic block and with poly(oxyalkylene) or polyester hydrophobic blocks, that most recent progress has been made in designing micelles that are capable of accommodating a range of water-insoluble guest molecules, and the reader is directed to many recent articles that review progress in this area (94,107, 112–123). Comparison of reported data with a view to the determination of those factors that are responsible for enhanced solubilization capacity is complicated by a lack of uniformity of the method of data presentation and often by the fact that saturation solubilities of the micelles were not determined. In addition, as already discussed, the method of preparation of the solubilized system and the state of ionization of the drug are important factors influencing solubilization capacity, which need to be known for a reliable comparison of data. Nevertheless, some generalizations have been possible for solubilization by copolymers with poly(oxyethylene) as the hydrophilic block and with poly(oxyalkylene) or polyester hydrophobic blocks (122). Table 9 shows the solubilization capacities of a selection of Pluronic polyols. In general, the enhancement ratios S/S_0 (where S is the solubility of the drug in the copolymer micelles expressed as milligram per gram of copolymer and S_0 is the solubility in aqueous solution under similar conditions) for solutions at 25°C are in the range of 1 to 3, with a maximum value of 6. This relatively low ability of the Pluronic polyols to solubilize water-insoluble drugs is in part a consequence of their limited micellization at room temperature. Although any micelles formed at ambient temperature may be large, they are few in number, and this is reflected in the poor solubilizing capacity. This effect is clearly demonstrated by Molpeceres et al. (124) in a study of the solubilization of cyclosporine A by Pluronic F68 in which solubilization was noted only at a temperature of 50°C, which corresponds to the lowest temperature at which micelles of this

Table 9 Solubilization Capacities of EPE Copolymers

Drug	T (°C)	S_0 (mg/dL)	Copolymer[a]	CMT (°C) (1 wt%)	Copolymer (wt%)	Experimental method	S (mg/g)	S/S_0[b]
Allopurinol	25	78	F127	24	2.5	SF	92	1.2
Camptothecin	25	0.4	F127	24	1	D	1.4	6
Clonazepam	25	0.1	F68	50	10	SF	0.3	3
Diazepam	25	3	F108	30	6	SF	6	2
Estradiol	25	0.4	F127	24	1	SF	1.9	5
Griseofulvin	25	1.0	P94	23	1	SF	2.2	2
			P123	16	1	SF	4.0	4
			F127	24	1	SF	3.2	3
Indomethacin	37	1.0	P85	30	5	SF	1.7	2
Ketoprofen	37	11	P85	30	5	SF	13.6	1.2
Lorezapam	25	4.8	F68	50	10	SF	16	3
Pyroxicam	30	8	F98	>30	1[c]	SE	13	2
	37	3.1	P85	30	5	SF	4.0	1.3
Tropicamide	25	560	F127	24	5	SF	790	1.4

[a]Pluronic notation: see Table 4.
[b]Solubility enhancement expressed as the ratio of S = solubility per g of copolymer (equivalent to solubility in 1 dL of 1 wt% copolymer solution) to S_0 = solubility in water.
[c]Concentration of F98 was assumed to be 1 wt%.
Abbreviations: D, dialysis; SF, shake flask; SE, solvent evaporation.
Source: From Ref. 122.

copolymer are first noted [critical micelle temperature (CMT)]. The data for solubilization of indomethacin, ketoprofen, and pyroxicam by Pluronic P85 included in Table 9, and that for griseofulvin by Pluronic P123, show that even at temperatures above the CMT, the solubilization capacity is poor.

A significant improvement in solubilization capacity is noted when the polypropylene block is replaced with more hydrophobic blocks formed from 1,2-butylene oxide, styrene oxide, and phenyl glycidyl ether, all of which have CMTs well below 25°C, and hence are fully micellized at room temperature. In general, the solubilization capacity for aromatic drugs such as carbamazepine, frusemide, griseofulvin, halofantrine, nabumetone, and spironolactone increased with the hydrophobicity of this block as indicated by the CMC value (122), in line with the predicted relationships between the solubilization capacity of block copolymer micelles and the compatibility of the solubilizate with the hydrophobic block that forms the micelle core (125). As with polyoxyethylated nonionic surfactants, there is an improvement in solubilization capacity with increase in the length of the hydrophobic block for copolymers of similar composition and architecture. For example, $E_{45}S_{10}$ is a better solubilizer of griseofulvin than $E_{45}S_8$, and $E_{17}B_{12}$ was reported to solubilize larger amounts of carbamazepine and spironolactone than $E_{11}B_8$ (98). Other workers reporting similar examples of this effect are Reketas et al. (126) and Crothers et al. (98). However, the most dramatic improvement in solubilizing capacity occurs when micelles are so large that a spherical core cannot be formed and highly elongated, probably wormlike micelles are formed (see sect. "Factors Influencing Micelle Properties"). For example, the enhancement ratio S/S_0 of $E_{17}S_8$, the micelles of which are wormlike with an aggregation number of about 240 (127), is reported to be between two to five times that of other diblock copolymers of styrene oxide (128). There is also evidence from experimental work on other systems (94) of enhanced solubilization when micelles are cylindrical rather than spherical.

Much higher solubilization capacities have been observed with polyester block copolymers having poly(caprolactone) (CL), poly(valerolactone) (PVL), and poly(DL-lactide) (L) hydrophobic blocks (Table 10). Very high S/S_0 ratios are noted with the CL block copolymers, although it should be noted that the values of this ratio are dependent on the precision of S_0 values, which are usually very low for the drugs involved. However, because the long-chain hydrophobic blocks of CL are very hydrophobic, it has not been possible to use simple shake-flask techniques to prepare the solubilized systems, and solubilization methods necessitating the use of organic cosolvents and dialysis techniques are required as indicated in the table. Hence, although it is possible to achieve much higher solubilization enhancement using copolymers based on CL blocks, this does necessitate more complex (and costly) solubilization techniques.

One of the problems associated with the use of micellar solutions for drug delivery is the large dilution experienced on administration, particularly when given orally or by intravenous injection, which may potentially lead to drug precipitation. The micellar systems of block copolymers generally have low CMCs and exhibit a slow rate of micelle dissociation; nevertheless, their stability may be further increased by chemical stabilization of the hydrophobic core. For example, core stabilization of the $E_{86}L_{49}$ copolymers described by Kim et al. (129) was achieved by polymerization of a methacryloyl group attached to the poly(lactic acid) block, providing drug carrier micelles with the potential to retain their integrity under all physiological conditions. Table 10 shows that it was possible to incorporate about 45 mg of paclitaxel per gram of polymerized copolymer, which is comparable to the drug loading achieved for this drug by Zhang et al. (130) in a micellar solution of conventional $E_{45}L_{18}$.

Table 10 Solubilization Capacities of Polyesters with Caprolactone, Valerolactone, and DL-lactide Hydrophobic Blocks

Drug	T (°C)	S_0 (mg/dL)	Copolymer	Copolymer (wt%)	Experimental method	S (mg/g)	S/S_0[a]
Cyclosporin A	–	2.3	$E_{114}CL_{44}$	1	CSE	104	45
17β-Estradiol	25	0.4	$E_{45}CL_{23}$	1	D	1900	4750
Ellipticine	–	0.015	$E_{114}CL_{35}$	1	D	325	22000
			$E_{114}L_{58}$			1.2	80
Dihydrotestosterone (androstanolone)	25	0.52	$E_{44}CL_{20}$	1	D	1300	2500
Indomethacin	25	0.094	$E_{114}CL_{27}$	1	D	350	3700
Paclitaxel	25	0.05	$E_{86}L_{49}$-X[b]	1	D	45	900
			$E_{45}VL_{20}$	10	SE	92	1800
			$E_{45}L_{18}$	0.04		20	400
Testosterone	25	2.3	$E_{50}L_{23}$	0.25	SF	7	3

[a]Solubility enhancement expressed as the ratio of S = solubility per gm of copolymer (equivalent to solubility in 1 dL of 1 wt% copolymer solution) to S_0 = solubility in water.
[b]$E_{86}L_{49}$-X micelles are core polymerized.
Abbreviations: SF, shake-flask method; SE, solvent evaporation method; D, dialysis method; CSE, cosolvent evaporation method.
Source: From Ref. 122.

PHASE PROPERTIES OF SURFACTANTS

As discussed in the previous section, there is frequently a transition from the typical spherical micelle structure to a more elongated or rodlike micelle as solution concentration is increased. At concentrations well above the CMC, more ordered structuring of the solution occurs, and liquid crystalline phases (or mesophases) separate out from the remainder of the solution. The liquid crystalline phases that occur on increasing the concentration of surfactant solutions are referred to as *lyotropic* liquid crystals; their structure is shown diagrammatically in Figure 25. A typical phase diagram is shown in Figure 26 for the polyoxyethylated nonionic surfactant $C_{12}E_6$ [$CH_3(CH_2)_{11}(OCH_2CH_2)_6OH$] (131). For a comprehensive description of the phase properties of ionic and nonionic surfactants, the reader should consult reviews by Laughlin (132), Attwood and Florence (1), Tiddy (133), Chernik (134), and Khan (135).

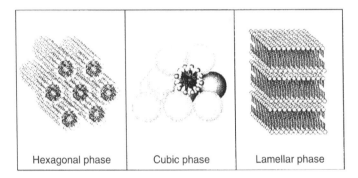

| Hexagonal phase | Cubic phase | Lamellar phase |

Figure 25 Diagrammatic representation of forms of lyotropic liquid crystals.

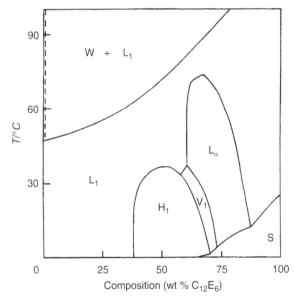

Figure 26 Phase diagram of the $CH_3(CH_2)_{11}(OCH_2CH_2)_6OH(C_{12}E_6)/H_2O$ system. L_1, isotropic micellar solution; W, very dilute surfactant solution; H_1, middle or hexagonal phase; L_α, neat or lamellar phase; V_1, normal bicontinuous cubic phase; S denotes the presence of solid. *Source*: From Ref. 131.

Hexagonal Phase

The hexagonal phase (or middle phase), H_1, is characterized by a hexagonal array of infinitely long, cylindrical micelles arranged in a hexagonal pattern, each micelle being surrounded by six others. The radius of the circular cross section is close to that of the extended length of the surfactant molecule. At even higher surfactant concentrations, a reversed (or inverted) hexagonal phase H_2 comprising hexagonally close-packed infinite water cylinders surrounded by polar heads of surfactant molecules, and a continuum of the hydrophobic parts may be observed. Several applications of the reversed hexagonal phase as a vehicle for drug delivery have been reported. For example, Norling et al. (136) have described their use in the development of a stable, sustained release formulation of an antimicrobial agent, metronidazole, to treat periodontol disease. Aqueous colloidal dispersions of reversed hexagonal phase have been prepared using either glyceryl monooleate (GMO, monoolein)/sunflower oil or GMO/retinyl palmitate surfactant mixtures sterically stabilized with a triblock polymer (Pluronic F127) in water (137). Such dispersions have been termed "hexosomes" (138).

Lamellar Phase

The lamellar phase (or neat phase), L_α, is built of bilayers of surfactant molecules alternating with water layers. This phase is symmetrical around the middle of the bilayer, and the normal and reversed phases are identical. Comparatively little work has been reported on the application of lamellar phases as such in drug delivery despite the fact that they provide favorable locations for the incorporation of both hydrophilic and lipophilic drugs and have the potential for controlling their release. Hydrophilic drugs can be solubilized within the interlamellar aqueous channels that can act as pores, the tortuosity of which is determined by the amount of free water and the orientation of the lamellae (139), whereas lipophilic drugs will be trapped in the lipophilic bilayers. In contrast, vesicles formed by dispersions of the lamellar phase of certain surfactants in an excess of water have been extensively studied, as discussed below.

Liposomes and Niosomes

The most extensively studied vesicular systems are those formed by phospholipids, which are referred to as *liposomes*, and to a lesser extent those formed from some nonionic surfactants, referred to as *niosomes*. The assembly into closed bilayers is rarely spontaneous, and vesicle formation usually involves the initial hydration of the surfactant at elevated temperature followed by size reduction involving some input of energy, usually sonication, to form a colloidal dispersion (140). Vesicles are consequently nonequilibrium structures, and will eventually revert to the lamellar phase. They are unilamellar or multilamellar spheroidal structures in which water-soluble drugs can be entrapped by intercalation in the aqueous layers, while lipid-soluble drugs can be solubilized within the hydrocarbon interiors of the bilayers (Fig. 27), thus providing potential vehicles for the solubilization and delivery of drugs (141).

Liposomes are usually formed by naturally occurring phospholipids such as lecithin (phosphatidyl choline). The net charge of the liposome can be varied by incorporation of, for example, a long-chain amine such as stearylamine (to give positively charged vesicles) or dicetyl phosphate (to give negatively charged species). The method of production of liposomes and their application as drug carriers have been extensively reviewed (140,142). Since liposomes can encapsulate drugs, proteins, and enzymes, the systems can

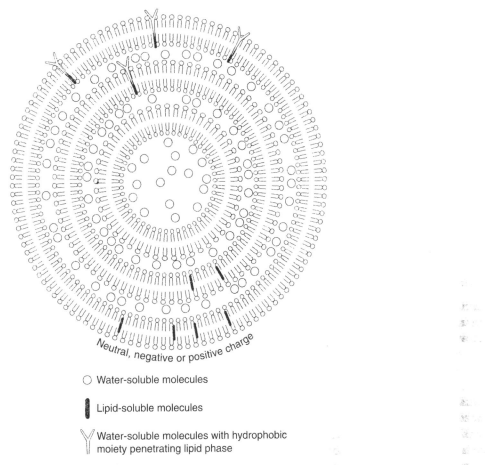

○ Water-soluble molecules

❙ Lipid-soluble molecules

⅄ Water-soluble molecules with hydrophobic
‖ moiety penetrating lipid phase

Figure 27 Diagrammatic representation of a liposome in which three bilayers of polar phospholipids alternate with aqueous compartments; water-soluble and lipid-soluble substances may be accommodated in the aqueous and lipid phases, respectively. Certain macromolecules can insert their hydrophobic regions into the lipid bilayers with the hydrophilic portions extending into water. *Source*: From Ref. 139.

be administered intravenously, orally, or intramuscularly to decrease toxicity, increase specificity of uptake of drug, and in some cases, to control release. Liposomes have several disadvantages as carriers to deliver drugs, however; they are, for example, liable to oxidative degradation, and must be stored and handled in a nitrogen atmosphere.

Niosomes have several advantages over liposomes for use in drug delivery, in particular, their more defined chemical nature, lower cost, and better stability. Although most naturally occurring phospholipids have dual hydrophobic chains, examples can be found of both single as well as double alkyl chain nonionic surfactant analogues that are able to form vesicles. Principal among vesicle-forming nonionic compounds are the alkyl ether lipids. These can be broadly divided into two classes on the basis of the nature of the hydrophilic head group: alkyl ethers in which the hydrophilic head group consists of repeat glycerol subunits, related isomers, or larger sugar molecules, and those in which the hydrophilic head groups consist of repeat ethylene oxide subunits. Alkyl esters, amides, and fatty acid and amino acid compounds also form vesicles. Often various additives, such as the wedge-shaped molecule cholesterol, must be included in the formulation to achieve the required CPP for formation of stable niosomes. The preparation and use of niosomes as drug carriers have been reviewed (143–145).

Cubic Phase

Micellar Cubic Phases

In some surfactant systems, another liquid crystalline state, the cubic phase, V_1, occurs between the hexagonal and lamellar phases. The most common type of cubic phase is the micellar cubic phase, which is a highly viscous phase formed by the close packing of small micelles of spherical or near-spherical shape. Reversed micellar–type cubic phases consist of globular water cores surrounded by the surfactant molecules. An interesting micellar cubic phase that has received considerable attention for its potential in drug solubilization and delivery is that formed by aqueous micellar solutions of $E_mP_nE_m$ copolymers, particularly the commercially available poloxamer, Pluronic F127 ($E_{106}P_{69}E_{106}$), which forms cubic phase gels at ambient temperature at a concentration of about 20 wt%.

Thermoreversible gelation of such compounds is of particular pharmaceutical interest. The gelation of concentrated solutions of F127 on cooling from a high temperature (hot gelation) or on heating from a low temperature (cold gelation) was described by Schmolka and Bacon (146). Figure 28 shows the gel diagram for aqueous solutions of F127, 18 wt% solutions of which form gels at 25°C; the C-shaped phase diagram showing sol-gel transition at both low and high temperatures is typical of many other block copolymer systems with pharmaceutical application. It is the gel formation on heating that is of most pharmaceutical interest; in principle a subcutaneously injected low viscosity solution containing solubilized drug will gel in situ as the temperature approaches body temperature, so providing a gel depot from which drug may be slowly released.

The reason for gelation on temperature increase can be seen by considering the micellization process. As mentioned in section "Micelle Formation in Aqueous Solution," micellization is entropy driven, that is, the standard entropy and enthalpy of micellization are both positive, reflecting the increased disorder of the water when the hydrophobic

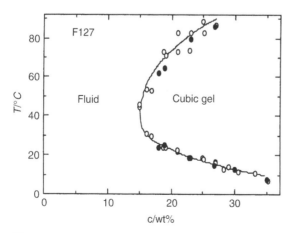

Figure 28 Gel boundary for aqueous solutions of copolymer F127. The filled circles are data points obtained by the tube inversion method for the mixture. The unfilled circles are data points from rheometry. *Source*: From Ref. 122.

block is removed to the micelle core: the hydrophobic effect. The value of the standard enthalpy of micellization is an indicator of the magnitude of the hydrophobic effect, and for $E_mP_nE_m$ copolymers in dilute solution the value is high, $\Delta_{mic}H° = 150$–350 kJ/mol (147,148). However, in more concentrated solution, the value is much lower (of the order of 20 kJ/mol for a 20 wt% solution), consistent with the poly(oxyethylene) blocks modifying the water structure and weakening the hydrophobic effect. The implication is that a poly(oxyethylene)-based surfactant may be incompletely micellized in a concentrated solution at 20°C even though it is well micellized in aqueous solutions at the same temperature at lower concentrations. However, because of the endothermic nature of the micellization process, the extent of micellization in the concentrated solution increases with temperature, and a packed micellar gel forms at a critical gelation temperature. While the low-temperature gel boundary is attributable to the formation of additional micelles, the copolymer is completely associated at the high-temperature boundary, and the mass concentration of micelles is constant. This upper boundary results from a reduction in micelle volume at constant concentration, a consequence of the negative temperature coefficient of solubility of poly(oxyethylene), which leads to contraction of the micelle corona. The physical chemistry of aqueous micellar gels of $E_mP_nE_m$ and related copolymers has been reviewed (147,149–151).

So far as gelation is concerned, diblock copolymers and triblock copolymers with oxyethylene terminal blocks of similar overall composition (E_mP_n and $E_mP_{2n}E_m$) behave in the same way, but copolymers with the reverse triblock architecture ($P_nE_{2m}P_n$) differ. As described by Mortensen et al. for copolymer $P_{15}E_{156}P_{15}$ (152), copolymer chains bridge between micelles to form transient networks in moderately concentrated solutions. At higher concentrations, the network fills the whole volume, and at high-enough concentrations an ordered gel is formed.

In addition to the extensive studies on the triblock copolymers of ethylene oxide and propylene oxide, the formation of cubic phase gels by triblock copolymers of ethylene oxide and other epoxides, notably 1,2-butylene oxide, styrene oxide, and phenyl glycidyl ether, has also been reported (150,153–155), and also by copolymers with diblock architecture (156,157). These studies have defined the general rules for controlling the gelation behavior by changing the hydrophobic block length; increasing the length of the hydrophobic block lowers the cold-gelation boundary and broadens the temperature range of the gel, while increasing the length of the hydrophilic block reduces the minimum concentration for gel formation (122).

Copolymers of ethylene oxide with poly(DL-lactide) and poly(caprolactone) blocks are much more hydrophobic than those with poly(propylene oxide) blocks. Block lengths required for satisfactory cold gelation of $CL_nE_mCL_n$ and $E_mCL_nE_m$ copolymers have been defined (158,159). An alternative approach has been to reduce the hydrophobicity of poly(lactide) blocks by copolymerization with glycolide (160–163), and copolymers of this type are available under the trade name Regel^{TM} (Protherics) (162). Others have used statistical polymerization of glycolide and CL to the same effect (164).

A more general approach to the control of gelation, avoiding the need for synthesis, is to use a mixture of two copolymers with different attributes, that is, to combine the satisfactory gelation characteristics of a micellar solution of one copolymer with the more favorable solubilization characteristics of micelles of another. For example, a micellar solution of $E_{137}S_{18}E_{137}$ is a good solubilizer for aromatic drugs (98), while a solution of $E_{62}P_{39}E_{62}$ (F87) has satisfactory gelation behavior, similar to that of F127 (165) but low solubilization capacity; a mixture of these two copolymers retains the gelation behavior of F87 while benefiting from the superior solubilization capacity of $E_{137}S_{18}E_{137}$ (166–168).

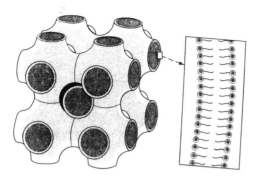

Figure 29 Structure of glyceryl monooleate–water bicontinuous cubic phase with inset showing the lipid bilayer. *Source*: Redrawn from Ref. 169.

Bicontinuous Cubic Phases

A more complex cubic phase, the bicontinuous cubic phase, occurs with some amphiphilic lipids such as glyceryl monooleate (monoolein, GMO) at high concentration (60–80%). The structure of this phase is unique and consists of a curved bicontinuous lipid bilayer extending in three dimensions, separating two networks of water channels with pores of about 5 nm diameter (169) (Fig. 29). The bicontinuous structure of the cubic phases enables solubilization of diverse molecules ranging from proteins to small-molecule drugs, and the tortuosity of the bicontinuous structure leads to diffusion-controlled release of the solubilizates (170). Reversed bicontinuous cubic phases formed by GMO have been widely studied as potential drug delivery vehicles for a wide variety of drugs with a range of physicochemical properties [see review by Drummond and Fong (171)]. On dilution of the bicontinuous cubic phases, the structures retain their integrity and coexist with excess water, forming a colloidal dispersion of cubic phase vesicles or *cubosomes* (172–175). Not surprisingly, these systems have been extensively investigated as controlled release vehicles (176–179).

REFERENCES

1. Attwood D, Florence AT. Surfactant Systems. London: Chapman and Hall, 1983.
2. Booth C, Attwood D. Macromol Rapid Commun 2000; 21:501–527.
3. Nace VM, ed. Nonionic Surfactants. Polyoxyalkylene Block Copolymers. Surfactant Science Series. Vol. 60. New York: Marcel Dekker, Inc., 1996:185–210.
4. Attwood D. Microemulsions. In Kreuter J, ed. Colloidal Drug Delivery Systems. New York: Marcel Dekker Inc., 1994.
5. Overbeek JThG. Proc Roy Dutch Acad Sci Ser 1986; B89 (1):61.
6. Florence AT, Attwood D. Physicochemical Principles of Pharmacy. 4th ed. London: Pharmaceutical Press, 2006:181.
7. Gaines GL. J Colloid Interface Sci 1977; 62:191.
8. Martin AS, Lawrence SJ, Rollet DA, et al. Eur J Phys 1993; 14:19.
9. Pethica BA. Thin Solid Films 1987; 152:3.
10. Schwartz DK. Surf Sci Rep 1997; 27:241.
11. Roberts GG. Adv Phys 1985; 34:475.
12. Swalen JD, Allara DL, Andrade JD, et al. Langmuir 1987; 3:932.
13. Reiss HE, Matsumoto M, Uyeda N et al. J Colloid Interface Sci 1976; 57:396.
14. Cadenhead DA, Phillips MC. J Colloid Interface Sci 1967; 24:491.
15. Dynarowicz-Łatka P, Dhanabalan A, Oliveira ON. Adv Colloid Interface Sci 2001; 91:221.
16. Bettarini S, Bonosi F, Gabrielli G, et al. Thin Solid Films 1992; 210/211:42.

17. Ganguly P, Paranjape DV, Sastry M, et al. Langmuir 1993; 9:487.
18. Laxhuber LA, Möhwald H. Langmuir 1987; 3:837.
19. Zasadzinski JA, Viswanathan R, Madsen L, et al. Science 1994; 263:1726.
20. Dhanabalan A, Prasanth Kumar N, Major S, et al. Thin Solid Films 1998; 327/329:787.
21. Schwartz DK, Viswanathan R, Zasadzinski JA. Phys Rev Lett 1993; 70:1267.
22. Dynarowicz-Łatka P, Dhanabalan A, Oliveira ON, Jr. J Phys Chem B 1999; 103:5992.
23. Peltonen L, Hirvonen J, Yliruusi J. J Colloid Interface Sci 2001; 239:134.
24. von Tscharner V, McConnell HM. Biophys J 1981; 36:409.
25. Lösche M, Möhwald H. Rev Sci Instr 1984; 5:1968.
26. Hénon S, Meunier J. J Rev Sci Instr 1991; 62:936.
27. Hönig D, Möbius D. J Phys Chem 1991; 95:4590.
28. Krüger P, Schalke M, Wang Z, et al. Biophys J 1999; 77:903.
29. Flanders BN, Vickery SA, Dunn RC. J Microsc 2001; 202:379.
30. Peng JB, Barnes GT, Gentle IR. Adv Colloid Interface Sci 2001; 91:163.
31. Peachey NM, Eckhardt CJ. Micron 1994; 25:271.
32. Balashev K, Jensen TR, Kjaer K, et al. Biochimie 2001; 83:387.
33. Vollhardt D. Morphology of monolayers at air-water interfaces. In: Somasundaran P, ed. Encyclopedia of Surface and Colloid Science; Vol 5, 2nd ed. New York: Taylor and Francis, 2006:4104–4118.
34. Hidalgo AA, Caetano W, Tabak M, et al. Biophys Chem 2004; 109:85.
35. Reiss HE, Swift HS. J Colloid Interface Sci 1978; 64:111.
36. Ghaicha L, Leblanc RM, Villamagna F, et al. Langmuir 1995; 11:585.
37. Li ZX, Lu JR, Fragneto G, et al. Colloids Surf A 1998; 135:277.
38. Schlossman DM, Mitrinovic DM, Zhang Z, et al. Synchrotron Radiat News 1999; 12:53.
39. Aratono M, Takanori T. Liquid-liquid interfacial films. In: Somasundaran P, ed. Encyclopedia of Surface and Colloid Science; Vol 5, 2nd ed. New York: Taylor and Francis, 2006:3436.
40. Lowy DA. Fatty acids at liquid-liquid interface. In: Somasundaran P, ed. Encyclopedia of Surface and Colloid Science; Vol 4, 2nd ed. New York: Taylor and Francis, 2006:2544–2556.
41. Zhao J, Brown W. Langmuir 1995; 11:2944; Zhao J, Brown W, Langmuir 1996; 12:1141.
42. Lin SY, Dong C, Hsu TJ, et al. Colloids Surf A 2002; 196:189.
43. Romero-Cano MS, Martín-Rodríguez A, Chauveteau G, et al. J Colloid Interface Sci 1998; 198:266.
44. Kuno H, Abe R. Kolloid Z 1961; 177:40; Abe R, Kuno H. Kolloid Z 1962; 181:70.
45. Corkill JM, Goodman JF, Tate JR. Trans Farad Soc 1966; 62:979.
46. Winnik MA, Bystryak MS, Odrobina E. Langmuir 2000; 16:6118.
47. Kronberg B, Käll L, Stenius P. J Dispersion Sci Technol 1981; 2:215.
48. Kronberg B, Stenius P, Igeborn G. J Colloid Interface Sci 1984; 102:418.
49. Steinby K, Silveston R, Kronberg B. J Colloid Interface Sci 1993; 155:70.
50. Romero-Cano MS, Martín-Rodríguez A, de las Nieves FJ. J Colloid Interface Sci 2000; 227:323.
51. Connor P, Ottewill RH. J Colloid Interface Sci 1971; 37:642.
52. Fuerstenau DW. J Phys Chem 1956; 60:981; Somasundaran P, Healy TW, Fuerstenau DW. J Phys Chem 1964; 68:3562; Somasundaran P, Fuerstenau DW. J Phys Chem 1966; 70:90.
53. Cosgrove T, Obey TM, Vincent B. J Colloid Interface Sci 1986; 111:409.
54. Cosgrove T, Crowley TL, Ryan K, et al. Colloids Surf A 1990; 51:255.
55. Bolze J, Hörner KD, Ballauff M. Colloid Polym Sci 1996; 274:1099.
56. Geffroy C, Cohen Stuart MA, Wong K, et al. Langmuir 2000; 16:6422.
57. Gilchrist VA, Lu JR, Keddie JL, et al. Langmuir 2000; 16:740.
58. Gilchrist VA, Lu JR, Staples E, et al. Langmuir 1999; 15:250.
59. Howse JR, Steitz R, Pannek M, et al. Phys Chem Chem Phys 2001; 3:4044.
60. Colombié D, Landfester K, Sudol ED, et al. J Colloid Interface Sci 1998; 202:554.
61. Martín-Rodriguez A, Jódar-Reyes AB. Adsorption of surfactants at polymer surfaces. In: Somasundaran P, ed. Encyclopedia of Surface and Colloid Science; Vol 1, 2nd ed. New York: Taylor and Francis, 2006:746–767.

62. Rouchotas C, Cassidy OE, Rowley G. Int J Pharm 2000; 195:1.

63. Nogami H, Nagai T, Wada S. Chem Pharm Bull 1970; 18:342.

64. Nogami H, Nagai T, Uchida H. Chem Pharm Bull 1969; 17:176.

65. Nogami H, Nagai T, Nambu N. Chem Pharm Bull 1970; 18:1643.

66. Nogami H, Sakurai S, Nagai T. Chem Pharm Bull 1975; 23:1404.

67. El-Masry S, Khalil SAH. J Pharm Pharmacol 1974; 26:243.

68. Khalil SAH, Iwuagwa M. J Pharm Sci 1978; 67:287.

69. Abe I, Kamaya H, Ueda I. J Pharm Sci 1990; 79:354.

70. Richards NE, Meakin BJ. J Pharm Pharmacol 1974; 26:166.

71. El-Masry S, Khalil SAH. J Pharm Pharmacol 1974; 26:243–248.

72. Saski W. J Pharm Sci 1963; 52:264.

73. Bauer G, Ullman E. Arch Pharm 1973; 306:86.

74. Mukerjee P. Adv Colloid Interface Sci 1967; 78:2480.

75. Zana R. Brief review on the chemical relaxation studies of micellar equilibria. In: Wyn-Jones E, ed. Chemical and Biological Applications of Relaxation Spectrometry. Dordrecht, Holland: D. Reidel Publishing Company, 1975: 133–138.

76. Gettins WJ, Wyn-Jones E, eds. Techniques and Applications of Fast Reactions in Solutions. Dordrecht, Holland: D. Reidel Publishing Company, 1979.

77. Aniansson EAG, Wall SN. J Phys Chem 1974; 78:1024; Aniansson EAG, Wall SN. J Phys Chem 1975; 79:857; Aniansson EAG, Wall SN, Almgren M, et al. J Phys Chem 1976; 80:905.

78. Zana R. Micellar systems: dynamics. In: Somasundaran P, ed. Encyclopedia of Surface and Colloid Science; Vol 5, 2nd ed. New York: Taylor and Francis, 2006:3703.

79. Maeda H. Thermodynamic analysis of micellar systems. In: Somasundaran P, ed. Encyclopedia of Surface and Colloid Science; Vol 8, 2nd ed. New York: Taylor and Francis, 2006:6221–6234.

80. Burchfield TE, Woolley EM. J Phys Chem 1984; 88:2149; Woolley EM, Burchfield TE. J Phys Chem 1984; 88:2155; Woolley EM, Burchfield TE. J Phys Chem 1985; 89:714; Woolley EM, Burchfield TE. Fluid Phase Equilib 1985; 20:225.

81. Mukerjee P, Ghosh AK. J Am Chem Soc 1970; 92:6403; Ghosh AK, Mukerjee P. J Am Chem Soc 1970; 92:6408–6413.

82. Attwood D. Colloidal properties of drugs. In: Aggregation Processes in Solution. Amsterdam: Elsevier Scientific Publishing Co., 1983: 211–240.

83. Attwood D. Adv Colloid Interface Sci 1995; 55:271.

84. Attwood D. Micellar drugs. In: Somasundaran P, ed. Encyclopedia of Surface and Colloid Science. Vol 5, 2nd ed. New York: Taylor and Francis, 2006:3675–3689.

85. Mukerjee P. J Pharm Sci 1974; 63:972.

86. Mukerjee P. In: van Olphen H, Mysels KJ, eds. Physical Chemistry: Enriching Topics from Colloid and Surface Science. La Jolla, California: Theorex, 1975:135–154.

87. Attwood D. J Pharm Pharmac 1972; 24:751; Attwood D, Udeala OK. J Pharm Pharmac 1975; 27:395; Attwood D. J Pharm Pharmac 1976; 28:407.

88. Attwood D, Agarwal SP, Waigh RD. J Chem Soc Farad 1980; 1(76):2187.

89. Attwood D. J Phys Chem 1976 80:1984.

90. Attwood D, Doughty D, Mosquera V, et al. J Colloid Interface Sci 1991 41:316; Attwood D, Blundell R, Mosquera V. J Colloid Interface Sci 1993; 157:50.

91. Attwood D, Waigh R, Blundell R, et al. Magn Reson Chem 1994; 32:468.

92. Attwood D. J Chem Soc Farad Trans 1983; 1, 79:2669.

93. Schott H. J Pharm Sci 1973; 62:162.

94. Allen C, Maysinger D, Eisenberg A. Coll Surf B 1999; 16:3.

95. Chaibundit C, Ricardo NMPS, Booth C, et al. Langmuir 2002; 18:4277.

96. Zhou Z, Chaibundit C, D'Emanuele A, et al. Int J Pharm 2008 354:82.

97. Chaibundit C, Sumanatrakool P, Chinchew S, et al. J Colloid Interface Sci 2005; 283:544.

98. Crothers M, Zhou Z, Ricardo NMPS, et al. Int J Pharm 2005; 293:91.

99. Henriksson U, Odberg L, Erikson JC, et al. J Phys Chem 1977; 81:76.

100. Reiss-Husson F, Luzzati V. J Phys Chem 1964; 69.

101. Hayashi S, Ikeda S. J Phys Chem 1980; 84:744.
102. Ismail AA, Gouda MW, Motawi MM. J Pharm Sci 1970; 59:220.
103. Collett JH, Koo L. J Pharm Sci 1975; 64:1253.
104. Tomida H, Yotsuyanagi T, Ikeda K. Chem Pharm Bull 1978; 26:2824.
105. Tomida H, Yotsuyanagi T, Ikeda K. Chem Pharm Bull 1978; 26:2832.
106. Wiedmann TS, Kamel L. J Pharm Sci 2002; 91:1743.
107. Aliabadi HM, Lavasanifar A. Expert Opin Drug Deliv 2006; 3:139.
108. Salib NN, Ismail AA, Geneidi AS. Pharm Ind 1974; 36:108.
109. Arnarson T, Elworthy PH. J Pharm Pharmacol 1980; 32:381.
110. Barry BW, El Eini DID. J Pharm Pharmacol 1976; 28:210.
111. Saettone MF, Giannaccini B, Delmonte G, et al. Int J Pharm 1988; 43:67.
112. Savic R, Eisenberg A, Maysinger D. J Drug Target 2006; 14:343.
113. Gaucher G, Dufresne MH, Sant VP, et al. J Control Release 2005; 109:169.
114. Kabanov AV, Batrakova EV, Alakhov VY. J Control Release 2002; 982:189.
115. Kabanov AV, Alakhov VY. Crit Rev Ther Drug Carrier Syst 2002; 19:1.
116. Torchilin VP. J Control Release 2001; 73:137.
117. Kwon GS, Kataoka K. Adv Drug Delivery Rev 1995; 16:295.
118. Liggins RT, Burt HM. Adv Drug Delivery Rev 2002; 54:191.
119. Kataoka K, Kwon GS, Yokohama M, et al. J Control Release 1993; 24:119.
120. Adams ML, Lavasanifar A, Kwon GS. J Pharm Sci 2003; 92:1343.
121. Chiappetta DA, Sosnik A. Eur J Pharm Biopharm 2007 66:303.
122. Attwood D, Zhou Z, Booth C. Expert Opin Drug Deliv 2007; 4:533.
123. Attwood D, Booth C. Solubilization of poorly soluble aromatic drugs by micellar solutions of amphiphilic block copoly(oxyalkylene)s. In:Tadros Th F, ed. Colloid Stability and Application in Pharmacy. Colloid and Interface Science Series. Vol 3, Weinheim: Wiley-VCH, 2007, pp. 61–68.
124. Molpeceres J, Guzman M, Bustamante P, et al. Int J Pharm 1996; 130:75.
125. Nagarajan R, Barry M, Ruckenstein E. Langmuir 1986; 2:210.
126. Reketas CJ, Mais SM, Crothers M, et al. Phys Chem Chem Phys 2001; 3:4769.
127. Yang Z, Crothers M, Attwood D, et al. J Colloid Interface Sci 2003; 263:312.
128. Crothers M, Zhou Z, Ricardo NMPS, et al. Int J Pharm 2005; 293:91.
129. Kim JH, Emoto K, Ijima M, et al. Adv Technol 1999; 10:647.
130. Zhang X, Jackson JK, Burt HM. Int J Pharm 1996; 132:195.
131. Mitchell DJ, Tiddy GJT, Waring L, et al. J Chem Soc Faraday Trans I 1983; 79:975.
132. Laughlin RG The Aqueous Phase Behavior of Surfactants. London: Academic Press, 1994.
133. Tiddy GJT. Phys Rev 1980; 57:1.
134. Chernik GC. Curr Opin Colloid Interface Sci 2000; 4:381.
135. Khan A. Curr Opin Colloid Interface Sci 1996; 1:614.
136. Norling T, Lading P, Engström S, et al. J Clin Periodontol 1992; 19:687.
137. Gustafsson J, Ljusberg-Wahren H, Almgren M, et al. Langmuir 1997; 13:6964.
138. Larsson K. Proc Int Symp Control Rel Bioact Mat 1997; 24:198.
139. Bodde HE, de Vringer T, Junginger HE. Prog Colloid Polym Sci 1986; 72:37.
140. New RRC, ed. Liposomes: A Practical Approach. Oxford: Oxford University Press, 1990.
141. Gregoriadis G. N Engl J Med 1976; 295:704.
142. Crommelin DJA, Schreier H. Liposomes. In: Kreuter J, ed. Colloidal Drug Delivery Systems. New York: Marcel Dekker, 1994:73–190.
143. Bouwstra JA, Hofland HEJ. Niosomes. In: Kreuter J, ed. Colloidal Drug Delivery Systems. New York: Marcel Dekker, 1994:191–217.
144. Uchegbu IF, Florence AT. Adv Colloid Interface Sci 1995; 58:1.
145. Uchegbu IF, Vyas SP. Int J Pharm 1998; 172:33.
146. Schmolka IR, Bacon LR. J Am Oil Chem Soc 1967; 44:559.
147. Chu B, Zhou ZK. Physical chemistry of polyoxyalkylene block copolymer surfactants. In: Nace VM, ed. Nonionic Surfactants, Poly(oxyalkylene) Block Copolymers, Surfactant Science Series. Vol 60. New York: Marcel Dekker, 1996:67–143.

148. Alexandridis P, Holzwarth JF, Hatton TA. Macromolecules 1994; 27:2414.

149. Mortensen K. Small-angle scattering studies of block copolymer micelles, micellar mesophases and networks. In: Alexandridis P, Lindman B, eds. Amphiphilic Block Copolymers. Amsterdam: Elsevier, 2000:191–220.

150. Hamley IW, Mai SM, Ryan AJ, et al. Phys Chem Chem Phys 2001; 3:2972.

151. Jones DS, Brown AF, Woolfson D. J Appl Polym Sci 2003; 87:1016.

152. Mortensen K, Brown W, Jørgensen E. Macromolecules 1994; 27:5654.

153. Taboada P, Velasquez G, Barbosa S, et al. Langmuir 2005; 21:5263.

154. Castelletto V, Hamley IW, Yuan XY, et al. Soft Matter 2005; 1:138.

155. Yang Z, Crothers M, Ricardo NMPS, et al. Langmuir 2003; 19:943.

156. Kelarakis A, Havredaki V, Booth C. Macromol Chem Phys 2003; 204:15.

157. Crothers M, Attwood D, Collett JH, et al. Langmuir 2002; 18:8685.

158. Bae SJ, Suh JM, Sohn YS, et al. Macromolecules 2005; 38:5260.

159. Hwang MJ, Suh JM, Bae YH, et al. Biomacromolecules 2005; 5:885.

160. Jeong B, Choi YK, Bae YH, et al. J Control Release 1999; 62:109.

161. Jeong B, Bae YH, Kim SW. Macromolecules 1999; 32:7064.

162. Zentner GM, Rathi R, Shih C, et al. J Control Release 2001; 72:203.

163. Lee DS, Shim MS, Kim SW, et al. Macromol Rapid Commun 2001; 22:587.

164. Huynh DP, Shim WS, Kim JH et al. Polymer 2006; 47:7918.

165. Harrison WJ, Aboulgasem GJ, Elathrem FAI, et al. Langmuir 2005; 21:6170.

166. Ricardo NMPS, Pinho MEN, Yang Z, et al. Int J Pharm 2005; 300:22.

167. Pinho MEN, Costa FMLL, Filho FBS, et al. Int J Pharm 2007; 328:95.

168. Hamley IW, Castelletto V, Ricardo NMPS, et al. Polym Int 2007; 56:88.

169. Shah JC, Sadhale Y, Chilukuri DM. Adv Drug Delivery Rev 2001; 47:229.

170. Anderson DM, Wennerström H. J Phys Chem 1990; 94:8683.

171. Drummond CJ, Fong C. Curr Opin Colloid Interface Sci 2000; 4:449.

172. Spicer PT. Cubosomes: bicontinuous cubic liquid crystalline nanostructured particles. In: Schwarz JA, Contescu C, Putyera K, eds. Encyclopedia of Nanoscience and Nanotechnology.. New York: Marcel Dekker, 2003:881–892.

173. Spicer PT. Curr Opin Colloid Interface Sci 2005; :274.

174. Engström S. Lipid Technol 1990; 2:42.

175. Gustafsson J, Ljusberg-Wahren H, Almgren M, et al. Langmuir 1997; 13:6964.

176. Barauskas J, Johnsson M, Tiberg F. Nano Lett 2005; 5:1615.

177. Garg G, Saraf S, Saraf S. Biol Pharm Bull 2007; 30:350.

178. Zhao X-Y, Zhang J, Zheng L-Q, et al. J Dispersion Sci Technol 2004; 25:795.

179. Esposito E, Cortesi R, Drechsler M, et al. Pharm Res 2005; 22:2163.

13

Tablet Dosage Forms

Murat Turkoglu
Department of Pharmaceutical Technology, Marmara University, Istanbul, Turkey

Adel Sakr
College of Pharmacy, University of Cincinnati, Cincinnati, Ohio, U.S.A.

INTRODUCTION

This chapter deals first with the main aspects of tablet dosage forms before addressing the process of manufacture and testing of these most popular drug delivery systems. *Per oral* tablets occupy the broadest and the most significant place among all pharmaceutical dosage forms. Taking one or two tablets a day with a glass of water is the easiest and the most acceptable way of administration of a drug to a patient. William Brockedon patented the first tablet press in 1843 to compress potash and lime tablets (1), thus paving the way for the modern manufacture of tablets.

Drugs are administered in a wide variety of doses. Tablets of *L-thyroxine*, for example, may contain as low as 25 µg drug. On the other hand, amoxicillin/clavulanic acid tablets contain 1 g of actives per tablet. These two extremes cover a 10,000-fold range of drug content. Tablets may be made in different sizes and shapes, and the drug substance may comprise 0.1% to 90% of a tablet bulk. From the point of view of ease of manufacture, tablet production, compared with other dosage forms, provides the highest output per manufacturing hour, and is the most economical, especially if one considers modern manufacturing methods involving processes such as the direct compression (DC) or fluidized-bed granulation.

While tabletting may appear from what has been said to be a facile process, it is often far from straightforward. Drug molecules show various differences in physical and chemical properties (2). These include differences in their crystalline structure, particle size, water solubility, dose, and sensitivity to hydrolysis or oxidation (3), topics discussed elsewhere in this book. Hence, every drug molecule must be treated as a unique entity for formulation. Drugs synthesized in the last 30 years have been increasingly showing limited water solubility, poor flow and compression properties, and sensitivity to moisture and heat. Preparing a tablet dosage form from such molecules is a challenge, since the market demands easy and cost-effective manufacturing, an acceptable dissolution rate, and of course high bioavailability, and mechanically strong tablets that resist fracture during packaging, transport, and ultimately, in patient use. Furthermore, the tablets must fulfill the requirements

481

for bioavailability and, eventually, bioequivalence. When considering all these factors, designing and manufacturing a successful tablet requires optimization of the formulation and processing parameters, which can be achieved by the application of a thorough knowledge of excipients, and the subsequent selection of the most suitable manufacturing process.

TYPES OF TABLETS AND TABLET DESIGN

Tablet design is based on the experience and knowledge of excipients, which are materials serving the purpose of making a *good tablet* when combined with a drug. The mechanical and chemical properties of excipients have the utmost importance, and the area is closely related to materials engineering as well as pharmacy. Expected properties of a modern tablet include mechanical strength suitable for coating, packaging, and transportation; an optimum size, shape, and color for identification; ease of swallowing; and, finally, fulfilling the pharmacopoeial requirements for drug content and release rates as well as stability and bioavailability.

Some of the pharmaceutical tablet types based on the way of administration or presentation to the patient are listed below (4–7):

1. Simple uncoated tablets
2. Coated tablets
3. Effervescent tablets
4. Buccal and sublingual tablets
5. Chewable tablets
6. Multilayered tablets
7. Sugarcoated tablets
8. Fast-disintegrating tablets
9. Vaginal tablets
10. Osmotic tablets
11. Controlled-release tablets
12. Multicomponent tablets

Simple Uncoated Tablets

The simplest form of a pharmaceutical tablet consists of a combination of a drug and some functional excipients compressed directly. This tablet should be formed by compression without difficulty using binders, disintegrants, and lubricants, and when used by a patient, it should disintegrate in the stomach and should of course be bioavailable. Such simple tablets are manufactured by mixing the drug and excipients in a V-shaped mixer and are compressed in a tablet press using dies and punches of suitable size.

Film-Coated Tablets

A tablet can be coated with a polymer film to provide greater ease of swallowing, protection against light or moisture, protection of the drug from gastric acidity, and modification or control of drug release rate. Identification of a formulation by color or logo is extremely important today not only for patient safety but also because of the problem of counterfeiting. Polymers and processes are available to achieve all of these properties.

Effervescent Tablets

Effervescent tablets are designed to dissolve or disperse quickly in water as a result of the release of carbon dioxide from the reaction between sodium bicarbonate and citric acid in the formulation. Such tablets are generally the largest tablets in terms of size and weight, with diameters up to 3 cm and weights of the order of 4 to 5 g. Although they are called tablets, the mode of administration is naturally indirect; the patients take the drug solution or suspension after dispersal. Their manufacture may require a low humidity environment, special tablet presses, and specialized lubrication for tablet ejection.

Buccal and Sublingual Tablets

These special tablets are designed for fast and complete drug action through dissolution in the buccal cavity or placement sublingually. As a result, the first pass effect may be avoided. Buccal tablets are used for hormone replacement therapy, for example, with methyl testosterone; sublingual tablets are frequently used for the delivery of isosorbide dinitrate and nitroglycerin.

Chewable Tablets

Sometimes a tablet is designed in such a way that it is chewable. This results in its disintegration. Chewable tablets have some advantages, among them being that a large dose of a drug can be formulated, since the tablets are not swallowed whole. Children can be convinced to take such medication, no water is required for administration, and the disintegration step for a tablet is actively achieved in the mouth before it dissolves in the gastric medium. Pediatric multivitamin or mineral formulas, aspirin, vitamin C 1000 mg, and vitamin A 50,000 units are usually formulated as chewable tablets.

Multilayered Tablets

Tablets can be designed and manufactured to have separate layers or a core tablet inside a tablet. In this way, two or more drugs can be kept separate in a single tablet. Such complicated systems have found limited applications over the years in the pharmaceutical industry, but there is a revival of interest in the use of combination dosage forms for the treatment of diseases such as AIDS, where multiple drugs are administered each day. Tablet presses with two or three hoppers are available for the purpose of preparing multilayered dose forms. These include the Colton 232, the Kilian Prescoter, and the Manesty DryCota machines (6). Recently, an excellent application potential was reported for compression coating (8), namely, the colonic delivery of drugs using a pectin-hydroxy propyl methyl cellulose (HPMC) combination, which was successful for the delivery of 5-aminosalycylic acid (5-ASA), and also for peptides such as nisin. This type of drug delivery system requires compression-coating equipment for mass production since a 100-mg core tablet containing the drug is surrounded by a pectin-HPMC mixture.

Sugarcoated Tablets (Dragees)

Before the development of film-coating processes, the major coating material was a sugarcoat. Tablets were sugarcoated for the very same reasons as film coating. These tablet types generally start with a seed or core tablet that contains the drug, and the

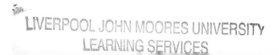

resultant coating process is a lengthy one using simple syrup, shellac, and talc, several layers of which are deposited onto the core tablet. Usually, a weight increase of as much as 100% to 300% is considered normal.

Fast-Disintegrating Tablets

This type of tablet is the newest addition to the family of tablets (9). The main reason for the development of such tablets is the potential for administration of small doses to the elderly or children who have difficulties in swallowing intact tablets. A tablet is administered by placing it on a spoon and adding some water, in two to four seconds the tablet completely disintegrates to granules that can be swallowed easily. Fast-disintegrating tablets are not only made out of special granules but can also be compressed using coated spherical pellets such as enteric-coated omeprazole pellets (10).

Vaginal Tablets

Tablets are made to be used for insertion into the vagina for treatment of local infections or hormone replacement therapy. For instance, ornidazole and micanazole nitrate combination and estradiol hemihydrate tablets are formulated as vaginal tablets. These tablets release the drugs slowly in 20 to 30 minutes.

TABLET FORMULATION DESIGN

Tablet formulation design starts with a predetermined value, which is the dose size. The amount of drug in a tablet can be a limiting step in formulation design. Tablet excipients can be classified on the basis of their functionality as listed below (2,4,5,9):

1. Fillers/diluents
2. Binders
3. Disintegrants
4. Lubricants
5. Glidants
6. Buffering agents
7. Sweeteners
8. Wetting agents
9. Coating agents
10. Matrix formers

Fillers/Diluents

Lactose

Fillers are used to arrive at a tablet of reasonable size when a drug forms a small portion of the formula, as in the case of 25 μg estradiol vaginal tablets. Depending on the physiological conditions and formulation, one needs a tablet of around 100 mg for ease of handling and administration, and therefore, fillers are used to increase bulk. Usually, α-lactose monohydrate is the first material to be considered (4,5,11–13). This water-soluble disaccharide is obtained from whey by crystallization and drying after cheese production. Lactose is a water-soluble diluent, 216 mg dissolving in 1-mL water. Using three different drying techniques, fluidized-bed methods, roller drying, and spray drying, α-lactose monohydrate, anhydrous β-lactose, and spray-dried lactose are obtained, respectively. The three different lactose grades differ considerably in their mechanical properties in relation to tabletting. For instance, anhydrous β-lactose shows a steep compression force–tablet crushing strength relation. On the other hand, α-lactose monohydrate and even spray-dried lactose are inferior grades in this respect. Spray drying of lactose forms partial amorphous structures, and that contributes to its better compressibility. Spray-dried lactose flows well because of its spherical granule shape. Therefore, the mechanical properties and the size distribution of lactose types must be known before making a selection out of many lactose grades. A partial list of excipients used in tablet manufacturing is following:

- Fillers/diluents used in tablet formulations (12)
  - Lactose (α-lactose monohydrate, anhydrite β-lactose, spray-dried lactose)
  - Microcrystalline cellulose (Avicel PH 101, Avicel PH 200, Emcocel)
  - Starch (Corn starch, partially hydrolyzed starch)
  - Dibasic calcium phosphate (Emcompress, Di-Tab)
  - Mannitol (Parteck, Delta M)
  - Sorbitol (Neosorb 60)
  - Calcium sulfate (Delaflo)
  - Compressible sucrose (Di-Pac, Des-tab, Nu-Tab)
- Binders used in tablet formulations (12)
  - Polyvinylpyrrolidone (PVP)
  - Sodium carboxymethyl cellulose
  - HPMC (Low molecular weight, 5 cps)
  - Starch paste
  - Simple syrup
- Lubricants and glidants used in tablet formulations (12)
  - Magnesium stearate
  - Stearic acid
  - Sodium stearyl fumarate
  - Hydrogenated vegetable oil
  - PEG 4000, 6000
  - Hexagonal boron nitride
  - DL-Leucine
  - Sodium lauryl sulfate
  - Glyceryl behenate
  - Sodium benzoate
  - Colloidal silicone dioxide
  - Talc
  - Starch
- Super disintegrants (12)
  - Sodium starch glycolate (Explotab)
  - Cross-linked PVP (Polyplasdone XL)
  - Cross-linked carboxymethyl cellulose (Ac-Di-Sol)

Starch

Starch has been used as a tablet/capsule excipient for a long time (4,5,12–14). Unlike lactose, starch has a multifunctional use in solid dosage forms. It serves as a filler/diluent as well as a disintegrant, and also as a binder in the form of starch paste. Depending on the region, starch can be obtained from corn, potatoes, wheat, or rice. It contains amylose and amylopectin units. Starch is not water soluble. For pharmaceutical purposes, starch does not flow well and cannot be compressed into strong compacts. Hence, partially pregelatinized starch is obtained by mechanical means such as rupturing the starch granules between hot rollers to render it partial water solubility. This contributes to its binding properties because of about 15% free amylopectin, 5% free amylose, and 80% unmodified starch. Starch normally has the highest equilibrium moisture content among all pharmaceutical excipients, that is to say, about 11% to 14%. In general, starch or modified starch does not have good mechanical properties for tabletting processes without the contribution of other plastic deformation-showing materials. On the other hand, starch is a good disintegrant in tablets, especially in the form of its semisynthetic derivative such as sodium carboxymethyl starch, which is extremely important. Its abundance and low cost make it a major pharmaceutical excipient.

Microcrystalline Cellulose

Since its introduction to the pharmaceutical industry in 1964 by FMC, microcrystalline cellulose (MCC) has revolutionized tablet formulation (4,5,12,15,16). MCC forms very strong compacts under even low compression pressures. It is obtained from wood pulp after controlled acid hydrolysis, which produces a high degree of crystallinity to the cellulose chains. After neutralization, filtering, and spray drying a white granular powder is obtained. MCC has at least nine different commercial grades (Avicel PH grades, FMC, U.S.A.) according to its average particle size (20 –180 μm), moisture content (1.5–5.0%), bulk density (0.25–0.44 g/mL), and volumetric flow (1.5–5.0 L/min) for applications ranging from wet granulation to direct compression. MCC shows a strong plastic deformation under pressure and a high dilution potential. Therefore, good compressibility can be matched with good flow only by selecting the right grade or making a wet granulation to a certain size and shape. As a diluent, it is used in combination with spray-dried lactose or dicalcium phosphate dihydrate during the DC tabletting to balance the cost or flow properties. In a compression force–crushing strength plot, MCC shows the steepest line among all excipients reaching 20-kg tablet crushing strength at about 750 kg.force. MCC is not water soluble but absorbs water. In a fluidized-bed granulation process, MCC requires the highest amount of water for the same granule size when compared to starch and lactose monohydrate.

Dicalcium Phosphate Dihydrate

This water-insoluble material is among the top five excipients in modern tablet formulations (4,5,12,13). The true density of dicalcium phosphate dihydrate is 2.3 g/mL, which makes it one of the heaviest pharmaceutical excipients per volume with a reported tapped density of 0.7 g/mL. Dicalcium phosphate anhydrous is also available. At 2000 kg.f compression, tablet crushing strength reaches a maximum of 100 N with this excipient. Therefore, its binding properties are inferior to those of MCC. The main mechanism of compaction of dicalcium phosphate is brittle fracture, creating new surfaces, which therefore shows much less lubricant sensitivity: This can be an advantage over plastically deforming materials such as MCC or some starches. Dicalcium phosphate dihydrate, like other inorganic salts, has a detrimental effect on tablet tooling.

Mannitol

Mannitol in various polymorphic forms is the main excipient of chewable tablets due to its negative heat of solution, which results in a pleasant mouth feel. A new mannitol grade, namely, δ-mannitol (Parteck, Delta M) has been reported to be superior to the other polymorphs such as α- or β-mannitol in terms of mechanical properties and chemical reactivity. Hence, tablets with higher crushing strengths can be manufactured. Mannitol is nonhygroscopic and shows a low reactivity with drug substances. Therefore, it has the potential to be utilized more in future tablet formulations.

Coprocessed Excipient Products

Some flexibility is necessary in the design of tablet formulations. Selecting each excipient depends on the physical and chemical properties of the drug, the drug dose, and the required final form and function of the tablet. There are however aids for the formulator. There are some coprocessed excipients containing usually a diluent and binder, and sometimes, even a disintegrant in a readymade granulation. Ludipress™ (BASF, Germany) contains α-lactose monohydrate, polyvinylpyrrolidone (PVP), and Kollidon CL. Cellactose 80™ (Meggle, Germany) contains α-lactose monohydrate and cellulose powder, Prosolv™ SMCC (JRS Pharma, Germany), silicified MCC, contains 98% MCC and 2% colloidal silicon dioxide, which provides a better granule flow and an opportunity for smaller and denser tablets upon direct compression. There are also coprocessed actives like ascorbic acid, thiamine, riboflavine, pyridoxine, paracetamol, and acetyl salicylic acid. For those drugs that are manufactured in huge volumes, the use of coprocessed excipients is efficient, since the small capacity of many pharmaceutical manufacturing plants for wet or dry granulation cannot deal with huge volumes.

Materials that contribute to plastic deformation, which means stronger compacts upon compression or forming a matrix such as methyl cellulose (MC), HPMC, hydoxy propyl cellulose (HPC), cellulose powder, gelatine, and mannitol are used.

Coprocessed products are so designed that by simple addition of the drug, compressed tablets may be produced. Using coprocessed active allows minimum excipient addition and manipulation.

Binders

Binders in tablet technology serve the purpose of binding small drug or excipient particles together to impart cohesiveness, and to form a granulate of a designed size range, usually larger than the initial material that flows freely and is also compressible, and eventually to be compressed into tablets or to be filled into capsules. A binder will help the tablet to remain intact after compression. Binders can be added as dry powders to form a matrix that will include the drug, as in the case of dry granulation or in direct compression. Sometimes, the binders are dissolved in liquids such as water or alcohol and then sprayed onto the powder mixture as with wet granulation. Materials such as MCC act as a binder/diluent in the case of direct compression. However, a polymer such as PVP is solely used as a binder. One of the commercial products of PVP is Kollidon™ (BASF), which has grades on the basis of molecular weight of the polymer: Kollidon K 25 (MW 28,000–34,000), K 30 (MW 44,000–54,000), and K 90 (MW 1,000,000–1,500,000) contain PVP of increasing molecular weights (4,5,17). PVP has some advantages over other binders: it is used in relatively small concentrations such as 1% to 5% to prepare a binder solution, it is soluble to above 10% in water, ethanol, and glycerol, which provides an opportunity for water-free granulation. One of the most significant advantages of PVP is its low viscosity (5–10 mPa.sec) even up to concentrations as high as 20% (w/v). A low-viscosity solution can easily be sprayed using peristaltic pumps during a fluidized-bed granulation. Starch paste has been a traditional binder, at concentrations between 5% and 10%. Starch is dispersed in cold water, and then slowly heated up to boiling with constant stirring. When a translucent paste is formed, it can be diluted with cold water. On the other hand, preparing a starch paste with modified starch will not require boiling, since it dissolves in warm water because of the free amylopectin. In modern granulation processes using high-shear mixers, starch paste finds few applications. HPMC, MC, HPC, and ethyl cellulose can be used as binders in tablet formulations. These cellulose-based binders perform as well as PVP in modern granulation processes. Hydrophilic polymers, especially of low molecular weight, for instance HPMC E6 (6 cP viscosity grade), can be dissolved in water to obtain a low-viscosity solution, and they bind well and contribute to plastic deformation during tabletting (18). The high-molecular weight grades of these cellulose-based materials can be used as matrix formers, and incorporated into formulations as dry binders. Ethyl cellulose is not water soluble, so it is used as an alcoholic solution. Materials such as PVP and HPMC have largely replaced other binders such as gelatine, sucrose, simple syrup, or acacia.

Disintegrants

Disintegrants serve the purpose of facilitating the disintegration of tablets into its components either after administration in the GI tract or just before administration, such as in the case of the fast-disintegrating tablets (4,5,9,12). Disintegrants may play an important role in the bioavailability of a drug in tablet dose forms. When disintegrants come into contact with water, they usually swell, as their cross-linked molecular structure, such as in amylose in starch or in cross-linked PVP, imbibes water and swells, providing the force to disperse the tablet. Depending on the formulation design, some tablets containing higher percentages of MCC may disintegrate readily during disintegration tests without an additional disintegrant. Addition of starches externally to the final granulation before tabletting is best justified for disintegration purposes. Starch is a "mild" tablet disintegrant. In the past, there was concern that tablet compression forces should not exceed certain limits or tablet crushing strengths 70 to 80 N because of the probability of prolonged disintegration times. However, with the advent of modern excipients, mechanically strong tablets with 200 to 300 N crushing strengths can be produced, and these tablets will disintegrate within five minutes or less using the super-disintegrants (4,12). Super-disintegrants are materials added to tablet formulations in a range of 1% to 5% to assure disintegration within 1 to 10 minutes. Among these are sodium carboxymethyl starch (Explotab™, Mendell, U.S.A.), cross-linked sodium carboxymethyl cellulose (Pharmacel™ XL, DMV, Netherlands), and cross-linked PVP (17) (Kollidon™ XL, BASF). The rank order of the degree of swelling in water in two minutes for those disintegrants has been reported to be sodium carboxymethyl starch > sodium carboxymethyl cellulose > L-HPC 11 > cross-linked PVP > starch > MCC.

Lubricants

Pharmaceutical lubricants are materials used in tablet formulations to reduce the friction between the lower punch and the die and the tablet (2,4,9,19,20). Friction damages both the tablet and the tablet press during the ejection cycle. Lubricants are a mechanical necessity, without which modern tablet manufacturing would be impossible. Glidants are materials that reduce interparticular friction, covering the particle surfaces with a thin layer, and as a result helping in better granule flow. Colloidal silicon dioxide, talc, and starch can be used as glidants; colloidal silicon dioxide is effective as low as 0.5% as a glidant. Lubricants are added to pharmaceutical granules just before the tabletting stage. Mixing the main granule mass with a lubricant has been an intensively investigated subject. Prolonged mixing with a surface-covering lubricant such as magnesium stearate negatively affects the binding capacity of a granule mass. Hence, tablet formation might be inhibited, unless the granule mass undergoes brittle fracture and creates new clean surfaces. Especially, materials exhibiting plastic deformation with a limited surface area would show a strong sensitivity to lubricants. Therefore, the specific surface area of a lubricant as well as the surface area of the granule mass are both important parameters in selecting lubricant type, concentration, and mixing times. Boundary lubricants will adhere on the metal surfaces of the tablet press, die, and punches and will form a boundary layer with the tablet. Alkaline stearates such as magnesium stearate are an example of a boundary lubricant. Magnesium stearate is still the most effective pharmaceutical lubricant. Its usual concentration range is between 0.1% and 2%, and its effectiveness shows a biphasic profile, a region of a fast reduction in friction up to 1 %, and a slower friction-reducing effect after 1%. Magnesium stearate reduces not only the lower punch ejection force by about 70% but also tablet tensile strength (21). Stearic acid is the second most important lubricant. It is not as effective as magnesium stearate, the minimum effective stearic acid concentration is about 1%, and it reduces the lower punch ejection force no more than 30%. This fatty acid is however useful when an alkaline ingredient in a tablet formula is undesirable. The hexagonal form of boron nitride (HBN) has been reported as a potential tablet lubricant (21). HBN is similar to graphite, which is soft and lubricious. This inorganic solid powder retains its ability to lubricate in extreme cold or heat. It was reported that boron nitride reduced the lower punch ejection force as efficiently as magnesium stearate, but its ability to reduce the tablet tensile strength is less than magnesium stearate. The result is mechanically stronger tablets. Therefore, there is a good potential for HBN to be used as a tablet lubricant. For effervescent tablets, water-soluble lubricants are required since insoluble alkaline lubricants would accumulate on the surface of final solution or form a cloudy solution with an alkaline taste, all of which is undesirable. Sodium lauryl sulfate, DL-leucine, or various PEGs can be used as water-soluble lubricants. Liquid paraffin and hydrogenated vegetable oil are also among the lubricants, but their effectiveness is lower than that of magnesium stearate and stearic acid.

TABLET-MANUFACTURING OPERATIONS

Once a tablet formulation is designed with drug, binder, disintegrant, diluent, pH buffer, lubricant, or a matrix former polymer, a manufacturing method must also be determined. The manufacturing method will depend on the dose of active ingredient, the limitations of drug substance such as heat sensitivity or water insolubility, availability of specialized equipment such as high-shear granulators or fluidized beds, the time frame for manufacturing, and the batch size (2,4,5,9). Certain manufacturing methods can be used interchangeably. On the other hand, sometimes a specific manufacturing method must be employed, for instance, passing the formulation three times through a roller compactor and compressing a 1500-mg formulation to produce a tablet of reasonable size. Therefore, deciding on a manufacturing method is a complex task that requires time, equipment, and formulation optimization, as well as a close collaboration between formulation scientists and process engineers. In general terms, there are three manufacturing processes for tablets: wet granulation, dry granulation, and direct compression as discussed below.

Wet Granulation

The purpose of wet granulation is to convert the drug and excipient mixture into granules that flow well into dies, and which are compressible into mechanically strong and acceptable tablets. Wet granulation has many subtypes. The classical traditional wet granulation operation consists of the following processes:

- Premixing drug with other ingredients using a V-shaped mixer
- Transferring the mixture into a *traditional low shear granulator* where a binder solution is added under a mechanical shear until a certain granule size and binding are obtained
- Wet sieving of granules through a desired screen size
- Drying of granules in a tray-oven dryer
- Dry sieving/milling of granules to a certain particle size distribution
- Adding a lubricant to the dry granules
- Compressing the granules into tablets

The wet granulation operation as described above has been used for more than 50 years in the pharmaceutical industry, and there is a great expertise on this area. However, introduction of new materials and equipment, changing manufacturing needs, and time limitations for manufacturing have brought new modifications to classical wet granulation. Two different modified wet granulation operations are summarized below.

Modification to traditional wet granulation I involves the following:

- Premixing drug with other ingredients using a V-shaped mixer or a high-shear mixer/granulator
- Transferring the mixture into a high-shear granulator where a binder solution is added, and a certain granule size is obtained in a very short time.
- Wet sieving of granules through a desired screen size may or may not be required because of very uniform and narrow particle size distribution
- Drying of granules in a *fluidized bed* or in a *microwave* dryer
- Alternatively, drying the wet mass in the same high-shear mixer/granulator.
- Dry sieving/milling of granules to a certain particle size distribution
- Adding a lubricant to dry granules
- Compressing the granules into tablets

Modification to traditional wet granulation II (4,22) involves the following:

- Premixing drug with other ingredients using a V-shaped mixer
- Transferring the mixture into a *fluidized-bed granulator* where a binder solution is sprayed until a certain granule size and simultaneous drying occur
- Dry sieving/milling of granules to a certain particle size distribution
- Adding a lubricant to dry granules
- Compressing the granules into tablets

On the basis of the modifications summarized above, traditional wet granulation has become a more feasible, time-saving, and economical operation. In a regular workday, many batches can be manufactured with a high reproducibility. The high-shear granulators and/or fluidized-bed granulators/dryers are at the center of these operations. Among the advantages of wet granulation are better drug content uniformity for low-dose drugs, better mechanical tablet properties such as high crushing strength, and low friability due to well-distributed binder molecules over the drug and diluent particles. Expensive equipment, limited batch capacity, and the need for drying are among the disadvantages of wet granulation operations.

Dry Granulation

Dry granulation is the method of producing granules without any solvent use or drying prior to tablet manufacturing. The flow and compressibility are attained by mechanical compression. A dry binder such as MCC or a polymer such as HPMC that will contribute to plastic deformation can be added to the mixture. In the past, before the availability of continuous roller compactors, compressing briquette tablets in specialized tablet presses and breaking those tablets into granules was the method of choice, but this operation produced dust and had other problems. Therefore, dry granulation was not a preferred way of manufacturing tablets. In modern application of dry granulation (23,24), counter-rotating steel rollers are used to apply pressure to the powder. The surface of these rollers can be smooth or grooved depending on the properties of the powder. The compressed product has a higher density upon processing between the rollers. Some formulations may require double or triple pass through roller compactor for maximum densification. The final product will require size reduction and sieving. Modern dry granulation using roller compactors is a straightforward, reproducible operation with few steps. Hence, it is a rapid and economical way of producing pharmaceutical granules. The selection and concentration of formulation ingredients as well as their mechanical properties are more critical in this process than in wet granulation.

The basic steps in dry granulation are

- premixing drug with other ingredients using a V-shaped mixer,
- transferring the mixture into a *roller compactor* using a closed-circuit vacuum equipment to prevent dust formation,
- milling/sieving of the resulting flakes or ribbons into granules,
- adding lubricant and/or disintegrant to granules, and finally
- compressing the granules into tablets

The operation parameters that affect the product properties as might be anticipated include roll pressure, speed, surface texture, and the gap between the rollers. The powders are fed to a roller compactor by a screw feeder under positive pressure. For those tablets that approach or exceed 1000 mg such as the 825-mg amoxicillin and 125-mg potassium clavulanate combination, dry granulation is the most feasible way of manufacture.

Direct Compression✷

As the name implies, this method involves no further processing of powders before tabletting. A formulation is well mixed to ensure uniform drug distribution, and after adding a lubricant, tablets are compressed (2,5,9). However, the requirements for flowability and compressibility must be met by the excipients or the drug substance requires to be coated or processed. Since direct compression involves only mixing and compressing steps, it is the most preferred way of making tablets, given appropriate choice of excipients.

Steps in direct compression are listed here.

- Premixing drug with other ingredients using a V-shaped mixer
- Adding a lubricant to the granules
- Mixing with lubricant 3 to10 minutes
- Compressing the granules

Availability of DC excipients does not guarantee the success of DC tabletting. The drug substance must also have appropriate compressibility and flowability if the drug represents more than one-third of tablet formulation. In that case, DC excipients may compensate for flowability and compressibility. If a drug powder with an insufficient flow and compressibility forms a large portion of a tablet, the DC method cannot be used. Active materials such as acetaminophen, amoxicillin, ascorbic acid, thiamine, and riboflavine have DC grades. The DC grades are produced by coprocessing the actives with polymers such as MC, hydroxypropyl MC, acrylates, or PVP through a spray-drying or fluidized-bed coating process. Direct compression requires the use of directly compressible excipients, and thus limits a formulator's ability for further processing. However, once a compressible formulation is designed, manufacturing is straightforward and simple. A pharmaceutical company that manufactures tablets only with DC method needs only powder-powder mixers and tablet presses, which means lower investment costs. MCC is the most important DC excipient. Other DC excipients include anhydrous β-lactose, spray-dried lactose, unmilled dicalcium phosphate dihydrate, pregelatinized starch, and mannitol DC.

TABLET PRESSES AND TOOLING

Tablets are compressed using a *compression station* consisting of a die, a lower punch, and an upper punch. Tablet presses can be divided into two classes: single-station reciprocating presses and multi-station rotary presses (25,26). The rotary tablet press comprises a compression unit, which is detachably mounted. The compression unit consists of a die table with punches, a feeding device for the granules to be compressed into the dies, and a tablet discharge device for removal of tablets. The capacity of rotary tablet presses is determined by the rotation speed of the turret and the number of stations on the press. For instance, a rotary tablet press with 30 stations and rotation speed of 60 rpm produces 108,000 tablets per hour. Rotary tablet presses can have die table rotation speeds between 25 and 120 rpm, and the number of stations may be as many as 90. During such high production rates, there are limits in tablet weight and diameter, which is usually between 11 and 13 mm, and the maximum fill depths are between 15 and 20 mm. With smaller number of stations such as 35, larger tablets of about 25 mm in diameter can be produced, resulting in a lower tablet output such as 88,000 tablets per hour. The tabletting cycle starts with the flow of granules into die cavity; this is called the *filling stage*. The next step is the *weight adjustment,* where the excess material is pushed outside the die by the lower punch, and the *compression stage* that involves the upper punch meeting the lower punch. The vertical movement of the lower punch pushing the tablet to the die surface accomplishes the *ejection stage*, and the cycle starts over again. The main differences between the single-station eccentric press and a rotary press are (9,25,26) the dwell time for punches and applied forces. The dwell times are very short for rotary presses in the range of 8 to 10 milliseconds, and much higher for single-station presses in the range of 250 milliseconds. The maximum applied forces are in the range of 50 to 100 kN for rotary presses and 15 to 50 kN for eccentric single-station presses. Hence, tablet formulations may be optimized by using small rotary presses instead of single-station presses to obtain a high correlation between laboratory scale and manufacturing scale operations. There are overall length standards for rotary tablet press punches. The American standard punches have an overall length of 133.35 mm (5.25″), compared with the European standard 133.60 mm (5.26″), while the Japanese norm is the same as the U.S. standard (27). The steel selection and manufacturing of dies and punches is a specialized area (28). According to industry standards, the steel for dies should conform to DIN 1.2550 standard that has a partial composition: 0.6% C,

1.87% W, 0.95% Cr, 0.33% Mn, and 0.16% V. Punch steel (DIN 1.2080) contains 1.96% C, 11.5% Cr, and 0.24% Mn. Since punches have to face abrasive wear, high tensile stresses, and compressional forces, the punch steel is harder and tougher. After giving the appropriate shape to the steel rods, a heat treatment step follows. Heat treatment involves preheating, heating, and hardening with a stepwise increase in temperature from 550°C to 1050°C in about 1.5 hours, then a cooling step in an oil bath and tempering at least three times at 520°C to 550°C for 6 hours to optimize mechanical properties. The next step for punch and dies is coating and surface treatment to provide resistance against wear and corrosion and to improve frictional properties (27,28). Hard chromium, titanium nitride, and chromium nitride coatings provide those properties. Therefore, the punches and dies for tablet presses are made from special steel alloys, but they can only be used after appropriate heat treatment and surface coating.

QUALITY CONTROL OF TABLETS

After manufacturing tablets, a series of tests are carried out to assure that they meet the specifications of pharmacopoeia or industry standards. These tests are as listed below:

- Crushing strength
- Disintegration
- Friability
- Dissolution
- Drug content uniformity
- Weight uniformity
- Weight and thickness

Some tablets are ready to be used after manufacture, while some need to be coated for further functional properties such as enteric coating or controlled-release coating.

Tablet Crushing Strength

Although tablet crushing strength is not an official test, it is one of the most important properties of a tablet, since it demonstrates the mechanical strength of a tablet for further operations, such as coating and blistering, and provides an idea of the robustness of a tablet till it reaches a patient. Tablet tensile strength can be calculated as follows (29,30):

$$\sigma = \frac{F}{A}$$

where σ is the tensile strength (N/mm^2), F is the fracture force (N), and A is the fracture plane (mm^2).

For a typical tablet shape, a splitting test for a cylinder, the equation becomes

$$\sigma = \frac{2F}{\pi d h}$$

where d is tablet diameter (mm) and h the tablet height (mm).

However, the fracture force that can be obtained by a diametrical crushing of a tablet is still a useful parameter. Under normal conditions, a tablet should have a minimum crushing force value of 90 N. Below that value, still pharmaceutically acceptable tablets can be manufactured but with borderline properties. For instance, a tablet with a crushing force of 120 N can be considered strong enough for a film-coating operation. Tablets with crushing strength values as high as 300 N are manufactured using modern excipients and equipment. Such tablets must still of course comply with the other requirements. European Pharmacopoeia (EP) lists the test under *Resistance of Crushing of Tablets* and recommends measurements on 10 tablets.

Tablet Disintegration Test

Tablets must be tested to ensure disintegration. The United States Pharmacopeia (USP) and EP have official standards, including descriptions of the apparatus type dimensions and test conditions (31,32). For instance, EP has two different types of apparatus, one for tablets that are 18 mm or smaller in size, *Apparatus A*, testing six tablets. Another for larger tablets, called *Apparatus B*, with a test with three tablets. The technical specifications of the apparatus, the test conditions, and evaluation criteria can be found in the USP or EP. A tablet is considered to have disintegrated when no residue remains on the screen of the apparatus that makes a reciprocating movement in a selected solution. The test is carried out at 37°C. The solutions used are distilled water, 0.1 N HCl, pH 6.8 buffer solutions, and the other USP buffer solutions. For instance, modified release coated tablets are kept in acid solution, and they should not disintegrate in two hours. Plain uncoated tablets should disintegrate in no longer than 15 minutes, whereas water-soluble film-coated tablets should disintegrate in less than 30 minutes. Disintegration is considered a prerequisite for dissolution, and in turn, for good bioavailability. Therefore, it is very important that a designed tablet will disintegrate within the time limits or will withstand without disintegration to protect the drug, for instance, in acid conditions sometimes up to five hours.

Tablet Friability Test

This test shows the strength of tablets against mechanical attrition. In EP 5.0, a tablet friability apparatus and test conditions are described (32). The procedure as follows: If the tablet target weight is less than 650 mg, 20 tablets are weighed. If the tablet target weight is more than 650 mg, 10 tablets are sufficient for the test. The drum is rotated 100 times and the tablets are weighed again. No more than 1% weight loss should occur due to breakage. Although 1% friability is permitted in the EP or USP, from the technological point of view it is considered too much. A good tablet formulation and an appropriate manufacturing process should result in tablets with 0% or maximally 0.5% friability. If 1% or higher friability occurs, formulation scientists and process engineers should correct the situation. Selecting appropriate binder and binder concentrations and compressing tablets with a crushing strength value of 90 N or more will result in tablets with low or no friability.

Tablet Dissolution Test

Since drug dissolution is a prerequisite for in vivo drug absorption, tablet dissolution tests have been one of the most important tablet quality control tests. The *paddle, basket,* and *flow-through cell* apparatus are all described in the USP or EP with great detail, and the technical drawings can be found in these compendia (31,32). The rotation speed, temperature, composition, and the volume of dissolution medium are specified and can change on the basis of the monograph of a drug or the dosage form. The sink conditions must be met during the test. Otherwise, the flow-through cell must be used for those drugs with a low solubility. During dissolution study, a temperature of 37°C ± 0.5°C must be maintained for tablets, and 50 rpm is the most frequently used rotation speed. The solutions used during dissolution tests are as follows: distilled water, pH 1.2, pH 6.8 buffer solutions, and the other USP or EP buffer solutions. Unless otherwise stated, 85% drug release is expected from tablets in 15 minutes or 30 minutes depending on the European or the U.S. regulations. For the extended release products, drug dissolution profile is given in the individual monograph of a drug.

Tablet Weight and Drug Content Uniformity

During tablet manufacturing, individual tablet weights may vary for many reasons, some resulting from the formulation and others from tooling and equipment. This variation must be within an acceptable range. The EP states that weight uniformity for 20 uncoated or film-coated tablets may deviate between 5% and 10% depending on the tablet weight (32). If tablet weight is 80 mg or less, maximum 10% deviation is permitted. For tablets with weights between 80 mg and 250 mg, 7.5%, and for those weighing more than 250 mg, a maximum 5% deviation is permitted. The production of uniform weight tablets is extremely important, and it can only be assured by a free granule flow, selecting the appropriate lubricant/glidant, and punches with tight working length tolerances. On the other hand, drug content uniformity test is based on the individual drug content of the selected number of tablets. According to the EP, 10 tablets are tested. The preparation complies if the individual content is between 85% and 115%. In case of noncompliance, the extension of the test can be found in the EP. Content uniformity test differs from the weight uniformity since the uniform distribution of a drug depends on the manufacturing method. Low-dose drugs, such as 100 µg drug per tablet, require special precautions during manufacture. For instance, dissolving the active in binder solution and spraying onto other excipients, mixing the drug by geometric dilution method during the granulation, and also preferring wet granulation to direct compression. The USP, 30th edition, 2007, requires more strict conditions for uniformity of dosage units on the basis of weight variation or content uniformity. The choice of applying the test depends on the dose and ratio of drug substance. More details are in the USP (31).

MECHANICS OF GRANULE COMPRESSION AND TABLET FORMATION

Tablets can be considered as composite materials. A typical tablet formulation may contain cellulose-based products, inorganic mineral materials, disaccharides, polysaccharides, esters of fatty acids, fatty acids, some organic acids, bases, and synthetic polymers with all kinds of different crystalline structures. Hence, a combination of different materials at different percentages forms a product with unique mechanical properties. Behavior of granules and pharmaceutical powders under compression has been the subject of intensive research (33–36). When two punches meet to compress a granule mass into a tablet, several processes occur simultaneously in a very short time. Consolidation of particles, decrease in porosity of powder column, and finally reaching the minimum volume, and then deformation or fragmentation occur. In the literature, three distinct cases were described for materials under pressure:

- Plastic deformation
- Elastic deformation
- Brittle fracture

The experimental procedure to determine the behavior of a pharmaceutical powder under pressure is well established. The Heckel equation (33,34) was first proposed for metal powders and later adopted for pharmaceutical powders. The equation provides information about the mechanism of compact formation and the magnitude of plastic deformation on the basis of slope. The decrease in porosity with pressure follows a first-order kinetics.

$$\ln \frac{1}{1-D} = kP + A$$

where D is the relative density, P is the applied pressure, k and A are the parameters that can be obtained experimentally.

In a plot of P versus $\ln 1/(1 - D)$, A is the intercept that is related to the die filling and consolidation of particles, whereas k is a measurement of plasticity. The steeper the k, the more plastic the deformation. In addition to the Heckel equation, some modifications of the Heckel equation were proposed, and also some other empirical powder compaction equations were developed such as the Cooper-Eaton and the Kawakita. For instance, in the Kawakita equation, the tapped density measurements are used instead of compaction pressures (37).

REFERENCES

1. Wilkinson L. William Brockedon, F.R.S. (1787–1854). Notes Rec R Soc Lond 1971; 26:65–72.
2. Davies P. Oral Solid Dosage FormsIn: Gibson M, ed. Pharmaceutical Preformulation and Formulation. Boca Raton, USA: Interpharm/CRC, 2004:379–458.
3. Gibson M. Aiding candidate drug selection: introduction and objectives. In: Gibson M, ed. Pharmaceutical Preformulation and Formulation. Boca Raton, FL: Interpharm/CRC, 2004: 15–95.
4. Kornchankul W, Parikh N, Sakr A. Correlation between wet granulation kinetic parameters and tablet characteristics. Pharm Ind 2001; 63:764–774.
5. Shangraw RF. Compressed tablets by direct compression. In: Lieberman HA, Lachman L, Schwartz JB, eds. Pharmaceutical Dosage Forms: Tablets. Vol 1, 2nd ed. New York: Marcel Dekker, 1989:195–246.
6. Gunsel WC, Dusel RG. Compression coated and layer tablets. In: Lieberman HA, Lachman L, Schwartz JB, eds. Pharmaceutical Dosage Forms: Tablets. Vol 1, 2nd ed. New York: Marcel Dekker, 1989:247–284.
7. Conine JW, Pikal MJ. Special tablets. In: Lieberman, Lachman, Schwartz, eds. Pharmaceutical Dosage Forms: Tablets. Vol 1, 2nd ed. New York: Marcel Dekker, 1989:329–366.
8. Ugurlu T, Turkoglu M, Soyogul O, et al. Colonic delivery of compression coated nisin tablets using pectin/HPMC polymer mixture. Eur J Pharm Biopharm 2007; 67:202–210.
9. Habib W, Khankari R, Hontz J. Fast-dissolve drug delivery systems. Crit Rev Ther Drug Carrier Syst 2000; 17:61–72.
10. Turkoglu M, Varol H, Çelikok M. Tableting and stability of enteric coated omeprazole pellets. Eur J Pharm Biopharm 2004; 57:279–286.
11. Lactose Products, DMV International, Veghel, The Netherlands. Available at: www.dmv-international.com/.
12. Rowe RC, Sheskey PJ, Owen SC, eds. Handbook of Pharmaceutical Excipients. 5th ed. London: Pharmaceutical Press, 2006.
13. Bolhuis GK, Chowhan ZT. Materials for direct compression. In: Alderborn G, Nyström C, eds. Pharmaceutical Powder Compaction Technology. New York: Marcel Dekker, 1996:419–500.
14. Spress, Pregelatinized Corn Starch, Grain Processing Corp., Muscatine, IA. Available at: www. grainprocessing.com.

15. Avicel PH. Microcrystalline Cellulose, FMC Corp., Philadelphia, PA. Available at: www. fmcbiopolymer.com.
16. Emcocel, Microcrystalline Cellulose, Mendell, Patterson, New York.
17. Kollidon Polyvinylpyrrolidone for the Pharmaceutical Industry. 6th ed. Germany: BASF, 2001.
18. Turkoglu M, Nirun E, Yeniyurt M. A modified laboratory size rotary fluidized-bed for pharmaceutical solid materials processing. Pharm Eng 1999; 19:70–77.
19. Bolhuis GK, Holzer AW. Lubricant sensitivity. In: Alderborn G, Nyström C, eds. Pharmaceutical Powder Compaction Technology. New York: Marcel Dekker, 1996:517–560.
20. Sinka IC, Cunningham JC, Zavaliangos A. The effect of wall friction in the compaction of pharmaceutical tablets with curved faces: a validation study of the Drucker-Prager cap model. Powder Technol 2003; 133:33–43.
21. Turkoglu M, Sahin I, San T. Evaluation of hexagonal boron nitride as a new tablet lubricant. Pharm Dev Technol 2005; 10:381–388.
22. Turkoglu M, He M, Sakr A. Evaluation of rotary fluidized-bed as a wet granulation equipment. Eur J Pharm Biopharm 1995; 41:388–394.
23. Turkoglu M, Aydin I, Murray M, et al. Modeling of roller compaction process using neural networks and genetic algorithms. Eur J Pharm Biopharm 1999; 48:239–245.
24. Chilsonator Brochure. The Fitzpatrick Company Europe, Belgium. Available at: www. fitzpatrick.be.
25. Krumme M, Schwabe L, Fromming KH. Development of computerised procedures for the characterisation of the tableting properties with eccentric machines. Die Pharmazie 1996; 51:315–323.
26. Fette Brochure, Wilhelm Fette GMBH, Germany, No:8083 (488 1 S). Available at: www.fette. com/.
27. Tablet Compression Tooling, I Holland Ltd., Nottingham, England. Available at: www. iholland.co.uk/.
28. Cihan G, Eke K, Gokyildiz MD, et al. Design and Improving the Quality of Materials Used in Pharmaceutical Tablet Manufacturing Dies and Punches [graduation thesis]. Istanbul, Turkey: Faculty of Chemical-Metallurgical Engineering, Istanbul Technical University, 2004.
29. Neville AM. Properties of Concrete. London: Pitman Publishing, 1981:549–552.
30. Olsson H, Nystrom C. Assessing tablet bond types from structural features that affect tablet tensile strength. Pharm Res 2001; 18:203–210.
31. The United States Pharmacopeia (USP). 30th Rev. United States Pharmacopeial Convention, Inc., Rockville, MD, 2007.
32. European Pharmacopoeia (EP). 5th ed. Directorate for the Quality of Medicines of the Council of Europe, Cedex, France, 2004.
33. Heckel RW. Density pressure relationship in powder compaction. Trans Metall Soc AIME 1961; 221:671–675.
34. Heckel RW. An analysis of powder compaction phenomena. Trans Metall Soc AIME 1961; 221:1001–1008.
35. Eriksson M, Alderborn G. The effect of particle fragmentation and deformation on the interparticulate bond deformation process during powder compaction. Pharm Res 1995; 12:1031–1039.
36. Hiestand EN. Principles tenets and notions of tablet bonding and measurements of strength. Eur J Pharm Biopharm 1997; 44:229–242.
37. Paronen P, Ilkka J. Porosity-pressure functions. In: Alderborn G, Nyström C, eds. Pharmaceutical Powder Compaction Technology. New York: Marcel Dekker, 1996:55–75.

14

Hard- and Soft-Shell Capsules

Larry L. Augsburger
University of Maryland, School of Pharmacy, Department of Pharmaceutical Sciences, Baltimore, Maryland, U.S.A.

HISTORICAL DEVELOPMENT AND ROLE AS A DOSAGE FORM

Capsules are solid dosage forms in which the drug substance is enclosed within either a hard or soft soluble shell. Generally the shells are formed from gelatin. The capsule may be regarded as "container" drug delivery system, which provides a tasteless/odorless dosage form without the need of a secondary coating step, as may be required for tablets. Swallowing is easy for most patients, since the shell is smooth and hydrates in the mouth, and the capsule often tends to float on swallowing in the liquid taken with it. Their availability in a wide variety of colors makes capsules aesthetically pleasing. There are numerous additional advantages to capsules as a dosage form, depending on the type of capsule employed.

Capsules may be classified as either *hard* or *soft* depending on the nature of the shell. Soft-gelatin capsules (sometimes referred to as "softgels") are made from a more flexible, plasticized gelatin film than that of hard-gelatin capsules. Most capsules of either type are intended to be swallowed whole; however, some soft-gelatin capsules are intended for rectal or vaginal insertion as suppositories. The majority of capsule products manufactured today are of the hard-gelatin type. One survey (1) has estimated that the use of hard-gelatin capsules to prepare solid dosage forms exceeds that of soft-gelatin capsules by about 10-fold.

The first capsule prepared from gelatin was a one-piece capsule that was patented in France by Mothes and DuBlanc in 1834 (2). Although the shells of these early capsules were not plasticized, such capsules would be classified today as "soft-gelatin capsules" on the basis of shape, contents, and other features. Intended to mask the taste of certain unpleasant-tasting medication, they quickly gained popularity primarily as a means for administering copaiba balsam, a drug popular at the time in the management of venereal disease (2). These capsules were made one at a time by hand by dipping leather molds in a molten gelatin mixture, filling with a pipette, and sealing with a drop of molten gelatin (3). Today, soft-gelatin capsules are prepared from plasticized gelatin by means of a plate process or, more commonly, by a rotary die process in which they are formed, filled, and sealed in a single operation. With few exceptions, soft-gelatin capsules are filled with solutions or suspensions of drugs in liquids that will not solubilize the gelatin shell. They are a completely sealed dosage form: the capsule cannot be opened without destroying the

499

capsule. Because liquid contents can be metered with high-quality pumps, soft-gelatin capsules are among the most accurate and precise of all solid oral dosage forms. Depending on the machine tooling, a wide variety of sizes and shapes are possible. Typical shapes include spherical, oval, oblong, tube, and suppository type; size may range from 1 to 480 minims (16.2 minims = 1 mL) (3).

Although the patent holders at first sold both filled and empty soft-gelatin capsules, the sale of empty shells was discontinued after 1837 (2). However, the demand that had been created for the empty capsules led to several attempts to overcome the patents, which, in turn, resulted in the development both of the gelatin-coated pill and the hard-gelatin capsule (2). The first hard-gelatin capsule was invented by J.C. Lehuby to whom a French patent was granted in 1846 (2). It resembled the modern hard-gelatin capsule in that it consisted of two, telescoping, cap and body pieces. In Lehuby's patent, the capsule shells were made of starch or tapioca sweetened with syrup, although later additions to the patent claimed carrageen (1847) and mixtures of carrageen with gelatin (1850) (2). The first person to describe a two-piece gelatin capsule made from gelatin was James Murdock, who was granted a British patent in 1848 and who is often credited as the inventor of the modern hard-gelatin capsule. Since, Murdock was a patent agent by profession, it has been suggested that he was actually working on behalf of Lehuby (2).

Unlike soft-gelatin capsules, hard-gelatin capsules are manufactured in one operation and filled in a completely separate operation. Originally, they were made by hand dipping greased metal pin-like molds into a molten gelatin mixture, drying the resultant films, stripping them from the pins, and joining the same two pieces together (2). Today, they are manufactured in a similar manner by means of a completely automated process. For human use, hard-gelatin capsules are supplied in at least eight sizes ranging in volumetric capacity from 0.13 to 1.37 mL. Typically, they are oblong shaped; however, some manufacturers have made modest alterations in that shape to be distinctive.

In further contrast to soft-gelatin capsules, hard-gelatin capsules typically are filled with powders, granules, or pellets. Modified-release granules or pellets may be filled without crushing or compaction, thus avoiding disruption of barrier coats or other possible adverse effects on the release mechanism. Although many manufacturers of hard capsule–filling equipment also have developed modifications to their machines, which would permit the filling of liquids or semisolid matrices, there are few commercial examples.

Filled hard-gelatin capsules are held together by interlocking bumps and grooves molded into the cap and body pieces, and the capsules may be additionally sealed by a banding process that places a narrow strip of gelatin around the midsection of the capsule where the two pieces are joined, or by a spray sealing process.

Additional advantages and attributes of both hard- and soft-shell capsules are discussed in the following sections.

Nongelatin Capsules

Capsules made from gelatin predominate; however, recent years have seen an increased interest and availability of nongelatin capsules. Such alternative shell compositions may satisfy religious, cultural, or vegetarian needs to avoid animal sources. Hard-shell capsules made from starch were developed by Capsugel, a Division of Pfizer, Inc. (Peapack, New Jersey, U.S.). These consist of two parts—fitted cap and body pieces that are made by injection molding the glassy mass formed when starch containing 13% to 14% water is heated, and then dried (4). Temperatures in the range of 140°C to 190°C reportedly produce masses that flow satisfactorily without degradation. The two parts are formed in separate molds. Unlike hard-gelatin capsules that are supplied with the caps and bodies prejoined, the two parts are supplied separately. The caps and bodies do not interlock and must be sealed together at the time of filling to prevent their separation. Capsugel has licensed this technology to West Pharmaceutical Services, Lionville, Pennsylvania, which uses the starch capsule in their TARGIT® technology for site-specific delivery to the colon. TARGIT is based on the application of enteric polymer coatings to the starch capsules (5).

Hard shells manufactured from hypromellose, the *United States Pharmacopeia–National Formulary* (USP-NF) official title for hydroxypropylmethylcellulose (HPMC), are also available, for example, Quali-V® (Qualicaps Inc., Whitsett, North Carolina, U.S.) and Vcaps® from Capsugel. Like hard-gelatin capsules, hard-shell HPMC capsules can be formed using a dipping technology. In the case of gelatin capsules, the shells are formed by the gelation (on cooling) of an aqueous gelatin composition that clings to the surface of mold pins (described in more detail later in this chapter). To use the dipping technology, certain additives must be added to HPMC to promote the formation of a gelling system. In one example, small quantities of carrageenan (lowers the thermal gelation temperature) and potassium chloride (promotes gelation) are added (6). In another example, the gelling system consists of gellan gum and potassium acetate (7). Both gellan gum and carrageenan are negatively charged polysaccharides; hence, the positively charged potassium cations promote gelation by reducing the electrostatic repulsion of the polysaccharide chains (7).

Nongelatin soft-shell capsules have also been introduced in recent years. For example, Catalent Pharma Solutions (Somerset, New Jersey, U.S.) has developed Vegicaps® Soft Capsules, the shells of which consist of modified starch, carrageenan, disodium phosphate, glycerin, and/or sorbitol (8). Another starch-based soft-shell capsule, VegaGels®, is available from Swiss Caps USA, Inc. (Miami, Florida, U.S.) (9). Both sources form and fill capsules in a rotary die process similar to that used to produce soft-gelatin capsules.

HARD-SHELL CAPSULES

Advantages

Powder-filled hard-shell capsules often have been assumed to have better bioavailability than tablets. Most likely, this assumption is derived from the fact that the shell rapidly dissolves and ruptures, which affords at least the potential for rapid release of the drug, together with the lack of use of a compaction process comparable to tablet compression in filling the capsules. However, capsules can be just as easily malformulated as tablets. There have been number of reports of bioavailability problems with capsules (10–13).

Powder-filled hard-shell capsules allow for a degree of flexibility of formulation not obtainable with tablets: Often they are easier to formulate because there is no requirement that the powders be formed into a coherent compact that must stand up to handling like tablets. However, it must be recognized that the problems of powder blending and homogeneity, powder fluidity, and lubrication in hard-capsule filling are similar to those encountered in tablet manufacture. The ability of such dry solids to be uniformly filled into a dosing-disc cavity or dosing tube is the determining factor in weight variation and, to a degree, content uniformity.

Modern capsule-filling technology makes possible the filling of various combinations of diverse systems, for example, beads/granules, tablets, liquid/semisolids, small soft-gelatin capsules, or even smaller hard-shell capsules into hard-shell capsules. Such multicomponent capsules offer many possibilities in dosage form design (14).

Incompatibilities can be overcome by separating problem ingredients within the same capsule; for example, one component could be filled as a coated pellet. Various modified or controlled drug delivery systems can be created by incorporating modified-release beads or granules. Immediate-release and sustained-release formulations of a drug can be included in the same capsule. In another possible configuration, two different drugs whose pharmacokinetic properties require different modified-release profiles can be filled into the same capsule as different species of beads. Indeed, capsules are ideally suited to the dispensing of granular or bead-type modified-release products since they may be filled without a compression process that could rupture the particles or otherwise compromise the integrity of any controlled-release coatings.

Traditionally the province of soft-shell capsules, the filling of liquids into hard-shell capsules, made feasible through improvements in encapsulation and sealing technology, has become a topic of substantial interest today. As will be discussed later, the liquid filling of capsules of either type offers numerous advantages, such as the ability to manage low melting point drugs, enhance the content uniformity of low-dose drugs, and enhance the bioavailability of poorly soluble, hydrophobic drugs.

Hard-shell capsules also may be used to advantage as unit-dose containers for delivering dry powder drugs by inhalation (15,16). Micronized drug with carrier powder is released for inhalation in dry powder inhaler (DPI) devices that either cut or puncture the shell walls (17). Such systems are used to deliver asthma and allergy drugs like sodium cromolyn, and may prove advantageous for delivering large, labile, biological molecules that are difficult to deliver by other means.

Hard-shell capsules are widely used in preliminary drug studies. Phase I development studies are often carried out with hard-shell capsule formulations because of their relative ease of formulation and manufacture, even though the final formulation often may be intended to be a compressed tablet. For conventional filling machines, fillers and other excipients are often needed, especially when doses are small in relation to capsule shell volumes. In a recent development, Capsugel has introduced a new filling machine, the Xelodose® microdosing system for the precise direct filling of doses as low as 100 mcg without the need for excipients (18). This development provides very broad flexibility for dispensing different doses for phase I clinical studies while minimizing the potential for interactions with excipients.

Hard-shell capsules also are uniquely suitable for blinded clinical tests. Bioequivalence studies of tablet formulations may be conveniently "blinded" by inserting tablets into opaque capsules, often along with an inert filler powder. Even capsule products may be disguised by inserting them into larger capsules.

Disadvantages

From a pharmaceutical manufacturing point of view, there is some disadvantage in the fact that output rates (e.g., capsules/hr) of even the fastest automatic capsule-filling machines are substantially slower than the rates at which modern high-speed production tablet presses can produce tablets, which is a factor that adds to the cost of capsule production. Another factor is the cost of the shells. Although hard-shell capsule products may thus tend to be more costly to produce than tablets, the relative cost-effectiveness of capsules and tablets must be judged on a case-by-case basis. This cost disadvantage diminishes as the cost of the active ingredient increases or when the tablets must be coated (19). Furthermore, it may be possible to avoid the cost of a granulation step by choosing encapsulation in lieu of tableting.

Highly soluble salts (e.g., iodides, bromides, chlorides) generally should not be dispensed in hard capsules. Their rapid release may cause gastric irritation because of the formation of a high drug concentration in localized areas. A somewhat related concern is that hard-gelatin capsules may become lodged in the esophagus where the resulting localized high concentration of certain drugs (doxycycline, potassium chloride, indomethacin, and others) may cause damage (20). Marvola (20) measured the force required to detach various dosage forms from isolated pig esophagus mounted in an organ bath and found that gelatin capsules tended to adhere more strongly than tablets. However, the detachment forces were greatly reduced for both after a water rinse (to simulate drinking) and when there was a slow continuous flow of artificial saliva. In an in vivo study, Hey et al. (21) studied the esophageal transit of barium sulfate tablets and gelatin capsules radiologically in 121 healthy volunteers. The subjects' position (standing or lying down) and the volume of water taken (25 or 100 mL) during swallowing were considered. The majority (60%) of the volunteers had some difficulty in swallowing one or more of the preparations: Many preparations were shown to adhere to the esophagus and to begin to disintegrate in the lower part of the esophagus. Delayed transit time occurred more frequently with large round tablets than with small tablets or capsules. In contrast to tablets, patient position or the volume of water taken had less influence on the passage of capsules. Despite their findings, Hey et al. did not prefer capsules because of their potential for esophageal adhesion. In general, it was recommended that patients should remain standing 90 seconds or more after taking tablets or capsules and that they should be swallowed with at least 100 mL water. In a study considering only the esophageal transit of barium sulfate–filled hard-gelatin capsules, Channer and Virjee (22) found that 26 of 50 patients exhibited sticking; however, only three of these patients were aware that a capsule had lodged in their esophagus. These investigators also concluded that drugs should be taken with a drink while standing. Evans and Roberts (23) compared barium sulfate tablets and capsules and found a greater tendency for esophageal retention with tablets than with capsules. Fell (24) pointed to the large difference in density between barium sulfate and typical pharmaceutical preparations as a complicating factor in drawing conclusions about any differences in esophageal retention between tablets and capsules from such studies.

Few studies have compared the mucosal adhesion of HPMC and gelatin hard-shell capsules. In an in vitro study, Ponchel and Degobert (25) compared the force required to detach gelatin and HPMC hard-shell capsules from isolated porcine esophageal mucosa. They found that the adhesiveness of the two types of capsules was comparable. But later a similar study revealed that the force required to detach HPMC capsules was significantly lower ($p < 0.001$) than that for gelatin capsules (26). On the basis of scintigraphic evidence gathered in a study of esophageal transit involving 11 human volunteers, Cole et al. (7) questioned the relevance of isolated tissue studies. They found the esophageal transit of HPMC and gelatin capsules to be quite rapid (<20 sec) in most cases, with no significant difference between the two types of capsules.

The Manufacture of Hard-Gelatin Capsules (27–30)

In all cases, the shells are manufactured by a dipping process in which sets of stainless steel mold pins are dipped into gelatin solutions, and the shells are formed by gelation on the pin surfaces. As previously noted, HPMC hard-shell capsules are also produced by a dipping process. The basic mechanical design of the equipment was developed about 50 years ago by Colton (27,28).

Shell Composition

Gelatin is the most important constituent of the dipping solutions, but other components may also be present (28–30).

Gelatin Gelatin is prepared by the hydrolysis of collagen obtained from animal connective tissue, bone, skin, and sinew. This long polypeptide chain yields on hydrolysis 18 amino acids, the most prevalent of which are glycine and alanine. Gelatin can vary in its chemical and physical properties depending on the source of the collagen and the manner of extraction.

There are two basic types of gelatin. Type A, which is produced by an acid hydrolysis, is manufactured mainly from pork skin. Type B gelatin, produced by alkaline hydrolysis, is manufactured mainly from animal bones. The two types can be differentiated by their isoelectric points (4.8–5.0 for type B and 7.0–9.0 for type A) and by their viscosity-building and film-forming characteristics.

Either type of gelatin may be used, but combinations of pork skin and bone gelatin are often used to optimize shell characteristics (27–29). Bone gelatin contributes firmness, whereas pork skin gelatin contributes plasticity and clarity.

The physicochemical properties of gelatin of most interest to shell manufacturers are the bloom strength and viscosity. Bloom strength is an empirical gel strength measure, which gives an indication of the firmness of the gel. It is measured in a Bloom gelometer, which determines the weight in grams required to depress a standard plunger a fixed distance into the surface of a 6.67%w/w gel under standard conditions. Gelatins which are produced from the first extraction of the raw materials have the highest bloom strength. Bloom strengths in the range of 150 to 280 g are considered suitable for capsules.

The viscosity of gelatin solutions is vital to the control of the thickness of the cast film. Viscosity is measured on a standard 6.67% w/w solution at 60°C in a capillary pipette, and is generally in the range of 30 to 60 mP.

Colorants Commonly, various soluble synthetic dyes ("coal tar dyes") and insoluble pigments are used. Commonly used pigments are the iron oxides.

Colorants not only play a role in identifying the product but may also play a role in improving patient compliance. Thus, the color of a drug product may be selected in consideration of the disease state for which it is intended. For example, Buckalew and Coffield (31) found in a panel test that four colors were significantly associated with certain treatment groups (white—analgesia, lavender—hallucinogenic effects, orange or yellow—stimulants and antidepressants).

Opaquing agents Titanium dioxide may be included to render the shell opaque. Opaque capsules may be employed to provide protection against light or to conceal the contents.

Preservatives When preservatives are employed, parabens are often selected.

Water Hot, demineralized water is used in the preparation of the dipping solution. Initially, a 30% to 40% w/w solution of gelatin is prepared in large stainless steel tanks. Vacuum may be applied to assist in the removal of entrapped air from this viscous preparation. Portions of this stock solution are removed and mixed with any other ingredients, as required, to prepare the dipping solution. At this point, the viscosity of the dipping solution is measured and adjusted. The viscosity of this solution is critical to the control of the thickness of the capsule walls.

Shell Manufacture

The Colton machine illustrated in Figure 1 is a fully automatic implementation of the dipping process. The steps are as follows:

1. Dipping (Fig. 2)— Pairs of stainless steel pins are dipped into the dipping solution to simultaneously form the caps and bodies. The pins are lubricated with a proprietary mold-release agent. The pins are at ambient temperature

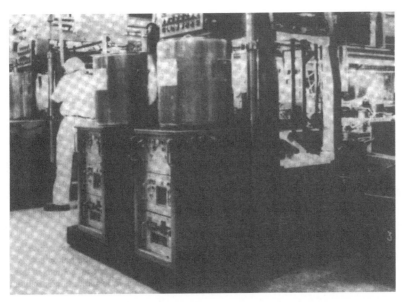

Figure 1 View of a hard-gelatin capsule manufacturing machine. *Source*: Courtesy of Elanco Qualicaps, formerly a Division of Eli Lilly Co., Indianapolis, Indiana, U.S.

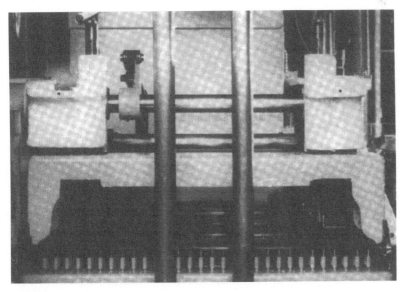

Figure 2 Dipping of pins in the manufacture of hard-gelatin capsules. *Source*: Courtesy of Elanco Qualicaps, formerly a Division of Eli Lilly and Co., Indianapolis, Indiana, U.S.

(about 22°C), whereas the dipping solution is maintained at a temperature of about 50°C in a heated, jacketed dipping pan. The length of time to cast the film has been reported to be about 12 seconds, with larger capsules requiring longer dipping times (29).

2. Rotation—After dipping, the pins are withdrawn from the dipping solution, and as they are done so, they are elevated and rotated two and a half times until they are facing upward. This rotation helps to distribute the gelatin over the pins uniformly and to avoid the formation of a bead at the capsule ends. After rotation, they are given a blast of cool air to set the film.

3. Drying—The racks of gelatin-coated pins then pass into a series of four drying ovens. Drying is done mainly by dehumidification by passing large volumes of dry air over the pins. Only a temperature elevation of a few degrees is permissible to prevent film melting. Drying must not be so rapid as to cause "case hardening" of the outer surface of the forming shells that would impede further moisture removal.

   Overdrying must be avoided as this could cause films to split on the pins due to shrinkage or at least make them too brittle for the later trimming operation. Underdrying will leave the films too pliable or sticky for subsequent operations.

4. Stripping—A series of bronze jaws (softer than stainless steel) strip the cap and body portions of the capsules from the pins.

5. Trimming (Fig. 3)—The stripped cap and body portions are delivered to collets in which they are firmly held. As the collets rotate, knives are brought against the shells to trim them to the required length.

6. Joining (Fig. 4)—The cap and body portions are aligned concentrically in channels, and the two portions are slowly pushed together.

The entire cycle takes about 45 minutes; however, about two-third of this time is required for the drying step alone.

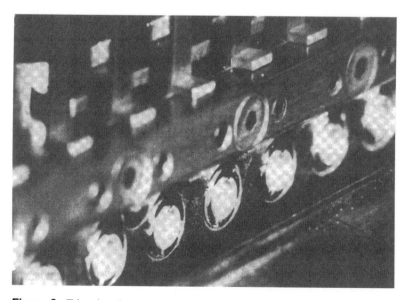

Figure 3 Trimming the newly cast and dried shells to proper length. *Source*: Courtesy of Elanco Qualicaps, formerly a Division of Eli Lilly and Co., Indianapolis, Indiana, U.S.

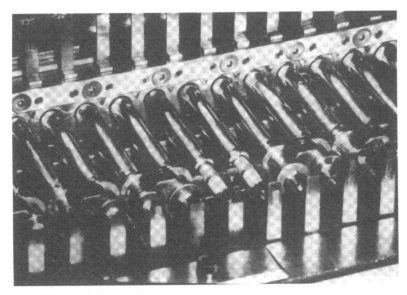

Figure 4 Joining caps and bodies. *Source*: Courtesy of Elanco Qualicaps, formerly a Division of Eli Lilly and Co., Indianapolis, Indiana, U.S.

Sorting

The moisture content of the capsules as they are ejected from the machine typically will be in the range of 15% to 18% w/w (28). Additional adjustment of moisture content toward the final desired specification will occur during the sorting step. During sorting, the capsules passing on a lighted moving conveyor are examined visually by inspectors. Any defective capsules spotted are thus manually removed. Defects are generally classified according to their nature and potential to cause problems in usage. The most serious of these defects are the ones that could cause stoppage of a filling machine such as imperfect cuts, dented capsules, or those with holes. Other defects may cause problems on usage, such as capsules with splits, long bodies, or grease inside. Many less important, cosmetic faults, which only detract from appearance, also may occur (small bubbles, specks in the film, marks on the cut edge, etc.).

Printing

In general, capsules are printed prior to filling. Empty capsules can be handled faster than filled capsules, and should there be any loss or damage to the capsules during printing, no active ingredients would be involved (27). Generally, printing is done on offset rotary presses having throughput capabilities as high as three or four million capsules per hour (27). Available equipment can print either axially along the length of capsules or radially around the circumference of capsules.

Sizes and Shapes

For human use, empty gelatin capsules are manufactured in eight sizes, ranging from 000 (the largest) to 5 (the smallest). The volumes and approximate capacities for the traditional eight sizes are listed in Table 1.

The largest capsule normally acceptable to patients is size 0. Size 0 and size 00 hard-gelatin capsules having an elongated body (e.g., 0E and 00E) also are available,

Table 1 Capsule Volumes and Estimated Fill Weights

Size	Volume (32)	Calculated fill weight (g) at powder density of 0.8 g/cm^3
000	1.37	1.096
00	0.95	0.760
0	0.68	0.544
1	0.50	0.400
2	0.37	0.296
3	0.30	0.240
4	0.21	0.168
5	0.13	0.104

which provide greater fill capacity without an increase in their respective diameters. Three larger sizes are available for veterinary use: nos. 10, 11, and 12, having approximate capacities of 30, 15, and 7.5 g, respectively.

Although the standard shape of capsules is the traditional, symmetrical, cylindrical shape, some manufacturers have employed distinctive proprietary shapes. Lilly's Pulvule$^®$ is designed with a characteristic body section that tapers to a bluntly pointed end. Glaxo Smith Kline's Spansule$^®$ capsules exhibit a characteristic taper at both the cap and body ends.

Sealing and Self-Locking Closures

Positive closures help prevent the inadvertent separation of capsules during shipping and handling. Such safeguards have become particularly important with the advent of high-speed filling and packaging equipment. This problem is particularly acute in the filling of noncompacted bead or granular formulations.

Hard-gelatin capsules are made self-locking by forming indentations or grooves on the inside of the cap and body portions. Thus when they are fully engaged, a positive interlock is created between the cap and body portions. Examples include Posilok$^®$ (Qualicaps, Inc., Whitsett, North Carolina, U.S.) and Coni-Snap$^®$ (Capsugel, Div. Pfizer Inc., Greenwood, South Carolina, U.S.). The rim of the body portion of Coni-Snap capsules is tapered to help guide the cap onto the body. In high-speed automatic capsule-filling machines, this feature can reduce or eliminate snagging or splitting of capsules. Both brands of locking capsules are preclosed by a prelock feature based on indentations formed further down on the cap that keeps the caps and body pieces of the empty capsules together during shipping and handling, but allows their easy separation for capsule filling. The Coni-Snap principle with prelock feature is illustrated in Figure 5.

Capsugel has also developed the Coni-Snap Supro$^®$ capsule (Fig. 6). Similar to Coni-Snap regarding locking mechanism and tapered body edge, this capsule differs in that it is short and squat, and the cap overlaps the body to a greater degree (33).

Hard-gelatin capsules may be made hermetically sealed by the technique of banding wherein a film of gelatin, often distinctively colored, is layered down around the seam of the cap and body. Banding currently is the single most commonly used sealing technique. Pfizer's Kapseal$^®$ is a trademark for banded capsules. In one popular modern banding process, the Hicapseal^{TM} machine (Qualicaps, Inc., Whitsett, North Carolina, U.S.) applies two thin layers of gelatin, one on top of the other. Banded capsules can provide an

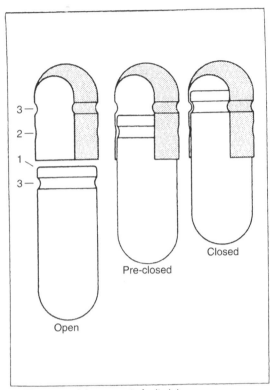

1 The tapered rim prevents faulty joins
2 These indentations prevent the pre-closed capsule
  from opening too early
3 These groovs lock the two halves together after filling
  (SNAP-FIT™ principle)

Figure 5 Coni-Snap mechanically locking capsule showing prelock feature. *Source*: Courtesy of Capsugel, a Division of Pfizer Inc., Greenwood, SC.

effective barrier to atmospheric oxygen (34). As shown in Table 2, the banding of Posilock® capsules resulted in about a 60-fold reduction in the rate of oxygen permeation. The greatest permeation occurred through the nonbanded, noninterlocking traditional capsules. These data suggest that most diffusion occurs through the interface between the cap and body. The experiment was carried out using a custom-built system in which nitrogen was flushed through capsules maintained in an oxygen-containing environment. Oxygen that permeated into the capsules was washed through by the nitrogen and detected in the effluent nitrogen by means of a coulombic (Oxtran®) detector.

Spot welding was once commonly used to lock the cap and body sections of bead-filled capsules together. In the thermal method, two hot metal jaws are brought into contact with the area where the cap overlaps the filled body (35).

Capsugel had proposed a low-temperature thermal method of hermetically sealing hard-gelatin capsules (35). The process involved immersion of the capsules for a fraction of a second in a hydroalcoholic solvent, followed by rapid removal of excess solvent, which is drained off, leaving traces in the overlapping area of the cap and body (held by capillary forces). Finally, the capsules are dried with warm air. A more recent adaptation of this approach has been introduced by Capsugel called Liquid Encapsulated Microspray Sealing (LEMS™) technology. This technology is employed in capsule-filling machines

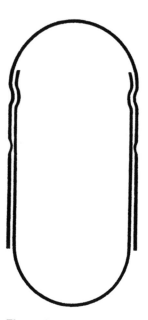

Figure 6 Coni-Snap Supro. *Source*: Courtesy of Capsugel, a Division of Pfizer Inc., Greenwood, SC.

Table 2 Oxygen Permeation Through Size 00 Gelatin Capsules

	Oxygen permeation rate (mL/24 hr)		
	Traditional nonlocking (not banded)	Locking[a] (not banded)	Locking[a] (banded[b])
Mean[c]	0.280	0.065	0.0011
Standard deviation	0.43	0.0029	0.0002

[a]Posilok.
[b]Capsules were banded using a tabletop Qualiseal[®] banding machine.
[c]Five replicates.
Source: Redrawn from Ref. 34.

specifically designed for the filling of liquids and semisolids into hard-gelatin capsules. The LEMS process involves the spraying of a mist of the hydroalcoholic solution onto the joint between the cap and the body. The fluid is drawn by capillarity into the interface between the cap and the body, excess fluids are removed by suction, and a gentle heat is applied to effect melting and fusion in the interface.

In the wake of several incidents of tampering with over-the-counter (OTC) capsules that occurred about 25 years ago, sometimes with fatal consequences, much thought was given as to how to make capsules safer (35). Logically, attention was focused on sealing techniques as possible means of enhancing the safety of capsules by making them tamper evident, so that they could not be tampered with without destroying the capsule or at least causing obvious disfigurement.

Storage, Packaging, and Stability Considerations

Finished hard-gelatin capsules normally contain an equilibrium moisture content of 13% to 16%. This moisture acts as a plasticizer and thus is critical to the physical properties of the shells. At lower moisture contents (<12%), shells become too brittle; at higher moisture contents (>18%), they become too soft (36,37). It is best to avoid extremes of temperature and to maintain a relative humidity of 40% to 60% when handling and storing capsules.

The bulk of the moisture in capsule shells is physically bound and can readily transfer between the shell and its contents, depending on their relative hygroscopicity (38,39). The removal of moisture from the shell could be sufficient to cause splitting or cracking, as has been reported for capsules filled with the deliquescent material, potassium acetate (40). Sodium cromolyn (cromoglycate) has been reported to act as a "sink" for moisture; that is, it continuously removed moisture from hard-gelatin shells, especially at higher temperatures (41). Conditions that favor the transfer of moisture to powder contents may lead to caking and retarded disintegration or other stability problems. It may be useful to prior equilibrate the shell and its contents to the same relative humidity within the acceptable range (42,43).

One issue that has received substantial attention in recent years is the loss of water solubility of gelatin shells, apparently as a result of sufficient exposure to high humidity and temperature or to trace reactive aldehydes (44). Such capsules frequently develop a "skin" or pellicle during dissolution testing, exhibit retarded dissolution, and may fail to meet USP drug dissolution specifications. This insolubilization of gelatin capsules is generally attributed to "gelatin cross-linking" (45). In one example, photoinstability compounded by humidity has been suggested as the explanation for the retarded dissolution of model compounds from hard-gelatin capsules containing certified dyes, particularly when FD & C Red No. 3 was incorporated in both the cap and the shell (46,47). The problem also has been attributed to the presence of trace aldehydes in excipients (48) as well as to the liberation of furfural from the rayon stuffing in packages (44). These results point to the need for appropriate storage conditions and moisture-tight packaging, as well as the need to exclude aldehydes. The issue is not new. The loss of water solubility on exposure of gelatin to elevated temperature and humidity was reported in 1968 to be "particularly disadvantageous in the case of gelatin desserts (49)." The phenomenon also has been reported to occur with gelatin-coated acetaminophen tablets (50). The inclusion of gastric enzymes in dissolution media tends to negate these effects (47,50,51); thus, the phenomenon may have little physiological significance.

In 1992, the Food and Drug Administration (FDA) formed the Gelatin Capsule Working Group to address this gelatin solubility problem (52). Composed of members of pharmaceutical industry trade associations, gelatin capsule manufacturers, USP, and academia, the working group developed a protocol to use stressed and unstressed capsules to determine if these in vitro changes in dissolution were reflected in in vivo performance. Both hard-gelatin and soft-gelatin capsules were stressed by exposure to formaldehyde. Bioequivalence studies comparing stressed and unstressed capsules of acetaminophen indicated that moderately stressed capsules that fail to meet dissolution specifications without enzymes were bioequivalent to unstressed capsules. Overstressed capsules that failed dissolution specifications with and without enzymes in the dissolution medium failed the bioequivalence test. On the basis of these data, the working group recommended that a second step (tier) be added to standard USP or New Drug Application/Abbreviated New Drug Application dissolution tests. The second tier incorporates enzymes in the dissolution medium. Thus, if the product fails the dissolution test in the absence of enzymes, but passes the test when enzymes are added to the dissolution medium, the product's performance is considered acceptable.

HPMC capsules generally have lower equilibrium moisture contents than gelatin capsules (4–6% for Qualicaps Inc.'s Quali-V capsules (53) and 5–7% for Capsugel's Vcaps (54)). Unlike the case with gelatin capsules, the moisture does not serve as a plasticizer, and HPMC capsules show better physical stability on exposure to extremely low humidities. For example, Nagata reported (55) that Quali-V® HPMC capsules did not become brittle and crack even when the moisture content was 1% or less. Because of their low moisture content, HPMC capsules may be more suitable than gelatin capsules for some moisture-sensitive drugs. HPMC capsules are also resistant to cross-linking with aldehydes (53–55).

The water vapor penetration rate and oxygen permeability of films of HPMC and gelatin have been studied (56). The water vapor penetration rate of an HPMC film was found to be substantially lower than that of a gelatin film (263 $g/M^2/24$ hr vs. 446 $g/M^2/$ 24 hr), but the oxygen permeability of the HPMC film was greater than that of the gelatin film, apparently due to the looser structure of the HPMC film. After three days, the concentration of oxygen in a chamber closed off by a gelatin film was 0.1% and that of the chamber closed off by a film of HPMC was 0.3% (56). Prior to testing, the air in the chamber was replaced with nitrogen so that initial oxygen concentration was 0%. On the basis of these data, it has been suggested that when oxygen-sensitive drugs are filled into HPMC capsules, either an antioxidant should be included in the formulation or special packaging, such as blister packs with aluminum foil should be employed to minimize oxygen permeation (55).

The Filling of Hard-Gelatin Capsules

Many of the essential features of modern automatic high-speed capsule-filling machines have their origins in simpler, manual filling devices developed in the latter part of the 19th century (57). In general, filling machines in use in the pharmaceutical industry have the following operations in common:

Rectification   The empty capsules are oriented so that all point to the same direction, that is, body end downward. In general, the capsules pass one at a time through a channel just wide enough to provide a frictional grip at the cap end. A specially designed blade pushes against the capsule and causes it to rotate about its cap end as a fulcrum. After two pushes (one horizontally and one vertically downward), the capsules will always be aligned body end downward, regardless of which end entered the channel first.

Separation of caps from bodies   This process also depends on the difference in diameters between cap and body portions. Here, the rectified capsules are delivered body end first into the upper portion of split bushings or split-filling rings. A vacuum applied from below pulls the bodies down into the lower portion of the split bushing. The diameter of the caps is too large to allow them to follow the bodies into the lower bushing portion. The split bushings are then separated to expose the bodies for filling.

Dosing of fill material   Various methods are employed, as described on the following pages.

Replacement of caps and ejection of filled capsules   The cap and body bushing portions are rejoined. Pins are used to push the filled bodies up into the caps for closure, and to push the closed capsules out of the bushings. Compressed air also may be used to eject the capsules.

These machines may be either semiautomatic or fully automatic. Semiautomatic machines such as the type 8 machines (e.g., Capsugel's Cap 8 machine) require an

Table 3 Selected Automatic Capsule-Filling Machines

Make/Model	Dosing principle	Motion	Rated[a] production capacity (capsules/hr)
Bosch[b]	Dosing disc		
GKF 400S		I	24,000
GKF 701		I	42,000
GKF 2500		I	150,000
IMA[c]	Dosator		
Zanasi 6		I	6,000
Zanasi 40		I	40,000
Matic 100		C	100,000
Matic 200		C	200,000
MG2[d]	Dosator		
Futura		C	48,000
G70		C	70,000
G140		C	140,000
G250		C	250,000

[a]On the basis of manufacturer/distributor literature.
[b]Bosch Packaging Technology, Minneapolis, Minnesota, U.S.
[c]IMA North America, Inc., Bristol, Pennsylvania, U.S.
[d]MG America, Inc., Fairfield, New Jersey, U.S.
Abbreviations: I, intermittent; C, continuous.

operator to be in attendance at all times. Depending on the skill of the operator, the formulation, and the size of capsule being filled, these machines are capable of filling as many as 120,000 to 160,000 capsules in an eight-hour shift. This output contrasts sharply with the output of fully automatic machines, some models of which are rated to fill that many capsules or more in one hour. Automatic capsule-filling machines may be classified as either intermittent or continuous motion machines. Intermittent machines exhibit an interrupted filling sequence as indexing turntables must stop at various stations to execute the basic operations described above. Continuous motion machines execute these functions in a continuous cycle. The elimination of the need to decelerate and accelerate from one station to the next makes greater machine speeds possible with continuous motion machines (58). Some representative automatic capsule-filling machines and their capacities are listed in Table 3. Although capsule-filling machines may vary widely in their engineering design, the main difference between them from a formulation design point of view is the means by which the formulation is dosed into the capsules.

Powder Filling

The types of filling machines available for filling hard-shell capsules and their operating principles have been the subject of a number of reviews (30,58–63). Four main dosing methods may be identified for powder filling:

Auger Fill Principle

At one time, nearly all capsules were filled by means of semiautomatic equipment wherein the powder is driven into the capsule bodies by a rotating auger, as exemplified by the type 8 machines (Fig. 7). The empty capsule bodies are held in a filling ring, which rotates on a turntable under the powder hopper. The fill of the capsules is primarily

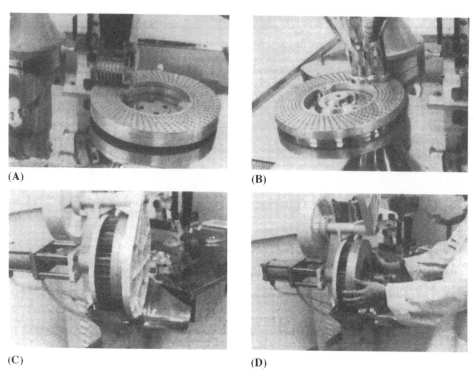

Figure 7 Type 8 semiautomatic capsule-filling machine. (**A**) "Sandwich" of cap and body rings positioned under rectifier to receive empty capsules. Vacuum is pulled from beneath the rings to separate caps from bodies. (**B**) Body ring is positioned under foot of powder hopper for filling. (**C**) After filling the bodies, the cap and body rings are rejoined and positioned in front of pegs. A stop plate is swung down in back of rings to prevent capsule expulsion as the pneumatically driven pegs push the bodies to engage the caps. (**D**) The plate is swung aside, and the pegs are used to eject the closed capsules.

volumetric. Because the auger mounted in the hopper rotates at a constant rate, the rate of delivery of powder to the capsules tends to be constant. Consequently, the major control over fill weight is the rate of rotation of the filling ring under the hopper. Faster rates produce lighter fill weights because bodies have a shorter dwell time under the hopper. Ito et al. (64) compared an experimental flat blade auger with an original screw auger and found that the screw auger provided greater fill weight (30–60% greater for a test lactose formulation) and smaller coefficients of weight variation (up to 50% smaller at the two fastest ring speeds). The formulation requirements of this type of machine have been the subject of only a limited number of reports. In general, the flow properties of the powder blend should be adequate to assure a uniform flow rate from the hopper. Glidants may be helpful. Ito et al. also studied the glidant effect of a colloidal silica using a Capsugel type 8 filling machine (64). They found that there was an optimum concentration of colloidal silica for minimum weight variation (approximately 0.5% for lactose capsules; approximately 1% for corn starch capsules). Employing a similar Elanco machine in a multivariate study involving several fillers, Reier et al. found that the presence of 3% talc as a glidant reduces weight variation compared with 0% talc (65). On the basis of a multiple stepwise regression analysis of their data, these investigators came to two important conclusions: (*i*) Average fill weight was dependent on machine speed, capsule size, and the formulation specific volume, in that order and (*ii*) weight variation was a function of machine speed, specific volume, flowability, and the presence of glidant, but independent of capsule size.

Lubricants, such as magnesium stearate and stearic acid, are also required. These substances facilitate the passage of the filling ring under the foot of the powder hopper and help prevent the adherence of materials to the auger.

Vibratory Fill Principle

The Osaka machines (Fig. 8) use a vibratory feed mechanism (66,67). The capsule bodies held in a rotating turntable pass under the powder held in a chamber. A perforated resin plate that is connected to a vibrator is positioned at the bottom of the chamber. The powder bed tends to be fluidized by the vibration of the plate; this action assists the flowing of the powder into the capsule bodies through holes in the resin plate (67). Fill weight is controlled by the vibrators and by setting the position of the bodies under the powder feed mechanism. The capsule bodies are supported on pins in holes bored through a disc plate. While they pass under the feed area, the pins may be set to drop the bodies to below the level of the disc, thereby causing overfill. However, the capsules are eventually pushed up so that their upper edges become level with the surface of the disc plate. When this occurs, the excess powder is forced out and eventually scraped off. This process affords some light compression of the powder against the resin plates and offers the opportunity to modify the fill weight. Weight variation has been related to the formulation flow properties. Kurihara and Ichikawa reported that the fill weight variation with model

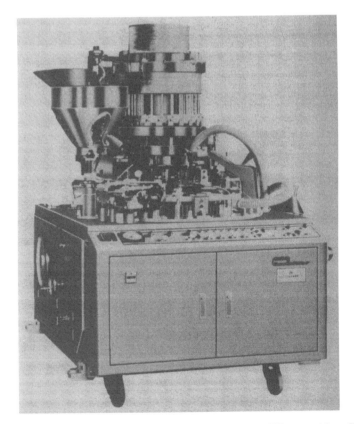

Figure 8 Osaka model R-18O automatic capsule-filling machine. Courtesy of Sharpley-Stokes Division, Pennwalt Corp. Warminster, Pennsylvania, U.S.

OCF-120 was more closely related to the minimum orifice diameter than to the angle of repose (66). Apparently, the minimum orifice diameter is a better analogy of the flowing of powder into capsule bodies than the static angle of repose. No systematic studies of the formulation requirements for this machine have been reported; however, typical stearate lubricants may be indicated to prevent the binding of push rods and guides.

Piston-Tamp Principle

Most capsules are filled on piston-tamp machines. These are fully automatic fillers in which pistons or tamping pins lightly compress the individual doses of powders into plugs (sometimes referred to as "slugs"), and eject the plugs into empty capsule bodies. The compression forces are low, often in the range of 50 to 150 N, or about 50- to 100-fold less than typical tablet compression forces. Hence, plugs are very soft compacts that often are not able to be recovered intact from the filled capsules.

There are two types of piston-tamp fillers: dosator machines and dosing-disc machines. In a survey of equipment used by pharmaceutical companies, Heda found that dosator machines are used in production slightly more frequently than dosing-disc machines (68). Interestingly, about 18% of the companies responding to the survey reported that they use both types of filling machines.

Dosing-disc machines This type of machine is exemplified by the Bosch GKF models (formerly Hofliger–Karg) and the Harro–Hofliger KFM models, among others (Fig. 9).

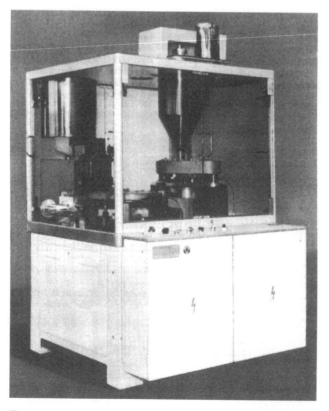

Figure 9 Hofliger Karg model GKF 1500 automatic capsule-filling machine. *Source*: Courtesy of Robert Bosch Corp., Packaging Machinery Division, South Plainfield, New Jersey, U.S.

(A)

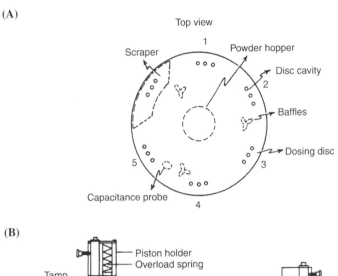

(B)

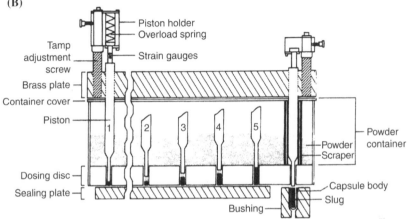

Figure 10 Illustration of the dosing-disc filling principle: (**A**) view looking down on the dosing disc; (**B**) side view (projected) showing progressive plug formation. Note the placement of strain gauges on the piston to measure tamping and plug ejection forces (see text). *Source*: From Ref. 70.

The dosing-disc-filling principle has been described (69,70) and is illustrated in Figure 10. The dosing disc, which forms the base of the dosing or filling chamber, has a number of holes bored through it. A solid brass "stop" plate slides along the bottom of the dosing disc to close off these holes, thus forming openings similar to the die cavities of a tablet press. The powder is maintained at a relatively constant level over the dosing disc. Five sets of tamping pins (e.g., Bosch GKF machines) compress the powder into the cavities to form plugs. The cavities are indexed under each of the five sets of tamping pins so that each plug is compressed five times per cycle. After the five tamps, any excess powder is scraped off as the dosing-disc indexes to position the plugs over empty capsule bodies where they are ejected by transfer pins. The dose is controlled by the thickness of the dosing disc (i.e., cavity depth), the powder bed depth, and the tamping pressure. The flow of powder from the hopper to the disc is auger assisted. A capacitance probe senses the powder level and activates an auger feed if the level falls to below the preset level. The powder is distributed over the dosing disc by the centrifugal action of the indexing rotation of the disc. Baffles are provided to help maintain a uniform powder level. However, working with a GKF model 330, Shah et al. (70) noted that a uniform powder bed height was not maintained at the first tamping station because of its nearness to the scrape-off device.

Kurihara and Ichikawa reported that variation in fill weight was closely related to the angle of repose of the formulation; however, a minimum point appeared in the plots of the angle of repose versus coefficient of variation of filling weight (66). Apparently, at higher angles of repose, the powders did not have sufficient mobility to distribute well under the acceleration of the intermittent indexing motion. At lower angles of repose, the powder was apparently too fluid to maintain a uniform bed. However, these investigators did not appear to make use of powder compression through tamping, and this complicates the interpretation of their results.

In a more recent study running model formulations having different flow properties on a GKF 400 machine, Heda found that Carr Compressibility Index values (CI%) should be 18<CI%<30 to maintain low weight variation (68). Poorly flowing powders (CI% > 30) were observed to dam up around the ejection station. The Carr Compressibility Index is calculated from the loose and tapped bulk density as follows (71):

$$CI\% = \frac{\rho_{\text{Tapped}} - \rho_{\text{Loose}}}{\rho_{\text{Tapped}}} \times 100 \qquad (1)$$

where ρ_{Tapped} and ρ_{Loose} are the tapped and loose bulk densities, respectively. Higher values indicate that the interparticulate cohesive and frictional interactions that interfere with powder flow are relatively more important. Thus flowability is inversely related to the CI% value.

Dosing disc machines generally require that formulations be adequately lubricated, for example, by adding magnesium stearate, to prevent powder from adhering to tamping pin faces and other metal surfaces, and to reduce friction between any sliding components with which the powder may come into contact. Some degree of compactibility is also important as coherent plugs appear to be desirable for clean, efficient transfer at ejection. However, there may be less of a dependence on formulation compactibility than that exists for dosator machines (61,68).

Harro–Hofliger produces a machine that is similar to Bosch GKF machines, except that it employs only three tamping stations. However, at each station, the powder in the dosing cavities is tamped twice before rotating a quarter turn to the next station. Another difference is that the powder in the filling chamber is constantly agitated to help in the maintenance of a uniform powder bed depth.

Dosator machines The dosator machines are exemplified by the Zanasi and MG2 machines pictured in Figures 11 and 12. Figure 13 illustrates the basic dosator principle. The dosator principle has been previously described (72,73). The dosator consists of a cylindrical dosing tube fitted with a moveable piston. The end of the tube is open, and the position of the piston is preset to a particular height to define a volume (again, comparable to a tablet press "die cavity") that would contain the desired dose of powder. In operation, the dosator is plunged down into a powder bed maintained at a constant preset level by agitators and scrapers. The powder bed height is generally greater than the piston height. Thus, as powder enters the open end, it is slightly compressed against the piston [sometimes termed "precompression" (72)]. While the dosator is at its lowest position in the powder bed, the piston is then caused to apply a tamping blow, thus further compressing the powder captured within the dosator. In the next step, the dosator, bearing the plug, is withdrawn from the powder hopper and is moved over to an empty capsule body where the piston is pushed downward to eject the plug. In Macofar machines, a bushing bearing the capsule body is rotated into position under the dosator to receive the ejected plug (74). For a given set of tooling and powder bed height, the setting of the initial piston height in the dosing tube determines the weight of a given formulation filled

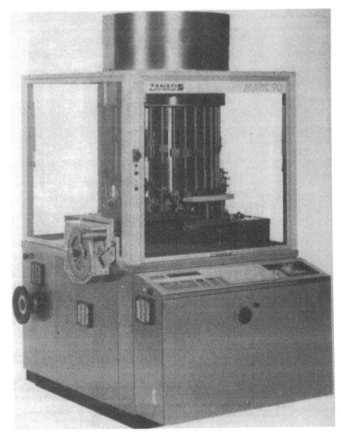

Figure 11 Zanasi Matic 90 automatic capsule-filling machine. *Source*: Courtesy of IMA North America, Inc., Fairfield, Connecticut, U.S.

into the capsules. For a given piston height setting, increasing or decreasing the height of the powder bed into which the dosator dips also can affect the fill weight.

In one of the earliest reports evaluating the Zanasi machine, Stoyle suggests that formulations should have the following characteristics for successful filling (73):

1. Fluidity is important for powder feed from the reservoir to the dipping bed and also to permit efficient closing in of the hole left by the dosator.
2. A degree of compactibility is important to prevent loss of material from the end of the plug during transport to the capsule shell.
3. Lubricity is needed to permit easy and efficient ejection of the plug.
4. Formulations should have a moderate bulk density. It was suggested that low bulk density materials or those that contain entrapped air may not consolidate well, and capping similar to what occurs in tableting may result.

The relationship between formulation *flow properties* and *weight variation* on Zanasi machines has been studied. For example, Irwin et al. (75) compared the weight variation of capsules filled on a Zanasi LZ-64 machine with formulations composed of different diluents and lubricants. The formulations had different flow properties, as judged by a recording flowmeter. Generally, it was found that the better the rate of flow, the more uniform the capsule fill weight was. Chowhan and Chow (76) compared the powder consolidation ratio with the coefficient of variation (relative standard deviation) of capsule weight and found a

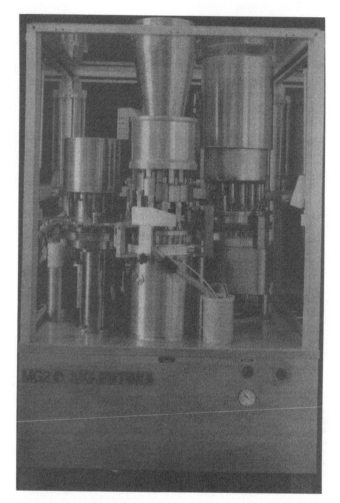

Figure 12 MG2 Futura automatic capsule-filling machine. Courtesy of MG America, Inc., Fairfield, New Jersey, U.S.

linear relationship for a test formulation containing 5% or 15% drug, 10% starch, 0.5% magnesium stearate, and lactose q.s. The capsules were filled on a Zanasi machine. Powder flow characteristics were inferred from the volume reduction (consolidation), which occurs when a series of loads are applied to the surface of the loosely packed powder bed in cylindrical containers. The powder consolidation ratio was the intercept of the plot of

$$\log \frac{V_0 - V}{V} \text{ versus } \frac{P}{P_0} \qquad (2)$$

where V_0 is initial powder volume, V the powder volume at a given surface pressure, P the surface pressure, and $P_0 = 1 \text{ kg/cm}^2$. Further work to assess the usefulness and limitations of this approach appears warranted.

The effect of *machine variables on fill weight and its uniformity* was evaluated by Miyake et al. (77) using a Zanasi Z-25. In general, they found that the filling mechanism was a compaction process. The following relationship was found to apply:

$$r = a(i) \log P_r + b(i) \qquad (3)$$

where r is the density ratio, $a(i)$ and $b(i)$ are constants, and P_r the compression ratio = $(H - L)/L$, where H is powder bed height and L the piston height (within the dosator).

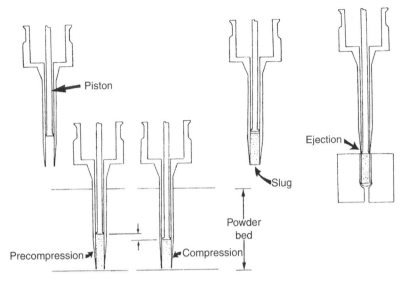

Figure 13 Dosator-filling principle. *Source*: From Ref. 83.

The quantitative retention of powder within the dosator during transfer from the powder bed to the capsule shell is essential to a successful filling operation. Applying hopper design theory, Jolliffe et al. (78,79) reported that powder retention requires a stable powder arch be formed at the dosator outlet, and this stable arch depends on the angle of wall friction. In general, there is an optimum angle of wall friction for which the compression force needed to ensure a stable arch is a minimum. That angle will be dependent on finish of the inner surface of the dosing tube as well as the properties of the powder. Generally, more freely flowing powders will require larger minimum compressive stresses than less freely flowing powders. But the rougher the surface, the lower the required minimum stress is likely to be. For example, Jolliffe and Newton showed that the rougher of two inner dosing-tube surfaces finishes promoted the formation of a stable arch by different size fractions of lactose by reducing the cohesive strength required within the powder plug for arching (79).

Heda (68) found that the optimum CI% for minimum weight variation for a Zanasi LZ-64 machine was between 25 and 35. Powders with high Carr Index values > 30 produced stronger plugs with lower weight variation. For more freely flowing powders having Carr Index values < 20, higher compression forces may improve powder retention in the dosator tube.

Nonpowder Filling

Modern automatic capsule-filling machines offer enormous flexibility in terms of what can be filled into hard-shell capsules. In addition to powder dosing, filling devices also are available that can feed beads or pellets, microtablets, tablets, and liquid or pasty materials into capsules. Often, these can be installed at different filling stations of the same machine such that capsules may be dosed from several different filling devices as they pass by each station before closure and ejection. Such arrangements could, for example, permit the dosing of several different tablets, different batches of beads (perhaps immediate-release and modified-release beads) or combinations of tablets, powder plugs, and beads into the same capsule.

Beads, pellets, etc., may be poured directly into the capsule body via gravity feed devices, which rely on the free-flowing nature of such materials. In this approach, capsules are filled to their volumetric capacity, and partial fills for multiple dosing are not possible. Modern automatic filling machines circumvent this issue by employing various indirect filling methods, that is, the required quantity of beads, granules, etc., is first fed to a separate, volumetric metering chamber of adjustable capacity, and then the measured volume of material is transferred to the capsule body. The metering chamber is usually filled by gravity (e.g., Bosch GKF); however, in certain machines (e.g., Zanasi), the chamber is a modified dosator that draws and holds the beads into its open end by means of vacuum. In general, the dose is determined by the size of the metering chamber. If blends of different bead batches or formulations are being dispensed, the uniformity of the dose dispensed depends upon the size, shape, and density of the particles, since differences in these properties may cause the pellets to segregate in hoppers and the feed mechanism. The development of electrostatic charges on beads or pellets also may cause separation of individual beads as well as problems in flowing and transferring from filling chambers. The addition of 1% talc to the beads may resolve this problem (80).

Typically, tablets are fed to the bodies through a tube and are simply released in the required number as the body passes beneath. Pumpable, liquid fills are dosed by conventional liquid-dispensing devices adapted for capsule filling.

Instrumented Capsule-Filling Machines and Their Role in Formulation Development

A major development in pharmaceutical technology has been the application of instrumentation techniques to tablet presses. The ability to monitor the forces that develop during the compaction, ejection, and detachment of tablets has brought about new insights into the physics of compaction, facilitated formulation development, and provided a means for the in-process control of tablet weight in manufacturing (81,82). In most cases, automatic capsule filling is carried out on dosator or dosing-disc machines, which resemble tableting to the degree that there are compression and ejection events. Given this similarity to tableting and the benefits that have accrued from instrumented tablet machines, it was only logical that similar instrumentation techniques be applied to these capsule-filling machines. Although both types of machines have been instrumented, most reports have been concerned with dosator machines (83).

Cole and May were the first investigators to report the instrumentation of an automatic capsule-filling machine (84,85). They bonded strain gauges to the piston of a Zanasi LZ-64 dosator. Because the dosators rotate from the plug formation station to the plug ejection station during capsule filling, this machine required modification by installation of a planetary gear system to prevent the continuous twisting of the cable connecting to the strain gauges during operation. Their work demonstrated for the first time that compression and ejection forces could be recorded during plug formation and ejection. They reported several important features of how the measured piston force varied with time: (*i*) an initial compression force that rose to a peak value as a result of the dosator having been plunged downward into the powder bed, (*ii*) a partial retention of this force during rotation of the dosator bearing the plug to the ejection station, and (*iii*) the development of a peak ejection force, that is, the force required to initiate the movement of the plug in ejection from dosing tube.

Small and Augsburger also reported on the instrumentation of the same model of Zanasi machine with strain gauges (72). Twisting of the connecting cable was avoided by connecting it to a low-noise mercury contact swivel mounted over the capsule hopper. This was a simpler arrangement than that employed by Cole and May (85) in that it

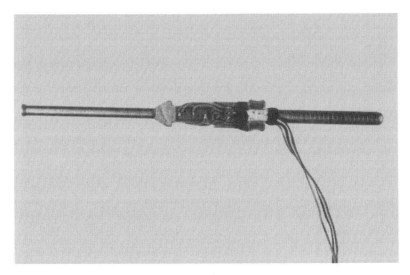

Figure 14 Strain gauges bonded to Zanasi piston. *Source*: From Ref. 72.

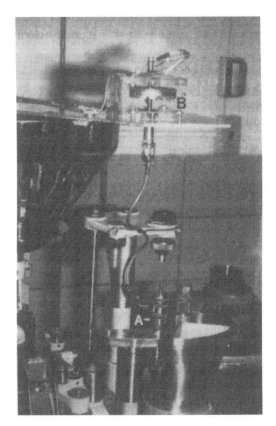

Figure 15 Instrumented Zanasi LZ-64 showing mercury swivel for signal removal: (**A**) dosator containing strain-gauged piston; (**B**) mercury swivel. *Source*: From Ref. 72.

permitted electrical contact to be maintained during experimental runs without the need for a planetary gear system nor any other machine modification. Figures 14 and 15 illustrate their instrumented piston and the mounting of the mercury swivel. In contrast to Cole and May, Small and Augsburger reported a two-stage plug formation (compression) trace: (72) (*i*) a precompression force that occurs when the dosator plunges downward into the powder bed and (*ii*) compression of the powder by the tamping of the piston at the bottom of dosator travel in the powder bed. Apparently, the earlier workers did not make use of this piston compression feature of the Zanasi-filling principle. Like Cole and May, Small and Augsburger also reported retention and ejection forces. The retention force, which apparently is a result of elastic recovery of the plug against the piston, was observed by Small and Augsburger only when running certain unlubricated materials. This phenomenon was not observed in their lubricated runs, apparently because the lubricant permits the plug to more readily slip to relieve any residual pressure (72). It is interesting to note that both teams of investigators reported instances of drag on the piston as it returns to the original position after ejection. This drag force, which may indicate inadequate lubrication, was manifested by the appearance of a negative force (i.e., a trace below the baseline) during retraction of the piston. Sample traces from Small and Augsburger appear in Figure 16.

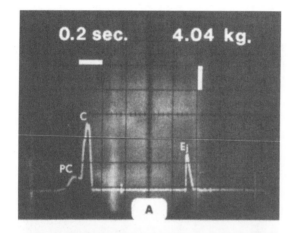

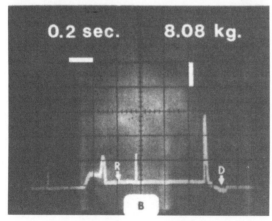

Figure 16 Typical force-time trace from an instrumented Zanasi LZ-64 automatic capsule-filling machine. *Abbreviations:* PC, precompression resulting from dipping of dosator into the powder bed; C, compression resulting from actual piston tamping; R, retention force; Ej, ejection; D, drag force developing during retraction of piston. *Source*: From Ref. 72.

Small and Augsburger (86) later reported a detailed study of the formulation lubrication requirements of the Zanasi LZ-64. Three fillers were studied (microcrystalline cellulose, pregelatinized starch, and anhydrous lactose). Powder bed height, piston height, compression force, and lubricant type and concentration were varied to determine their effects on ejection force. Generally, anhydrous lactose exhibited higher lubrication requirements than either pregelatinized starch or microcrystalline cellulose. Comparing several concentrations of magnesium stearate, minimum ejection forces were recorded at 1% with anhydrous lactose, 0.5% with microcrystalline cellulose, and 0.1% with pregelatinized starch. The magnitude of the ejection force was affected by machine-operating variables. After precompression, ejection force was found to increase with the compression force. However, at a given compression force, ejection force also increases with an increase in either the piston height or the powder bed height. Increases in the piston height increases frictional resistance to ejection because it results in longer plugs with greater contact area with the inner surface of the dosing tube. For a given piston height, increases in the powder bed height appears to increase the frictional resistance to ejection by increasing the amount of compression that occurs at precompression. Figure 17 is typical. These results suggest the possibility of manipulating machine-operating variables

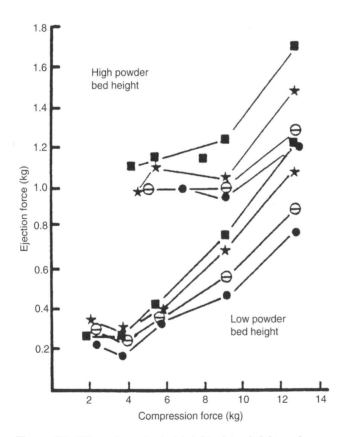

Figure 17 Effect of powder bed height, piston height, and compression force on plug ejection force in an instrumented Zanasi LZ64 automatic capsule-filling machine (pregelatinized starch lubricated with 0.005% magnesium stearate). Note that the first point of each curve is precompression. Piston height (mm): ■, 15; ★, 14; ⊖, 13; ●, 12. *Source*: From Ref. 86.

to reduce the amount of lubricant needed in the formulation. As will be discussed later in this chapter, hydrophobic lubricants like magnesium stearate potentially can interfere with the wetting of powders and, thereby, retard drug dissolution.

Mehta and Augsburger (87) later reported the mounting of a linear variable displacement transducer (LVDT) on the previously instrumented Zanasi LZ-64 machine (72). This device allows the measurement of piston travel (displacement) during compression and ejection. From the simultaneous measurement of piston travel and ejection force, ejection force versus displacement curves were plotted. These plots are of interest because the area under the curve is a measure of the work or energy of ejection. In a preliminary study, the work of ejection of several formulations differed even though their peak ejection forces were comparable, suggesting that work measurement may be more informative of lubrication than peak ejection force alone (88).

Greenberg (89) used strain gauges to instrument a larger Zanasi machine (model AZ-60). This intermittent motion machine employs three groups of eight dosators. Two instrumented pistons were installed in two dosators in one group. The system was unique in that a high-quality 10-pole slip ring was used to avoid twisting of the cables. Botzolakis (90) later described the successful replacement of the previously reported mercury swivel with a 10-pole gold contact slip ring assembly.

Piezoelectric transducers have also been used to instrument automatic capsule-filling machines. Mony et al. (91) instrumented a Zanasi model RV-59 by fitting a piezoelectric load cell to the upper end of a piston. This system can only register a force when the upper end of the piston is in actual contact with the compression or ejection knobs. Therefore, this instrumentation provides a measure only of overall compression and ejection forces and does not permit the detection of precompression, retention, or piston retraction drag forces. Moreover this instrumentation adds the force required to compress the piston retraction spring to any forces measured. No attempt to correct their data for this variable was reported. Rowley et al. (92) reported the mounting of a small piezoelectric load cell to the ejection knob of a Zanasi LZ-64 machine to monitor ejection force. This approach suffers from the same disadvantages as that of Mony et al.; however, these latter investigators did report subtracting out the force required to compress the dosator spring from their measurements. This correction was obtained by making a "blank" run with an empty dosator.

The instrumentation of a dosing-disc machine was first reported by Shah et al. (70). Two pistons of a model GKF 330 (Hofliger and Karg)-filling machine were instrumented using strain gauges to enable simultaneous monitoring of either two of the tamping stations or one tamping station and ejection (Figs. 10 and 18). This preliminary study revealed the complexity of the interaction of the various tamping stations on the final fill weight. Using additional instrumented pistons and microprocessor-controlled data acquisition techniques, Shah et al. (93) later evaluated seven compaction parameters and concluded that, aside from station no. 1, all tamping stations and all piston positions within a station contribute equally to plug formation. The nearness of station no. 1 to the scrape-off bar results in nonuniform powder bed height and a high degree of compression force variability. Model calculations suggesting that fill weight could be achieved for some formulations with only three tamps were supported by experiments in which fill weight was determined as a function of tamping force and the number of tamps for typical lubricated fillers. The effects of tamping force and multiple tamping on drug dissolution also were investigated using this equipment (94). Cropp et al. (95) later installed displacement transducers on the machine previously instrumented by Shah et al. (93) to further study the multiple tamping effect and to assess the role of overload spring tension on the fill weights obtained. More recently, Podczeck (96,97) reported the instrumentation

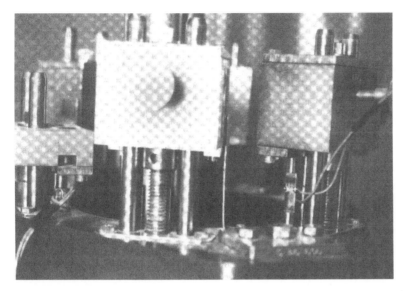

Figure 18 Strain-gauged pistons mounted in a Hofliger Karg model 330 automatic capsule-filling machine. *Source*: From Ref. 70.

of a Bosch GKF 400S dosing-disc machine using a prototype pneumatic tamping head fitted with a piezoelectric force transducer. The pneumatic system, which replaces the overload springs normally mounted over the tamping pins, is fitted with a feedback switch valve and provides a potential means for feedback control of fill weight during continuous running of the machine.

Instrumentation has also been developed to measure the mechanical strength of plugs. Greenberg may be the first investigator to report the measurement of plug "hardness" (89). A pneumatically driven piston, moving at a controlled rate, was brought against the plug held in a narrow channel. A ring indicator registered the highest force developed as the plug fails. Hardness values were generally under 0.1 N. Later, others report measuring the plug mechanical strength using a three-point flexure test (93,98,99). In this test, the plug is supported at each end, and a blunt-edged blade mounted on the moving head of a bench-type tensile strength tester is lowered at a slow, controlled rate against the unsupported midpoint of the plug to cause it to fail. When tested in this manner, the maximum breaking force for plugs is generally up to 1 N.

Capsule-Filling Machine Simulation

The development of programmable compaction simulators was a significant development in tableting research. Since they can be programmed to effectively simulate the action of production rotary tablet presses at their operating speeds under controlled laboratory conditions; require only small quantities of material; and provide independent control over compressive force, punch position, and punch speed, compaction simulators offer substantial advantages over using instrumented tablet presses in research and development (100). Clearly, the programmable simulation of automatic capsule-filling machines similarly would be advantageous in the design and development of capsule formulations, and several researchers have taken important steps toward that end.

It could be argued that researchers have been simulating capsule filling under laboratory conditions for a number of years. Generally this simulation involved using the dosing mechanism that had been removed from an actual machine to make plugs. For example, Stewart et al. (101) reported research using a Zanasi dosator fitted to a moveable crosshead. Veski and Marvola (102) reported the use of an MG2 dosing tube mounted on a digital balance with piston fitted to a manually operated lever system. Such approaches allow for the convenient study of plug formation using small quantities of material, but programmability to simulate the action of different machines at their operating speeds is not possible.

Jolliffe et al. (103) reported the development of an MG2 capsule-filling simulator. This simulator employs the filling turret of a model G-36 machine and a drive mechanism that allows the normal up and down motion of the dosators, but without the usual turret rotation. One dosator was employed that was instrumented by bonding strain gauges to the piston. Additionally, displacement transducers were fitted to permit measurement of piston movement relative to the dosator and dosator movement relative to the turret. Jolliffe and Newton (104) used this simulator to study the effects of changes in compression ratio on fill weight variation and compression and ejection stresses for four size fractions of lactose. Generally, the ranges of compression ratio over which uniform weights could be obtained with minimum tamping pressure was found to be far greater for the finely divided, cohesive powders than for the coarser, freely flowing size fractions. Fine, cohesive powders have greater void volumes and, therefore, are capable of greater volume reduction than free-flowing powders. This system was later used by Jolliffe and Newton to study the role of dosator nozzle inner wall texture on plug retention, that is, the ability of the formed plug to be carried in the dosator without loss of material during machine operation (105). Tan and Newton used this system to study the relationship between powder flow parameters, fill weight, and weight variation (106), to explore further the relationship between powder retention and dosator inner wall texture (107–109), and to study the effect of compression on fill weight and weight variability (110) and plug density (111).

Britten and Barnett fitted the dosator mechanism from a Macofar MT13-2 capsule-filling machine with pneumatic cylinders (112). One pneumatic cylinder brings the bowl bearing the powder bed to the dosator (simulating the dipping action leading to precompression), and separate pneumatic cylinders provide piston compression and plug ejection. The speeds of these three cylinders are adjustable through flow control valves. LVDTs monitor the movement of the bowl and piston. Semiconductor strain gauges are mounted on the piston and on the outer surface of the dosator tube to measure both the tamping pressure and the radial pressure on the plug. The analog signals from the transducers are digitized and stored by a microprocessor-controlled data acquisition system, and the data are downloaded to a PC for further manipulation (113). Capable of maximum dosator and pistons speeds of 500 and 600 mm/sec, respectively, this system is only able to attain about 75% of the full range of speeds attainable with the Macofar MT13-2 (113). However, this range nearly covers the full range of speeds of the Zanasi AZ-20, a machine that employs a similar dosator mechanism (113). Using this system, Britten et al. were the first to report the direct measurement of residual radial plug pressures (114). In a study of the relationship between the residual radial pressure and compression pressure, they found that pregelatinized starch (unlubricated) exhibited much greater elasticity than lubricated lactose. It was also found for these two materials that plug weight or density was not affected by the ejection rate, but that faster precompression speeds lead to reduced plug weight, possibly because powder tended to be pushed ahead of the nozzle, rather than enter it (114). Later, using the same simulator, Tattawasart and Armstrong (115) conducted a three-factor Box–Behnken study of the effects of compression pressure, piston height, and lubricant concentration on various properties of lactose plugs. As learned from earlier studies with microcrystalline cellulose, pregelatinized starch, and lactose using an instrumented dosator machine (86), ejection pressure was found to be dependent both on piston compression pressure and piston height. But, interestingly, it was found that these relationships with compression pressure and piston height held even when ejection pressure was normalized for differences in plug length. Moreover, magnesium stearate concentration had no significant effect on plug weight, weight uniformity, porosity, and length. A level of 0.5% magnesium stearate was found to be suitable lubrication for lactose.

More recently, Heda et al. reported the simulation of plug formation using a programmable Mand tablet compaction simulator (99). The simulator was fitted with tooling machined to match a no. 1 tamping pin and a special deep die to accommodate different capsule plug lengths. Plug formation at different constant punch speeds of 1, 10, and 100 mm/sec was studied. Although the simulator was capable of running at much higher speeds, tamping pin speed was limited to 100 mm/sec in this preliminary study, a speed that slightly exceeds the reported tamping pin movement of a GKF 330 dosing-disc machine. This study revealed that certain powder compression equations (e.g., the pressure-density relationships of Kawakita and Heckel and the Shaxby–Evans' exponential relationship) can be applied to plug formation and demonstrated the potential for programmable capsule machine simulation.

Design of Powder-Filled Hard-Shell Capsule Formulations

Like any dosage form, the capsule can be viewed as a *drug delivery system* since the choice of excipients and the principles involved in the design of the dosage form can affect the rate and amount of drug delivered to the site of action. Clearly, the initial design criterion of the dosage form must be to make the drug optimally available for absorption in a manner consistent with intended use (e.g., immediate release or modified release). However, the dosage form must be designed also to meet a number of other criteria. These include stability, manufacturability, and patient acceptability. Both the shell and its contents must exhibit physical and chemical stability. Not only must the drug substance be stable, but the rate and extent of drug release also must be stable. The formulation also should allow for efficient, cost-effective production of the required batch sizes and provide for accuracy and uniformity of drug content from one capsule to the next within acceptable limits. Patient acceptability is also an important design criterion as this encourages patent compliance with the prescribed dosing. As much as possible, the dosage form should have an attractive appearance, including color, be of a size easily swallowed, and not have any unpleasant odor or taste. As discussed previously, the capsule easily meets these criteria. However, as much as possible, capsule sizes that are difficult to swallow should be avoided.

Often these design criteria involve *competitive requirements*. What is best for meeting one criterion may be counterproductive in meeting another criterion. For example, certain excipients such as the hydrophobic stearate lubricants are important for efficient manufacture, yet they have the potential to retard the release of drug from an immediate-release formulation. The design of a dosage form thus frequently requires the optimization of formulation and process variables in a way that best meets all design criteria.

This section addresses the design of immediate-release powder formulations for hard-shell capsules. In general, powder formulations for encapsulation should be developed in consideration of the particular filling principle involved. The requirements imposed on the formulation by the filling process, such as lubricity, compressibility and/

or compactibility, and fluidity can vary between machine types. Furthermore, the interplay between formulation variables and process variables may be expected to influence drug release. This seems particularly evident in the case of those machines that form compressed plugs.

Rupture and Dissolution of Shell to Expose and Release Capsule Contents

Bioavailability from capsules first requires that shells rupture and/or dissolve to expose and release contents to body fluids. When immersed in a dissolution fluid at 37°C, hard-gelatin capsules can be seen to rupture first at the shoulders of the cap and body where the gelatin shell is the thinnest (116,117). As the dissolution fluid penetrates the capsule contents, the powder mass begins to disintegrate and deaggregate from the ends. HPMC shells rupture more slowly than gelatin shells, and different grades and compositions of HPMC capsules may behave differently.

HPMC capsules have been shown to disintegrate more slowly than gelatin capsules, but HPMC shells dissolve and disperse more uniformly from capsule surfaces (6,118,119). In one study, Missaghi and Fassihi compared HPMC capsules (carrageenan and K^+ gelling system) with standard gelatin capsules (119). The capsules were filled with powdered cellulose mixed with 0.5% magnesium stearate. The HPMC capsules disintegrated more slowly than gelatin capsules in various media using the USP disintegration test method, and the HPMC shells were seen to disperse in a more uniform pattern than gelatin capsule shells. The disintegration times varied according to the media (119). For example, the mean disintegration time ($\pm$ standard deviation) of HPMC capsules in diluted hydrochloric acid (pH = 1.5) was 151.7 ($\pm$ 16.8) seconds, whereas in a potassium phosphate buffer (pH = 6.8), it was 270.0 ($\pm$ 26) seconds. In those same media, the disintegration time of gelatin capsules was 34.0 ($\pm$ 3.6) seconds and 53.3 $\pm$ (6.6) seconds, respectively. The shorter disintegration time of gelatin at pH 1.5 was thought to be due to its greater solubility at that pH, whereas the slower disintegration of HPMC capsules in the buffer was attributed to the K^+ ions increasing the gel strength of the carrageenan in the shell walls (119).

Using real-time dissolution spectroscopy to estimate rupture time, El-Malah et al. found that the in vitro rupture time of HPMC capsules depended on not only the dissolution medium but also the grade of the capsule, and was independent of capsule size (120). Pharmaceutical and nutritional grade HPMC capsules (Quali-V) were compared. Rupture time was based on the time of detection of Labrosol (caprylocaproyl macroglycerides, Gattefossé) released from the capsules in standard USP type II dissolution apparatus at 37°C using a fiber-optic probe. The shortest rupture times were found for gelatin capsules, which ranged from 1.1 to 1.5 minutes in simulated gastric fluid (SGF) and from 1.3 to 2.1 minutes in simulated intestinal fluid (SIF). The corresponding rupture times for pharmaceutical grade HPMC capsules were 2.85 to 3.75 minutes in SGF and 6.15 to 10.5 minutes in SIF. But still longer times were found for the nutritional grade of HPMC: 3.6 to 4.8 minutes (SGF) and 9.67 to 11.25 minutes (SIF). The longer rupture times of HPMC capsules in SIF was attributed to its higher salt concentration, particularly K^+ ions. Differences in such factors as the grade or molecular weight of HPMC, any additives employed, and/or the process used to produce the capsules were suggested as possible explanations for the differences found in the rupture times of the two grades of HPMC capsules.

Chiwele et al. showed that in media at a pH $\leq$ 5.8, HPMC capsules dissolved rapidly and independently of temperature between 10°C and 55°C, whereas gelatin capsules generally did not dissolve at temperatures below 30°C (6). On the basis of these observations, they proposed that HPMC capsules could be administered with either warm or cold drinks and gelatin capsules preferably should be given with a warm drink. But, since the shell dissolution of both capsule types was prolonged and more variable when tested in a pH 6.8 phosphate buffer, they suggested that capsule formulations should not be taken with carbonated cola-type drinks (6).

These reported longer in vitro rupture or disintegration times for HPMC capsules should not be assumed to necessarily lead to meaningful in vivo or bioavailablity differences. For example, Cole et al. conducted in vitro dissolution tests and an in vivo evaluation of ibuprofen bioavailability in a study comparing HPMC capsules (gellan gum and K^+ gelling system) and standard gelatin capsules (7). The in vitro dissolution tests revealed that acid conditions and the presence of K^+ cations slowed the opening of HPMC capsules, but there was no difference between these HPMC capsules and gelatin capsules when tested in water. A four-way crossover biostudy was conducted with 11 healthy human subjects in fed and fasted state. The in vivo opening times (determined by scintigraphy) of the HPMC capsules also were longer, but bioavailability studies revealed no significant differences in maximum plasma concentration (C_{max}) or area under the plasma concentration-time curve (AUC). Tuleu et al. conducted a scintographic study comparing the disintegration of HPMC capsules (carrageenan and K^+ gelling system) with standard gelatin capsules filled with a lactose-based mixture in eight healthy fasted male subjects (121). The study showed that all capsules disintegrated rapidly in the stomach and revealed small but statistically insignificant differences in their in vivo disintegration times. The mean and ranges for the disintegration times were as follows: HPMC, 9 minutes (6–11 minutes); and gelatin, 7 minutes (3–13 minutes). In another study, Hankanen et al. investigated the preparation of sustained-release formulations of ibuprofen by mixing the drug with different amounts of various molecular weight grades of HPMC powder as the diluent (26). The mixtures were filled in HPMC capsules (Quali-V) and standard gelatin capsules (Coni-Snap). The capsules were administered either orally or rectally to two groups of eight healthy human subjects. Hankanen et al. reported no marked difference in bioavailability between the HPMC or gelatin capsules either orally or rectally and concluded that the two shell materials can be regarded as interchangeable from a biopharmaceutical viewpoint (26).

The Role of Excipients and the Impact of Formulation and Process Variables on Drug Release

It is apparent that once capsule contents are exposed by shell rupture and dissolution, the efficiency by which the drug will be released will depend on the wettability of the powder mass, the rapidity with which fluid penetrates the powder, the rate of disintegration and deaggregation of the contents, and the nature of the primary drug particles. These processes, in turn, can be significantly affected by the design of the formulation and the mode of filling. Such factors as the amount and choice of fillers and lubricants, the inclusion of disintegrants or surfactants, and the degree of plug compaction can have a profound effect on drug release.

Active Ingredient

The dose of the drug and its solubility are important considerations in the design of the formulation. The amount and type of active ingredient influence capsule size and the nature and amount of excipients to be used in the formulation. Larger-dose drugs that must be granulated to produce tablets may be more easily direct-filled into hard-shell capsules with proper choice of excipients.

Dissolution of the drug in gastrointestinal fluids must occur before absorption can occur, and drugs having sufficiently high water solubility often exhibit few formulation problems. For drugs of low water solubility, the absorption rate may be governed by the dissolution rate, that is, exhibit *dissolution rate–limited absorption*. In such cases, if dissolution occurs too slowly, absorption efficiency may suffer. Possible drug instability in gastrointestinal fluids is another concern for slowly dissolving drugs that can affect their bioavailability.

The solubility of a drug should be considered together with its dose. Even a poorly soluble drug can completely dissolve under physiological conditions if its dose is sufficiently small. Thus, a *dose solubility volume*, that is, the volume required to dissolve the dose of the drug, is a more useful tool to judge potential solubility problems than solely the equilibrium solubility of the drug. Amidon et al. (122) defined a drug as having "high solubility" if the largest human dose is soluble in 250 mL (or less) of water throughout the physiological pH range of 1 to 8 at 37°C. A drug is considered a "low-solubility" drug if more than 250 mL of water is required to dissolve the largest dose at any pH within that range at 37°C. The reference volume estimate of 250 mL is the assumed minimum initial gastric volume available. This volume is based on the volume of water recommended for ingestion during the administration of a dosage form in a typical bioequivalence study protocol (123).

Bioavailability depends not only on having the drug in solution but also on the drug's permeability. A jejunal permeability of at least 2 to 4×10^{-4} cm/sec, measured in human subjects by intubation, is considered "high permeability" (122). For many drugs and other substances, this permeability corresponds to a fraction absorbed of 90% or better. Amidon et al. (122) thus proposed a Biopharmaceutics Classification System (BCS) for drugs on the basis of the above definitions of these two parameters. Table 4 defines the BCS and includes some drugs representative of each class.

The BCS makes an important contribution to the rational formulation of both drug products and regulatory policy. Since the BCS gives formulation scientists the ability to estimate the likely contribution of dissolution rate, solubility, and intestinal permeability to oral drug absorption, it provides a basis for estimating the risk of encountering bioavailability problems. Because of their high solubility and permeability, class I drugs are expected to exhibit few bioavailability problems. However, class II drugs (low solubility and high permeability) are prone to exhibit dissolution rate–limited absorption. On the other hand, class III drugs (high solubility and low permeability) are likely to exhibit permeation rate–limited absorption. Class IV drugs (low solubility and low permeability) present serious obstacles to bioavailability, and some may best be formulated in solubilized form, such as a parenteral or liquid-filled or semisolid-filled

Table 4 Biopharmaceutics Classification System (122–128)

Solubility	High permeability (fraction absorbed ≥ 90%)	Low permeability (fraction absorbed < 90%)
High solubility (≤250 mL required to dissolve the largest dose in pH range 1–8 at 37°C)	I. Metoprolol tartrate Propranolol HCl	II. Piroxicam Naproxen
Low solubility (>250 mL required to dissolve the largest dose in pH range 1–8 at 37°C)	III. Ranitidine Cimetidine	IV. Furosemide Hydrochlorothiazide

soft- or hard-shell capsule formulation. Clearly, the early recognition of the BCS class into which the drug falls will provide important guidance in making formulation decisions.

The FDA applied the BCS in a regulatory guidance entitled "Immediate Release Solid Oral Dosage Forms; Scale-Up and Post Approval Changes: Chemistry, Manufacturing, and Controls; In Vitro Dissolution testing; In Vivo Bioequivalence Documentation" (129). Also known by its acronym, SUPAC-IR, this guidance defines levels of postapproval changes and recommends tests and other requirements needed to document that product quality and performance had not changed after certain minor changes in manufacturing (batch size, equipment, process or site) or product composition (levels of excipients) were made to an approved product. Postapproval changes are often needed to update processes through the use of newer, more efficient equipment and methods, to change site of manufacture as a result of mergers and acquisitions, or to change scale of manufacture in response to product demand. SUPAC-IR deals with these changes by defining three levels of changes. Level I changes are those that are unlikely to have any detectable impact on product quality and performance. Level 2 changes are those that could have significant impact on product quality and performance. Level 3 changes are those that are likely to have significant impact on quality and performance. As the level changes from 1 to 3, the rigor of testing and filing requirements needed to justify the change increases. For certain changes, the tests and filing requirements depend on the biopharmaceutic classification of the drug. Along with certain other requirements, dissolution testing may be used to justify level 1 and 2 compositional changes, that is, drug dissolution from the changed product and the original product should be similar. However, the rigor of the dissolution test to be used depends on the risk of bioavailability problems as represented by the drug's BCS class (class IV excluded). High solubility–high permeability drugs require the least rigorous dissolution test. More rigorous dissolution testing is required for high solubility–low permeability drugs, and the most rigorous dissolution testing is required for low solubility–high permeability drugs. Level 3 composition and process changes require human bioequivalence tests to justify the change. In a more recent guidance that addresses BCS, FDA broadened this policy to permit the use of dissolution testing as a surrogate for human bioavailability testing for rapidly dissolving immediate-release products of high solubility–high permeable drugs that are not considered by FDA to be narrow therapeutic index drugs (128). That guidance also changed the pH range in which to determine the drug's solubility volume from 1 to 7.5. For the purposes of this guidance, *rapidly dissolving* is defined as not less than 85% of labeled content dissolving in not more than 30 minutes in 900 mL (or less) of each of three vehicles: SGF USP (without enzymes), pH 4.5 buffer and pH 6.8 buffer, or SIF USP (without enzymes). Either USP dissolution apparatus I at 100 rpm or USP apparatus II at 50 rpm may be used.

Drugs of low water solubility are often micronized to increase their dissolution rate. Particle size reduction increases the surface area per unit weight of the drug, thereby increasing the surface area available from which dissolution can occur. For instance, Fincher et al. (130) studied the different particle size fractions of sulfathiazole administered in capsules to dogs, and found that the smallest particle size gave the highest blood level. Also, Bastami and Groves (131) reported that reducing the particle size of sodium phenytoin improved the dissolution rate from capsules containing 100 mg of the drug and 150 mg lactose. There are, however, practical limitations to this approach. Micronized particles with high surface to mass ratios may tend to aggregate owing to surface cohesive interaction, thereby reducing the surface area effectively available for dissolution. Newton and Rowley (132) found that at equivalent bed porosities, larger particle size fractions of a poorly soluble drug, ethinamate, gave better dissolution from capsules of the pure drug than smaller particle sizes. They attributed this result to the smaller particle size fractions having reduced *effective* surface area for dissolution owing to their aggregation. The compaction of fine particles into capsules also reduces the bed permeability and generally retards dissolution (132).

From a manufacturing point of view, a compromise may have to be struck between small particle size and good flow properties. Small particles in general are more poorly flowing than larger particles. Surface cohesive and frictional interactions, which oppose flow properties, are more important in smaller particle size powders because of their larger specific surface areas. One possible way to both reduce the effects of aggregation of fine particles and enhance flow properties is granulation. When micronized ethinamate was granulated in a simple moist process with isopropanol, bed permeability and drug dissolution from capsules were greatly enhanced compared with that of the micronized powder (128). See the section "Hydrophilization and Granulation" for additional comments on the role of granulation in capsules.

Fillers

Fillers (diluents) are often needed to increase the bulk of the formulation. The most common capsule diluents are starch and lactose. Inorganic salts appearing in capsule formulations include, among others, magnesium and calcium carbonate and calcium phosphate. Fillers modified to enhance their flowability and compactibility for direct compaction tableting are particularly advantageous in developing formulations for automatic capsule-filling machines. Examples include pregelatinized starch (Starch[®] 1500[a]), spray-processed (monohydrate) lactose (Fast-Flo[®] Lactose[b]), direct compression grade (anhydrous) lactose (Sheffield[TM] Anhydrous DT[c]), agglomerated (monohydrate) lactose (Pharmatose[®] DCL 15[d]), and unmilled dicalcium phosphate dihydrate (Emcompress[®e]).

Formulations intended to be run on dosator machines may sometimes benefit from the greater compactibility of microcrystalline cellulose (e.g., Avicel[®,f] Emcocel[®g]), particularly when the drug makes up a relatively large amount of the capsule content and the quantity of excipient that can be added is limited. In these machines it is essential to prevent powder loss from the open end of the dosing tube during plug transfer from the powder bed to ejection into the capsule body. The failure to have a cohesive plug may also cause loss due to a "blow off" of powder owing to displaced air as the plug is ejected into the shell. As previously pointed out, a degree of compactibility is also important in formulations for dosing-disc machines. Using a Zanasi AZ-5 dosator machine, Patel and Podceck (133) studied several microcrystalline celluloses and concluded that medium and coarse particle size grades can be considered "good" excipients for capsules. Of the eight sources and types tested, Avicel[®] PH 101, Avicel[®] PH103, Microcel[®], and Emcocel[®] appeared to be the most suitable sources for capsule filling. Recently, a silicified grade of

---

[a]Colorcon Inc., West Point, Pennsylvania, U.S.

[b]Sheffield[TM] Pharma Ingredients, Norwich, New York, U.S.

[c]Sheffield[TM] Pharma Ingredients, Norwich, New York, U.S.

[d]DMV North America, Delhi, New York, U.S.

[e]JRS Pharma LP, Patterson, New York, U.S.

[f]FMC Corp., Food and Pharmaceutical Products Div., Philadelphia, Pennsylvania, U.S.

[g]DMV North America, Delhi, New York, U.S.

microcrystalline cellulose and original microcrystalline cellulose were evaluated and found to be good plug formers when tested in tablet compaction simulator adapted to produce capsule plugs at piston compression forces and speeds found in some capsules-filling machines (134). Several grades of ProSolv® silicified microcrystalline cellulose (SMCC) and a comparable control grade of standard microcrystalline cellulose-produced plugs having higher maximum breaking force than either anhydrous lactose or Starch® 1500 when tested under similar compression conditions. SMCC is an intimate physical mixture of microcrystalline cellulose and 2% colloidal silicon dioxide produced through a coprocessing technique. The reader is referred to Bolhuis and Armstrong (135) for additional information on SMCC and other tableting fillers modified for direct compaction.

From a drug dissolution point of view, formulators may need to consider the solubility of both the filler and the drug. Generally, poorly soluble drugs benefit from the use of soluble fillers (e.g., lactose) or hydrophilic fillers (e.g., microcrystalline cellulose), which can enhance the wettability of capsule contents and may help disintegration as well. For instance, Newton et al. (136) demonstrated that the dissolution of poorly soluble ethinamate from capsules improved greatly when the concentration of lactose in the formulation was increased to 50%. But formulators may need to observe caution when large amounts of soluble fillers are used in combination with some soluble drugs because the dissolution of the filler may interfere with the dissolution of the drug. For example, Withey and Mainville (137) found that the inclusion of 80% lactose in the formulation severely retarded dissolution of soluble chloramphenicol from capsules. There was little or no effect on dissolution when up to 50% lactose was included. It was suggested that dissolution of the lactose occurs more rapidly and that chloramphenicol dissolution is retarded because of the high concentration of lactose already in solution. The effect that a filler can have on bioavailability was graphically illustrated when Australian physicians noted an increase in the number of patients exhibiting phenytoin toxicity while using a particular sodium phenytoin capsule product (138). This occurrence coincided with the manufacturer changing the filler from calcium sulfate to lactose and was the result of increased bioavailability when lactose was the filler. Bastami and Groves (131) reported that the in vitro dissolution of phenytoin may not be complete in the presence of calcium sulfate and suggested the formation of an insoluble calcium salt of the drug.

It has also been reported that lactose at a concentration of 50% enhanced the dissolution of phenobarbital (free acid form) from capsules, but had no effect on the dissolution of the water-soluble sodium phenobarbital (139). On the other hand, cornstarch at 50% slowed the dissolution of sodium phenobarbital and improved the dissolution of the free acid; however, the effect in either case was dependent on the moisture content of the starch (139). The t_{50} (time required for 50% drug dissolution) for 50:50 phenobarbital/cornstarch capsules decreased from 28 to 9 minutes as the starch moisture content increased from 1.2% w/w to 9.5% w/w. This compares to a t_{50} of 25 minutes for the drug alone. Drug dissolution also improved in the 50:50 sodium phenobarbital/cornstarch mixtures with increased moisture; however, even at the highest moisture content (13.5%), t_{50} was still about double that of the drug alone (4.9 minutes vs. 2.5 minutes).

The intrinsic dissolution rates of selected fillers are compared in Table 5 (140). Anhydrous lactose, which is predominantly the more soluble β-lactose, exhibits nearly twice the intrinsic dissolution rate of the α-lactose monohydrate. Of particular interest is the pH-dependent solubility of some fillers that show dramatically reduced intrinsic dissolution rates under less acidic conditions. The use of such fillers is of potential

Table 5 Intrinsic Dissolution Rates of Selected Fillers, mg/min cm^2 at 37°C

Anhydrous lactose
  Purified water—21.9
Lactose monohydrate
  Purified water—12.4
Dicalcium phosphate, dihydrate
  0.1M HCl—6.27
  0.01M HCl—0.90
Anhydrous dicalcium phosphate
  0.1M HCl—5.37
  0.01M HCl—0.69
Calcium sulfate dihydrate
  0.1M HCl—1.15
  0.01M HCl—0.75

Source: From Ref. 140.

concern in populations that exhibit achlorhydria, such as the elderly. In such cases, disintegration and dissolution could be substantially delayed.

Glidants

Glidants are finely divided dry powders added to formulations in small quantities to improve their flow properties. Glidant particles of sufficiently fine particle size have been observed to adsorb onto the surfaces of the bulk powder particles. Glidants are thought to act at particle surfaces to enhance the fluidity of the formulation (or bulk powder) by one or more of several possible mechanisms (141,142): (*i*) reducing roughness by filling surface irregularities, (*ii*) reducing attractive forces by physically separating the bulk powder particles, (*iii*) modifying electrostatic charges, (*iv*) acting as moisture scavengers, and (*v*) serving as ball bearings between bulk powder particles. Usually, there is an optimum concentration for best flow. For the colloidal silicas, often this is less than 1%. The optimum concentration varies with the glidant and may be related to the concentration just needed to coat the host particles (134,143). Exceeding this concentration will usually result in either no further improvement in flow or, even, a worsening of flow. Glidants include the colloidal silicas, cornstarch, talc, and magnesium stearate. York (142) reported the following order of effectiveness for two powder systems: fine silica > magnesium stearate > purified talc.

Lubricants

Capsule formulations usually require lubricants just as do tablet formulations. Lubricants ease the ejection of plugs, reduce filming on pistons and adhesion of powder to other metal surfaces, and reduce friction between sliding surfaces in contact with powder. The same lubricants are used in both tablet and capsule formulations. Lubricants are generally added last in the manufacturing process because they exert their function at particle surfaces.

The most effective lubricants are the hydrophobic stearates, such as magnesium stearate, calcium stearate, and stearic acid. Magnesium stearate is the most widely used lubricant (144,145). Lubricants proposed as being less hydrophobic such as hydrogenated vegetable oils, polyethylene glycols (PEGs), and sodium stearyl fumarate are less effective in this application (145).

High concentrations of hydrophobic lubricants such as magnesium stearate in a formulation can retard drug release by coating particles and making formulations more hydrophobic (136,146–148). But overmixing even low concentrations of laminar lubricants (e.g., magnesium stearate, calcium stearate) also can be a problem. Laminar lubricants are said to be "mixing sensitive." That is, under the rigors of mixing, the particles delaminate, that is, shear readily when subjected to a tangential force, to form a hydrophobic film on the surfaces of host particles (149–151). The extent of coating of host particles by the hydrophobic lubricant thus also depends on the intensity and duration of mixing. If blended for a sufficient length of time, even a low level of addition of a laminar lubricant can retard wetting and drug dissolution (148). Formulators are thus careful not to add too much of such lubricants nor to mix for too long. Generally, the appropriate level of lubricant is added last and blended for a minimum amount of time, usually two to five minutes.

The mixing and delamination of lubricants like magnesium stearate does not end when a blender is stopped. The powder handling mechanism of the filling machine can cause additional mixing and shearing of the formulation. For example, Desai et al. (152) reported overmixing of magnesium stearate in the hopper of an MG2 dosator machine. During operation of the machine, the powder in the hopper is continuously mixed with a rotating blade. Compared with initial dissolution profiles (before running the machine), the dissolution of three drugs was markedly reduced after running the machine for 30 minutes when the magnesium stearate level was 1%. When the level of magnesium stearate was reduced to 0.25%, lubrication was adequate and dissolution was satisfactory over the 30-minute filling run. Replacement of magnesium stearate with the more hydrophilic lubricants Stear-O-Wet (magnesium stearate coprocessed with the wetting agent sodium lauryl sulfate) and sodium stearyl fumarate also resulted in satisfactory dissolution. Ullah et al. (153) encountered a related problem when scaling up the batch size of cefadroxil monohydrate capsules. The formulation was initially developed on a small-scale Zanasi LZ-64 dosator machine with a blend containing 1% magnesium stearate. On scale-up to a GKF 1500 production dosing-disc machine, the capsules exhibited significantly slower dissolution than those produced on the Zanasi machine. They attributed their observation to additional shearing of the formulation during the tamping step, which resulted in increased coating of drug particles with magnesium stearate. Using a laboratory scale mixer/grinder to simulate the shearing action of the filling machine, a reduced level of 0.3% magnesium stearate was selected for scale-up to 570 and 1100 kg (full production) size batches. Dissolution was found satisfactory for both scale-up batch sizes.

When contemplating the transfer of formulations between dosator and dosing-disc machines, formulators should consider that formulations for these two types of machines may require different levels of lubrication. The report by Ullah et al. (153), which describes experiences encountered in the scale-up of a smaller batch to larger batches, is particularly interesting in that it also describes the transfer of a formulation from a dosator machine to a dosing-disc machine. Although the greater shearing action that occurs in powder bed when mixing larger (scaled-up) masses may in part have contributed to their observations, the suggestion that shearing due to the tamping action in the dosing-disc machine was a factor contributing to slower drug dissolution also points to a possible important difference in the lubrication requirements of formulations for the two types of filling machines. As part of a larger effort aimed at addressing several possible formulation requirement differences between these machine types, Heda et al. (154) compared the plug ejection forces of model formulations containing 0.25%, 0.50% and 1.0% magnesium stearate filled using equivalent plug compression forces of 100 and

200 N on instrumented capsule-filling machines of both types. The batch size, blending method, and mixing time were identical for the model formulations. Heda et al. observed that plug ejection forces were consistently lower when the model formulations were run on a Höfliger & Karg GKF 400 machine than on a Zanasi LZ-64 machine. These data suggested a possible twofold difference in the level of magnesium stearate required for running these formulations on this equipment. The observations of Heda et al. could be related to greater shearing of magnesium stearate in the dosing-disc machine, as proposed by Ullah et al. (153). A greater coverage of particle surfaces with magnesium stearate could not only cause plugs to be sufficiently hydrophobic to slow dissolution but also result in better lubricated plugs requiring lower ejection forces. For the interested reader, a more comprehensive discussion of the issues involved in scaling-up capsule formulations and their transfer between dosator and dosing-disc machines is available (155).

Magnesium stearate on particle surfaces can also reduce particle cohesiveness and soften plugs. There is evidence to suggest that this phenomenon can lead to unexpected enhanced drug dissolution in certain instances. Consider the work of Stewart et al. (101) who found that the effect of magnesium stearate concentration on the dissolution of a model low-dose drug, riboflavin, from capsules was dependent in some manner on the type of filler. As previously described, the capsules were filled using the dosator of a Zanasi machine that had been fitted to a moveable crosshead. They found that the soluble fillers they had tested exhibited the anticipated slowed dissolution with increasing magnesium stearate levels. However, the trends with insoluble fillers were not so predictable. In some cases insoluble fillers were only slightly affected by the concentrations of magnesium stearate studied. For others, such as microcrystalline cellulose, there appeared to be an ideal *intermediate* lubricant concentration at which the dissolution rate was maximized. Following up on this work, Mehta and Augsburger found that the mechanical strength of microcrystalline cellulose–based plugs produced in a dosator was reduced by the amount of lubricant used, and this appeared to be beneficial to drug dissolution (98). Hydrochlorothiazide was the tracer drug used for dissolution testing. These investigators compared the time for 60% of the drug content to dissolve (t_{60}) and plug breaking force for two fillers lubricated with magnesium stearate concentrations ranging from 0.05% to 0.75%. Batch size, blending method, and mixing time were the same in all cases. The instrumented Zanasi filling machine they used permitted standardization of the plug compression force so that only the lubrication concentration effect was studied. With microcrystalline cellulose–based plugs, t_{60} decreased from 55 to 12 minutes as the magnesium stearate concentration was increased progressively from 0.015% to 0.75%. At the same time, plug-breaking force dramatically decreased from 84 g for plugs containing 0.05% magnesium stearate down to about 2.0 g for plugs containing 0.75% magnesium stearate. With the lactose-based formulation, t_{60} increased slightly with the lubricant level from 12 to 18 minutes, while plug-breaking force decreased slightly, although not significantly ($p = 0.05$), from 18 to 13 g. For the microcrystalline cellulose case, it was suggested that the increase in hydrophobicity with increase in magnesium stearate level may be more than offset by reduced plug cohesiveness in the concentration range studied, which probably led to better moisture penetration and plug disintegration. Yet, dissolution was markedly slowed when the magnesium stearate concentration was 2%, suggesting that the hydrophobic effect of the lubricant eventually becomes overwhelming at higher levels (98). This dual effect of magnesium stearate has also been noted in Nakagwu's study of the dissolution of rifampicin from hard-gelatin capsules (156). These investigators varied both the concentration of magnesium stearate and the blending time. Up to a limit, lengthening the blending time of magnesium stearate was found to *increase* the rate of rifampicin dissolution. This effect, which was most noticeable at lower lubricant concentrations, was attributed to reduced cohesiveness of the formulation resulting from the longer lubricant-mixing times.

Disintegrants

Traditional tablet disintegrants are often found in modern capsule formulations. Their inclusion in formulations promotes the disintegration and deaggregation of capsule contents to release primary drug particles, thereby promoting rapid drug dissolution. Early studies of the role of disintegrants in capsule formulations usually involved hand-filled capsules and often led to mixed results (147,157,158). The loose-packed contents of capsules filled by methods that afford little compression provide little structure for disintegrants to expand against to effect disintegration. However, the advent of filling machines, which compress capsule contents, together with the development of newer disintegrants, which have superior swelling and/or moisture absorbing properties, appear to warrant serious consideration of disintegrants in modern capsule formulations. These newer disintegrants, which have been called "super disintegrants," (159,160) include croscarmellose sodium, type A (e.g., AcDiSol[®h]), sodium starch glycolate (e.g., Primojel[®, i] Explotab[®j]) and crospovidone (e.g., Polyplasdone[®] XL[k]). For instance, Botzolakis et al. (161) compared various levels of these newer disintegrants against 10% starch and 0% disintegrant as controls in dicalcium phosphate–based capsules filled on an instrumented Zanasi LZ-64 at a uniform compression force. In most cases, the dissolution

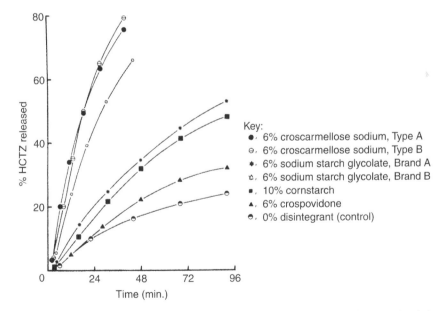

Figure 19 Effect of disintegrants on hydrochlorothiazide dissolution from hard-gelatin capsules (filler, dicalcium phosphate; lubricant, 1% magnesium stearate). *Source*: From Ref. 161.

---

[h]FMC Corp., Food and Pharmaceutical Products Div., Philadelphia, Pennsylvania, U.S.

[i]Generichem Corp., Totowa, New Jersey, U.S.

[j]JRS Pharma LP, Patterson, New York, U.S.

[k]ISP Corp., Wayne, New Jersey, U.S.

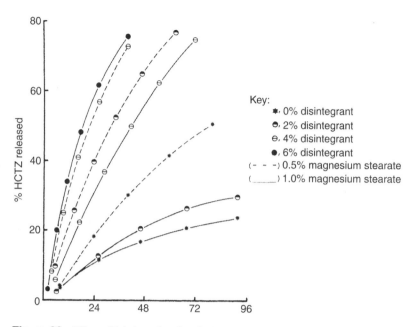

Figure 20 Effect of lubricant level on hydrochlorothiazide dissolution from hard-gelatin capsules (filler, dicalcium phosphate; disintegrant, croscarmellose sodium, type A). *Source*: From Ref. 161.

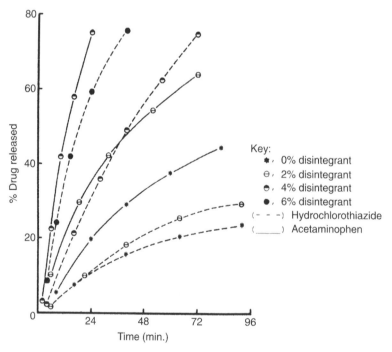

Figure 21 Effect of croscarmellose sodium (type A) on drug dissolution from hard-gelatin capsules (filler, dicalcium phosphate; lubricant, 1% magnesium stearate). *Source*: From Ref. 161.

rate of hydrochlorothiazide was dramatically enhanced over the controls (Fig. 19). The data plotted in Figures 20 and 21 demonstrate that disintegrant efficiency is concentration dependent. Although the typical use levels of super disintegrants in direct compression tablets are in the range of 2% to 4%, the most effective disintegrants required 4% to 6% for fast dissolution from capsules. Figures 20 and 21 also point up the importance of drug

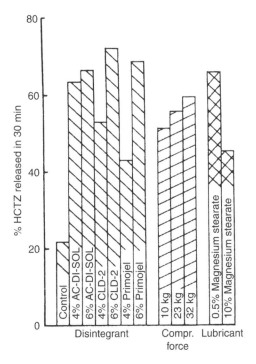

Figure 22 Averaged effect of disintegrant, lubricant, and compression force on hydrochlorothiazide dissolution from dicalcium phosphate–based capsules. *Source*: From. Ref. 162.

solubility and magnesium stearate level. When magnesium stearate was reduced (l.0–0.5%) or when a more soluble drug (acetaminophen) was substituted for hydrochlorothiazide, less croscarmellose was needed to exert a similar effect on dissolution (161).

In a later study (162) the effect of disintegrants on hydrochlorothiazide dissolution from both water-soluble (anhydrous lactose) and water-insoluble (dicalcium phosphate) fillers was compared for different lubricant levels and plug compression forces (instrumented Zanasi LZ-64 machine). Statistical analysis of this multivariable study revealed all main factors and their interactions to be significant. However, by averaging the results for each factor over all conditions, the relative magnitude of each main factor could be assessed, as in Figures 22 and 23. Although the disintegrants were effective in promoting drug dissolution from both fillers, the effect was much less dramatic with lactose. This finding is not surprising since the lactose-based capsule without disintegrant is already a fast-releasing formulation. Soluble fillers tend to dissolve rather than disintegrate. A beneficial effect of increasing the tamping force is also apparent, though the effect was much more evident with the dicalcium phosphate–based capsules. As compression force increases, plug porosity may decrease, possibly making the swelling action of disintegrants more effective. Again, the retardant effect on dissolution of the hydrophobic lubricant is evident; however, it is apparent that the soluble lactose-based formulation is much less profoundly affected.

The multiple compression (tamping) that occurs in dosing-disc machines has been shown to slow dissolution, but that effect may be minimized by the inclusion of a super disintegrant. In the absence of any disintegrant, Shah et al. found that the dissolution of hydrochlorothiazide from capsules was slower after two and again after three tamps at a given plug compression force compared with capsules filled using a single tamp at the same compression force (94). This difference was greatest when the plug compression

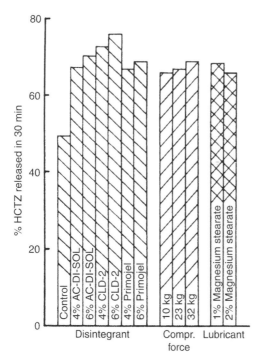

Figure 23 Averaged effect of disintegrant, lubricant, and compression force on hydrochlorothiazide dissolution from anhydrous lactose–based capsules. *Source*: From Ref. 162.

force was 200 N than when it was 100 N. But the addition of 4% of croscarmellose to the formulation essentially eliminated the effects of multiple tamping or compression force on dissolution (94).

Surfactants

Surfactants may be included in capsule formulations to increase the wetting of the powder mass and enhance drug dissolution. The "water-proofing" effect of hydrophobic lubricants may be offset by the use of surfactants. Numerous studies have reported the beneficial effects of surfactants on disintegration and deaggregation and/or drug dissolution (132,136,146,158). Botzolakis demonstrated enhanced liquid uptake into capsule plugs due to surfactants (90). The most common surfactants employed in capsule formulations are sodium lauryl sulfate and sodium docusate. Levels of 0.1% to 0.5% are usually sufficient.

Ong et al. (163) found that several hydrophilic anionic, nonionic, or cationic surfactants can alleviate the deleterious effect of magnesium stearate overmixing on dissolution from capsules when added with the lubricant in a ratio as low as 1 part surfactant:5 parts lubricant (w/w). These successful surfactants were sodium *N*-lauroyl sarcosinate, sodium stearoyl-2-lactylate, sodium stearate, poloxamer 188, cetylpyridinium chloride, and sodium lauryl sulfate. The lipophilic surfactant, glyceryl monostearate, did not alleviate the magnesium stearate–mixing effect. A reduction in surfactant particle size was shown to enhance effectiveness, particularly in the case of those surfactants with low solubility and slow dissolution rate.

The effectiveness of surfactants in overcoming the hydrophobic effect of magnesium stearate may not be a result solely of an increase in the wetting properties of the bulk phase. Compared with putting the surfactant in the dosage form, Botzolakis (90) and Wang and Chowhan (164) found that adding an equivalent amount of surfactant to the dissolution medium was not effective. The possible impact of the surfactant at particle surfaces in the microenvironment around the dissolving particles where local concentrations are high should be considered. In addition to the wetting effect, surfactants at concentrations exceeding the critical micelle concentration can increase drug solubility, thereby resulting in a greater effective concentration gradient. The situation is complex, since drug solubilization within micelles also reduces the effective rate of drug diffusion (165). Another possible contributing mechanism for the role of surfactants has been proposed by Ong et al. (163) and Wang and Chowhan (164). On the basis of order of mixing studies and scanning electron microscopy of powder mixtures, these investigators suggest that surfactants and magnesium stearate may interact strongly enough with each other to inhibit the magnesium stearate and drug-excipient interactions that cause reduced dissolution.

Hydrophilization and Granulation

Another approach to improving the wettability of poorly soluble drugs is to treat the drug with a solution of a hydrophilic polymer. Lerk et al. (166) reported that both wettability of the powder and the rate of dissolution of hexobarbital from hard-gelatin capsules could be greatly enhanced if the drug were treated with methylcellulose or hydroxyethylcellulose. In this process, called hydrophilization, a solution of the hydrophilic polymer was spread onto the drug in a high-shear mixer, and the resultant mixture dried and screened. No benefit was accrued when the drug and polymer were merely dry blended. No other excipients were included, and the capsules were loosely packed by hand. Lerk et al. (167) later treated phenytoin by hydrophilization with methylcellulose and compared the pure and treated drug compressed into plugs at 120 N to simulate a tamping machine. The plugs were manually filled into hard-gelatin capsules. The treated phenytoin was found to dissolve and be absorbed (in human subjects) considerably faster than the untreated drug. However, there were no lubricants or fillers, etc., included in these capsules as may be required for actual filling. The beneficial effect of hydrophilization on disintegration of benylate from hard-gelatin capsules was demonstrated in vivo in human subjects by external scintigraphy (168).

The benefits of hydrophilization can be expected whenever powders are wet granulated with typical binders such as pregelatinized starch, hydroxypropyl methylcellulose, and polyvinyl pyrrolidone, which form a hydrophilic film on particle surfaces.

Powders for encapsulation may be granulated to reduce bulk, enhance flow, reduce agglomeration of fine particles or their adhesion to metal surfaces, and improve the content uniformity of low-dose drugs. Wet granulation provides for the addition of a liquid phase (binder solution or solvent) in which a very low-dose drug may be dissolved and which facilitates its uniform dispersion throughout the mass. When the moist agglomerates formed by the granulation process are dried, the drug is "locked" in the granules, thereby preventing its segregation in subsequent handling steps. Granulation is thus a form of ordered mixing. The potential adverse effect of temperature and exposure to water on the stability of some drugs may limit the application of wet granulation. In such cases, dry granulation by the older slugging process or the more contemporary roller compaction process can be used to accomplish most of the objectives of granulation, although such dry processes do not inherently provide for the addition of the drug in solution or hydrophilization. Of course, the liquid addition of low-dose drugs to form an ordered mix also may be accomplished by dissolving the drug in a solvent, spraying the solution onto a filler in an appropriate mixing device, and evaporating the solvent.

Systematic Formulation Development and Analysis of Critical Variables

More and more, pharmaceutical scientists are adopting systematic approaches to the design, formulation, and optimization of dosage forms. New understandings of biopharmaceutic principles, for example, the Biopharmaceutical Drug Classification System, coupled with software-driven optimization and decision-making tools, have given pharmaceutical scientists the ability to make logical and deliberate formulation design decisions. Among the tools employed by formulation scientists today are multivariate analysis and response surface methodology (125,169) and artificial intelligence (170–173).

Response Surface Analysis of Piroxicam Capsules

One example of the application of response surface analysis to powder-filled capsules is the study of critical formulation variables for 20 mg piroxicam capsules (125). Piroxicam is a BCS class II drug (low solubility and high permeability). A review of this study is particularly informative and useful because it links in vitro outcomes (i.e., dissolution) with in vivo outcomes in human subjects. A *resolution V* central composite (face centered) experimental design was implemented in which five formulation (independent) variables were studied at each of three levels. Thirty-two batches of capsules were manufactured in which these variables and their levels were varied. Batch size varied from 5 to 7 kg, depending on the bulk densities of the blends. The five variables studied and their levels appear in Table 6.

The effect of piroxicam particle size was evaluated by comparing the piroxicam powder as received, termed "unmilled," with the same lot of piroxicam that was remilled, termed "milled." The remilling of piroxicam substantially reduced its particle size and increased its specific surface area from 1.79 to 4.91 M^2/g. The capsules were filled using a Zanasi LZ-64 automatic capsule-filling machine instrumented to monitor plug compression force. The capsules were filled with a consistent compression force.

Table 6 Piroxicam Study Experimental Design

Variable	Level		
	Low	Medium	High
Sodium lauryl sulfate	0%	0.5%	1.0%
Magnesium stearate	0.5%	1.0%	1.5%
Magnesium stearate blending time	2 min	10 min	18 min
Filler: percent lactose in binary mixtures with microcrystalline cellulose	0%	50%	100%
Percent milled (4.91 M^2 g) piroxicam in binary mixtures with unmilled (1.79 M^2 g) piroxicam	0%	50%	100%

Colloidal silica (glidant) and sodium starch glycolate (disintegrant) were fixed at 0.1% and 5%, respectively, in all batches.
Source: Redrawn from Ref. 125.

Dissolution profiles (percent piroxicam dissolved vs. time) were obtained using methods described in the USP XXIII monograph for piroxicam capsules. On the basis of the data analysis, the percent lactose and an interaction between piroxicam particle size and sodium lauryl sulfate level were the most important variables affecting the percent of piroxicam dissolved at 10 minutes. However, the predominant variable affecting the percent dissolved in 45 minutes was the wetting agent, sodium lauryl sulfate, which was followed closely by piroxicam particle size. The apparent reduced significance of the level of lactose at 45 minutes may be due to its complete dissolution by then. Interestingly, the magnesium stearate level and its blending time were either not significant or among the least significant factors affecting piroxicam dissolution. This observation can be largely explained by the ability of sodium lauryl sulfate to overcome the hydrophobicity of magnesium stearate. In addition, the water solubility of lactose and the disintegrant, sodium starch glycolate, may also help overcome any hydrophobic lubricant effects.

The plotting of response surfaces permits visualization of the effects of various levels of the independent variables. For example, the response surfaces in Figure 24 reveal that the ability of sodium lauryl sulfate to enhance the percent dissolved in 10 minutes is most apparent when piroxicam is unmilled. The sodium lauryl sulfate level has comparatively little effect on 10-minute dissolution when the drug is milled and presumably more rapidly dissolving because of its larger specific surface area.

All piroxicam batches were manufactured in compliance with Good Manufacturing Practices, and three formulation having *fast*, *moderate*, and *slow* dissolution were chosen for comparison to a lot of the innovator's product in a human bioavailability study (125). The resulting pharmacokinetic data provided still another opportunity to examine the effects of formulation variables. To explore the relationship between the in vitro

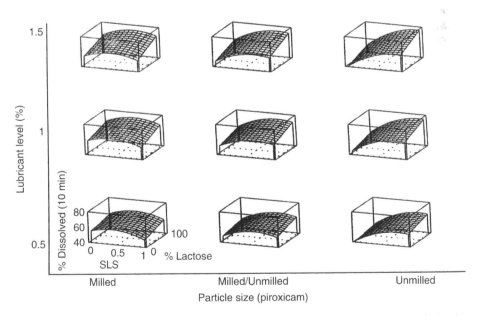

Figure 24 Response surfaces for the effect of formulation variables on percent of piroxicam dissolving from capsules in 10 minutes. *Source*: From Ref. 125.

Table 7 Apparent Permeability and Dissolution Rates for Piroxicam Capsules

Formulation	Apparent permeability rate constant, $k_p^1 \pm SE, hr^{-1}$	First-order dissolution rate constant, $k_d \pm SE, hr^{-1}$	$\alpha = \frac{k_p^1}{k_d}, \pm SE$
Fast (Q45^a = 95)	7.26 ± 1.12	8.10 ± 0.60	0.896 ± 0.138
Moderate (Q45 = 87)	7.17 ± 1.10	4.66 ± 0.10	1.54 ± 0.24
Innovator (Q45 = 80)	10.7 ± 2.6	3.13 ± 0.20	3.42 ± 0.84
Slow (Q45 = 65)	11.3 ± 3.8	1.75 ± 0.05	6.50 ± 2.17
Mean	9.00 ± 1.14		

^{a}Percent of labeled content dissolving in 45 minutes.
Abbreviation: SE, standard error.
Source: From Refs. 125 and 127.

dissolution of piroxicam from these capsules and in vivo absorption, Polli (127) used the following previously described (174) deconvolution-based model.

$$F_a = \frac{1}{f_a}\left(1 - \frac{\alpha}{\alpha - 1}(1 - F_d) + \frac{1}{\alpha - 1}(1 - F_d)^\alpha\right) \qquad (4)$$

In this equation, F_a is the fraction of the dose of the drug absorbed in time t, and f_a is the fraction of the total amount of drug absorbed at $t = \infty$; α is the ratio of the apparent first-order permeation rate constant, k_p^1, to the first-order dissolution rate constant, k_d, and F_d is the fraction of the dose dissolved in time t. The model makes a number of assumptions: apparent first-order permeability, first-order dissolution under sink conditions, drug is stable in the gastrointestinal lumen or at the gastrointestinal wall, identicalness of in vitro and in vivo dissolution profiles, and the absence of a lag time for permeation or dissolution. Nevertheless, this model does provide some useful and interesting information. Of particular interest is the term α. If $\alpha \gg 1$, the permeation rate constant is much greater than the dissolution rate constant and drug absorption is expected to be dissolution rate limited. If $\alpha \ll 1$, the reverse is true, and the rate-limiting step to absorption is intestinal permeation. The values of α for the *slow*, *moderate*, and *fast* formulations and a lot of the *innovator* products are given in Table 7.

These results are consistent with a BCS class II drug showing dissolution rate–limited absorption. An examination of the data for the *slow*, *moderate*, and *innovator* formulations in Table 7 indicate that piroxicam absorption is generally dissolution rate limited (i.e., $\alpha > 1$). Indeed, for the *slow* formulation, $\alpha = 6.50$, indicating dissolution was about several-fold dominating over permeability in controlling overall piroxicam absorption. The data in Table 7 also point to the role of formulation. The *fast* capsule was formulated using the milled piroxicam, 1% sodium lauryl sulfate, and lactose, which promoted dissolution such that $k_d \cong k_p^1$. Indeed, because of *formulation design*, the *fast* product is slightly more permeability rate limited than dissolution rate limited (i.e., α is slightly less than 1), overcoming piroxicam's biopharmaceutic properties.

It is interesting that the in vitro dissolution test (USP) was more sensitive to the piroxicam formulation variables than the biodata. Despite their differences in dissolution rate, the *fast*, *moderate* and *slow* products were found bioequivalent to each other and to the lot of *Innovator* products studied (125). It is possible that the formulation variables studied either did not affect in vivo dissolution or the differences were not discernable because of the long biological half-life of piroxicam (175).

Artificial Intelligence Applications for Formulation Support

One form of artificial intelligence, called a knowledge-based system (KB) or expert system (ES), is a computer program that attempts to capture the expertise of specialists who have knowledge and experience in a well-defined domain (area). Such systems are designed to simulate the expert's problem-solving process. In rule-based systems, the knowledge is often represented as a set of rules that express the relationship between pieces of information in the form of conditional statements that specify actions to be taken or advice to be followed. As applied here, the user enters certain information about the properties of the drug (e.g., dose, solubility, particle size, flow properties, BCS classification) and any specific user requirements (e.g., preferred excipients, method of manufacture, capsule size), and the expert system returns a suggested formulation. Well-designed expert systems can shorten development time, result in simpler formulations, provide the rationale for the formulation design, serve as a teaching tool for novices, and accumulate and preserve the knowledge and experience of experts who may leave the laboratory through retirement, change of employer, or other reason. However, an ES can only deal with situations that have been anticipated and must, therefore, be designed to handle every contingency. One example is Capsugel's CAPEX® expert system, a centralized system that incorporates worldwide industrial experience and expertise in support of powder formulations for hard-shell capsules (171). The decision trees and production rules that make up this expert system were developed from three databases: historical data collected from published literature, knowledge acquired from industrial experts, and information developed through statistically designed laboratory experiments. Another example is a customized, in-house expert system for hard-shell capsule formulations that incorporates the policies and practices of the Sanofi Research Center that was developed by Bateman et al. (172).

A neural network (NN) is a computer program that attempts to simulate certain functions of the human brain, for example, learning or abstracting from experience and generalizing. In essence, NN programs are computational models. By the introduction of data, NNs are *trained* to recognize patterns in the data. Depending on the training data selected, pattern recognition models for specific domains (or fields), such as tablet formulation, granulation, and capsule formulation and others may be created. The training data may be newly developed in the laboratory on the basis of historical data. Such models make it possible for formulators to generalize for future cases or situations within certain limits, such as predicting drug dissolution from a hydrophilic matrix capsule system (170), predicting tablet hardness and friability (176), and modeling bimodal drug delivery (177) or other desired delivery system outcomes. One limitation of NN models is that their effectiveness is limited by the training data itself.

A hybrid of a NN with an expert system has been developed for capsule formulation support (178,179). The system was created with the objective of developing capsule formulations that would meet desired drug dissolution criteria for BCS class II (i.e., low solubility, high permeability) drugs. The hybrid system consists of three modules: a *decision module* (expert system), a *prediction module* (NN), and a *control module*. The *decision module* produces a proposed formula based on certain input data and user requirements. The *prediction module* predicts the dissolution performance of the proposed formula. The *control module*, driven by any difference there might be between the desired dissolution rate and the predicted dissolution rate of the proposed formula, controls the optimization of dissolution. In practice, the control module inputs the formula generated by the decision module to the prediction module, computes the predicted dissolution rate, and then requests the user's acceptance of the current formula based on that predicted dissolution performance. If the user finds the prediction acceptable, the control module terminates the formulation development process. But, if the predicted dissolution rate is not acceptable to the user, the control module will offer him or her a set of available parameter adjustments (e.g., excipient choices and levels) for improving the dissolution rate. This process can be iterated until a satisfactory formula is found or the user ends the optimization. The prototype hybrid system demonstrated good predictability for the model compound, piroxicam. On the basis of the success of this prototype, the system was modified by Wilson et al. to make it more generalized, and the generalized version was found to have good predictability for six different BCS class II drugs whose solubilities varied over a broad range (180). Wilson et al. later found that a Bayesian network (BN), another form of artificial intelligence that has the potential to help formulation development, could successfully model the cause-effect relationships between the variables used in the generalized expert network (181).

Capsules Filled with Liquids and Semisolid Matrices

Traditionally the domain of soft-gelatin capsules, today both soft- and hard-shell capsules may be filled with liquids or semisolid matrices. Perhaps the main reason soft-gelatin capsules became the historical standard for liquid-filled capsules was the inability to prevent leakage from hard-gelatin capsules. The advent of self-locking capsules, such sealing techniques as banding and liquid sealing, and the development of high resting state viscosity fills have made liquid/semisolid-filled hard-shell capsules a feasible dosage form today (182). Semisolid matrices generally consist of high proportions of solid material dispersed in a liquid phase. Often the solid is a waxy or fatty substance requiring that the formulation be filled into the capsule as a melt; in other instances, a liquid formulation may be thickened by the addition of an excipient such as colloidal silicon dioxide to form a thixotropic gel (183). Thixotropic gels exhibit shear thinning when agitated and thus are pumpable. Yet, when agitation stops, the system rapidly reestablishes a gel structure. Several significant technological and drug delivery advantages may be derived from liquid/semisolid-filled capsules (184–189).

Content Uniformity

In liquid/semisolid-filled capsules, the drug is a liquid or at least dissolved, solubilized, or suspended in a liquid, pumpable vehicle. The liquid fill is metered into individual capsules via high-precision pumps, thereby achieving a much higher degree of reproducibility than is possible with the powder or granule flow and feed required for the manufacture of tablets and dry filled capsules. Moreover, a higher degree of homogeneity is possible in liquid systems than can be achieved in powder blends. This latter point is especially important in dealing with potent, low-dose drugs that represent only a minor component of overall blends.

In powder-filled capsules and tablets, the precision blending of drugs and excipients and the prevention of their unblending during subsequent handling and operations are of paramount importance to achieving of acceptable content uniformity in the finished product. But the problems encountered in achieving that goal in powder blends could be substantial (190). There is the statistical sampling problem of assuring that each portion of the blend that is delivered to the capsule contains within allowable variation the desired amount of drug. This is a critical problem when the dose is so low that the active is effectively a very minor or trace component of the blend. Moreover, there are a number of technological problems that make difficult the attainment and maintenance of acceptable blend homogeneity (190). Particles of different size and density tend to segregate. Surface frictional and cohesive interactions can cause particles to aggregate and resist the differential movement of particles needed to achieve good mixing. Even the time of mixing in the blender is critical, and the optimum blend time needs to be determined. Blending for too long (i.e., overmixing) can cause some blends to demix in the blender due to differences in particle size, shape, or density or the agglomeration of cohesive active particles. In the most critical of low-dose cases, traditional blending may be abandoned, and the drug may be introduced by methods such as liquid addition, that is, spraying a solution of the drug onto fillers followed by drying. Another possible alternative described previously in the "Hydrophilization and Granulation" section is to carry out a wet granulation procedure in which the drug is dissolved in the binder solution.

These types of problems can be eliminated in liquid/semisolid-filled capsules where the drug substance may be dissolved or solubilized in the liquid vehicle. No dry blend of discrete particles can be truly homogenous, but a true solution, if formed, is a homogeneous molecular dispersion.

Drug Dissolution and Bioavailability

Another major problem faced by formulation scientists that can be addressed by liquid/semisolid matrix capsules is poor drug aqueous solubility, which can lead to variable and poor bioavailability. Formulating the drug substance in solution or solubilized form essentially eliminates dissolution of the solid as a rate-limiting step. Even when the drug cannot be solubilized, it could be delivered as a dispersion of micronized or nanometer-sized particles in a suitable vehicle that promotes rapid dispersion of capsule contents and dissolution. For example, Hom and Miskel (191,192) compared the in vitro dissolution rates of 20 drugs from soft-gelatin capsules and tablets. The drugs were either dissolved in PEG 400 or suspended in polyols or nonionic surfactants. In all cases, more rapid dissolution occurred from the capsules. Similarly, single-dose studies in human subjects comparing the sedative temazepam as a powder-filled hard-gelatin capsule and as a PEG solution in soft-gelatin capsules revealed higher and earlier peak plasma levels from the PEG formulation, although there was no significant difference in their total availabilities (193). In still another example, digoxin dissolved in a vehicle consisting of PEG 400, ethanol, propylene glycol, and water and filled in soft-gelatin capsules produced higher mean plasma levels in human subjects during the first seven hours after administration than either an aqueous solution or commercial tablets (194). The areas under the 14-hour plasma concentration curves were also greater for the soft-gelatin capsule compared with the solution or tablets.

Today, much interest is being focused on both hard- and soft-shell capsules as vehicles for lipid-based drug delivery systems (LBDDSs) designed to improve the dissolution and bioavailability of poorly soluble, hydrophobic drug substances. These systems deliver the drug essentially dissolved or solubilized in a lipid phase. Lipid-based systems can overcome the problems of poor aqueous drug solubility, but exactly how the absorption of poorly soluble, hydrophobic drug substances is enhanced by lipids is not fully understood (195).

LBDDSs are complex compositions of three main classes of components: lipids, surfactants, and cosolvants (196). The lipid component may be a single lipid or a blend of fatty materials. The most important lipids in this application are fatty acids or their derivatives (e.g., mono-, di- and triglycerides, propylene glycol esters). These can be either solid or liquid at room temperature, depending on such factors as their chain length and degree of unsaturation of the fatty acid chains. Lipid-based formulations frequently also include a surfactant (emulsifier) to assist in the breakup and dispersion of the capsule content in gastrointestinal fluids. Typically, these are nonionic surfactants (e.g., polyoxyl 40 stearate, polysorbate 80, and sorbitan monopalmitate) of varying hydrophilic-lipophilic balance (HLB). Lipid-based systems may also include cosolvants (e.g., alcohol, PEG 400, propylene glycol) if needed to help solubilize the drug substance. Self-emulsifying lipid-based systems are unique compositions of drug, lipid, emulsifier, and perhaps a small quantity of cosolvent that spontaneously emulsify in the presence of water with only gentle agitation, as may occur when delivered to the aqueous content of gastrointestinal tract where digestive motility provides the gentle agitation (196). These systems can form emulsions (particle size > about 0.15 μm) if the ratio of surfactant to lipid is < 1, and microemulsions (particle size < about 0.15 μm) if the ratio is > 1 (197). The efficiency of "self-emulsification" appears strongly correlated with the HLB of the surfactant, with HLB values of 12 to 15 generally considered to have good efficiency (198).

Solving Other Formulation Problems

Liquid/semisolid matrix–filled capsules of both types can provide a practical solution to the problems of formulating liquid material, materials with low melting point, and hygroscopic substances. Materials that are liquid under room temperatures may require the addition of substantial amounts of dry powder excipients to convert them to free-flowing powders. The sorption of moisture under ambient conditions may make hygroscopic, deliquescent solids sticky and poor flowing. These materials also often require the addition of substantial amounts of excipient powder to convert them to free-flowing materials suitable for dry solid dosage forms. Some low melting solids may soften and become sticky during tablet compression and stick to punch faces without the addition of excipients, a problem that is often difficult for formulators to resolve.

Smith et al. demonstrated that ibuprofen, which has a low melting point and is thermostable, could be successfully filled into hard-gelatin capsules as a melt using 10% or less of such excipients as AcDiSol, maize starch, arachis oil, stearic acid, beeswax, and others (199). These excipients afforded a wide range in dissolution performance depending on the excipient and its level of addition. The hydrophobic excipients like stearic acid slowed dissolution; whereas disintegrants increased the dissolution rate. Doelker et al. reported the successful filling of four liquid or deliquescent drugs (benzonatate, nicotinic acid, chloral hydrate, paramethadione) in hard-gelatin capsules using Gelucire® excipients (glycerides and other fatty acid esters available with different HLB values) as the vehicle or matrix (200). The drugs were incorporated in the melted vehicle before pouring into the capsules. Dissolution performance was comparable to the tested equivalent marketed as soft-gelatin products. Bowtle et al. developed a successful stable semisolid matrix hard-gelatin capsule product of the highly hygroscopic antibiotic vancomycin HCl by incorporating the drug in polyethylene glycol 6000 (201).

Many volatile drugs and drugs subject to atmospheric oxidation may also be formulated satisfactorily in liquid/semisolid-filled capsules. Soft-gelatin capsules are hermetically sealed as a natural consequence of the manufacturing process. Hom et al. (202) have shown that the soft-gelatin shell can be an effective barrier to oxygen. As discussed earlier in this chapter, when sealed, hard-gelatin capsules also are effective barriers to oxygen. Richardson and Stegemann compared freeze etchings of soft-gelatin and hard-gelatin shells taken from a scanning electron microscope (186). They suggested that the larger channels they found in the soft-gelatin shell (apparently created by the plasticizer) may expose contents to more oxygen.

Handling in Manufacture

The reduced dustiness and lack of a compression stage in manufacture of liquid and semisolid formulations decreases the risk of cross contamination in manufacturing areas and possible exposure of technicians to toxic drugs.

Soft-shell capsules (3,203,204)

Soft-gelatin capsules are available in a wide variety of sizes and shapes suitable for oral, rectal, and vaginal administration. Specialty capsules in tube form (e.g., ophthalmics, ointments) or bead form (various cosmetics) may also be produced.

Shell composition (3) Like hard-gelatin shells, the basic component of soft-gelatin shells is gelatin; however, the shell has been plasticized, by the addition, most usually, of glycerin or sorbitol, and sometimes, combinations of these. Other components may include dyes, opacifiers, preservatives, and flavors. The ratio of dry plasticizer to dry gelatin determines the "hardness" of the shell and can vary from 0.3 to 1.0 for a very hard shell to 1.0 to 1.8 for a very soft shell. Lower ratios in the range of about 0.3 to 0.5 are generally used when capsules are to be filled with oily vehicles; intermediate ranges of about 0.4 to 0.6 for oily vehicles that include a surfactant, and still higher ratios of about 0.6 to 1.0 are used when fully water-miscible vehicles are used. Up to 5% sugar may be included to give a "chewable" quality to the shell. The basic gelatin formulation from which the plasticized films are cast most usually consists of one part gelatin, one part water, and 0.4 to 0.6 part plasticizer. The typical residual shell moisture content of finished capsules will be in the range of 6% to 10%.

Formulation (3,205) Soft-shell capsule formulations generally involve liquid rather than powder technology. Materials are generally formulated to produce the smallest possible capsule consistent with maximum stability, therapeutic effectiveness, and manufacture efficiency (3).

Soft-shell capsules may contain a single liquid, a combination of miscible liquids, a solution of a drug in a liquid, or a suspension of a drug in a liquid. Liquids are limited to those that do not have an adverse effect on the gelatin walls. The pH of the liquid can be between 2.5 and 7.5. Liquids with more acid pH would tend to cause leakage by hydrolysis of the gelatin. Liquids with pH > 7.5 and aldehydes decrease shell solubility by tanning (cross-linking) the gelatin. Aqueous emulsions cannot be filled because inevitably water will be released, which will affect the shell. Bauer and Dortunc (206) have proposed nonaqueous emulsions for both soft- and hard-shell capsules. In general, the emulsions were composed of a hydrophilic liquid such as PEG 400 and a triglyceride oil as the lipophilic liquid. Other liquids that cannot be encapsulated include water (>5% of contents) and low molecular weight alcohols such as ethyl alcohol, which diffuse readily through conventional soft-gelatin capsule shell walls. Modification of the shell composition may help retain low molecular weight volatile compounds. Working with soft-gelatin films, Moreton and Armstrong found that the rate of diffusion of ethanol through soft-gelatin films could be significantly reduced by replacing the glycerin plasticizer with the higher polyols such as xylitol, sorbitol, and lycasin (hydrogenated corn syrup) (207).

Traditionally, the types of vehicles used in soft-gelatin capsules have fallen into two main groups:

1. Water immiscible, volatile or more likely nonvolatile liquids such as vegetable oils, aromatic and aliphatic hydrocarbons (mineral oil), medium-chain triglycerides and acetylated glycerides.
2. Water miscible – nonvolatile liquids such as low molecular weight PEG (PEG 400 and 600) that are hydrophilic and readily mix with water and accelerate dissolution of dissolved or suspended drugs.

Glycerin and propylene glycol can be encapsulated, but only at low concentrations (5–10%), because of the tendency of these substances to migrate into and soften the shell.

Suspensions are formed when drug substances cannot be dissolved in the vehicle. It is a common practice to micronize (colloid mill) all materials during the preparation of a suspension and to include suspending agents to prevent sedimentation and promote homogeneity. The suspending agent depends on the type of vehicle. Typical suspending agents for group 1 oily bases and their concentration as a percentage of base are beeswax (5%), paraffin wax (5%), animal stearates (1–6%). Suspending agents for nonoily group 2 bases include carbowaxes such as PEG 4000 and 6000 (1–5%), solid nonionics (10%), or solid glycol esters (10%).

Historically, the group 1 vehicles, particularly vegetable oils and medium-chain triglycerides, were common in soft-gelatin capsules. Vehicles of the class 2 type, especially PEG 400 and 600, have become popular in more recent years as a means of addressing the bioavailability problems of poorly soluble drugs. Most recently, a substantial interest in delivering complex lipid-based delivery systems in capsules has developed that is aimed at improving the dissolution and bioavailability of poorly soluble, hydrophobic drugs.

In general, all liquids used for filling must flow by gravity at a temperature of 35°C or less. The sealing temperature of gelatin films is 37°C to 40°C.

Compatibility and Stability Concerns

There is a more intimate contact between the shell and its liquid contents than exists with dry-filled hard-gelatin capsules, which increases the possibility of interactions. For instance, chloral hydrate formulated with an oily vehicle exerts a proteolytic effect on the gelatin shell; however, the effect is greatly reduced when the oily vehicle is replaced with PEG (3). A number of excipients used in soft-gelatin capsules, such as plasticizers, PEGs, polysorbates, and others, are known to undergo auto oxidation to form higher molecular weight aldehydes, which can lead to loss of gelatin aqueous solubility through cross-linking (45). The migration of formaldehyde from the polyethylene glycol fill of soft-gelatin capsules into shells has been studied by near-infrared (NIR) spectrophotometry (208).

Drugs can migrate from an oily vehicle into the shell, and this has been related to their water solubility and their partition coefficient between water and the nonpolar solvent (209). Studying 4-hydroxybenzoic acid as an encapsulated solution, Armstrong et al. found that most transfer to the shell occurred during drying subsequent to manufacture; however, after completion of drying, only a combined 89% of the original amount of solute could be found in the shell and contents (207). It was thus considered that some of the solute may migrate to the outer shell surface where it can be lost by erosion or washing (207).

The possible migration of a drug into the shell must be considered in the packaging of topical products in soft-gelatin tubelike capsules as this could affect drug concentration in the ointment, etc., as applied (3). For other products such as oral capsules or suppository capsules, both the shell and the contents must be considered in judging drug content when migration occurs. It is interesting that drug in the shell may provide for an initial dissolution of drug prior to shell rupture. In one study, when shell migration was negligible, there was a definite lag time in drug dissolution from encapsulated oily solution, indicating that rupture of the shell had to occur before solute release (207). The larger the proportion of drug in the shell, the more overall drug release was dependent on the dissolution of the shell.

One physical parameter of finished capsules measured in stability studies is "softness." Whereas this parameter traditionally has been measured subjectively, Vemuri (210) has reported the objective measurement of this property by compression of individual capsules between the platens of a physical testing machine.

Manufacture (3,203)

Several different processes may be used to manufacture soft-gelatin capsules.

Plate process The oldest commercial process, this semiautomatic, batch process has been supplanted by more modern, continuous processes. Equipment for the plate process is no longer available. In general, the process involved (*i*) placing the upper half of a plasticized gelatin sheet over a die plate containing numerous die pockets, (*ii*) application of vacuum to draw the sheet into the die pockets, (*iii*) filling the pockets with liquid or paste, (*iv*) folding the lower half of the gelatin sheet back over the filled pockets, and (*v*) inserting the "sandwich" under a die press where the capsules are formed and cut out.

Rotary die process The first continuous process is the rotary die process, which was invented in 1933 by R.P. Scherer. Apart from its being a continuous process, the rotary die process reduced manufacturing losses to a negligible level and content variation to ± 1% to ±3% range, both major problems with earlier processes. In this process, the die cavities are machined into the outer surfaces of two rollers (i.e., die rolls). The die pockets on the left-hand roller form the left side of the capsule; the die pockets on the right-hand roller form the right side of the die capsule. The die pockets on the two rollers match as the rollers rotate. Two plasticized gelatin ribbons (prepared in the machine) are continuously and simultaneously fed with the liquid or paste fill between the rollers of the rotary die mechanism. The forceful injection of the feed material between the two ribbons causes the gelatin to swell into the left- and right-hand die pockets as they converge. As the die rolls rotate, the convergence of the matching die pockets seals and cuts out the filled capsules. The process is illustrated in Figure 25 and an actual machine is pictured in Figure 26.

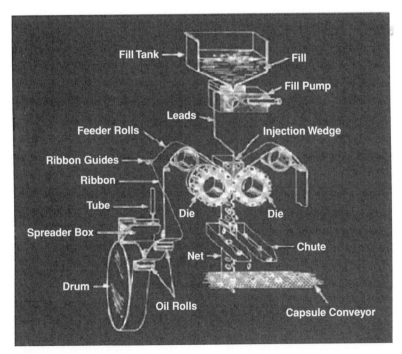

Figure 25 Illustration of the rotary die process. (Courtesy of Scherer, RP North America, Clearwater, FL.)

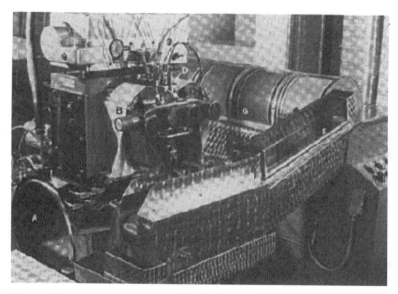

Figure 26 Rotary die machine. (**A**) Ribbon casting drum; (**B**) ribbon; (**C**) filling leads; (**D**) injection mechanism; (**E**) rotary die; (**F**) capsule wash; (**G**) infrared dryer. (Courtesy of Scherer, RP North America, Clearwater, FL.)

Accogel process A continuous process for the manufacture of soft-gelatin capsules filled with powders or granules was developed by Lederle Laboratories in 1949. In general, this is another rotary process involving (*i*) a measuring roll, (*ii*) a die roll, and (*iii*) a sealing roll. The measuring roll rotates directly over the die roll, and the pockets in the two rolls are aligned with each other. The powder or granular fill material is held in the pockets of the measuring roll under vacuum. A plasticized sheet is drawn into the die pockets of the die roll under vacuum. As the measuring roll and die rolls rotate, the measured doses are transferred to the gelatin-lined pockets of the die roll. The continued rotation of the filled die converges with the rotating sealing roll where a second gelatin sheet is applied to form the other half of the capsule. Pressure developed between the die roll and sealing roll seals and cuts out the capsules.

Bubble method Truly seamless, one-piece soft-gelatin capsules can be made by a "bubble method" (202). A concentric tube dispenser simultaneously discharges the molten gelatin from the outer annulus and the liquid content from the inner tube. The liquids are discharged into chilled oil as droplets that consist of a liquid medicament core within a molten gelatin envelop. The droplets assume a spherical shape under surface tension forces, and the gelatin congeals on cooling. The finished capsules then must be degreased and dried.

Frequently, soft-gelatin capsule manufacture is contracted out to a limited number of firms having the necessary filling equipment and expertise.

Hard-Shell Capsules

Most hard-shell-filling machine manufacturers have developed models capable of filling liquids and semisolids; this technology can be brought in-house, thus avoiding the necessity of having to contract the work outside to a specialty house (182).

The formulation of liquid/semisolid matrices for hard-shell capsules has been discussed (211). Generally, the fill material must be pumpable. A high resting state viscosity is not an absolute formulation prerequisite if capsules are banded and the contents have a viscosity of about 100 cP to prevent leakage from the mechanically interlocked capsules prior to banding. Powdered drugs may be dissolved or suspended in thixotropic or thermal setting systems.

As with soft-gelatin capsules, any materials filled into hard capsules must not dissolve, alter, or otherwise adversely affect the integrity of the shell. The materials that may be used as carriers for the drug cover a wide range of chemical classes and melting points. These include vegetable oils, hydrogenated vegetable oils, various fats such as carnauba wax and cocoa butter, and PEGs (molecular weights 200–20,000), and others. In general, the more lipophilic the contents, the slower the release rate; thus, by selecting excipients with varying HLB, it may be possible to achieve varying release rates (211).

The more hygroscopic lower molecular weight grades of PEG, for example, PEGs 400 and 600, may exhibit compatibility problems with hard-gelatin shells: lower molecular weight PEGs are more suitable for soft-gelatin capsules because of the presence of the plasticizer in the shell wall (212). Qualicaps has developed a grade of gelatin capsules made from gelatin and PEG 4000 for use with hygroscopic formulations or moisture-sensitive ingredients (6).

Like soft-gelatin capsules, the development of aldehydes in PEG by auto oxidation that can lead to gelatin cross-linking, loss of capsule aqueous solubility, and reduced in vitro dissolution rate in the absence of enzymes is a concern. In some formulations, PEG may be adequately stabilized by adding butylated hydroxyanisole (BHA) and water to the fill composition. Stein and Bindra added BHA and water to fill compositions consisting of "compound A" and some higher molecular weight PEGs and found good dissolution stability compared with unstabilized formulations after three months storage under stress conditions of 40°C (75% relative humidity) and 50°C (humidity not controlled) for the PEG 1450-3350 matrix (213). However, the use of HPMC shells is another alternative for developing dissolution-stable PEG formulations. The dissolution of similarly stressed formulations in HPMC shells was stable and the HPMC shells exhibited less tendency to deform during filling with the hot melt (213). The HPMC capsule formulations exhibited slower initial dissolution than gelatin, attributed to slower disintegration of the shell, but complete dissolution (defined as >95%) was reached within 30 minutes (213).

Barak found that the insoluble nonsteroidal anti-inflammatory agent (NSAID), etodolac could be satisfactorily formulated in hard-gelatin capsules as a melt dispersion using lipid-based carriers with solubilizing properties (214). The drug was dispersed in Gelucire® 44/14 (mixture of saturated polyglycolized glycerides with an HLB value of 14), TPGS® (water-soluble derivative of vitamin E having an HLB value of 13.2), or a mixture of these. In all cases, the dissolution rate from these systems was dramatically faster than that of the pure drug. Under ambient (25°C/60% relative humidity) and stress storage (40°C/75% relative humidity) conditions for six months, etodolac was found chemically stable in the formulations, but dissolution slowed (but was still substantially faster than pure drug), possibly due to the formation of etodolac microcrystals and absorption of water by the carrier vehicles. It was concluded that shelf life should be acceptable if moisture-resistant packaging is used (214). Shen and Zong found the bioavailability in beagle dogs of water-insoluble atorvastatin to be significantly increased when administered as a self-microemulsifying lipid-based mixture in Licaps® (starch hydrolysate) hard-shell capsules (198).

For thixotropic systems, the liquid excipient is often thickened with colloidal silicas. In one example (211), the liquid active clofibrate was formulated as a thermal-setting system by adding 30% (on the basis of total weight) PEG 20,000. In another example (211), vitamin E was filled as a thixotropic system by adding approximately 6% each (on the basis of total weight) beeswax and fumed silicon dioxide.

FURTHER READING

Podczeck F, Jones BE, eds.Pharmaceutical Capsules. 2nd ed. London: The Pharmaceutical Press, 2004.

REFERENCES

1. Delaney R. Surveying consumer preferences. Pharm Exec 1982; 2(3):34.
2. Jones BE, Turner TD. A century of commercial hard gelatin capsules. Pharm J 1974; 213:614–617.
3. Stanley JP. Capsules II. Soft gelatin capsules. In: Lachman L, Leiberman HA, Kanig JL, eds. The Theory and Practice of Industrial Pharmacy. 2nd ed. Philadelphia: Lea & Febiger, 1976: 404–420.
4. Eith L, Stepto RFT, Wittwer F, et al. Injection-moulded drug-delivery systems. Manuf Chem 1987; 58(1):21.
5. Watts P, Smith A. TARGIT™ technology: coated starch capsules for site-specific drug delivery into the lower gastrointestinal tract. Expert Opin Drug Deliv 2005; 2(1):159–167.
6. Chiwele I, Jones BE, Podczeck F. The shell dissolution of various empty hard capsules. Chem Pharm Bull (Tokyo) 2000; 48(7):951–956.
7. Cole ET, Scott RA, Cade D, et al. In vitro and in vivo pharmacoscintigraphic evaluation of ibuprofen hypromellose and gelatin capsules. Pharm Res 2004; 21(5):793–798.
8. Brochure. Advanced softgel solutions to pharmaceutical formulation challenges, Catalent Pharma Solutions. Available at: http://www.catalent.com/drug/oral/vegicaps.pdf. Accessed January 23, 2008.
9. Brochure. VegaGels® Technical Information. Available at: http://www.swisscaps.com/downloads/VegaGels_Broschuere_2005.pdf. Accessed January 23, 2008.
10. Mortada LM, Ismail FA, Khalil SA. Correlation of urinary excretion with in vitro dissolution using four dissolution methods for ampicillin capsules. Drug Dev Ind Pharm 1985; 11:101–130.
11. Arnold K, Gerber N, Levy G. Absorption and dissolution studies on sodium diphenylhydantoin capsules. Can J Pharm Sci 1970; 5(4):89–92.
12. Aguiar AJ, Wheeler LM, Fusari S, et al. Evaluation of physical and pharmaceutical factors involved in drug release and availability from chloramphenicol capsules. J Pharm Sci 1968; 57:1844–1850.
13. Glazco AJ, Kinkel AW, Alegnani WC, et al. An evaluation of the absorption characteristics of different chloramphenicol preparations in normal human subjects. Clin Pharmacol Ther 1968; 9: 472–474.
14. Innercap—Multi Phase Capsules. Available at: http://www.innercap.com/index.cfm?fuseaction =site.multiphase. Accessed January 23, 2008.
15. Jones BE. Hard, two-piece capsules and pulmonary drug delivery. Pharm Form and Quality 2004; 6(5):52–53.
16. Jones BE. Quali-V-I: a new key for dry powder inhalers. Drug Deliv Technol 2003; 3(6):52–57.
17. Chavan V, Dalby R. Effect of rise in simulated inspiratory flow rate and carrier particle size on powder emptying from dry powder inhalers. AAPS PharmSci 2(2): article 10.
18. Brochure. Introducing the New Xelodose®S. Capsugel Div. Pfizer, Inc. Available at: http://www.capsugel.com – Xcelodose S brochure.pdf. Accessed December 10, 2007.
19. A study of physician attitudes toward capsules and other pharmaceutical product norms. Elanco Products Co., Div. Eli Lilly & Co., Indianapolis, Indiana, 1971, El-0004.
20. Marvola M. Adherence of drug products to the oesophagus. Pharmacy Int 1982; 3:294–296.

21. Hey H, Jorgensen F, Hasselbach H, et al. Oesophageal transit of six commonly used tablets and capsules. Br Med J 1982; 285(11):1717–1719.

22. Channer KS, Virjee J. Effect of posture and drink volume on the swallowing of capsules. Br Med J 1982; 285(11):1702.

23. Evans T, Roberts GM. Where do all the tablets go? Lancet 1976; 2(Oct.-Dec.):1237–1239.

24. Fell JT. Esophageal transit of tablets and capsules. Am J Hosp Pharm 1983; 40:946–948.

25. Ponchel G, Degobert G. Capsules dures d'hydroxypropyl méthylcellulose: une alternative à la gélatine, étude comparative de leur adhésivité. STP Pharma Practiques 1999; 9:12–17.

26. Honkanen O, Laaksonen P, Marvola J, et al. Bioavailability and in vitro oesophageal sticking tendency of hydroxypropyl methylcellulose capsule formulations and corresponding gelatine capsule formulations. Eur J Pharm Sci 2002; 15:479–488.

27. Martyn GW Jr. Production history of hard gelatin capsules from molding through filling. Presented at Symposium on Modern Capsule Manufacturing, Society of Manufacturing Engineers, Philadelphia, Pennsylvania, January 31, 1978.

28. Jones BE. The manufacture of hard gelatin capsules. Chem Eng (London) 1982; 380:174–177.

29. Lappas LC. The manufacture of hard gelatin capsules.Presented to Research and Development Section, The American Drug Manufacturers Association, Atlantic City, New Jersey, October 8, 1954.

30. Jones BE. Hard gelatin capsules and the pharmaceutical formulator. Pharm Technol 1985; 9(9):106–108, 110, 112.

31. Buckalew LW, Coffield KE. An investigation of drug expectancy as a function of capsule color and size and preparation form. J Clin Psychopharmacol 1982; 2:245–248.

32. General worldwide specifications for Capsugel hard gelatin capsules. Revised November 29, 1999. Bulletin BAS-203-E. Capsugel, Div. Pfizer, Inc., Greenwood, South Carolina, 1999.

33. Coni-Snap®—the hard gelatin capsule with the advantages that matter. Bulletin BAS-112-E, USA. Capsugel, Div. Pfizer, Inc., Greenwood, South Carolina, 1982.

34. Shah R, Augsburger LL. Oxygen permeation in banded and non-banded hard gelatin capsules (abstr). Pharm Res 1989; 6:S–55.

35. Wittwer F. New developments in hermetic sealing of hard gelatin capsules. Pharm Manuf 1985; 2(6):24–29.

36. Scott D, Shah R, Augsburger LL. A comparative evaluation of the mechanical strength of sealed and unsealed hard gelatin capsules. Int J Pharm 1992; 84:49–58.

37. Murthy KS, Ghebre-Sellassie I. Current perspectives on the dissolution stability of solid oral dosage forms. J Pharm Sci 1993; 82:113–126.

38. Ito K, Kaga S-I, Takeya Y. Studies on hard gelatin capsules I. Water vapor transfer between capsules and powders. Chem Pharm Bull 1969; 17:1134–1137.

39. Strickland WA Jr, Moss M. Water vapor sorption and diffusion through hard gelatin capsules. J Pharm Sci 1962; 51:1002–1005.

40. Anon. Incompatibilities in prescriptions IV. The use of inert powders in capsules to prevent liquefaction due to deliquescence. J Am Pharm Assoc Sci Ed 1940; 29:136.

41. Bell JH, Stevenson NA, Taylor JE. A moisture transfer effect in hard gelatin capsules of sodium cromoglycate. J Pharm Pharmacol 1973; 25(suppl):96P–103P.

42. Kontny MJ, Mulski CA. Gelatin capsule brittleness as a function of relative humidity at room temperature. Int J Pharm 1989; 54:79–85.

43. Zografi G, Grandolfi GP, Kontny MJ, et al. Prediction of moisture transfer in mixtures of solids: transfer via the vapor phase. Int J Pharm 1988; 42:77–88.

44. Schwier JR, Cooke GG, Hartauer KJ, et al. Rayon: a source of furfural—a reactive aldehyde capable of insolubilizing gelatin capsules. Pharm Technol 1993; 17(5):78–79.

45. Digenis GA, Gold TB, Shah VP, et al. Cross-linking of gelatin capsules and its relevance to their in vivo-in vitro performance. J Pharm Sci 1994; 83(7):915–921.

46. Murthy KS, Enders NA, Fawzi MB. Dissolution stability of hard-shell products. Part I: the effect of exaggerated storage conditions. Pharm Technol 1989; 13(3):72–86.

47. Murthy KS, Reisch RG Jr., Fawzi MB. Dissolution stability of hard-shell capsule products. Part II: the effect of dissolution test conditions on in vitro drug release. Pharm Technol 1989; 13(6):53–58.

48. Mohamad H, Renoux R, Aiache S, et al. Etude de la stabilite biopharmaceutique des medicaments application a des gelules de chlorohydrate de tetracycline I. Etude in vitro. STP Pharma 1986; 2(17):531–535.

49. Marks EM, Tourtellotte D, Andus A. The phenomenon of gelatin insolubility. Food Technol 1968; 22:1433–1436.

50. Dahl T, Sue ILT, Yum A. The effect of pancreatin on the dissolution performance of gelatin-coated tablets exposed to high-humidity conditions. Pharm Res 1991; 8:412–414.

51. Mohamad H, Aiche J-M, Renoux R, et al. Etude de la stabilite biopharmaceutique des medicaments application a des gelules de chlorohydrate de tetracycline. IV. Etude complimentaire in vivo. STP Pharma 1986; 3(5):407–411.

52. Aikman M, Augsburger L, Berry I, et al. Collaborative development of two-tiered dissolution testing for gelatin capsules and gelatin-coated tablets using enzyme-containing media. Pharmacop Forum 1998; 24(5):7045–7050.

53. Jones BE. Quali-V® Hard Capsules—A New Tool for the Formulator. The Drug Delivery Companies Report. Autumn/Winter 2003, pp. 56–59. Available at: http://www.drugdeliveryreport.com/articles/ddcr_w2003_article10.pdf. Accessed February 12, 2008.

54. Brochure. Vcaps-Pharma. Available at: http://www.capsugel.com/pdf/Vcaps-Pharma-Brochure.pdf. Accessed February 12, 2008.

55. Nagata S. Advantages to HPMC capsules: a new generation's hard capsule. Drug Deliv Technol 2002; 2(2):34–39.

56. Nagata S. Cellulose capsules—an alternative to gelatin. In: Chiellini E, Sunamoto J, Migliaresi C, et al., eds. Biomedical Polymers and Polymer Therapeutics. New York: Kluer Academic/Plenum Publishers, 2001:53–62.

57. Jones BE. Evolution of the technology for filling two-piece hard capsules with powders. Tablets & Capsules 2006; 4(1):10–20.

58. Cole G. Capsule filling. Chem Eng (London) 1982; 382:473–473.

59. Augsburger LL. Powdered dosage forms. In: Dittert LW, ed., Sprowl's American Pharmacy. 7th ed. Philadelphia, Pennsylvania: JB Lippincott, 1974:301-343.

60. Clement H, Marquart HG. The Mechanical Processing of Hard Gelatin Capsules. News Sheet 3/70, Capsugel, A.G., CH-4000, Basel, Switzerland.

61. Ridgway K, Callow JAB. Capsule-filling machinery. Pharm J 1973; 212:281–285.

62. Anon. A look at capsules. Manuf Chem Aerosol News 1977; 48(7):26.

63. Hostetler V, Bellard JQ. Capsules I. Hard capsules. In: Lachman L, Lieberman HA, Kanig JL, eds. The Theory and Practice of Industrial Pharmacy. 2nd ed. Philadelphia, PA: Lea & Febiger, 1976:389-404.

64. Ito K, Kaga S-I, Takeya Y. Studies on hard gelatin capsules II. The capsule filling of powders and effects of glidant by ring filling machine-method. Chem Pharm Bull 1969; 17:1138–1145.

65. Reier G, Cohn R, Rock S, et al. Evaluation of factors affecting the encapsulation of powders in hard gelatin capsules I. Semi-automatic capsule machines. J Pharm Sci 1968; 57:660–666.

66. Kurihara K, Ichikawa I. Effect of powder flowability on capsule filling weight variation. Chem Pharm Bull 1978; 26:1250–1256.

67. Osaka R-180 Brochure, Osaka Automatic Machine Mfg Co., Osaka 591, Japan.

68. Heda P. A *Comparative Study of the Formulation Requirements of Dosator and Dosing Disc Encapsulators. Simulation of Plug Formation, and Creation of Rules for an Expert System for Formulation Design* [dissertation]. Baltimore, MD: University of Maryland; 1998.

69. GKF, Filling and Sealing Machine for Hard Gelatin Capsules, Hofliger + Karg, Brochure HK/GKF/4/82-2E, Robert Bosch Corp., Packaging Machinery Div., So. Plainfield, New Jersey.

70. Shah KB, Augsburger LL, Small LE, et al. Instrumentation of a dosing disc automatic capsule filling machine. Pharm Technol 1983; 7(4):42–54.

71. Wells JI. Pharmaceutical Preformulation: The Physicochemical Properties of Drug Substances. Chichester, England: Ellis Horwood Ltd, 1988:209–210.

72. Small LE, Augsburger LL. Instrumentation of an automatic capsule filling machine. J Pharm Sci 1977; 66:504–509.

73. Stoyle LE Jr. Evaluation of the zanasi automatic capsule machine. Proceedings of the Industrial Pharmacy Section, A.Ph.A. Presented at the 113th Annual Meeting, Dallas, Texas, April, 1966.

74. Macofar Mod. MT 13-1 and 13-2 Brochure, Macofar s.a.s., Bologna, Italy.

75. Irwin GM, Dodson GJ, Ravin LJ. Encapsulation of clomacron phosphate I. Effect of flowability of powder blends, lot-to-lot variability, and concentration of active ingredient on weight variation of capsules filled on an automatic capsule filling machine. J Pharm Sci 1970; 59: 547–550.

76. Chowhan ZT, Chow YP. Powder flow studies I. Powder consolidation ratio and its relationship to capsule-filling weight variation. Int J Pharm 1980; 4:317–326.

77. Miyake Y, Shimoda A, Jasu T, et al. Packing properties of pharmaceutical powders into hard gelatin capsules. Yakuzaigaku 1974; 34:32–37.

78. Jolliffe IG, Newton JM, Walters JK. Theoretical considerations of the filling of pharmaceutical hard gelatine capsules. Powder Technol 1980; 27:189–195.

79. Jolliffe IG, Newton JM. Practical implications of theoretical consideration of capsule filling by the dosator nozzle system. J Pharm Pharmacol 1982; 34:293–298.

80. Chopra R, Podczeck F, Newton JM, et al. The influence of pellet shape and film coating on the filling of pellets into hard shell capsules. Eur J Pharm Biopharm 2002; 53:327–333.

81. Schwartz JB. The instrumented tablet press: uses in research and production. Pharm Technol 1981; 5(9):102–132.

82. Marshall K. Instrumentation of tablet and capsule filling machines. Pharm Technol 1983; 7(3): 68–82.

83. Augsburger LL. Instrumented capsule filling machines: development and application. Pharm Technol 1982; 6(9):111–112, 114, 117–119.

84. Cole GC, May G. Instrumentation of a hard shell encapsulation machine. J Pharm Pharmacol 1972; 24(suppl):122P.

85. Cole GC, May G. The instrumentation of a zanasi LZ/64 capsule filling machine. J Pharm Pharmacol 1975; 27:353–358.

86. Small LE, Augsburger LL. Aspects of the lubrication requirements for an automatic capsule-filling machine. Drug Dev Ind Pharm 1978; 4:345–372.

87. Mehta AM, Augsburger LL. Simultaneous measurement of force and displacement in an automatic capsule filling machine. Int J Pharm 1980; 4:347–351.

88. Mehta AM, Augsburger LL. Quantitative evaluation of force displacement curves in an automatic capsule filling machine. Presented to the IPT Section, A.Ph.A. Academy of Pharmaceutical Sciences, 128th Annual A.Ph.A. Meeting, St. Louis, Missouri, March-April, 1981.

89. Greenberg R. Effects of AZ-60 filling machine dosator settings upon slug hardness and dissolution of capsules. Proceedings of the 88th National Meeting. Am Inst Chem Engrs, Session 11, Philadelphia, Pennsylvasnia, June 8-12, 1980 (Fiche 29).

90. Botzolakis JE. *Studies on the Mechanism of Disintegrant Action in Encapsulated Dosage Forms* [PhD dissertation]. Baltimore, MD: University of Maryland, 1985.

91. Mony C, Sambeat C, Cousin G. Interet des measures de pression dans la formulation et le remplissage des gelules. Newsheet, 1977. Capsugel A.G., Basel, Switzerland.

92. Rowley DJ, Hendry R, Ward MD, et al. The instrumentation of an automatic capsule filling machine for formulation design studies. Presented at 3rd International Conference on Powder Technology, Paris, 1983.

93. Shah KB, Augsburger LL, Marshall K. An investigation of some factors influencing plug formation and fill weight in a dosing disk-type automatic capsule-filling machine. J Pharm Sci 1986; 75:291–296.

94. Shah KB, Augsburger LL, Marshall K. Multiple tamping effects on drug dissolution from capsules filled on a dosing-disk type automatic capsule filling machine. J Pharm Sci 1987; 76: 639–645.

95. Cropp JW, Augsburger LL, Marshall K. Simultaneous monitoring of tamping force and piston displacement (F-D) on an Hofliger-Karg capsule filling machine. Int J Pharm 1991; 71:127–136.

96. Podczeck F. The development of an instrumented tamp-filling capsule machine: I. instrumentation of a Bosch GKF 400S machine. Eur J Pharm Sci 2000; 10:267–274.
97. Podczeck F. The development of an instrumented tamp-filling capsule machine: II. Investigations of plug development and tamping pressure at different filling stations. Eur J Pharm Sci 2001; 12:515–521.
98. Mehta AM, Augsburger LL. A preliminary study of the effect of slug hardness on drug dissolution from hard gelatin capsules filled on an automatic capsule filling machine. Int J Pharm 1981; 7:327–334.
99. Heda PK, Muller FX, Augsburger LL. Capsule filling machine simulation I: low force compression physics relevant to plug formation. Pharm Dev Technol 1999; 4(2):209–219.
100. Celik M, Marshall K. Use of a compaction simulator system in tablet research. Drug Dev Ind Pharm 1989; 15:758–800.
101. Stewart AG, Grant DJW, Newton JM. The release of a model low-dose drug (riboflavine) from hard gelatin capsule formulations. J Pharm Pharmacol 1979; 31:1–6.
102. Veski P, Marvola M. Design and use of equipment for simulation of plug formation in hard gelatin capsule filling machines. Acta Pharm Fennica 1991; 100:19–25.
103. Jolliffe IG, Newton JM, Cooper D. The design and use of an instrumented MG2 capsule filling machine simulator. J Pharm Pharmacol 1982; 34:230–235.
104. Jolliffe IG, Newton JM. An investigation of the relationship between particle size and compression during capsule filling with an instrumented MG2 simulator. J Pharm Pharmacol 1982; 34:415–419.
105. Jolliffe IG, Newton JM. The effect of dosator nozzle wall texture on capsule filling with the MG2 simulator. J Pharm Pharmacol 1983; 35:7–11.
106. Tan SB, Newton JM. Powder flowability as an indication of capsule filling performance. Int J Pharm 1990; 61:145–155.
107. Tan SB, Newton JM. Influence of capsule dosator wall texture and powder properties on the angle of wall friction and powder-wall adhesion. Int J Pharm 1990; 64:227–234.
108. Tan SB, Newton JM. Capsule filling performance of powders with dosator nozzles of different wall texture. Int J Pharm 1990; 66:207–211.
109. Tan SB, Newton JM. Minimum compression stress requirements for arching and powder retention within a dosator nozzle during capsule filling. Int J Pharm 1990; 63:275–280.
110. Tan SB, Newton JM. Influence of compression setting ratio on capsule fill weight and weight variability. Int J Pharm 1990; 66:273–282.
111. Tan SB, Newton JM. Observed and expected powder plug densities obtained by a capsule dosator nozzle system. Int J Pharm 1990; 66:283–288.
112. Britten JR, Barnett MI. Development and validation of a capsule filling machine simulator. Int J Pharm 1991; 71: R5–R8.
113. Britten JR, Barnett MI, Armstrong NA. Construction of an intermittent-motion capsule filling machine simulator. Pharm Res 1995; 12:196–200.
114. Britten JR, Barnett MI, Armstrong NA. Studies on powder plug formation using a simulated capsule filling machine. J Pharm Pharmacol 1996; 48:249–254.
115. Tattawasart A, Armstrong NA. The formation of lactose plugs for hard shell capsule fills. Pharm Dev Technol 1997; 2:335–343.
116. Ludwig A, Van Ooteghem M. Disintegration of hard gelatin capsules. Part 2: disintegration mechanism of hard gelatin capsules investigated with a stereoscopic microscope. Pharm Ind 1980; 42:405–406.
117. Ludwig A, Van Ooteghem M. Disintegration of hard gelatin capsules. Part 5: the influence of the composition of the test solution on disintegration of hard gelatin capsules. Pharm Ind 1981; 43: 188–190.
118. Podczeck F, Jones BE. The in vitro dissolution of theophylline from different types of hard shell capsules. Drug Dev Ind Pharm 2002; 28:1163–1169.
119. Missaghi S, Fassihi R. Evaluation and comparison of physicomechanical characteristics of gelatin and hypromellose capsules. Drug Dev Ind Pharm 2006; 32(7):829–838.

120. El-Malah Y, Nazzai S, Bottom CB. Hard gelatin and hypromellose (HPMC) capsules: estimation of rupture time by real-time dissolution spectroscopy. Drug Dev Ind Pharm 2007; 33(1):27–34.
121. Tuleu C, Khela MK, Evans DF, et al. A scintigraphic investigation of the disintegration behavior of capsules in fasting subjects: a comparison of hypromellose capsules containing carageenin as a gelling agent and standard gelatin capsules. Eur J Pharm Sci 2007; 30(3–4): 251–255.
122. Amidon GL, Lennernas H, Shah VP, et al. A theoretical basis for a biopharmaceutic drug classification: the correlation of in vitro drug product dissolution and in vivo bioavailability. Pharm Res 1995; 12:413–420.
123. Hussain AS. Classifying your drug: the BCS guidance. In: Amidon GL, Robinson JR, Williams RL, eds. Scientific Foundations for Regulating Drug Products. Arlington, VA: AAPS Press, 1997:197–204.
124. Rekhi GS, Eddington ND, Fossler MJ, et al. Evaluation of in vitro release rate and in vivo absorption characteristics of four metoprolol tartrate immediate release tablet formulations. Pharm Dev Technol 1997; 2(1):11–24.
125. Piscitelli DA, Bigora S, Propst C, et al. The impact of formulation and process changes on in vitro dissolution and bioequivalence of piroxicam capsules. Pharm Dev Technol 1998; 3(4): 443–452.
126. Eddington ND, Ashraf M, Augsburger LL, et al. Identification of formulation and manufacturing variables that influence in vitro dissolution and in vivo bioavailability of propranolol hydrochloride tablets. Pharm Dev Technol 1998; 3(4):535–547.
127. Polli JE. Analysis of in vitro–in vivo data. In: Amidon GL, Robinson JR, Williams RL, eds. Scientific Foundations for Regulating Drug Products. Arlington, VA: AAPS Press, 1997:335–351.
128. Waiver of in vivo bioavailability and bioequivalence studies for immediate release solid oral dosage forms based on a biopharmaceutics classification system. Center for Drug Evaluation and Research, Food and Drug Administration, Issued 8/2000, Posted 8/31/2000. http://www.fda.gov/cder/guidance/index.htm.
129. Immediate release solid oral dosage forms; Scale-up and post approval changes: chemistry, manufacturing, and controls; *In vitro* dissolution testing; *In vivo* bioequivalence documentation, November, 1995. Center for Drug Evaluation and Research, Food and Drug Administration. Available at: http://www.fda.gov/cder/guidance/index.htm.
130. Fincher JH, Adams JG, Beal MH. Effect of particle size on gastrointestinal absorption of sulfisoxazole in dogs. J Pharm Sci 1963; 54:704–708.
131. Bastami SM, Groves MJ. Some factors influencing the in vitro release of phenytoin from formulations. Int J Pharm 1978; 1:151–164.
132. Newton JM, Rowley G. On the release of drug from hard gelatin capsules. J Pharm Pharmacol 1970; 22:163S–168S.
133. Patel R, Podczeck F. Investigation of the effect of type and source of microcrystalline cellulose on capsule filling. Int J Pharm 1996; 128:123–127.
134. Guo M, Muller FX, Augsburger LL. Evaluation of the plug formation process of silicified microcrystalline cellulose. Int J Pharm 2002; 233(1-2):99–109.
135. Bolhuis GK, Armstrong NA. Excipients for direct compression—an update. Pharm Dev Technol 2006; 11(1):111–124.
136. Newton JM, Rowley G, Tornblom JFV. The effect of additives on the release of drug from hard gelatin capsules. J Pharm Pharmacol 1971; 23:452–453.
137. Withey RJ, Mainville CA. A critical analysis of a capsule dissolution test. J Pharm Sci 1969; 58: 1120–1126.
138. Tyrer JH, Eadie MJ, Sutherland JM, et al. Outbreak of anticonvulsant intoxication in an Australian city. Br Med J 1970; 4:271–273.
139. York P. Studies of the effect of powder moisture content on drug release from hard gelatin capsules. Drug Dev Ind Pharm 1980; 6:605–627.
140. Koparkar AD, Augsburger LL, Shangraw RF. Intrinsic dissolution rates of tablet filler-binders and their influence on the dissolution of drugs from tablet formulation. Pharm Res 1990; 7: 80–86.

141. Augsburger LL, Shangraw RF. Effect of glidants in tableting. J Pharm Sci 1966; 55:418–423.

142. York P. Application of powder failure testing equipment in assessing effect of glidants on flowability of cohesive pharmaceutical powders. J Pharm Sci 1975; 64:1216–1221.

143. Sadek HM, Olsen JL, Smith HL, et al. A systematic approach to glidant selection. Pharm Technol 1982; 6(2):43–62.

144. Shangraw RF, Demarest DA Jr. A survey of current industrial practices in the formulation and manufacture of tablets and capsules. Pharm Technol 1993; 17:32–44.

145. Jones B. Two-piece gelatin capsules: excipients for powder products, European practice. Pharm Tech Eur 1995; 7(10):25–34.

146. Newton JM, Rowley G, Tornblom JFV. Further studies on the effect of additives on the release of drug from hard gelatin capsules. J Pharm Pharmacol 1971; 23:156S–160S.

147. Samyn JC, Jung WY. In vitro dissolution from several experimental capsules. J Pharm Sci 1970; 59:169–175.

148. Murthy KS, Samyn JC. Effect of shear mixing on in vitro drug release of capsule formulations containing lubricants. J Pharm Sci 1977; 66:1215–1219.

149. Miller TA, York P. Pharmaceutical tablet lubrication. Int J Pharm 1988; 41:1–19.

150. Shah AC, Mlodozeniec AR. Mechanism of surface lubrication: influence of duration of lubricant-excipient mixing on processing characteristics of powders and properties of compressed tablets. J Pharm Sci 1977; 66:1377–1381.

151. Bolhuis MR, Lerk CF. Film forming of tablet lubricants during the mixing process of solids. Acta Pharm Technol 1977; 23:13–20.

152. Desai DS, Rubitski BA, Varia SA, et al. Physical interactions of magnesium stearate with starch-derived disintegrants and their effects on capsule and tablet dissolution. Int J Pharm 1993; 91:217–226.

153. Ullah I, Wiley GJ, Agharkar SN. Analysis and simulation of capsule dissolution problem encountered during product scale-up. Drug Dev Ind Pharm 1992; 18:895–910.

154. Heda PK, Muteba K, Augsburger LL. Comparison of the formulation requirements of dosator and dosing disc automatic capsule filling machines. AAPS PharmSci 2002; 4(3):article 17. Available at: http://www.aapsj.org/view.asp?art=ps040317.

155. Augsburger LL. Practical considerations in scaling up hard shell capsule formulations. In: Levin M, ed., Pharmaceutical Process Scale-Up. 2nd ed. New York: Marcel Dekker Inc, 2005:409–433.

156. Nakagwu H. Effects of particle size of rifampicin and addition of magnesium stearate in release of rifampicin from hard gelatin capsules. Yakugaku Zasshi 1980; 100:1111–1117.

157. Shah PT, Moore WE. Dissolution behavior of commercial tablets extemporaneously converted to capsules. J Pharm Sci 1970; 59:1034–1036.

158. Goodhart FW, McCoy RH, Ninger FC. New in vitro disintegration and dissolution test method for tablets and capsules. J Pharm Sci 1973; 62:304–310.

159. Shangraw RF, Mitrevej A, Shah M. A new era of tablet disintegrants. Pharm Technol 1980; 4(10): 49–57.

160. Shangraw RF, Wallace JW, Bowers FM. Morphology and functionality of tablet excipients for direct compression: Part II. Pharm Technol 1981; 5(10):44–60.

161. Botzolakis JE, Small LE, Augsburger LL. Effect of disintegrants on drug dissolution from capsules filled on a dosator-type automatic capsule-filling machine. Int J Pharm 1982; 12:341–349.

162. Botzolakis JE, Augsburger LL. The role of disintegrants in hard-gelatin capsules. J Pharm Pharmacol 1984; 37:77–84.

163. Ong JTH, Chowhan ZT, Samuels GJ. Drug-excipient interactions resulting from powder mixing VI. Role of various surfactants. Int J Pharm 1993; 96:231–242.

164. Wang LH, Chowhan ZT. Drug-excipient interactions resulting from powder mixing V. Role of sodium lauryl sulfate. Int J Pharm 1990; 60:61–78.

165. Corrigan OI, Healy AM. Surfactants in pharmaceutical products and systems. In: Swarbrick J, Boylan JC, eds., Encyclopedia of Pharmaceutical Technology. Vol 14. New York: Marcel Dekker, 1996:295–331.

166. Lerk CF, Lagas M, Fell JT, P Nauta. Effect of hydrophilization of hydrophobic drugs on release rate from capsules. J Pharm Sci 1978; 67:935–939.

167. Lerk CF, Lagas M, Lie-A-Huen L, et al. In vitro and in vivo availability of hydrophilized phenytoin from capsules. J Pharm Sci 1979; 68:634–637.

168. Lagas M, de Wit HJC, Woldring MG, et al. Technetium labelled disintegration of capsules in the human stomach. Pharm Acta Helv 1980; 55:114–119.

169. Hogan J, Shue P-I, Podczeck F, et al. Investigations into the relationship between drug properties, filling, and the release of drugs from hard gelatin capsules using multivariate statistical analysis. Pharm Res 1996; 13:944–949.

170. Hussain AS, Yu X, Johnson RD. Application of neural computing to pharmaceutical product development. Pharm Res 1991; 8:1248–1252.

171. Lai S, Podczeck F, Newton JM, et al. An expert system to aid the development of capsule formulations. Pharm Tech Eur 1996; 8(Oct.):60–65.

172. Bateman SD, Verlin J, Russo M, et al. The development of a capsule formulation knowledge-based system. Pharm Technol 1996; 20(3):174–184.

173. Peng Y, Augsburger LL. Expert systems and other AI applications. In: Augsburger LL, Hoag SW, eds. Pharmaceutical Dosage Forms: Tablets. 3rd ed. Vol 2, New York: Taylor and Francis, 2008:137–172.

174. Polli JE, Crison JR, Amidon GL. Novel approach to the analysis of in vitro–in vivo relationships. J Pharm Sci 1996; 85:753–760.

175. Hicks TA, Patel B, Augsburger LL, et al. The effect of relative magnitudes of absorption and elimination half-lives on the decision of Cmax-based bioequivalence (abstr). American Association of Pharmaceutical Scientists. Presented at the 8th Annual meeting, Orlando, FL, November 1993.

176. Kuppuswamy R, Shah R, Anderson SR, et al. Practical limitations of tableting indices. Pharm Dev Technol 2001; 6(4):505–520.

177. Ghaffari A, Addollahi H, Khoshayand MR, et al. Performance comparison of neural network training algorithms in modeling of bimodal drug delivery. Int J Pharm 2006; 327(1-2):126–138.

178. Guo M, Kalra G, Wilson W, et al. A prototype intelligent hybrid system for hard gelatin capsule formulation development. Pharm Technol 2002; 26(9): 44–60.

179. Kalra G, Peng Y, Guo M, et al. A hybrid intelligent system for formulation of BCS Class II drugs in hard gelatin capsules. Proceedings, International Conference on Neural Information Processing, Singapore, November 2002, Vol 4, pp. 1987–1991, November 18–22, 2002.

180. Wilson W, Peng Y, Augsburger LL. Generalization of a prototype intelligent hybrid system for hard gelatin capsule formulation development. AAPS PharmSciTech 2005; 6(3):E449–E457. Available at: http://www.aapspharmscitech.org/view.asp?art=pt060356.

181. Wilson WI, Peng Y, Augsburger LL. Comparison of statistical analysis and Bayesian networks in the evaluation of dissolution performance of BCS Class II model drugs. J Pharm Sci 2005; 94:2764–2776.

182. Francois D, Jones BE. Making the hard capsule with the soft center. Manuf Chem Aerosol News 1979; 50(3):37, 38, 41.

183. Walker SE, Ganley JA, Bedford K, et al. The filling of molten and thixotropic formulations into hard gelatin capsules. J Pharm Pharmacol 1980; 32:389–393.

184. Berry IR. Improving bioavailability with soft gelatin capsules. Drug Cosmet Ind 1983; 133(3): 32, 33, 102, 105–108.

185. Seager H. Soft gelatin capsules: a solution to many tableting problems. Pharm Technol 1985; 9(9):84, 86, 88, 90, 92, 94, 96, 98, 100, 102, 104.

186. Cole ET. Liquid-filled hard-gelatin capsules. Pharm Technol 1989; 13(9):124–140.

187. Richardson M, Stegemann S. Capsule filling. Tablets & Capsules 2007; 5(1):12–18.

188. Nink F. Liquid-filled capsules. Tablets & Capsules 2007; 5(6):44–49.

189. Cole ET, Cade D, Benameur H. Challenges and opportunities in the encapsulation of liquid and semi-solid formulations for oral administration. Adv Drug Deliv Rev 2008; 60(6):747–756.

190. Garcia TP, Prescott JK. Blending and blend uniformity. In: Augsburger LL, Hoag SW, eds. Pharmaceutical Dosage Forms: Tablets. 3rd ed. Vol 1,. New York: Taylor and Francis, 2008:111–174.

191. Hom FS, Miskel JJ. Oral dosage form design and its influence on dissolution rates for a series of drugs. J Pharm Sci 1970; 59:827–830.

192. Hom FS, Miskel JJ. Enhanced drug dissolution rates for a series of drugs as a function of dosage form design. Lex Sci 1971; 8(1):18–26.

193. Fuccella LJ, Bolcioni G, Tamassia V, et al. Human pharmacokinetics and bioavailability of temazepam administered in soft gelatin capsules. Eur J Clin Pharmacol 1977; 12:383–386.

194. Johnson BF, Bye C, Jones G, et al. A completely absorbed oral preparation of digoxin. Clin Pharmacol Ther 1976; 19:746–757.

195. Hauss DJ. Lipid-based systems for oral drug delivery: bioavailability of poorly water soluble drugs. Am Pharm Rev 2002; 5(4):88–93.

196. Cannon JB, Long MA. Emulsions, microemulsions, and lipid-based drug delivery systems for drug Solubilization and delivery – part II: oral applications. In: Liu R, ed. Water-Insoluble Drug Formulation. 2nd ed. Boca Raton, Florida: CRC Press, 2008:227–254.

197. Gao P, Charton M, Morozowich W. Speeding development of poorly soluble/poorly permeable drugs by SEDDS/S-SEDDS formulations and prodrugs (Part II). Pharm Rev 2006; 9(4):16, 18, 19–23.

198. Shen H, Zhong M. Preparation and evaluation of self-microemulsifying drug delivery systems (SMEDDS) containing atorvasten. J Pharm Pharmacol 2006; 58(9):1183–1191.

199. Smith A, Lampard JF, Carruthers KM, et al. The filling of molten ibuprofen into hard gelatin capsules. Int J Pharm 1990; 59:115–119.

200. Doelker C, Doelker E, Buri P, et al. The incorporation and in vitro release profiles of liquid, deliquescent or unstable drugs with fusible excipients in hard gelatin capsules. Drug Dev Ind Pharm 1986; 12(10):1553–1565.

201. Bowtle WJ, Barker NJ, Wodhams J. A new approach to vancomycin formulation using filling technology for semisolid matrix capsules. Pharm Technol 1988; 12(6):86–97.

202. Hom FS, Veresh SA, Ebert WR. Soft gelatin capsules II. Oxygen permeability study of capsule shells. J Pharm Sci 1975; 64:851–857.

203. Muller G. Methods and machines for making gelatin capsules. Manuf Chem 1961; 32:63–66.

204. Berry IR. One-piece, soft gelatin capsules for pharmaceutical products. Pharm Eng 1985; 5(5):15–19.

205. Ebert WR. Soft elastic gelatin capsules: a unique dosage form. Pharm Technol 1977; 1(10):44–50.

206. Bauer KH, Dortunc B. Non-aqueous emulsions as vehicles for capsule filling. Drug Dev Ind Pharm 1984; 10:699–712.

207. Moreton RC, Armstrong NA. The effect of film composition on the diffusion of ethanal through soft gelatin films. Int J Pharm 1998; 161(1):123–131.

208. Gold TB, Buice RG Jr, Lodder RA, et al. Detection of formaldehyde-induced crosslinking in soft eleastic gelatin capsules using near-infrared spectrophotometry. Pharm Dev Technol 1998; 3(2):209–214.

209. Armstrong NA, James KC, Pugh WKL. Drug migration into soft gelatin capsule shells and its effect on the in-vitro availability. J Pharm Pharmacol 1984; 36:361–365.

210. Vemuri S. Measurement of soft elastic gelatin capsule firmness with a universal testing machine. Drug Dev Ind Pharm 1984; 10:409–424.

211. The hard capsule with the soft center. Elanco Products Co., Div. Eli Lilly and Co., Indianapolis, Indiana.

212. Stegemann S. Hard Gelatin Capsules Today and Tomorrow. 2nd ed. Capsugel Library, BAS 192 E, 2002:19.

213. Stein D, Bindra DS. Stabilization of hard gelatin capsule shells filled with polyethylene glycol matrices. Pharm Dev Technol 2007; 12(1):71–77.

214. Barak NS. Etodolac-liquid-filled dispersion into hard gelatin capsules: an approach to improve dissolution and stability of etodolac formulation. Drug Dev Ind Pharm 2006; 32:865–876.

15

Parenteral Products

James C. Boylan
Pharmaceutical Consultant, Gurnee, Illinois, U.S.A.

Steven L. Nail
School of Pharmacy, Purdue University, West Lafayette, Indiana, U.S.A.

INTRODUCTION

The first official injection (morphine) appeared in the *British Pharmacopoeia* (BP) of 1867. It was not until 1898 when cocaine was added to the BP that sterilization was attempted. In the United States, the first official injections may be found in the *National Formulary* (NF), published in 1926. Monographs were included for seven sterile glass-sealed ampoules. The NF and the *United States Pharmacopeia* (USP) published chapters on sterilization as early as 1916, but no monographs for ampoules appeared in USP until 1942. The current USP contains monographs for over 500 injectable products (1).

Parenteral administration of drugs by intravenous (IV), intramuscular (IM), or subcutaneous (SC) routes is now an established and essential part of medical practice. Advantages for parenterally administered drugs include the following: rapid onset, predictable effect, predictable and nearly complete bioavailability, and avoidance of the gastrointestinal (GI) tract and, hence, the problems of variable absorption, drug inactivation, and GI distress. In addition, the parenteral route provides reliable drug administration in very ill or comatose patients.

The pharmaceutical industry directs considerable effort toward maximizing the usefulness and reliability of oral dosage forms in an effort to minimize the need for parenteral administration. Factors that contribute to this include certain disadvantages of the parenteral route, including the frequent pain and discomfort of injections, with all the psychological fears associated with "the needle," plus the realization that an incorrect drug or dose is often harder or impossible to counteract when it has been given parenterally (particularly intravenously), rather than orally.

In recent years, parenteral dosage forms, especially IV forms, have enjoyed increased use. The reasons for this growth are many and varied, but they can be summed up as (*i*) new and better parenteral administration techniques, (*ii*) an increasing number of drugs that can be administered only by a parenteral route, (*iii*) the need for simultaneous administration of multiple drugs in hospitalized patients receiving IV therapy, (*iv*) new forms of nutritional therapy, such as IV lipids, amino acids, and trace metals, and (*v*) the extension of parenteral therapy into the home.

Many important drugs are available only as parenteral dosage forms. Notable among these are numerous biotechnology drugs, insulin, several cephalosporin antibiotic products, and drugs such as heparin, protamine, and glucagon. In addition, other drugs such as lidocaine hydrochloride and many anticancer products are used principally as parenterals.

Along with this growth in the use of parenteral medications, the hospital pharmacist has become a very knowledgeable, key individual in most hospitals, having responsibility for hospital-wide IV admixture programs, parenteral unit-dose packaging, and often, central surgical supply. By choice, expertise, and responsibility, the pharmacist has accumulated the greatest fund of information about parenteral drugs—not only their clinical use but also their stability, incompatibilities, methods of handling and admixture, and proper packaging. More and more nurses and physicians are looking to the pharmacists for guidance on parenteral products.

To support the institutional pharmacist in preparing IV admixtures (which typically involves adding one or more drugs to large-volume parenteral fluids), equipment manufacturers have designed laminar flow units, electromechanical compounding units, transfer devices, and filters specifically adaptable to a variety of hospital programs.

The nurse and physician have certainly not been forgotten by manufacturers. A wide spectrum of IV and IM administration devices and aids have been made available in recent years for bedside use. Many innovative practitioners have made suggestions to industry that have resulted in product or technique improvements, particularly in IV therapy. The use of parenteral products is growing at a very significant rate in nonhospital settings, such as outpatient surgical centers and homes. The reduction in costs associated with outpatient and home care therapy, coupled with advances in drugs, dosage forms, and delivery systems, has caused a major change in the administration of parenteral products (2).

ROUTES OF PARENTERAL ADMINISTRATION

The major routes of parenteral administration of drugs are SC, IM, and IV. Other more specialized routes are intrathecal, intracisternal, intra-arterial, intraspinal, intraepidural, and intradermal (ID). The ID route is not typically used to achieve systemic drug effects. The major routes will be discussed separately. Definitions of the more specialized routes, along with additional information concerning needle sizes, volumes typically administered, formulation constraints, and types of medication administered, are summarized in Table 1.

The Subcutaneous Route

Lying immediately under the skin is a layer of fat, the superficial fascia, which lends itself to safe administration of a great variety of drugs, including vaccines, insulin, scopolamine, and epinephrine. SC injections are usually administered in volumes up to 2 mL using ½- to 1-in. 23-gauge (or smaller) needles. Care must be taken to ensure that the needle is not in a blood vessel. This is done by lightly pulling back on the syringe plunger (aspiration) before making the injection. If the needle is inadvertently located in a blood vessel, blood will appear in the syringe, and the injection should not be made. The injection site may be massaged after injection, to facilitate drug absorption. Drugs given

Table 1 Parenteral Routes of Drug Administration

Routes	Usual volume (mL)	Needle commonly used	Formulation constraints	Types of medication administered
Primary parental routes				
SVPs				
SC	0.5–2	5/8 in., 23 gauge	Need to be isotonic	Insulin, vaccines
IM	0.5–2	1½ in., 22 gauge	Can be solutions, emulsions, oils, or suspensions, isotonic preferably	Nearly all drug classes
IV	1–1000	Veinpuncture 1½ in., 20–22 gauge	Solutions, emulsions, and liposomes	Nearly all drug classes
LVPs	101 and larger (infusion unit)	Venoclysis 1½ in., 18–19 gauge	Solutions and some emulsions	Nearly all drug classes (see precautionary notes in text)
Other parenteral routes				
Intra-arterial: directly into an artery (immediate action sought in peripheral Area)	2–20	20–22 gauge	Solutions and some emulsions	Radiopaque media, antineoplastics, antibiotics
Intrathecal (intraspinal; into spinal canal)	1–4	24–28 gauge	Must be isotonic	Local anesthetics, analgesics; neurolytic agents
Intraepidural (into epidural space near spinal column)	6–30	5 in., 16–18 gauge	Must be isotonic	Local anesthetics, narcotics, a_2-agonists, steroids
Intracisternal: directly into caudal region of the brain between the cerebellum and the medulla oblongata			Must be isotonic	
Intra-articular: directly into a joint, usually for a local effect there, as for steroid anti-inflammatory action in arthritis	2–20	1.5–2 in., 18–22 gauge	Must be isotonic	Morphine, local anesthetics, steroids, NSAIDs, antibiotics

(Continued)

Table 1 Parenteral Routes of Drug Administration (*Continued*)

Routes	Usual volume (mL)	Needle commonly used	Formulation constraints	Types of medication administered
Intracardial: directly into the heart when life is threatened (epinephrine stimulation in severe heart attack)	0.2–1	5 in., 22 gauge		Cardiotonic drugs, calcium
Intrapleural: directly into the pleural cavity or a lung (also used for fluid withdrawal) Diagnostic testing	2–30	2–5 in., 16–22 gauge		Local anesthetics, narcotics, chemotherapeutic agents
ID	0.05	1/2–5/8 in., 25–26 gauge	Should be isotonic	Diagnostic agents

Abbreviations: SC, subcutaneous; IM, intramuscular; IV, intravenous; ID, intradermal; LVPs, large-volume parenterals; SVPs, small-volume parenterals; NSAIDs, nonsteroidal anti-inflammatory drugs.

by this route will have a slower onset of action than by the IM or IV routes, and total absorption may also be less.

Sometimes dextrose or electrolyte solutions are given subcutaneously in amounts from 250 to 1000 mL. This technique, called hypodermoclysis, is used when veins are unavailable or difficult to use for further medication. Irritation of the tissue is a danger with this technique. Administration of the enzyme hyaluronidase can help by increasing absorption and decreasing tissue distention. Irritating drugs and vasoconstrictors can lead to abscesses, necrosis, or inflammation when given subcutaneously. Body sites suitable for SC administration include most portions of the arms and legs plus the abdomen. When daily or frequent administration is required, the injection site can, and should, be continuously changed or rotated, especially by diabetic patients self-administering insulin.

The Intramuscular Route

The IM route of administration is second only to the IV route in rapidity of onset of systemic action. Injections are made into the striated muscle fibers that lie beneath the SC layer. The principal sites of injection are the gluteal (buttocks), deltoid (upper arm), and vastus lateralis (lateral thigh) muscles. The usual volumes injected range from 0.5 to 2.0 mL, with volumes up to 4.0 mL sometimes being given (in divided doses) in the gluteal or thigh areas (Table 1). Again, it is important to aspirate before injecting to ensure that the drug is not administered intravenously. Needles used in administering IM injections range from 1 to 1½ in. and 19 to 22 gauge, the most common being 1½ in. and 22 gauge.

The major clinical problem arising from IM injections is muscle or neuron damage, the injury normally resulting from faulty technique, rather than the medication. Most injectable products can be given intramuscularly, with a normal onset of action from 15 to 30 minutes. As a result, numerous dosage forms are available for this route of administration: solutions, oil-in-water (o/w) or water-in-oil (w/o) emulsions, suspensions (aqueous or oily base), colloidal suspensions, and reconstitutable powders. Those product forms in which the drug is not fully dissolved generally result in slower, more gradual drug absorption, a slower onset of action, and sometimes longer-lasting drug effects.

Intramuscularly administered products typically form a "depot" in the muscle mass from which the drug is slowly absorbed. The peak drug concentration is usually seen within one to two hours. Factors affecting the drug-release rate from an IM depot include the compactness of the depot (the less compact and more diffuse, the faster the release), the rheology of the product, concentration and particle size of drug in the vehicle, nature of the solvent or vehicle, volume of the injection, and tonicity and physical form of the product.

Needleless injector systems are sometimes used to administer drugs by either the IM or SC routes. In needleless injector systems, the drug formulation is propelled by pressure from a cylinder of compressed CO_2 through an orifice, creating a thin stream of liquid that penetrates the skin. The depth of penetration is determined by the size of the orifice used, which in turn determines whether the drug is administered intramuscularly or subcutaneously. Advantages of needleless injector systems include elimination of the "fear of needles," elimination of needlestick injuries to health care workers, and, in the case of mass immunization programs, lower cost of administration. Limitations of these systems include higher cost for patient-specific drug administration. Also, the incidence of irritation at the site of injection is somewhat higher for needleless injector administration, because the formulation is dispersed to a greater extent in the tissue at the site of injection relative to bolus injection via a needle.

The Intravenous Route

IV medication is injected directly into a vein either to obtain an extremely rapid and predictable response or to avoid irritation of other tissues. This route of administration also provides maximum availability and assurance in delivering the drug to the site of action. However, a major danger of this route of administration is that the rapidity of absorption makes effective administration of an antidote very difficult, if not impossible, in most instances. Care must often be used to avoid administering a drug too rapidly by the IV route, because irritation or an excessive drug concentration at sensitive organs such as the heart and brain (drug shock) can occur. The duration of drug activity is dependent on the initial dose and the distribution, metabolism, and excretion properties (pharmacokinetics) of the drug. For most drugs, the biological half-life is independent of the initial dose because the elimination process is first order. Thus, an IV drug with a short half-life would not provide a sustained blood level. The usual method of administration for drugs with short half-lives is to use continuous IV drip (IV infusion). IV injections (venipuncture) normally range from 1 to 1000 mL and are given with either a 19- to 20-gauge 1-in. needle, with an injection rate of 1 mL/10 sec for volumes up to 5 mL and 1 mL/20 sec for volumes over 5 mL. Only drugs in aqueous solutions, hydroalcoholic solutions, some emulsions, and liposomal formulations are to be given by the IV route.

Large proximal veins, such as those located inside the forearm, are most commonly used for IV administration. Because of the rapid dilution in the circulating blood and the general insensitivity of the venous wall to pain, the IV route may be used to administer drugs that would be too irritating to give by other routes (e.g., nitrogen mustards), provided that proper dosing procedures are employed. The risk of thrombosis is increased when extremities such as the wrist or the ankle are used for injection sites or when potentially irritating IV products are used, with the risk further increasing in patients with impaired circulation.

The IV infusion of large volumes of fluids (100–1000 mL) has become increasingly popular. This technique, called *venoclysis*, utilizes products known as large-volume parenterals (LVPs). It is used to supply electrolytes and nutrients, restore blood volume, and prevent tissue dehydration. Various parenteral drug solutions can be conveniently added to the LVP solutions as they are being administered, or before administration, to provide continuous and prolonged drug therapy as well as to administer a dilute solution of drugs where either the drug itself or the formulation is too irritating to administer at the concentration used in the formulation provided by the manufacturer. Such drug additions to LVPs have become very common in hospitals. The combination of parenteral dosage forms to be administered as a unit product is known as an IV admixture. Pharmacists practicing such IV additive product preparation must be very knowledgeable to avoid physical and chemical incompatibilities in the modified LVP, creation of therapeutic incompatibilities with other drugs, compromising sterility through breaches of aseptic technique, or addition of extraneous particulate matter.

Commonly administered LVPs include such products as Lactated Ringers Injection USP; Sodium Chloride Injection USP (0.9%), which replenish fluids and electrolytes; Dextrose Injection USP (5%), which provides fluid plus nutrition (calories); or various combinations of dextrose and saline. In addition, numerous other nutrient and ionic solutions are available for clinical use, the most popular of which are solutions of essential amino acids or lipid emulsions. These solutions are modified to be hypertonic, isotonic, or hypotonic to aid in maintaining fluid, nutritional, and electrolyte balance in a particular patient according to need. Indwelling needles or catheters are required in LVP administration. Care must be taken to avoid local or systemic infections or thrombophlebitis owing to faulty injection or administration technique.

IV infusions can be administered through peripheral veins, typically in the forearm, or through a central line that is surgically implanted in the subclavian vein. Another option for IV infusion that is becoming more popular is the peripherally inserted central catheter (PICC), where the catheter is fed through an incision in a peripheral vein to a large central vein near the heart. Central IV lines are commonly used for administration of very hypertonic formulations that would be excessively irritating to a peripheral vein, and for administration of *vesicants*, or drugs that are damaging to tissue. Introduction of the formulation into an area of high blood flow provides rapid dilution and minimizes irritation.

Other Parenteral Routes

Other more specialized parenteral routes are listed and described briefly in Table 1. The intra-arterial route involves injecting a drug directly into an artery. This technique is not simple and may require a surgical procedure to reach the artery. It is important that the artery not be missed, since serious nerve damage can occur to the nerves lying close to arteries. Doses given by this route should be minimal and given gradually, since, once injected, the drug effect cannot be neutralized. As shown in Table 1, the intra-arterial route is used to administer radiopaque contrast media for viewing an organ, such as the heart or kidney, or to perfuse an antineoplastic agent at the highest possible concentration to the target organ.

The intrathecal route is employed to administer a drug directly into the cerebrospinal fluid at any level of the cerebrospinal axis. This route is used when it is not possible to achieve sufficiently high plasma levels to accomplish adequate diffusion and penetration into the cerebrospinal fluid. This is not the same route used to achieve spinal anesthesia, for which the drug is injected within the dural membrane surrounding the spinal cord, or in extradural or epidural anesthesia (caudal or sacral anesthesia), for which the drug is deposited outside the dural membrane and within the body spinal caudal canals. Parenteral products administered by the intrathecal, intraspinal, and intracisternal routes must be formulated at physiological pH, be isotonic, and not contain antimicrobial preservatives to minimize the probability of nerve damage.

ID administration involves injection into the skin layer. This route is largely limited to injection of materials to detect hypersensitivity reactions for diagnostic purposes. It is important that the product per se be nonirritating. Volumes are normally given at 0.05 mL/dose, and the solutions are isotonic. ID medication is usually administered with a ½ - or 5/8-in., 25- or 26-gauge needle, inserted at an angle nearly parallel to the skin surface. Absorption is slow and limited from this site since the blood vessels are extremely small, even though the area is highly vascular. The site should not be massaged after the injection of allergy test materials. Skin testing includes not only allergens, such as pollens or dust, but also microorganisms, as in the tuberculin or histoplasmin skin tests.

SPECIALIZED LARGE-VOLUME PARENTERAL AND STERILE SOLUTIONS

LVPs designed to provide fluid (water), calories (dextrose solutions), electrolytes (saline solutions), or combinations of these materials have been described. Several other specialized LVP and sterile solutions are also used in medicine and will be described here, even though two product classes (peritoneal dialysis and irrigating solutions) are not parenteral products.

Hyperalimentation Solutions

Parenteral hyperalimentation involves administration of large amounts of nutrients (e.g., carbohydrates, amino acids, lipids, and vitamins) to maintain a patient who is unable to take food orally for several weeks at caloric intake levels of 4000 kcal/day or more. Earlier methods of parenteral alimentation, which involved IV administration of nutrients through a peripheral vein, were not typically able to maintain patients without weight loss and gradual deterioration in physical condition because, to administer sufficient calories at acceptable volumetric flow rates, the infusion solution must be hypertonic. Development of the technique of subclavian vein cannulation in the early 1950s paved the way for effective parenteral nutrition, since the infused fluid is rapidly diluted by the high blood flow in the subclavian vein. Hyperalimentation formulations commonly consist of mixtures of dextrose, amino acids, and lipids (usually soybean oil, safflower oil, or mixtures of the two) containing added electrolytes, trace metals, and vitamins. The method permits administration of life-saving or life-sustaining nutrients to comatose patients or to patients undergoing treatment for esophageal obstruction, GI diseases (including cancer), ulcerative colitis, and other disease states. As general perioperative support, parenteral nutrition is generally indicated whenever a patient is to take nothing by mouth for periods of five days or longer.

Cardioplegia Solutions

Cardioplegia solutions are LVP solutions used in heart surgery to help prevent ischemic injury to the myocardium during the time the blood supply to the heart is clamped off and during reperfusion, as well as to maintain a bloodless operating field and to make the myocardium flaccid. Cardioplegia solutions are typically electrolyte solutions where the electrolyte composition is intended to maintain diastolic arrest. These solutions are usually admixed by pharmacists in a hospital IV admixture program and are administered cold to cool the myocardium and minimize metabolic activity. Cardioplegia solutions are usually slightly alkaline and hypertonic to compensate for metabolic acidosis and to minimize reperfusion injury resulting from tissue edema.

Peritoneal Dialysis Solutions

The sterile peritoneal dialysis solutions are infused continuously into the abdominal cavity, bathing the peritoneum, and are then continuously withdrawn. The purpose of peritoneal dialysis is to remove toxic substances from the body or to aid and accelerate the excretion function normal to the kidneys. The process is employed to counteract some forms of drug or chemical toxicity as well as to treat acute renal insufficiency. Peritoneal dialysis solutions contain glucose and have an ionic content similar to normal extracellular fluid. Toxins and metabolites diffuse into the circulating dialysis fluid through the peritoneum, and are removed. At the same time, excess fluid is removed from the patient if the glucose content renders the dialysis solution hyperosmotic. An antibiotic is often added to these solutions as a prophylactic measure.

Irrigating Solutions

Irrigating solutions are intended to irrigate, flush, and aid in cleansing body cavities and wounds. Although certain IV solutions, such as normal saline, may be used as irrigating solutions, solutions designed as irrigating solutions should not be used parenterally. Since irrigating solutions used in treatment of serious wounds infuse into the bloodstream to some degree, they must be sterile, pyrogen-free, and made and handled with the same care as parenteral solutions.

FORMULATION OF PARENTERAL PRODUCTS

A successful therapeutic response following parenteral administration of a drug requires an adequate concentration of drug at the site of action. The IV route is characterized by the absence of an absorption step, and a major consideration in formulation of drugs for IV administration is assuring adequate solubility of the drug in the solution administered, while minimizing the probability of precipitation of the drug at the site of injection. IM and SC administration, however, require absorption of the drug from the site of injection. This absorption process is determined by physicochemical properties of the drug, the formulation used, and physiological factors such as extent of vascularity at the site of injection, distribution of fat in the tissue, amount of exercise, and condition of the tissue. With an IM suspension, drug dissolution is usually the rate-limiting step in the absorption of the drug at the injection site (3). The absorption of the drug following IM administration is greatly influenced by the physicochemical properties of the drug.

The Active Drug

A thorough evaluation of properties of the active drug or drugs is essential for developing a stable and safe parenteral dosage form. The physical and chemical factors that may significantly affect the development of a parenteral dosage form are discussed in chapter 7 and by Motola and Agharkar (4). Important properties include solubility and rate of solution. The most important factor affecting dissolution is the aqueous solubility of the drug itself (5), but other factors that can be important are the physical state of the drug (i.e., crystalline or amorphous), particle size, and perhaps formulation pH.

Crystal Characteristics

Many dry solid parenteral products, such as the cephalosporins, are prepared by sterile crystallization techniques. Control of the crystallization process to obtain a consistent and uniform crystal form, habit, density, and size distribution is particularly critical for drug substances to be utilized in sterile suspensions. For example, when the crystallization process for sterile ceftazidime pentahydrate was modified to increase the density and reduce the volume of the fill dose, the rate of dissolution increased significantly.

To obtain a uniform product from lot to lot, strict adherence to the procedures developed for a particular crystallization must be followed, including control of pH, rates of addition, solvent concentrations and purity, temperature, and mixing rates. Each crystallization procedure has to be designed to ensure sterility and minimize particulate contamination. Changes, such as using absolute ethyl alcohol instead of 95% ethanol during the washing procedure, can destroy the crystalline structure if the material being crystallized is a hydrate structure.

Drugs that associate with water to produce crystalline forms are called hydrates. Water content of the hydrate forms of sodium cefazolin as a function of relative humidity is seen in Figure 1. As shown in the figure, the sesquihydrate is the most stable structure when exposed to extreme humidity conditions (6). This figure also shows the importance of choosing the proper combination of hydrate and humidity conditions when designing a manufacturing process or facility.

Chemical Modification of the Drug

Improvement of the properties of a drug may be achieved by the chemical modification of the parent drug. The preparation of an ester, salt, or other modification of the parent structure may be employed with parenteral drugs to increase stability, alter drug solubility, enhance depot action, avoid formulation difficulties, and, possibly, decrease pain on injection. The modified drug that converts back to the active parent structure is defined as a prodrug. This conversion usually occurs within the body system or, for some drugs that are formulated as dry powders, on reconstitution. The preparation of prodrugs is becoming a common practice with many types of drugs. Examples of antibiotic prodrugs include benzathine penicillin, procaine penicillin, metronidazole phosphate, and chloramphenicol sodium succinate. Prodrugs are also common for injectable steroids such as methylprednisolone (formulated as methylprednisolone sodium succinate) and hydrocortisone (formulated as hydrocortisone sodium succinate).

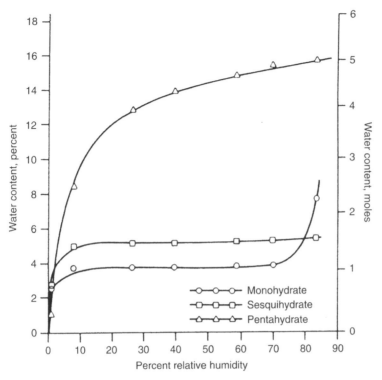

Figure 1 Water content versus relative humidity for hydrate forms of sodium cefazolin.

The preparation of salts of organic compounds is one of the most important tools available to the formulator. Compounds for both IM and IV solutions may require high solubility for the drug to be incorporated into acceptable volumes for bolus administration (Table 1). Sodium and potassium salts of weak acids and hydrochloride and sulfate salts of weak bases are widely used in parenterals requiring highly soluble compounds, on the basis of their overall safety and history of clinical acceptance.

If the solubility of a drug is to be reduced to enhance stability or to prepare a suspension, the formulator may prepare water-insoluble salts. A classic example is procaine penicillin G, the decreased solubility (7 mg/mL) of which, when compared with the very soluble penicillin G potassium, is utilized to prepare stable parenteral suspensions. Another alternative to preparing an insoluble drug is to use the parent acidic or basic drug and to buffer the pH of the suspension in the range of minimum solubility.

Polymorphism

The literature lists numerous examples of polymorphism, that is, the existence of several crystal forms of a given chemical that exhibit different physical properties (7). The conversion of one polymorph to another may cause a significant change in the physical properties of the drug and in critical quality attributes of drug products.

Studies of polymorphs in recent years have pointed out the effects of polymorphism on solubility and, more specifically, on dissolution rates. The aspect of polymorphism that is of particular concern to the parenteral formulator is physical stability of the product (8). Substances that form polymorphs must be evaluated so that the form used is stable in a particular solvent system. Physical stresses that occur during suspension manufacture may also give rise to changes in crystal form (9).

pH and pK

Profiles of pH versus solubility and pH versus stability are needed for solution and suspension formulations to help assure physical and chemical stability as well as to maximize or minimize solubility. This information is also valuable for predicting the compatibility of drugs with various infusion fluids.

In summary, the physical and chemical data that should be obtained on the drug substance include the following:

- Molecular structure and weight
- Melting point
- Thermal profile
- Particle size and shape
- Hygroscopicity potential
- Ionization constant
- Light stability
- Optical activity
- pH solubility profile
- pH stability profile
- Polymorphism potential
- Solvate formation

Added Substances (Excipients) in Parenteral Formulations

To provide efficacious and safe parenteral dosage forms, added substances must frequently be incorporated into the formula to maintain pharmaceutical stability, control product attributes, ensure sterility, or aid in parenteral administration. These substances include antioxidants, antimicrobial agents, buffers, bulking materials, chelating agents, inert gases, solubilizing agents, and protectants. In parenteral product development work, any additive to a formulation must be justified by a clear purpose and function. In addition, every attempt should be made to choose added substances that are accepted by regulatory agencies throughout the world, since most pharmaceutical development is international in scope. Because of the extensive pharmacological and toxicological data required to obtain approval for any new additive, most formulators continue to depend on materials already used in marketed parenteral products.

Some of the most commonly used added substances are listed in Table 2. Pharmacists involved in IV admixture programs must be aware of the types of additives that may be present in the products being combined, since the source of incompatibility between different drugs mixed in solution may be the excipients present. For example, drug formulations containing the preservative benzalkonium chloride, which is positively charged, are commonly incompatible with products containing anionic drugs and excipients.

Antioxidants

Salts of sulfur dioxide, including bisulfite, metasulfite, and sulfite, are the most common antioxidants used in aqueous parenterals. These antioxidants maintain product stability by being preferentially oxidized and gradually consumed over the shelf life of the product.

Table 2 Classes and Examples of Parenteral Additives

Additive class	Examples	Usual concentration (%)
Antimicrobials	Benzalkonium chloride	0.01
	Benzyl alcohol	1–2
	Chlorobutanol	0.25–0.5
	Metacresol	0.1–0.3
	Butyl *p*-hydroxybenzoate	0.015
	Methyl *p*-hydroxybenzoate	0.1–0.2
	Propyl *p*-hydroxybenzoate	0.2
	Phenol	0.25–0.5
	Thimerosal	0.01
Antioxidants	Ascorbic acid	0.01–0.05
	Cysteine	0.1–0.5
	Monothioglycerol	0.1–1.0
	Sodium bisulfite	0.1–1.0
	Sodium metabisulfite	0.1–1.0
	Tocopherols	0.05–0.5
Buffers	Acetates	1–2
	Citrates	1–5
	Phosphates	0.8–2.0
Bulking agents	Lactose	1–8
	Mannitol	1–10
	Sorbitol	1–10
	Glycine	1–2
Chelating agents	Salts of ethylenediaminetetraacetic acid	0.01–0.05
Protectants	Sucrose	2–5
	Glucose	2–5
	Lactose	2–5
	Maltose	2–5
	Trehalose	2–5
	HSA	0.1–1.0
Solubilizing agents	Ethyl alcohol	1–50
	Glycerin	1–50
	Polyethylene glycol	1–50
	Propylene glycol	1–50
	Lecithin	0.5–2.0
Surfactants	Polyoxyethylene	0.1–0.5
	Sorbitan monooleate	0.05–0.25
Tonicity-adjusting agents	Dextrose	4–5
	Sodium chloride	0.5–0.9

Abbreviation: HSA, Human serum albumin.

Irrespective of which salt is added to the solution, the antioxidant moiety depends on the final concentration of the thio compound and the final pH of the formulation (10). While undergoing oxidation reactions, sulfites may be converted to sulfates and other species. Sulfites can also react with certain drug molecules (e.g., epinephrine).

Sulfite levels are determined by the reactivity of the drug, the type of container, single- or multiple-dose use, container headspace, use of inert gas purge, and expiration dating period to be employed. Upper limits for sulfite levels are specified in most pharmacopoeias. Allowances on upper limits are made for concentrated drugs that are diluted extensively before use.

Sulfites have been reported to cause allergic reactions in some asthmatics. If possible, alternative antioxidants should be considered or the product should be manufactured and packaged in a manner such as to eliminate or minimize the concentration of bisulfite required. Deoxygenation of the makeup water, maintaining the solution under a nitrogen atmosphere throughout the manufacturing process, and purging the filled vials with an inert gas may significantly reduce the amount of antioxidant required.

Antimicrobial Agents

A suitable preservative system is required in all multiple-dose parenteral products to inhibit the growth of microorganisms accidentally introduced during withdrawal of individual doses. Preservatives may be added to single-dose parenteral products that are not terminally sterilized as a sterility assurance measure, that is, to prevent growth of any microorganisms that could be introduced if there were any inadvertent breach of asepsis during filling operations. However, the inclusion of a preservative in single-dose parenteral products must be weighed against the need to develop formulations that are acceptable to regulatory bodies worldwide. Inclusion of a preservative can be a difficult challenge, given the wide range of viewpoints concerning which preservatives are acceptable, and when it is appropriate to include them in a formulation. Partly because of this, there is a trend in parenteral product development to eliminate preservatives wherever practical to do so. This may require added measures in manufacturing to improve sterility assurance, such as using barrier technology to provide positive separation of personnel from product during aseptic filling and transfer steps.

The formulation scientist must be aware of interactions between preservatives and other components of a formulation that could compromise the efficacy of the preservative. For example, proteins can bind thimerosal, reducing preservative efficacy. Partitioning of preservative into a micellar phase or an oil phase (in an emulsion) can also reduce the effective concentration of preservative available for bactericidal or bacteriostatic action. Preservative efficacy testing should be done on the proposed formulation to assure an effective preservative concentration.

Several investigators have published research on incompatibilities of preservatives with rubber closures and other packaging components, particularly polymeric materials (11). Again, challenging the product with selected microorganisms to measure bacteriostatic or bactericidal activity is necessary, including evaluation of efficacy as a function of time throughout the anticipated shelf life of the product.

More subtle effects of preservatives on injectable formulations are possible. Formulation of insulin is an illustrative case study. Insulin is usually formulated as a multiple-dose vial, since individual dosage varies among patients. Preservation of zinc insulin with phenol causes physical instability of the suspension, whereas methylparaben does not. However, the presence of phenol is required for obtaining protamine insulin crystals (9).

Buffers

Many drugs require a certain pH range to maintain product stability. As discussed previously, drug solubility may also be strongly dependent on the pH of the solution. An important aid to the formulator is the information contained in a graph of the solubility

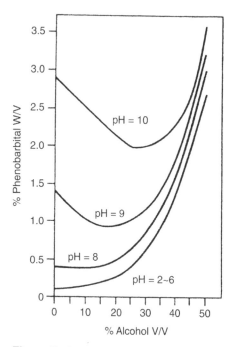

Figure 2 Solubility of phenobarbital as a function of pH and alcohol concentration. *Source*: From Ref. 5.

profile of the drug as a function of pH (Fig. 2). The product can then be buffered to approach maximum or minimum solubility, whichever is desired.

Parenteral products should be formulated to possess sufficient buffer capacity to maintain proper product pH. Factors that influence pH include product degradation, container and stopper effects, diffusion of gases through the closure, and the effect of gases in the product or in the headspace. However, the buffer capacity of a formulation must be readily overcome by the biological fluids; thus, the concentration and ratios of buffer ingredients must be carefully selected.

Buffer systems for parenterals consist of either a weak base and the salt of a weak base or a weak acid and the salt of a weak acid. Buffer systems commonly used for injectable products are acetates, citrates, and phosphates (Table 2). Amino acids are being increasingly used as buffers, especially for polypeptide injectables.

Chelating Agents

Chelating agents are added to complex and, thereby, inactivate metals such as copper, iron, and zinc that generally catalyze oxidative degradation of drug molecules. Sources of metal contamination include raw material impurities; solvents, such as water, rubber stoppers, and containers; and equipment employed in the manufacturing process (12). The most widely used chelating agents are edetate disodium derivatives and salts. Citric and tartaric acids are also employed as chelating agents.

Inert Gases

Another means of enhancing the product integrity of oxygen-sensitive medicaments is by displacing the air in the solution with nitrogen or argon. This technique may be made more effective by first purging with nitrogen or boiling the water to reduce dissolved oxygen. The container is also purged with nitrogen or argon before filling and may also be topped off with the gas before sealing.

Glass-sealed ampoules provide the most impervious barrier for gas transmission. A butyl rubber stock is used with rubber-stoppered products that are sensitive to oxygen because it provides better resistance to gas permeation than other rubber stocks.

Solubilizing Agents and Surfactants

Drug solubility can be increased by the use of solubilizing agents, such as those listed in Table 2, and by nonaqueous solvents or mixed solvent systems, to be discussed shortly. When using solubilizing agents, the formulator must consider their effect on the safety and stability of the drug.

A surfactant is a surface-active agent that is used to disperse a water-insoluble drug as a colloidal dispersion. Surfactants are used for wetting and preventing crystal growth in a suspension. They are used quite extensively in parenteral suspensions for wetting powders and providing acceptable syringability. They are also used in emulsions and for solubilizing steroids and fat-soluble vitamins.

Tonicity Adjustment Agents

It is important that injectable solutions that are to be given intravenously are isotonic, or nearly so. Because of osmotic pressure changes and the resultant exchange of ionic species across red blood cell membranes, nonisotonic solutions, particularly if given in quantities larger than 100 mL, can cause hemolysis or crenation of red blood cells (owing to hypotonic or hypertonic solutions, respectively). Dextrose, sodium chloride, or potassium chloride is commonly used to achieve isotonicity in a parenteral formula.

Protectants

A protectant is a substance that is added to a formulation to protect against loss of activity caused by some stress that is introduced by the manufacturing process or to prevent loss of active ingredients by adsorption to process equipment or primary packaging materials. Protectants are used primarily in protein formulations, liposomal formulations, and vaccines. For example, cryoprotectants and lyoprotectants are used to inhibit loss of integrity of the active substance resulting from freezing and drying, respectively. Compounds that provide cryoprotection are not necessarily the same as those that provide lyoprotection. Polyethylene glycol protects lactate dehydrogenase and phosphofructokinase from damage by freezing, but does not protect either protein from damage by freeze-drying. Compounds such as sucrose and trehalose are effective lyoprotectants for both proteins (13). Effective cryo- and lyoprotectants must be determined on a case-by-case basis, but sugars and polyhydroxy compounds are usually the best candidate compounds. These same types of compounds also tend to markedly improve the stability of proteins against inactivation by thermal denaturation.

Another type of protectant is used to prevent loss of active substance—again, usually a protein and usually present at a very low concentration—by adsorption to materials or equipment in the manufacturing process or to components of the primary package. In manufacturing, particular attention should be given to adsorption of the active entity to filters (especially nylon) and to silicone tubing used for transfer operations. For packaging materials, rubber closures and other polymeric materials should be examined carefully for adsorptive potential. The same consideration applies to infusion equipment, particularly considering that most materials in modern IV infusion therapy—plastic bags, infusion sets, and in-line filters—are polymeric.

Human serum albumin (HSA) may be used as a protectant against adsorptive loss of proteins present at low concentrations. HSA is present at higher concentration than the active substance, and is preferentially adsorbed, coating the surface of interest and preventing adsorption of the drug. For example, insulin is subject to adsorptive loss to hydrophobic materials. Addition of 0.1% to 1.0% HSA has been reported to prevent this adsorptive loss (9).

Vehicles

Aqueous Vehicles

Water for injection (WFI) is the most widely used solvent for parenteral preparations. The USP requirements for WFI and purified water have been recently updated to replace the traditional wet and colorimetric analytical methods with the more modern and cost-effective methods of conductivity and total organic carbon. WFI must be prepared and stored in a manner to ensure purity and freedom from pyrogens. The most common means of obtaining WFI is by the distillation of deionized water. This is the only method of preparation permitted by the European Pharmacopoeia (EP). In contrast, the United States and the Japanese Pharmacopeias also permit reverse osmosis to be used. The USP has also recently broadened its definition of source water to include not only the U.S. Environmental Protection Agency National Primary Drinking Water Standards but also comparable regulations of the European Union and Japan.

Microorganisms, dissolved organic and inorganic substances, and foreign particles are the most common contaminants found in water. Inorganic compounds are commonly removed by distillation, reverse osmosis, deionization, or a combination of these processes. Membrane and depth filters are used to remove particulate contaminants, and charcoal beds may be used to remove organic materials. Filtration, chilling or heating, or recirculation of water is used to reduce microbial growth and to prevent pyrogen formation that will occur in a static deionization system. To inhibit microbial growth, WFI must be stored at either 5°C or 60°C to 90°C if it is to be held for over 24 hours.

The USP also lists sterile WFI and bacteriostatic WFI, which, unlike WFI, must be sterile. Higher levels of solids are allowed in these vehicles because of the possible leaching of glass constituents into the product during high-temperature sterilization and subsequent storage. Bacteriostatic WFI USP must not be placed in containers larger than 30 mL. This is to prevent the administration of large quantities of bacteriostatic agents (such as phenol) that could become toxic if large volumes of solution are administered. Other aqueous vehicles that may be used in place of sterile WFI or bacteriostatic WFI for reconstitution or administering drugs include dextrose (5%), sodium chloride (0.9%), and a variety of other electrolyte and nutrient solutions, as noted earlier.

Nonaqueous and Mixed Vehicles

A nonaqueous solvent or a mixed aqueous/nonaqueous solvent system may be necessary to stabilize drugs, such as the barbiturates, that are readily hydrolyzed by water, or to improve solubility (e.g., digitoxin). Nonaqueous solvents must be carefully screened and tested to ensure that they exhibit no pharmacological action, are nontoxic and nonirritating, and are compatible and stable with all ingredients of a formulation.

A major class of nonaqueous solvents is the fixed oils. The USP (1) recognizes the use of fixed oils as parenteral vehicles and lists their requirements. The most commonly used oils are corn oil, cottonseed oil, peanut oil, and sesame oil. Because fixed oils can be quite irritating when injected and may cause sensitivity reactions in some patients, the oil used in the product must be stated on the label.

Sesame oil is the preferred oil for most of the official injections in oil. This is because it is the most stable (except in light) and, thus, will usually meet the official requirements. Fixed oils must never be administered intravenously and are, in fact, restricted to IM use.

The USP usually does not specify any oil but states that a suitable vegetable oil can be used. The main use of such oils is with the steroids, with which they yield products that produce a sustained-release effect. So same oil has also been used to obtain slow release of fluphenazine esters given intramuscularly (14). Excessive unsaturation of oil can produce tissue irritation. The use of injections in oil has diminished somewhat in preference to aqueous suspensions, which generally have less irritating and sensitizing properties. Benzyl benzoate may be used to enhance steroid solubility in oils if desired.

Water-miscible solvents are widely used in parenterals to enhance drug solubility and to serve as stabilizers. The more common solvents include glycerin, ethyl alcohol, propylene glycol, and polyethylene glycol 300. Examples of injectable products formulated with nonaqueous solvents are diazepam injection USP and phenytoin sodium USP. Mixed solvent systems do not exhibit many of the disadvantages observed with the fixed oils, but may also be irritating or increase toxicity, especially when present in large amounts or in high concentrations. A solution containing a high percentage of ethanol will produce pain on injection.

The formulator should be aware of the potential of nonaqueous solvents in preparing a solubilized or stable product that may not have been otherwise possible. The reader is directed to comprehensive reviews of nonaqueous solvents for additional information (15,16).

Parenteral Dosage Forms

Solutions

Most injectable products are solutions. Solutions of drugs suitable for parenteral administration are referred to as *injections*. Although usually aqueous, they may be mixtures of water with glycols, alcohol, or other nonaqueous solvents. Many injectable solutions are manufactured by dissolving the drug and any excipients, adjusting the pH, sterile filtering the resultant solution through a 0.22-μm membrane filter, and, when possible, autoclaving the final product. Most solutions have a viscosity and surface tension very similar to water, although streptomycin sulfate injection and ascorbic acid injection, for example, are quite viscous.

Sterile filtration, with subsequent aseptic filling, is common because of the heat sensitivity of many drugs. Those drug solutions that can withstand heat should be terminally autoclave sterilized after filling, since this best assures product sterility.

LVPs and small-volume parenterals (SVPs) containing no antimicrobial agent should be terminally sterilized. It is common practice to include an antimicrobial agent in SVPs, which cannot be terminally sterilized or is intended for multiple-dose use. The general exceptions are products that pass the USP Antimicrobial Preservative Effectiveness Test (1) because of the antimicrobial activity of the active ingredient, vehicle, pH, or a combination of these. For example, some barbiturate products have a pH of 9 to 10 and a vehicle that includes propylene glycol and ethanol.

Injections and infusion fluids must be manufactured in a manner that will minimize or eliminate extraneous particulate matter. Parenteral solutions are generally filtered through 0.22-μm membrane filters to achieve sterility and remove particulate matter. Prefiltration through a coarser filter is often necessary to maintain adequate flow rates, or to prevent clogging of the filters during large-scale manufacturing. A talc or carbon filtration aid (or other filter aids) may also be necessary. If talc is used, it should be pretreated with a dilute acid solution to remove surface alkali and metals.

The formulator must be aware of the potential for binding when filtering protein solutions. Because of the cost of most protein materials, a membrane that minimizes protein adsorption to the membrane surface should be used. Typical filter media that minimize this binding include hydrophilic polyvinylidene difluoride and hydroxyl-modified hydrophilic polyamide membranes (17). Filter suppliers will evaluate the compatibility of the drug product with their membrane media and also validate bacterial retention of the selected membrane.

The total fluid volume that must be filled into a unit parenteral container is typically greater than the volume that would contain the exact labeled dose. The fill volume is dependent on the viscosity of the solution and the retention of the solution by the container and stopper. The USP provides a procedure for calculating the fill dose that is necessary to ensure the delivery of the stated dose. It also provides a table of excess volumes that are usually sufficient to permit withdrawal and administration of the labeled volume.

Suspensions

One of the most difficult parenteral dosage forms to formulate is a suspension. It requires a delicate balance of variables to formulate a product that is easily resuspended and can be ejected through an 18- to 21-gauge needle through its shelf life. To achieve these properties, it is necessary to select and carefully maintain particle size distribution, ζ-potential, and rheological properties, as well as the manufacturing steps that control wettability and surface tension. The requirements for, limitations in, and differences between the design of injectable suspensions and other suspensions have been previously summarized (18–20).

A formula for an injectable suspension might consist of the active ingredient suspended in an aqueous vehicle containing an antimicrobial preservative, a surfactant for wetting, a dispersing or suspending agent, and perhaps a buffer or salt.

Two basic methods are used to prepare parenteral suspensions: (*i*) sterile vehicle and powder are combined aseptically or (*ii*) sterile solutions are combined and the crystals formed in situ. Examples of these procedures may be illustrated using penicillin G procaine injectable suspension USP and sterile testosterone injectable suspension USP.

In the first example, procaine penicillin, an aqueous vehicle containing the soluble components (such as lecithin, sodium citrate, povidone, and polyoxyethylene sorbitan monooleate) is filtered through a 0.22-μm membrane filter, heat sterilized, and transferred into a presterilized mixing-filling tank. The sterile antibiotic powder, which has previously been produced by freeze-drying, sterile crystallization, or spray-drying is aseptically added to the sterile solution while mixing. After all tests have been completed on the bulk formulation, it is aseptically filled.

An example of the second method of parenteral suspension preparation is testosterone suspension. Here, the vehicle is prepared and sterile filtered. The testosterone is dissolved separately in acetone and sterile filtered. The testosterone-acetone solution is aseptically added to the sterile vehicle, causing the testosterone to crystallize. The resulting suspension is then diluted with sterile vehicle, mixed, the crystals allowed to settle, and the supernatant solution siphoned off. This procedure is repeated several times until all the acetone has been removed. The suspension is then brought to volume and filled in the normal manner.

The critical nature of the flow properties of parenteral suspensions becomes apparent when one remembers that these products are frequently administered through 1-in. or longer needles having internal diameters in the range of only 300 to 600 µm. In addition, microscopic examination shows a very rough interior needle surface, further hindering flow. The flow properties of parenteral suspensions are usually characterized on the basis of *syringeability* or injectability. The term "syringeability" refers to the handling characteristics of a suspension while drawing it into and manipulating it in a syringe. Syringeability includes characteristics such as ease of withdrawal from the container into the syringe, clogging and foaming tendencies, and accuracy of dose measurement. The term "injectability" refers to the properties of the suspension during injection; it includes such factors as pressure or force required for injection, evenness of flow, aspiration qualities, and freedom from clogging. The syringeability and injectability characteristics of a suspension are closely related to viscosity and particle characteristics.

Emulsions

An emulsion is a dispersion of one immiscible liquid in another. This inherently unstable system is made possible through the use of an emulsifying agent, which prevents coalescence of the dispersed droplets. Parenteral emulsions have been used for several purposes, including (*i*) w/o emulsions of allergenic extracts (given subcutaneously) and (*ii*) o/w sustained-release depot preparations (given intramuscularly). Formulation options are severely restricted through a very limited selection of stabilizers and emulsifiers, primarily owing to the dual constraints of autoclave sterilization and parenteral injection. Additionally, unwanted physiological effects (e.g., pyrogenic reaction and hemolysis) have further limited the use of IV emulsions.

An increasingly popular class of IV emulsions is lipid emulsions. These preparations have been available in Europe and the United States for over 25 years. Fat is transported in the bloodstream as small droplets called chylomicra. Chylomicra are 0.5 to 1.0 µm spheres consisting of a central core of triglycerides and an outer layer of phospholipids. IV fat emulsions usually contain 10% oil, although they may range up to 20% (Table 3). These emulsions yield triglycerides that provide essential fatty acids and calories during total parenteral nutrition of patients who are unable to absorb nutrients through the gastrointestinal tract. The products commercially available in the United States range from 0.1 to 0.5 µm and have a pH of 5.5 to 8 (blood plasma has a pH of 7.4). Glycerol is commonly added to make the product isotonic. IV lipid emulsions are usually administered in combination with dextrose and amino acids. Drugs are generally not added to these admixtures, with common exceptions being heparin, insulin, and ranitidine.

Dry Powders

Many drugs are too unstable—physically or chemically—in an aqueous medium to allow formulation as a solution, suspension, or emulsion. Instead, the drug is formulated as a dry powder that is reconstituted by addition of water before administration. The reconstituted product is usually an aqueous solution; however, occasionally it may be an aqueous suspension (e.g., ampicillin trihydrate and spectinomycin hydrochloride are sterile powders that are reconstituted to form a sterile suspension).

Table 3 IV Fat Emulsions Composition in % (w/v)

Component (g/100 mL)	Intralipid[a]		Liposyn II[b]		Infonutrol[c]		Lipofundin[d]	Liphysan[e]	
	10%	20%	10%	20%	10%	20%	10%	10%	15%
Soybean oil	10	20	5	10					
Safflower oil			5	10					
Cottonseed oil					15	10		10	15
Egg phospholipids	1.2	1.2	1.2	1.2					
Soybean phospholipids					1.2		1.2		
Soybean lecithin								1.5	2
Glycerol	2.25	2.25	2.25	2.25					
Glucose					4				
Sorbitol							5	5	5
piuronic F-68					0.3				
DL-α-Tocopherol								0.05	0.05
WFI, q.s.	100 mL		100 mL		100 mL	100 mL		100 mL	

[a] Kabi-Vitrum A.G., Stockolm, Sweden.
[b] Abbott Laboratories, North Chicago, Illinois, U.S.
[c] Astra-Hewlett, Sodertaye, Sweden.
[d] Braun, Melsunger, West Germany.
[e] Egic, L, Equilibre Biologique S.A., Loiret, France.
Abbreviations: IV, intravenous; WFI, water for injection.

Dry powders for reconstitution as an injectable product may be produced by several methods: filling the product into vials as a liquid and freeze-drying, aseptic crystallization followed by powder filling, and spray-drying followed by powder filling. A brief discussion of each follows.

Freeze-drying The most common form of sterile powder is freeze-dried or lyophilized powder. The advantages of freeze-drying are that (*i*) water can be removed at low temperature, avoiding damage to heat-sensitive materials; (*ii*) if freeze-drying is done properly, the dried product has a high specific surface area, which facilitates rapid, complete rehydration (or "reconstitution") of the solid, and (*iii*) from an operations point of view, freeze-dried dosage forms allow drug to be filled into vials as a solution. This makes control of the quantity filled into each vial more precise than filling drug into vials as a powder. In addition, since drug is filled as a solution, there is minimal concern with dust containment, cross-contamination, and potential worker exposure to hazardous drugs.

Despite the advantages of freeze-drying, some limitations must be kept in mind.

1. Some drugs, particularly biological systems such as proteins, liposomal systems, and vaccines, are damaged by freezing, freeze-drying, or both. Although the damage can often be minimized by using protective agents in the formulation, the problem is still substantial.

2. Often the stability of a drug in the solid state depends on its physical state [i.e., crystalline or amorphous (8)]. If freeze-drying produces an amorphous solid and

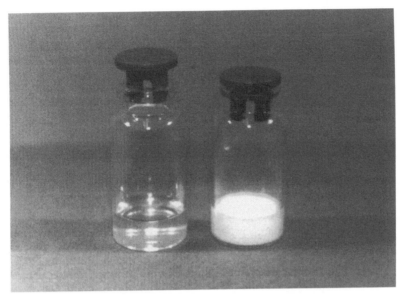

Figure 3 Vials typically used for lyophilization showing slotted stopper in the open and closed positions.

the amorphous form is not stable, then freeze-drying will not provide an acceptable product.
3. Freeze-drying is a relatively expensive drying operation. Although this is not an issue for many high-cost drug products, it can be an issue for more cost-sensitive products.

In freeze-drying, a solution is filled into vials, a special slotted stopper is partially inserted into the neck of the vial (Fig. 3), and trays of filled vials are transferred to the freeze-dryer. The solution is frozen by circulation of a fluid, such as silicone oil, at a temperature in the range of $-35°$ C to about $-45°$C through internal channels in the shelf assembly. When the product has solidified sufficiently, the pressure in the freeze-dry chamber is reduced to a pressure less than the vapor pressure of ice at the temperature of the product, and heat is applied to the product by increasing the temperature of the circulating fluid. Under these conditions, water is removed by sublimation of ice, or a phase change from the solid state directly to the vapor state without the appearance of an intermediate liquid phase. The phase diagram in Figure 4 illustrates the difference between freeze-drying and conventional drying methods, during which drying takes place by a phase change from the liquid state to the vapor state. Freeze-drying takes place below the triple point of water, at which solid, liquid, and vapor all coexist in equilibrium. As freeze-drying proceeds, a receding boundary can be observed in the vial as the thickness of the frozen layer decreases. This phase is called *primary drying*, during which ice is removed by direct sublimation through open channels created by prior sublimation of ice. After primary drying, additional drying is necessary to remove any water that did not freeze during the freezing process, but instead remained associated with the solute. This is called *secondary drying*, and consists of water removal by diffusion and desorption of water from the partially dried solid phase. The phases of a typical freeze-dry cycle—freezing, primary drying, and secondary drying—are illustrated by means of a plot of shelf temperature, chamber pressure, and product temperature in Figure 5.

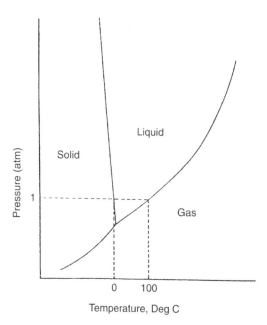

Figure 4 Phase diagram of water.

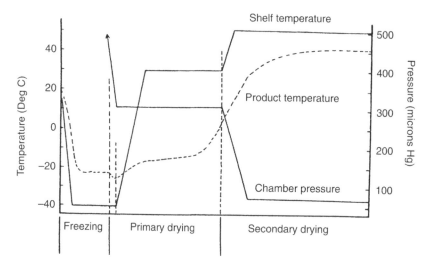

Figure 5 Process variables during a representative freeze-dry cycle.

The most important objective in developing a freeze-dried product is to assure that critical quality attributes are met initially and throughout the shelf life of the product. Examples of critical quality attributes are recovery of original chemical or biological activity after reconstitution, rapid and complete dissolution, appropriate residual moisture level, and acceptable cake appearance. In addition, process conditions should be chosen to maximize process efficiency, that is, those conditions that minimize drying time without adversely affecting product quality. The driving force for sublimation is the vapor pressure of ice, and the vapor pressure of ice is highly temperature-dependent, as shown below:

Temperature (°C)	Vapor pressure (mmHg)
−40	0.096
−30	0.286
−20	0.776
−10	1.950
0	4.579

Therefore, freeze-drying should be carried out at the highest allowable product temperature that maintains the appropriate attributes of a freeze-dried product. This temperature depends on the nature of the formulation. Process development and validation requires characterizing the physical state of the solute, or solutes, that result from the freezing process and identifying a maximum allowable product temperature for the primary drying process (21,22).

The term "eutectic temperature" is often misused in reference to freeze-drying. A eutectic mixture—an intimate mixture of ice and crystals of solute that melts as if it were a single, pure compound—is present only if the solute crystallizes when the solution is frozen. Eutectic melting can often be detected by thermal analysis, such as differential scanning calorimetry (DSC) (23,24). An example of a eutectic system is neutral glycine in water. The presence of a eutectic mixture is indicated by a melting endotherm in the DSC thermogram of the solution (Fig. 6) in addition to the melting endotherm for ice. In this example, the theoretical maximum allowable product temperature during primary drying is the eutectic melting temperature at −3.5°C. In practice, the product temperature should be maintained a few degrees below this temperature to assure that melting does not occur

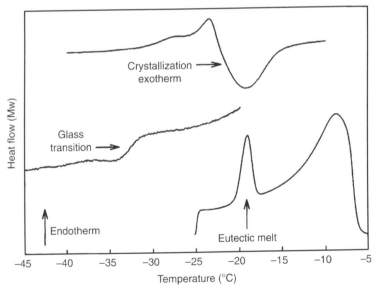

Figure 6 DSC thermograms showing representative thermal transitions in frozen solutions. The top thermogram is for a mannitol solution and is characteristic of a metastable glass-forming system. *Abbreviation*: DSC, differential scanning calorimetry.

during the process. Examples of some other common solutes that form eutectics, along with the eutectic temperature, are as follows (24):

Solute	Eutectic temperature (°C)
Calcium chloride	−51.0
Citric acid	−12.2
Mannitol	−1.0
Potassium chloride	−10.7
Sodium carbonate	−18.0
Sodium chloride	−21.5
Sodium phosphate, dibasic	−0.5

However, many solutes do not crystallize during the freezing process, but instead form a glassy mixture with unfrozen water. Examples include sugars, such as sucrose, lactose, and maltose, polymers, and many drugs. In this case, no eutectic mixture is formed. Instead, the freeze concentrate becomes more concentrated and viscous as the temperature decreases, and ice crystals grow. This process continues until a temperature is reached at which the viscosity of the freeze concentrate increases dramatically with only a small change in temperature, and ice crystal growth ceases on a practical time scale. This temperature is a glass transition temperature (called T'_g) and is an important characteristic of amorphous systems. Below the glass transition temperature, the freeze concentrate exists as a rigid glass. Above the glass transition temperature, the freeze concentrate behaves as a viscous liquid. The significance of the glass transition temperature of the freeze concentrate is that it is closely related to the *collapse temperature* in freeze-drying. If drying is carried out above the collapse temperature, the freeze concentrate will flow and lose the microstructure established by freezing once the supporting structure of ice crystals is removed. Collapse can be observed in a variety of forms, from a slight shrinkage of the dried cake (where the cake has pulled away from the wall of the vial) to total loss of any cake structure. An example of collapse is shown in Figure 7.

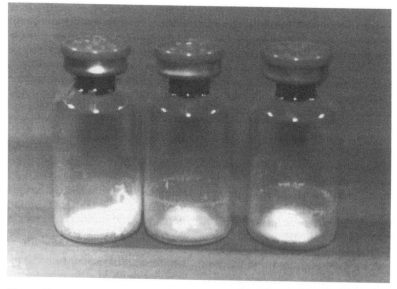

Figure 7 Collapse is characteristic of amorphous materials and can occur either during the freeze-dry process or during storage.

The glass transition of solutes that remain amorphous during and after the freezing process can often be seen in the DSC thermo gram as a shift in the baseline toward higher heat capacity. This is illustrated in the DSC thermogram of sucrose solution in Figure 6, in which the glass transition is observed at $-34^\circ C$ glass transition (T'_g) values of some other solutes common to freeze-drying are as follows (25):

Solute	Glass transition (T'_g)
Dextran	-9
Gelatin	-10
Glucose	-43
Lactose	-32
Maltose	-32
Polyvinylpyrrolidone	-24
Sorbitol	-48

Some solutes may form a metastable amorphous phase initially on freezing, and then crystallize when the material is heated. Mannitol, a common bulking agent in freeze-dried formulations, is an example of a solute that can, depending on the cooling rate during freezing, form a metastable amorphous system initially, then crystallize from the glass as the system is heated to above the glass transition temperature of the freeze concentrate. The DSC thermogram of a frozen mannitol solution is shown in Figure 6, where the exotherm indicates crystallization. Crystallization of mannitol during heating is believed to be the underlying cause of vial breakage in mannitol-based formulations (25).

Solutes that form metastable glassy systems upon freezing can sometimes be induced to crystallize by *thermal treatment,* or *annealing,* in the freeze-dry process. The product is first frozen to perhaps $-4^\circ C$, then heated to a temperature above the glass transition temperature, held for a few hours, and then cooled before starting the drying process. Some cephalosporins have been shown to crystallize during annealing steps (26). In addition, annealing has been shown to improve both the rate and the vial-to-vial uniformity of primary drying (27).

In general, crystallization of the solute is desirable in terms of freeze-drying properties, as well as quality attributes of the final product, for several reasons. First, when the solute crystallizes, nearly all the water is present as ice in the frozen matrix, and it is removed by direct sublimation during primary drying. Therefore, there is little water to be removed by secondary drying. This improves process efficiency, since water removed during secondary drying must be removed primarily by the process of diffusion, rather than by bulk flow. Second, eutectic temperatures are usually higher than collapse temperatures, which allows higher product temperatures and more efficient drying. Eutectic temperatures of most organic compounds are in the range of $-1^\circ C$ to about $-12^\circ C$, whereas collapse temperatures commonly are $-30^\circ C$ or lower. Third, the chemical and physical stability of a compound in crystalline form is generally better than that of the same compound in an amorphous form (8,28). This can be a critical aspect of determining the feasibility of a freeze-dried dosage form.

While crystallinity of a drug is generally desirable for freeze-drying, it is often important for excipients to remain amorphous. In particular, disaccharides (such as sucrose and trehalose) are important as formulation additives to stabilize proteins against damage caused by freezing, freeze-drying, or both. However, to be effective stabilizers, it is essential for these compounds to remain amorphous both during freeze-drying and during subsequent storage.

An understanding of the effect of formulation on freeze-drying behavior is important to the pharmaceutical scientist involved in the development of freeze-dried products. Mixtures of components should be expected to behave differently from single-component systems. For example, a compound that crystallizes readily from aqueous solution when it is the only solute present may not crystallize at all when other solutes are present. For solutes that remain amorphous on freezing, the glass transition temperature is affected by the presence of other solutes. Subtle variations in the composition of the formulation, such as changes in ionic strength or pH, may have a significant effect on the physical chemistry of the freezing and freeze-drying processes.

Many drugs are present in a dose too small to form a well-defined freeze-dried cake, and must be formulated with a *bulking agent,* the purpose of which is to provide a dried matrix in which the active ingredient is dispersed. Common bulking agents are mannitol, lactose, glycine, and mixtures of these compounds. Buffers are commonly used, such as sodium or potassium phosphate, acetate, citrate, tris-hydroxymethyl-aminomethane (THAM), or histidine. Formulations of proteins, liposomes, or cells generally require the presence of a *protectant*, or a substance that protects the active compound from damage by freezing, drying, or both. Disaccharides, such as sucrose and trehalose, are, in general, the most effective protectants (29). The use of maltose and lactose, also disaccharides, should be approached with caution, since they are both reducing sugars.

In addition to the effects of formulation factors on freeze-drying behavior, it is important for the pharmaceutical scientist to understand basic principles of heat and mass transfer in freeze-drying (30,31). Because of the high heat input required for sublimation (670 cal/g), transfer of heat from the heated shelf to the sublimation front is often the rate-limiting step in the coupled heat and mass transfer process. There are three basic mechanisms for heat transfer: conduction, convection, and radiation. *Conduction* is the transfer of heat by molecular motion between differential volume elements of a material. *Convection* is the transfer of heat by bulk flow of a fluid, either from density differences (natural convection) or because an external force is applied (forced convection). Because of the relatively low pressures used in freeze-drying, convection is probably not a large contributing factor in heat transfer. Heat transfer by *thermal radiation* arises when a substance, because of thermal excitation, emits radiation in an amount determined by its absolute temperature. Of these mechanisms, heat transfer by conduction is the most important. It takes place through a series of resistances—the bottom of the vial, the frozen layer of product, the metal tray (if used), and the vapor phase caused by lack of good thermal contact between the vial and the shelf. The thermal conductivity of the vapor phase at the pressures used in freeze-drying is dependent on pressure in the chamber. Therefore, to maintain consistent drying conditions from batch to batch, it is as important to control the chamber pressure as to control shelf temperature (32). In addition, changes in the geometry of the system that affect heat transfer will also affect process consistency. Examples include changing from molded to tubing vials, changing the depth of fill in the vials, and changing from trays with metal bottoms to those without bottoms. Thermal radiation is a small, but significant, contributor to the total quantity of heat transferred to the product. This can be a significant issue in scale-up of cycles from pilot dryers to production-scale equipment.

Mass transfer in freeze-drying refers to the transfer of water vapor from the sublimation front through open channels in the partially dried layer, created by prior sublimation of ice, through the headspace of the vial, past the lyostopper, through the chamber, to the condenser.

The reader is referred to basic studies of mass transfer in freeze-drying by Pikal et al. for in-depth treatment of the theoretical and practical aspects of mass transfer

(30,33). Briefly, the rate-limiting step in mass transfer is transfer of water vapor through the partially dried matrix of solids. Resistance of the dried layer increases in a more or less continuous fashion as the depth of the dried layer increases, and the resistance also increases with the concentration of solids in the dried layer. Other factors can also affect the resistance of the dried layer, such as the method of freezing; faster freezing tends to create a higher resistance in the dried layer.

Mass transfer of the "unfrozen" water through a glassy phase during secondary drying occurs more slowly than bulk flow of water vapor by direct sublimation, since no open channels are present in the glassy phase. The high resistance of the solid material to mass transfer is why secondary drying can be the most time-consuming phase of the freeze-dry cycle for amorphous solutes containing a large percentage of unfrozen water. According to studies reported by Pikal et al., shelf temperature is the most critical process variable affecting the rate of secondary drying and final moisture level (33). Chamber pressure has no measurable influence on secondary drying kinetics.

The quantity of residual water is frequently a critical product characteristic relative to chemical and physical stability of freeze-dried products, particularly amorphous solids. Water acts as a plasticizer of the solid material, lowering the glass transition temperature. A low glass transition temperature relative to the storage temperature can result in physical instability, such as cake shrinkage or collapse, or accelerated rates of chemical reactions leading to instability. Often a small change in moisture content can result in a large change in the glass transition temperature; therefore, careful consideration of appropriate limits on residual moisture is often an important part of the product development process.

Aseptic crystallization and dry powder filling Aseptic crystallization is primarily used for manufacture of sterile aqueous suspensions. However, if the physical form of the drug is critical to quality of the final product, better control over physical form can be attained by aseptic crystallization, because a large variety of organic solvents can be used to control the crystallization process. In aseptic crystallization, the drug is dissolved in a suitable solvent, and sterile filtered through an appropriate membrane filter. A second solvent—a sterility filtered nonsolvent for the drug—is then added at a controlled rate, causing crystallization and precipitation of the drug. The crystals are collected on a funnel, washed if necessary, and dried by vacuum drying. After drying, it may be necessary to mill or blend the drug crystals. The powder is then transferred to dry powder–filling equipment and filled into vials. Although simple in principle, there are obvious drawbacks to this approach. Batch-to-batch variability in crystal habit and crystal size and the resulting variability in physical properties can be troublesome for consistent product quality. Maintenance of asepsis between sterile crystallization and filling of the powder is a challenge during material handling and will usually result in decreased sterility assurance. Also, since the drug is filled into vials as a powder, maintenance of fill weight uniformity is generally more troublesome than when filling with a liquid.

Spray-drying A solution of drug is sterile filtered and metered into the drying chamber, where it passes through an atomizer that creates an aerosol of small droplets of liquid (Fig. 8). The aerosol comes into contact with a stream of hot sterile gas—usually air. The solvent evaporates quickly, allowing drug to be collected as a powder in the form of uniform hollow spheres. The powder is then filled into vials using conventional powder-filling equipment. Spray-drying may be more economical than freeze-drying, but challenges in the use of this technique include sterile filtration of very large volumes of air, constructing and maintaining a spray dryer that can be readily sterilized, aseptic

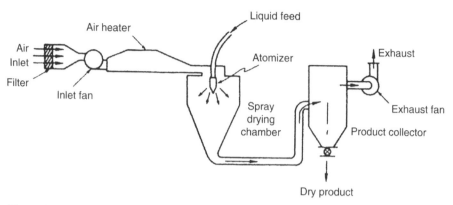

Figure 8 Schematic drawing of spray dryer.

transfer of powder from the spray dryer to the powder-filling line, and precise control of the drying conditions to prevent overheating of the product while providing adequate drying. Probably because of these limitations, the technique is not widely used.

Protein Formulations

The first biotechnology-derived therapeutic agent to be approved by the Food and Drug Administration (FDA) in the United States was human insulin (Humulin®, Eli Lilly and Company, Indianapolis, Indiana, U.S.) in 1982. The number of such products has grown steadily since then. This growth is expected to continue during the next decade. Because biotechnology-derived pharmaceuticals are generally proteins and glycoproteins, they require special consideration in formulation and processing.

Special problems with formulation and processing of proteins arise from the hierarchy of structural organization of proteins. In addition to primary structure (the amino acid sequence), proteins have secondary structure (interactions between peptide bonds, resulting in helical or sheetlike structures), tertiary structure (folding of chain segments into a precise three-dimensional arrangement), and, in some, quaternary structure (association of individual protein subunits into a multimeric structure). Disruption of this higher-order structure can lead to loss of the biologically active, or native conformation, which, in turn, causes physical instability, which may accelerate reactions that are characteristic of chemical instability of proteins.

Loss of the native conformation of a protein generally exposes hydrophobic amino acid residues that are normally buried on the inside of the self-associated structure and are shielded from the aqueous environment. This leads to association between the exposed hydrophobic residues of neighboring proteins (aggregation) or between these exposed residues and hydrophobic surfaces that the protein may encounter either in the manufacturing process or in the primary package.

Seemingly subtle aspects of processing may be critical in manufacturing pharmaceutical dosage forms of proteins. For example, vigorous agitation of a protein solution can cause foaming, generating a large air/water interface that is an excellent site for denaturation, aggregation, and perhaps precipitation of protein. Loss of protein by adsorption to surfaces, such as tubing and filters used in manufacturing, can result in subpotent product. Other potentially critical factors in maintenance of the native structure during processing include temperature, pH, the presence of organic solvents, and ionic strength of the formulation.

Disruption of the native structure of a protein can also contribute to chemical instability by accelerating the rates of a variety of degradation routes, including deamidation, hydrolysis, oxidation, disulfide exchange, β-elimination, and racemization.

Formulation strategies for stabilization of proteins commonly include additives such as other proteins (e.g., serum albumin), amino acids, and surfactants to minimize adsorption to surfaces. Modification of protein structure to enhance stability by genetic engineering may also be feasible, as well as chemical modification such as formation of a conjugate with polyethylene glycol.

Most proteins are not sufficiently stable in aqueous solution to allow formulation as a sterile solution. Instead, the protein is freeze dried and reconstituted before use. Development of a freeze-dried protein formulation often requires special attention to the details of the freezing process (potential pH shifts and ionic strength increase with freezing) as well as to potential loss of activity with drying. Formulation additives, such as sugars and polyhydroxy compounds, are often useful as cryoprotectants and lyoprotectants. Residual moisture may also be critical to the stability of the dried preparation (34).

Novel Formulations

A summary of sustained- and controlled-release parenteral dosage forms is included in volume 2, chapter 1. This subject is also covered extensively by Chien (35).

Concepts in drug delivery that have received increasing attention include drug carrier systems, implants, IV infusers, and implantable infusion pumps. Carrier systems include microspheres, liposomes, monoclonal antibodies, and emulsions. Drugs are incorporated into these systems to increase the duration of drug action, and to provide selective delivery of the drug to a specific target site or organ. Implants are used for the same reason. Unwanted side effects and adverse reactions are usually reduced because of selective delivery, which also results in a lower concentration of drug required to achieve the desired therapeutic effect. Infusion pumps provide a delivery system with uniform, continuous flow. A specific dose of a drug, such as insulin, may be administered to a patient on a continual or intermittent basis.

PACKAGING

Container components for parenteral products must be considered an integral part of the product because they can dramatically affect product stability, potency, toxicity, and safety. Parenteral dosage forms, especially solutions, usually require more detailed evaluation of packaging components for product compatibility and stability than do other pharmaceutical dosage forms. Common container components in direct contact with the product include various types of glass, rubber, plastic, and stainless steel (needles), all of which may react with the drug. Maintenance of microbiological purity and product stability, adaptability to production operations and inspections, resistance to breakage and leakage, and convenience of clinical use are factors that must be evaluated when selecting the container.

Parenteral packaging includes ampoules, rubber-stoppered vials and bottles, plastic bags and bottles, glass and plastic syringes, and syringe-vial combinations. Glass containers have traditionally achieved widespread acceptability for parenteral products because of their relative inertness. In recent years, hospital preference for unit-dose and clinical convenience has resulted in an increase in products packaged in disposable syringes and the development of polyvinyl chloride, polyester, and polyolefin plastic containers for IV fluids. Package systems, such as dual chamber plastic containers and Add-Vantage, have been developed for combining unstable mixtures of drugs and solutions. Several antibiotics that are unstable in solution are now available as frozen products in plastic containers. All these systems are designed for convenience and cost efficiency as well as minimizing the potential of contamination when preparing the admixture. Parenteral packaging materials are discussed in chapter 17.

STABILITY

A formal stability program is needed to assure that all critical attributes of any drug product are maintained throughout the shelf life of the product. A validated stability-indicating assay is essential to measure chemical or biological activity, and acceptance criteria should be established before initiating stability studies. Particular attention should be given to developing a detailed protocol for a stability study before preparing stability samples, including assays to be performed, storage conditions, and sampling intervals.

In general, expiration dating is based on the estimated time required for the active compound to reach 90% to 95% of labeled potency at the specified storage temperature. However, other considerations may limit the shelf life of the product. For example, the shelf life of products containing a preservative may be determined by adsorption of preservative to a rubber closure or another elastomeric component of the container-closure system. The drug substance itself may be subject to physical instability such as adsorption. The stability program should include placing enough units at the specified storage conditions to allow inspection of a statistically valid number of units to verify acceptable appearance of the product, such as the development of haze or discreet particulate matter in solution products, as well as to check for discoloration or any other physical attribute that would result in unacceptable pharmaceutical elegance. Formulation pH is often a critical attribute that must be monitored during a stability study, since pH may be affected both by chemical reactions in solution or by interactions between the formulation and the container-closure system.

Sterile powders may require special attention to identify which tests are required to assure adequate physical and chemical stability. The stability of many dried products is often sensitive to small differences in the amount of residual water present, requiring monitoring of residual moisture by Karl Fisher titration or loss on drying. This is particularly important for protein formulations. Special efforts may be needed to minimize the residual moisture in rubber stoppers, since water vapor can transfer from the closure to the powder during prolonged storage. Reconstitution time—the amount of time required after addition of diluent until all solids are dissolved—should be measured routinely. For freeze-dried products, cake shrinkage with time is not uncommon. This may be accompanied by discoloration, increased reconstitution time, or crystallization of one or more components of the formulation. The physical state of the drug—crystalline or amorphous—has an important influence on stability, particularly for cephalosporins. Periodic examination of stability samples by X-ray diffraction may be valuable to identify changes in physical state of either drug or excipients that could influence critical quality attributes. For some solid dosage forms subject to oxidative degradation, it is critical to exclude oxygen from the vial headspace. The headspace of selected vials should be analyzed periodically for oxygen. Many freeze-dried powders are stoppered under vacuum or an inert gas. Testing selected vials during the stability study for presence of vacuum in the headspace of the vial is a useful method of verifying container-closure integrity.

Sterile suspensions can be challenging with respect to physical stability, and this should be reflected in the stability protocol. Examples of physical stability issues for suspensions include (*i*) caking, which causes poor resuspendability; (*ii*) changes in the particle size distribution, particularly growth of large crystals of drug, which can cause poor syringeability; and (*iii*) polymorphic transformations, which can result in changes in dissolution characteristics and, therefore, the bioavailability of the drug.

For parenteral emulsions, the formulation scientist must be particularly aware of changes in particle size distribution of the oil phase. Droplet coalescence results in increased droplet size. As a general rule, average droplet size should be less than 1 μm. Droplet sizes of more than 6 μm can cause blockage of capillaries (capillary emboli).

STERILIZATION METHODS

Five sterilization processes are described in the USP: steam, dry heat, filtration, gas, and ionizing radiation. All are commonly used for parenteral products, except gas and ionizing radiation, which are widely used for devices and surgical materials. To assist in the selection of the sterilization method, certain basic information and data must be gathered. This includes determining (*i*) the nature and amount of product bioburden and (*ii*) whether the product and container-closure system will have a predominantly moist or dry environment during sterilization. Both these factors are of critical importance in determining the conditions (time and temperature) of any sterilization method chosen.

The natural bioburden in a well-maintained pharmaceutical parenteral manufacturing plant is quite low, often to the point that it is difficult to isolate and propagate plant bioburden for sterilization studies. Nevertheless, it is still important to characterize the microbiological bioburden in the process, and then monitor it at regular intervals.

For sterilization purposes, microorganisms can be categorized into three general categories: (*i*) easy to kill with either dry or moist heat, (*ii*) susceptible to moist heat but resistant to dry heat (e.g., *Bacillus subtilis*), or (*iii*) resistant to moist heat but susceptible to dry heat (e.g., *Clostridium sporogenes*). Organisms such as *B. subtilis* and *C. sporogenes* are often used as biological indicators because they are spore formers of known heat resistance. When used in a known concentration, they will be killed at a reproducible rate. In this manner, when a product has a low bioburden, biological indicator organisms can be used at a concentration of 1×10^3 in kill studies to simulate 10^6 kills of natural (environmental) bioburden. Processing and design of container-closure systems for individual products must be reviewed carefully to ascertain whether moist or dry conditions predominate, particularly in difficult-to-reach inner portions of closures. The use of biological indicators in validating parenteral container-closure systems has been reviewed by Akers and Anderson (36).

The USP also recommends the use of biological indicators, whenever possible, to monitor all sterilization methods except sterile filtration. Biological indicators are generally of two types. If a product to be sterilized is a liquid, microorganisms are added directly to carefully identified representative samples of the product. When this is not practical, as with solids or equipment to be sterilized, the culture is added to strips of filter paper. The organism chosen varies with the method of sterilization.

Sterilization tests are performed to verify that an adequate sterilization process has been carried out. Validation of the sterilization cycle also gives assurance of process integrity. Sterility is not assured simply because a product passes the USP sterility test. As outlined in the USP, the sterility test is described in considerable detail, including procedures for sampling, general conditions of the test, and specific procedures for testing solids and liquids. In addition, guidelines for the design of an aseptic work environment are outlined in some detail. Sample limitations, plus the impossibility of cultivating and testing all viable microorganisms that may be present, affect the reliability of sterility tests. Because of these problems, it is necessary to monitor and test sterilization equipment continuously. The reader is referred to Akers and Anderson for a review of validation of sterile products (36).

Sterilization by Steam

When drug solutions and containers can withstand autoclaving conditions, this method is preferred to other sterilization methods because moist heat sterilizes quickly and inexpensively. However, judgment must be exercised, and experiments run to ensure that the solution and container are permeable to steam. Oils and tightly closed containers, for example, are not normally sterilizable by steam.

Autoclave steam sterilization is a well-established and widely used procedure. Normally, steam enters through the top of the chamber (Fig. 9). Being lighter than air, it remains at the top of the chamber, but steadily and continuously drives the air out of the chamber through the bottom vent throughout the sterilization cycle. The velocity of steam entering the autoclave, the efficiency of water separation from incoming steam, the size of the drain, and the amount of vacuum applied are all factors that must be controlled to obtain efficient and reproducible steam sterilization in an autoclave. The reader is referred to a review by Leuthner (37) for a more thorough discussion of the theory and practice of steam sterilization.

With the widespread use of flexible packaging for LVP products, the use of steam sterilization has increased. Compared with the traditional LVP glass bottles closed with rubber stoppers, flexible LVP plastic containers (polyvinyl chloride, polyester, or polyolefin) offer autoclaving advantages. Specifically (*i*) a larger surface area is available for heating per unit volume of liquid; (*ii*) if held in a "flattened" position during

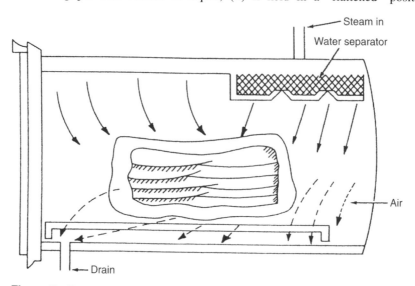

Figure 9 Gravity displacement steam sterilizer.

sterilization, the heat penetration depth required is reduced, resulting in a more uniform thermal mapping of the contents; and (*iii*) shorter heat-up and cooldown periods are required. The net effect is to allow a much shorter sterilization cycle for LVP products packaged in flexible containers, thus exposing the product to less heat, less potential for degradation, and reduced manufacturing costs.

Sterilization by Dry Heat

Dry heat is widely used to sterilize glassware and equipment parts in manufacturing areas for parenteral products. It has good penetration power and is not as corrosive as steam. However, heat-up time is slow, necessitating long sterilization periods at high temperatures. It is important to allow sufficient circulation around the materials to be sterilized. Metal cans are often used to contain the parts or containers that are to be sterilized.

The two principal methods of dry-heat sterilization are infrared and convection hot air. Infrared rays will sterilize only surfaces. Sterilization of interior portions must rely on conduction. Convection hot-air sterilizers are normally heated electrically and are of two types: gravity or mechanical. In gravity convection units, a fan is used to promote uniformity of heat distribution throughout the chamber.

Dry-heat processes kill microorganisms primarily through oxidation. The amount of moisture available to assist sterilization in dry-heat units varies considerably at different locations within the chamber and at different time intervals within the cycle. Also, the amount of heat available, its diffusion, and the environment at the spore/air interface all influence the microorganism kill rate. Consequently, cycles tend to be longer and hotter than would be expected from calculations to ensure that varying conditions do not invalidate a run. In general, convection dry-heat sterilization cycles are run above 160°C (38).

Sterilization by Ethylene Oxide

Ethylene oxide (ETO), a colorless gas, is widely used as a sterilant in hospitals and industry for items that cannot be sterilized by steam. It is often diluted with carbon dioxide, or sometimes fluorocarbons, to overcome its flammable and explosive nature. The mechanism by which ETO kills microorganisms is by alkylation of various reactive groups in the spore or vegetative cell. One of the more resistant organisms to ETO is *B. subtilis* var *niger* (*globigii*). It is the USP biological indicator for monitoring the effectiveness of ETO sterilization cycles. Several factors are important in determining whether ETO is effective as a sterilizing gas: gas concentration, temperature, humidity, spore water content, and substrate for the microorganisms. ETO should be present at a concentration of about 500 mL/L for maximum effectiveness. Once gas concentration is not a limiting factor, the inactivation rate of spores by ETO doubles for each 10°C rise in temperature. Relative humidity plays an important role in that the sensitivity of spores to ETO largely depends on the water content of the spore.

A "typical" ETO sterilization cycle is shown in Figure 10. As discussed at the beginning of this section, it is important to determine and monitor the bioburden level of the product entering the sterilizer. Also, the load configuration in the sterilizer is important in achieving uniform and reliable sterilization. Unfortunately, commercially available biological indicators used in ETO sterilization are often unreliable. Hopefully, progress will be made in this field in the years ahead.

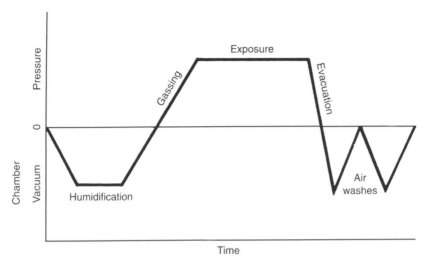

Figure 10 ETO sterilization cycle. *Abbreviation*: ETO, Ethylene Oxide.

Unlike other methods, it is necessary to posttreat the product, either through vacuum purging or by allowing the product to remain at ambient conditions for a time, to allow removal of residual ETO and ethylene chlorhydrin/ethylene glycol by-products before use by the consumer. In addition, in 1984 the U.S. Occupational Safety and Health Agency (OSHA) lowered the maximum permissible operator eight-hour exposure level from 50 to 1 ppm in air (on a time-weighted average) (39).

Sterilization by Filtration

Only in the past 30 years filters have become sufficiently reliable to use them on a wide scale to sterilize injectable solutions. Even now it is prudent to use filtration to sterilize only those products that cannot be terminally sterilized.

Filters are of two basic types: depth and membrane. Depth filters rely on a combination of tortuous pathway and adsorption to retain particles or microorganisms. They are made from materials such as diatomaceous earth, inorganic fibers, natural fibers, and porcelain. They carry a nominal rating, that is, a particle size above which a certain percentage of particles is retained. The major advantage of depth filters is their ability to retain large quantities of particles, including many below the nominal rating of the particular filter. Disadvantages of depth filters include grow-through and reproduction of microorganisms, tendency of the filter components to slough during line surges, and retention of some liquid in the filter. Membrane filters rely on sieving and, to a lesser degree, absorption to prevent particles from passing. Although all pores in a membrane filter are not of the same size, nevertheless, the filter can retain all particles larger than the stated size.

Similar to depth filters, membrane filters are made from a variety of materials, although filters made from cellulose ester derivatives are by far the most common. The advantages of membrane filters include no retention of product, no media migration, and efficiency independent of flow-rate pressure differential. The major disadvantages are low capacity before clogging and the need to prewash the filters to remove surfactants. Given the advantages and disadvantages of each type of filter, when large quantities of liquids are to be sterile filtered, such as in industrial applications, it is very common to use a relatively coarse-depth filter (1–5 mm) to remove the great majority of particles and, subsequently, use a membrane filter to remove the remaining particles and micro-organisms down to a predetermined size (0.22 μm).

Filter cartridges are used for filtering large volumes of solution or more viscous products because of the large surface area that is available through the pleated design. Hydrophobic filters are also available for sterile filtering of gases and solvents (40).

CLINICAL CONSIDERATIONS IN PARENTERAL PRODUCT DESIGN

Sterility, freedom from pyrogens, and acceptably low level of extraneous particulate matter are critical quality attributes of all injectable products. Additional critical quality attributes depend on the clinical use of the product. For example, for IV, IM, and SC routes, isotonicity and physiological pH (7.4) are always desirable to minimize potential irritation upon injection. Other factors may preclude this, however. If the required dose of drug must be administered in a small volume, it may not be feasible to formulate an isotonic solution. Likewise, solubility or stability considerations may preclude formulation at physiological pH. This explains why formulation pH for injectable drugs varies from about pH 2 to about pH 11.

However, for certain routes of injection, such as intrathecal, intraocular, or into any part of the brain, isotonicity and physiological pH are critical to minimize potential nerve damage. Absence of preservatives is also critical for these routes of administration for the same reason.

The effect of isotonicity on reducing pain on injection is somewhat uncertain, although it may at least reduce tissue irritation. Pain on injection may occur during and immediately following the injection, or it may be a delayed or prolonged type of pain that becomes more severe after subsequent injections. The actual cause of the pain is often unknown and varies significantly among patients. In some cases, pain may be reduced by minor formulation changes, such as adjusting tonicity and pH, or by adding an anesthetic agent such as benzyl alcohol or lidocaine hydrochloride. In other cases, pain is attributable to the drug, and pain reduction is more difficult or impossible to resolve. Pain, soreness, and tissue inflammation are often encountered in parenteral suspensions, especially those containing a high concentration of solids.

Thrombophlebitis, an inflammation of the venous walls, may occur during IV infusion and may be related to the drug being infused, pH or tonicity of the formulation, the administration technique, the device being used for the infusion (i.e., a needle or a catheter), the duration of the infusion, and the extent to which the administration device is mechanically stabilized (41). It is difficult to define the relative importance of each because of the interplay of all these variables. Irritation caused by the drug or the formulation can be minimized by observing published limits on the volumetric rate of infusion. The observance of proper technique should also be emphasized, including selection of the appropriate infusion device, venipuncture technique, stabilization of the catheter, and changing the administration device at appropriate time intervals.

The formulator should be aware of the clinical use of a drug when designing the dosage form. Specific examples are pediatric-dosage forms and unit-dosage forms, including disposable syringes and special packages for hospital, office, or home administration. Hospital packages can take several forms, depending, for example, on whether the package is to be unit-dose, reconstituted by a nurse, a bulk container for use in the pharmacy, or administered as a secondary "piggyback" IV container.

Drugs that affect tissue properties, particularly blood flow at the absorption site, may be used to control the rate of absorption. Reduced drug absorption may be achieved

Table 4 Maximum Amounts of Added Substances
Permitted in USP Injectable Products

Substance	Maximum
Mercury compounds	0.01
Cationic surfactants	0.01
Chlorobutanol	0.5
Cresol	0.5
Phenol	0.5
Sulfur dioxide	0.2
or sodium bisulfite equivalent	0.2
or sodium sulfite equivalent	0.2

Abbreviation: USP, United States Pharmacopeia.

physiologically with an IM preparation by incorporating epinephrine, which causes a local constriction of blood vessels at the site of injection. Increased muscular activity may enhance drug absorption because of increased drug flow.

When preparing preparations for IV and IM use, the formulator must be aware of the effect of added substances when unusually large doses of the drug are administered. Although the USP limits the use of some added substances (Table 4), these types of problems cannot always be anticipated. The USP urges special care when administering more than 5 mL (1). When effects do become apparent, the formulator should consider additional dosage sizes or formulation changes. Sometimes, during the life of a drug product, new uses and larger doses make the original formula unsatisfactory. When this happens, a new dosage form should be designed and the appropriate cautionary statements placed on the respective labels. The precautions, problems, hazards, and complications associated with parenteral drug administration are discussed extensively by Duma and Akers (42).

The preparation of a new drug substance or dosage form for evaluation in clinical trials (CTs) must meet the same regulatory requirements and controls as a marketed product. The current Good Manufacturing Practice (cGMP) requirements for CT products are outlined by FDA and are discussed in chapter 20.

Toxicity Studies

In toxicity studies, acute toxicity tests are usually carried out in the rat, mouse, cat, and dog. Subacute toxicity studies for IM products are performed by giving SC injections to rats and IM injections to dogs. In IV studies, the rat-tail vein or a front leg is used. Deliberate overdosing usually "washes out" metabolism differences between species. In dogs, it is common to give an IV dose 5 times that intended for humans. In rats this is increased to 10 times.

Irritation studies are done in rabbits. Each rabbit serves as its own control. The concentration selected for the irritation studies is that intended for humans.

Clinical Evaluation

Clinical evaluation of the dosage form is the most expensive and critical phase of product development. All that has been done before this point has been done in an effort to ensure a safe and reliable product for the clinician.

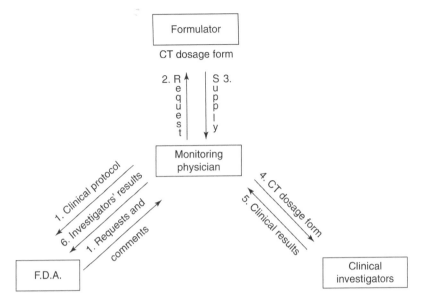

Figure 11 CT scheme. *Abbreviation*: CT, clinical trial

A drug company normally assigns one of its staff physicians as "monitoring" physician for the CT program. The monitoring physician has the key role in the conduct of the CT program (Fig. 11). He or she coordinates the establishment of clinical protocols, awarding of grants, gathering and "in-house" evaluation of clinical data, and preparation of the FDA submission.

The monitoring physician must first establish what the clinical protocol is going to be. With injectable products, this involves both a clinical pharmacology safety test and a dose-ranging study in humans. These studies are normally a single IM injection in several patients. Depending on the drug, clinical studies may proceed eventually to controlled double-blind studies. Care must be exercised to involve a sufficient number of patients to make the studies statistically meaningful. If the intention is to claim treatment of several clinical conditions for the product, each must be evaluated separately. Throughout the course of the studies, there is a continuing dialogue between the FDA and the monitoring physician.

When the clinical program has been approved by a peer review committee, and filed with FDA, the monitoring physician requests a sufficient amount of material from the formulator to initiate the clinical program. Before the dosage form is released to the custody of the monitoring physician, the new drug substance and the formulated product must be thoroughly evaluated to ensure proper potency, purity, and safety. Stability studies must also be initiated so that if the product becomes subpotent or physically unstable during the course of the CT, it can be recalled before any harm can result to the patients in the study.

After release of CT material, the monitoring physician supplies it to the clinical investigators with whom the clinical program has previously been discussed. As the clinical investigators use the product, they begin sending reports to the monitoring physician, who evaluates them and sends them to the FDA. Although the concept shown in Figure 11 is oversimplified, it does convey the principal framework under which the CTs are conducted.

QUALITY ASSURANCE

The terms "quality assurance" and "quality control" are sometimes used interchangeably, but there is an important difference. Quality control generally refers to testing of raw materials, packaging components, and final product for conformance to established requirements. Quality assurance is a term that includes quality control, but has broader meaning to include written operating procedures, personnel training, record keeping, and facility design and monitoring. The philosophy of a quality assurance program is to build quality into the product, rather than to rely only on final product testing to cull out defective product.

Although principles of quality control and quality assurance are important to all pharmaceutical dosage forms, they are especially critical when considering the unique attributes of parenteral dosage forms—sterility, absence of pyrogens, and freedom from extraneous particulate matter. Quality control is generally divided into three areas: raw materials, in-process controls, and product specifications. However, numerous attributes for a product have to be considered throughout all phases of development, evaluation, production, and storage to guarantee good quality.

The factors necessary to achieve quality in a product during the developmental stage have been discussed. The formulator of a new product must consider the manufacturing process to be used for full-scale production of the product. Many new product failures or deficiencies occur because of inability to resolve or foresee production-related problems, rather than to poor product development per se. Therefore, the scientist involved in the development of a product must be involved in development of its manufacturing process and testing. Standards must be carefully established for all raw materials and packaging components used in the product so that the quality of the product will be maintained. Trial production runs should be performed on a new product for stability testing and process evaluation.

Regulatory and Compendial Requirements

The manufacture and sale of parenteral products is regulated by federal and state laws, as well as by the USP. Federal drug regulations are discussed in detail in chapter 20. The USP provides specifications, test procedures, standards, etc. for parenteral products and their packaging components. In addition to individual monographs, the USP limits the use of certain additives (Table 4), the size of multiple-dose containers to 30 mL, and requires a suitable preservative to be added to containers intended for multiple use.

The cGMP regulations are guidelines that the FDA requires a pharmaceutical manufacturer to meet. Compliance with the cGMPs is a prerequisite for the approval of NDAs, INDs, and antibiotic forms. General areas in which GMP guidelines must be established and adhered to include

- Organization and personnel
- Buildings and facilities
- Control of drug components, packaging, and materials
- Production and process control
- Equipment
- Packaging and labeling control
- Holding and distribution
- Laboratory control
- Records and reports

Parenteral formulation and the preparation of parenterals for CT use obviously require adherence to cGMPs. A development group that generates CT materials should have guidelines and written procedures covering such areas as equipment (validation, maintenance, and cleaning), environmental monitoring, instruments (maintenance and calibration), housekeeping, documentation, training, and material handling and storage. Sterilization methods, aseptic processing, and filling techniques and methods must be validated to assure product sterility and quality. *Validation* is the process of proving that a process or equipment does what it is supposed to do within the established limits. All individuals performing an aseptic process must periodically pass a test to verify their aseptic technique.

Monitoring Programs

Process Facilities

Continual evaluation of manufacturing processes is necessary to maintain good manufacturing practices. Facilities, buildings, and equipment used in the production of parenteral products must be specially designed for this purpose. Factors to be considered when designing a new plant include environmental conditions, workflow, equipment, choice of materials, personnel, organization, process, documentation, production hygiene, and process controls (43,44). Thorough planning and engineering of a parenteral facility will not only help maintain the quality of the manufactured products but will also simplify cleanup and maintenance requirements. Contamination of a product is minimized by maintaining a clean facility.

Production Areas

Production areas can be separated into seven general classes: cleanup area, preparation area for packaging materials, preparation area for drug products, sterilization facilities, aseptic filling and processing areas, sorting and product holding areas, and a labeling section.

The exact identity of all packaging components, the bulk and filled product, labels, and so on, must be carefully maintained. The production ticket must be written so that it is easily understood and followed by the appropriate production personnel. All procedures should be clearly outlined, and limits established for all operators (e.g., "heat water to 35–45°C" or "autoclave sterilize for 15–20 minutes at 121–124°C").

All production processes, such as ampoule washing and sterilization, solution filtration, equipment setup and operation, sorting, and freeze-drier cleaning and operation, should be covered in detail in a procedure manual to ensure that all operations are understood as well as carried out properly and uniformly. Cleaning, sterilization, sterile filtration, filling, and aseptic processing operations must be validated.

Personnel

People are the principal source of contamination in clean room operations. All personnel involved throughout the development and production of a parenteral product must be aware of the factors that influence the overall quality of a product as well as the factors on which they directly impinge. It is of particular importance that production personnel be properly trained so that human error is minimized. They should be made aware of the use of the products with which they are involved and the importance of following all procedures, especially proper aseptic techniques. Procedures must be set up to verify that the product is being manufactured as intended. After manufacture of a batch, production tickets must be carefully checked, sterilization charts examined, and labels verified for correctness and count.

Environmental Monitoring

Control of environmental factors is important to product quality. Air quality and air movement, care and maintenance of the area, and personnel movement and attire are of particular importance.

The air quality in preparation and aseptic areas can be one of the greatest sources of product contamination. However, this problem can be minimized by use of the equipment currently available to provide clean air essentially free from microorganisms and dirt particles. Depth-type filters, electrostatic filters, and dehumidification systems are used to remove the major portion of the airborne contaminants. Air for aseptic areas is then passed through high-efficiency particulate air (HEPA) filters, which remove 99.97% of all particles 0.3 μm or larger. To prevent outside air from entering aseptic areas, a positive pressure is maintained relative to corridors.

A laminar flow enclosure provides a means for environmental control of a confined area for aseptic use. Laminar flow units utilize HEPA filters, with the uniform movement of air along parallel lines. The air movement may be in a horizontal or vertical direction and may involve a confined area, such as a workbench or an entire room. Laminar flow modules are suspended above filling lines, vial- and stopper-washing equipment, and other processes to provide an aseptic and particulate-free environment.

Regardless of the methods used to obtain a clean air environment, unless the parenteral operator is made completely aware of the limits of laminar flow; uses careful, planned movements; and is wearing proper clothing; he or she can be a source of product contamination. Operator movement within aseptic rooms should be minimized. The rooms must be disinfected regularly and thoroughly before setting up for aseptic operation.

Commonly used environmental monitoring techniques include the following:

Passive air sampling Petri dishes containing microbiological growth media are placed in aseptic areas for specified lengths of time, the "settling plates" are then incubated, and colonies are counted and identified. This is a qualitative test, since there is no way of knowing the volume of air represented by a given number of colonies.

Active air sampling Active air sampling provides quantitative data because air at a known flow rate is impacted on a strip of nutrient media, followed by incubation of the nutrient strips, and enumeration of colonies. Common active air–sampling instruments include the slit-to-agar impact sampler and the centrifugal (Reuter) sampler.

Air-classification measurement Electronic airborne particle–monitoring instruments count and size particulate matter in the sampled air with no consideration of whether the particles are viable or nonviable. Air classification is defined as the number of particles per cubic foot of air that are larger than 0.5 μm in diameter. Climet and HIAC-Royco are common instruments for airborne particulate monitoring.

Surface monitoring Contact (or Rodac) plates of growth media are applied to surfaces such as benchtops, walls, and personnel and then incubated. Colony-forming units (CFUs) are counted and identified.

Differential pressure measurement Differential manometers are instruments that measure the difference in pressure between two adjacent rooms. Cleaner environments must have a higher pressure than adjacent, less clean environments to prevent flow of relatively dirty air into the cleaner environment. This differential pressure must be monitored and controlled.

Product Testing and Evaluation

Quality control testing and evaluation is involved primarily with incoming raw materials, the manufacturing process, and the final product. Testing of incoming raw materials includes routine testing on all drugs, chemicals, and packaging materials.

Process controls include daily testing of WFI (USP), conformation of fill doses and yields, checking and approving intermediate production tickets, and checking label identity and count. Finished product control includes all the tests necessary to ensure the potency, purity, and identity of the product. Parenteral products require additional tests, which include those for sterility, pyrogens, clarity, and particulate analysis, and for glass-sealed ampoules, leaker testing.

Sterility Testing

The purpose of a sterility test is to determine the probable sterility of a specific batch. The USP lists the procedural details for sterility testing and the sample sizes required (1). The USP official tests are the direct (or culture tube inoculation) method and the membrane filtration method.

The interpretation of sterility results is divided into two stages by the USP relative to the type of sterility failure if one occurs. If sterility failure of the test samples occurred because of improper aseptic technique, or as a fault of the test itself, stage 1 may be repeated with the same sample size. Sample size is doubled in a stage 2 testing, which is performed if microbial growth is observed in stage 1, and there is no reason to believe that the test was invalid. The only absolute method to guarantee the sterility of a batch would be to test every vial or ampoule.

There is a probability of nonproduct-related contamination in the order of 10^{-3} when performing the sterility test because of the aseptic manipulations necessary to carry out the procedure. This level is comparable with the overall efficiency of an aseptic operation. Confidence in the sterility test is dependent on the fact that the batch has been subjected to a sterilization procedure of proved effectiveness. Records of all sterility tests as well as temperature recordings and records from autoclaves, ovens, or other equipment used during the manufacturing process must be maintained. All sterilizing equipment must be validated to ensure that the proper temperatures are obtained for the necessary time period. These validations are obtained by the use of thermocouples, chemical and biological indicators, sealed ampoules containing culture medium with a suspension of heat-resistant spores, and detailed sterility testing.

Pyrogen Testing

Pyrogenic substances are primarily lipid polysaccharide products of the metabolism of microorganisms; they may be soluble, insoluble, or colloidal. Pyrogens produced by gram-negative bacilli are generally the most potent. Minute amounts of pyrogens produce a wide variety of reactions in both animals and humans, including fever, leukopenia, and alterations in blood coagulation. Large doses can induce shock and eventually death.

Pyrogens readily contaminate biological materials because of their ability to withstand autoclaving as well as to pass through many filters. Several techniques are used to remove them from injectable products. The ideal situation is one in which no pyrogens are present in the starting materials. This is achieved by strict control of the cleanliness of equipment and containers, distillation of water, and limited processing times. In general, pyrogens may be destroyed by being subjected to prolonged heating. Other pyrogen-removal techniques, which are generally less effective or applicable, include ultrafiltration, absorption or adsorption, chemical (oxidation), aging, or a combination of these.

One pyrogen test is a qualitative biological test based on the fever response of rabbits. If a pyrogenic substance is injected into the vein of a rabbit, a temperature elevation will occur within three hours. Many imitative medical agents will also cause a fever.

A preferred method for the detection of pyrogens is the limulus amebocyte lysate (LAL) test. A test sample is incubated with amebocyte lysate from the blood of the horseshoe crab, *Limulus polyphemus*. A pyrogenic substance will cause a gel to form. This is a result of the clottable protein from the amebocyte cells reacting with the endotoxins. This test is more sensitive, more rapid, and easier to perform than the rabbit test.

Leaker Testing and Sealing Verification

Ampoules that have been sealed by fusion must be tested to ensure that a hermetic seal was obtained. The leaker test is performed by immersing the ampoules in a dye solution, such as 1% methylene blue, and applying at least 25 in. (64 cm) of vacuum for a minimum of 15 minutes. The vacuum on the tank is then released as rapidly as possible to put maximum stress on weak seals. Next, the ampoules are washed. Defective ampoules will contain blue solution.

Another means of testing for leakers is a high-frequency spark test system developed by the Nikka Densok Company of Japan, which detects pinholes in ampoules. Some advantages of this system include higher inspection accuracy, higher processing speed, and eliminating the possibility of product contamination (45).

Bottles and vials are not subjected to such a vacuum test because of the flexibility of the rubber closure. However, bottles that are sealed under vacuum may be tested for vacuum by striking the base of the bottle sharply with the heel of the hand to produce a "water hammer" sound. Another test is the spark test, in which a probe is applied outside the bottle. When it reaches the air space of the bottle, a spark discharge occurs if the headspace is evacuated.

The microbiological integrity of various packages, such as vials and stoppers, disposable syringes, and plastic containers, should be determined. A microbiological challenge test is performed by filling the package with a sterile medium, and then exposing the sealed container to one of the following tests that is appropriate for the package system: (*i*) static-aerosol challenge, (*ii*) static-immersion challenge, (*iii*) static-ambient challenge, or (*iv*) dynamic-immersion challenge. The static-immersion challenge test is used commonly with new package combinations. The sealed containers are periodically challenged by immersion into a suspension of challenge organisms. Storing the containers at 5°C or 40°C to 50°C, or both, before immersion provides additional stress.

Clarity Testing and Particulate Analysis

Clarity is defined as the state or quality of being clear or transparent to the eye. Clarity is a relative term subject to the visual acuity, training, and experience of the sorter. Clarity specifications are not given in the USP, other than to state that all injections be subjected to visual inspection.

Instruments that measure scattered light, such as the Photo-Nephelometer (Coleman Instruments, Oak Brook, Illinois, U.S.), are used to evaluate and set clarity standards for parenteral preparations. It is not possible to establish an overall standard value for all products (e.g., 30 nephelos) because the value itself is relative and influenced by many factors, including concentration, aging, stopper extracts, and the solubility characteristics of the raw materials. Nephelometer readings are insensitive to contamination by large (visible) particulates.

Particulate matter is defined in the USP as extraneous, mobile, undissolved substances, other than gas bubbles, unintentionally present in parenteral solutions. Test methods and limits for particulates are stated in the USP for large-volume injections and small-volume injections.

The development of sorting standards is the responsibility of the manufacturer. Parenteral solutions are sorted for foreign particles, such as glass, fibers, precipitate, and floaters. The sorter also checks for any container deficiency and improper dose volume when feasible. All products containing clear solutions should be inspected against a black and sometimes a white background using a special light source. Although manual visual inspection is the most common means of inspection, electronic particle detection equipment and computer-controlled electrooptic systems are replacing manual inspection and using a light source or camera, or both, positioned behind, above, or below the units being inspected.

The significance of particulate contamination in all parenteral preparations and devices has received much attention. Although it has not been established that particles can cause toxic effects, the pharmaceutical industry, the medical profession, hospital pharmacists, and the FDA all realize the importance of reducing particulate levels in all parenteral products and devices.

Sources of particulate matter include the raw materials, processing and filling equipment, the container, and environmental contamination. Several methods have been developed for identifying the source of particulates in a product so that they may be eliminated or reduced. The most effective method is that of collecting the particulates on a membrane filter and identifying and counting them microscopically. However, this method is time consuming and not adaptable to in-line inspection. Several video image projection methods for in-line detection of particles have been developed that provide potential for mechanizing inspection. Electronic particulate counters have been applied to parenterals because of the rapidity at which they do particulate analysis. Their main disadvantages are the lack of differentiation of various types of particulates, including liquids such as silicones, and the fact that particle size is measured differently from microscopic analysis. The USP tests for particulate matter in injections utilize both the microscopic and light obscuration methods (1).

Labeling

The package and, in particular, the labeling for parenteral dosage forms are integral and critical parts of the product. The labeling must be legible, and clearly identify the drug, its concentration, handling or storage conditions, and any special precautions. The dose or concentration must be prominently displayed when other concentrations of the same drug are marketed. Proper labeling is difficult with the space limitation dictated by small containers used for many parenteral products. Smaller containers have become increasingly popular because of the unit-dose concept.

REFERENCES

1. The United States Pharmacopeia. 24th ed. U.S. Pharmacopeial Convention, Rockville, MD, 2000.
2. Turco S. Sterile Dosage Forms. 4th ed. Philadelphia: Lea & Febiger, 1994.
3. Feldman S. Physicochemical factors influencing drug absorption from the intramuscular site. Bull Parenter Drug Assoc 1974; 28:53–63.
4. Motola S, Agharkar SN. Preformulation research of parenteral medications. In: Avis KE, Lieberman HA, Lachman L, eds. Pharmaceutical Dosage Forms: Parenteral Medications, Vol 1, 2nd ed. New York: Marcel Dekker, 1992:115–172.
5. Lin KS, Anschel J, Swartz CJ. Parenteral formulations IV: solubility considerations in developing a parenteral dosage form. Bull Parenter Drug Assoc 1971; 25:40–50.
6. Engel G, Pfeiffer R. Unpublished data. Indianapolis, IN: Eli Lilly & Co.
7. Haleblian JK. Characterization of habits and crystalline modification of solids and their pharmaceutical applications. J Pharm Sci 1975; 64:1269–1288.
8. Pikal MJ, Lukes AL, Lang JE, et al. Quantitative crystallinity determinations for beta-lac-tam antibiotics by solution calorimetry: correlations with stability. J Pharm Sci 1978; 67:767–773.
9. Brage L. Galenics of Insulin. New York: Springer-Verlag, 1982:41.
10. Schroeder LC. Sulfurous acid salts as pharmaceutical anti-oxidants. J Pharm Sci 1961; 50:891–901.
11. Lachman L, Sheth PB, Urbanyi T. Lined and unlined rubber stoppers for multiple-dose vial solutions. J Pharm Sci 1964; 53:211–218.
12. Motola S, Clawans C. Identification and surface removal of incompatible group II metal ions from butyl stoppers. Bull Parenter Drug Assoc 1972; 26:163–171.
13. Carpenter JF, Prestrelski SJ, Anchordoguy TJ, et al. Interactions of stabilizers with proteins during freezing and drying. In: Cleland JL, Langer R, eds. Formulation and Delivery of Peptides and Proteins. ACS Symposium Series 567. Washington DC: American Chemical Society, 1994:134–147.
14. Freyfuss J, Shaw JM, Ross JJ Jr. Fluphenazine enanthate and fluphenazine decanoate: intramuscular injection and esterification as requirements for slow-release characteristics in dogs. J Pharm Sci 1976; 65:1310–1315.
15. Spiegel AJ, Noseworthy MM. Use of nonaqueous solvents in parenteral products. J Pharm Sci 1963; 52:917–927.
16. Hem SL, Bright DR, Banker GS, et al. Tissue irritation evaluation of potential parenteral vehicles. Drug Dev Commun 1974–1975; 1:471–477.
17. Pitt A. Protein adsorption to microporous filtration membranes. J Parenter Sci Technol 1987; 41:110–114.
18. Akers MJ, Fites AL, Robison RL. Formulation design & development of parenteral suspensions. J Parenter Sci Technol 1987; 41:88–96.
19. Boylan JC. Bull Parenter Drug Assoc 1965; 19:98.
20. Boylan JC, Robison RL. Rheological stability of a procaine penicillin G suspension. J Pharm Sci 1968; 57:1796–1797.
21. MacKenzie AP. The physicochemical basis for the freeze-drying process. Dev Biol Stand 1977; 36:51–67.
22. Franks F. Freeze drying: from empiricism to predictability. Cryo Lett 1990; 11:93–110.
23. Nail SL, Gatlin LA. Freeze Drying: Principles and Practice. In: Avis KE, Lieberman HA, Lachman L, eds. Pharmaceutical Dosage Forms: Parenteral Medications. 2nd ed, Vol 2. New York: Marcel Dekker, 1992:163–234.
24. Her LM, Nail SL. Measurement of glass transitions in frozen solutions by differential scanning calorimetry. Pharm Res 1994; 11:54–59.
25. Williams NA, Lee Y, Polli GP, et al. The effects of cooling rate on solid phase transitions and associated vial breakage occurring in frozen mannitol solutions. J Parenter Sci Technol 1986; 40:135–141.

26. Gatlin LA, DeLuca PP. Kinetics of a phase transition in a frozen solution. J Parenter Drug Assoc 1980; 34:398–408.
27. Searles JA, Carpenter JF, Randolph TW. Primary drying rate heterogeneity during pharmaceutical lyophilization. Am Pharm Rev 2000; 3:6–24.
28. Oguchi T. Freezing of drug/additive binary systems II. Relationship between decarboxylation behavior and molecular states of p-aminosalicylic acid. Chem Pharm Bull 1989; 37:3088–3091.
29. Crowe J, Crowe L, Carpenter J. Are freezing and dehydration similar stress vectors? A comparison of modes of interaction of biomolecules with stabilizing solutes. Cryobiology 1990; 27:219–231.
30. Pikal MJ, Shah S, Senior D, et al. Physical chemistry of freeze drying: measurement of sublimation rates of frozen aqueous solutions by a microbalance technique. J Pharm Sci 1983; 72:635–650.
31. Pikal MJ, Roy ML, Shah S. Mass and heat transfer in vial freeze-drying of pharmaceuticals: role of the vial. J Pharm Sci 1984; 73:1224–1237.
32. Nail SL. The effect of chamber pressure on heat transfer in the freeze drying of parenteral solutions. J Parenter Drug Assoc 1980; 34:358–368.
33. Pikal MJ, Shah S, Roy ML, et al. The secondary drying stage of freeze drying: drying kinetics as a function of shelf temperature and chamber pressure. Int J Pharm 1990; 60:203–217.
34. Ahern TJ, Manning MJ. Stability of Protein Pharmaceuticals. Part A: Chemical and Physical Pathways of Protein Degradation. New York: Plenum Press, 1992.
35. Chien YW. Novel Drug Delivery Systems: Fundamentals, Developmental Concepts, Biomedical Assessments. New York: Marcel Dekker, 1982:219–292.
36. Akers MJ, Anderson NR. Sterilization Validation. In: Nash RA, Wachter AH, eds. Pharmaceutical Process Validation. 3rd ed. New York: Marcel Dekker, 2003:83–158.
37. Leuthner EJ. In: Swarbrick J, Boylan J, eds. Autoclaves and Autoclaving, Encyclopedia of Pharmaceutical Technology. Vol 1. New York: Marcel Dekker, 1988:393–414.
38. Groves FM, Groves MJ. In: Swarbrick J, Boylan J, eds. Dry Heat Sterilization and Depyrogenation, Encyclopedia of Pharmaceutical Technology. Vol 4. New York: Marcel Dekker, 1991:447–484.
39. Reich RR, Burgess DJ. In: Swarbrick J, Boylan J, eds. Ethylene Oxide Sterilization, Encyclopedia of Pharmaceutical Technology. Vol 5. New York: Marcel Dekker, 1992:315–336.
40. Meltzer TH. In: Swarbrick J, Boylan J, eds. Filters and Filtration, Encyclopedia of Pharmaceutical Technology. Vol 6. New York: Marcel Dekker, 1992:51–91.
41. Turco SJ. Therapy Hazards Assoc. Parenter Bull Parenter Drug Assoc 1974; 28:197–204.
42. Duma RJ, Akers MJ, Turco SJ. Parenteral Drug Administration: Routes, Precautions, Problems, Complications, and Drug Delivery Systems. In: Avis KE, Lieberman HA, Lachman L, eds. Pharmaceutical Dosage Forms: Parenteral Medications. 2nd ed, Vol 1. New York: Marcel Dekker, 1992:17–58.
43. Hempel HE. Large scale manufacture of parenterals. Bull Parenter Drug Assoc 1976; 30:88–95.
44. Blackmer RA. Sterile operations facility. J Parenter Sci Technol 1984; 38:183–189.
45. Akers MJ. In: Robinson JR, ed. Parenteral Quality Control: Sterility Pyrogen, Particulate, and Package Integrity Testing. Vol 1. New York: Marcel Dekker, 1985:207–209.

Index

An environmentally friendly book printed and bound in England by www.printondemand-worldwide.com

PEFC Certified

This product is
from sustainably
managed foresss
and controlled
sources

www.pefc.org

PEFC/16-33-415

MIX
Paper from
responsible sources
FSC® C004959

This book is made entirely of sustainable materials; FSC paper for the cover and PEFC paper for the text pages.

#0291 - 111013 - C0 - 254/178/35 [37] - CB